INTERACTIVE AND INTEGRATIVE CARDIOLOGY

ANNALS OF THE NEW YORK ACADEMY OF SCIENCES
Volume 1080

INTERACTIVE AND INTEGRATIVE CARDIOLOGY

Edited by Samuel Sideman, Rafael Beyar, and Amir Landesberg

Published by Blackwell Publishing on behalf of the New York Academy of Sciences
Boston, Massachusetts
2006

Library of Congress Cataloging-in-Publication Data

Larry and Horti Fairberg Cardiac Workshop (4th : 2006 : Charleston, S.C.) Interactive and integrative cardiology / edited by Samuel Sideman and Rafael Beyar.
  p. ; cm. – (Annals of the New York Academy of Sciences, ISSN 0077-8923 ; 1380)
  Includes bibliographical references and index.
  ISBN-13: 978-1-57331-651-4 (alk. paper)
  ISBN-10: 1-57331-651-2 (alk. paper)
  1. Heart cells–Congresses. 2. Heart–Physiology–Congresses. 3. Heart–Pathophysiology–Congresses. I. Sideman, S. II. Beyar, Rafael. III. New York Academy of Sciences. IV. Title. V. Series.
  [DNLM: 1. Heart–physiology–Congresses. 2. Calcium Channels –physiology–Congresses. 3. Heart Diseases–therapy–Congresses. 4. Models, Cardiovascular–Congresses. 5. Myocytes, Cardiac–physiology–Congresses. W1 AN626YL v.1380 2006 / WG 202 L334i 2006]

QP114.C44L37 2006
612.1'7–dc22
                                                                    2006019884

The *Annals of the New York Academy of Sciences* (ISSN: 0077-8923 [print]; ISSN: 1749-6632 [online]) is published 28 times a year on behalf of the New York Academy of Sciences by Blackwell Publishing, with offices located at 350 Main Street, Malden, Massachusetts 02148 USA, PO Box 1354, Garsington Road, Oxford OX4 2DQ UK, and PO Box 378 Carlton South, 3053 Victoria Australia.

Information for subscribers: Subscription prices for 2006 are: Premium Institutional: $3850.00 (US) and £2139.00 (Europe and Rest of World).
Customers in the UK should add VAT at 5%. Customers in the EU should also add VAT at 5% or provide a VAT registration number or evidence of entitlement to exemption. Customers in Canada should add 7% GST or provide evidence of entitlement to exemption. The Premium Institutional price also includes online access to full-text articles from 1997 to present, where available. For other pricing options or more information about online access to Blackwell Publishing journals, including access information and terms and conditions, please visit www.blackwellpublishing.com/nyas.

Membership information: Members may order copies of the *Annals* volumes directly from the Academy by visiting www.nyas.org/annals, emailing membership@nyas.org, faxing 212-888-2894, or calling 800-843-6927 (US only), or +1 212 838 0230, ext. 345 (International). For more information on becoming a member of the New York Academy of Sciences, please visit www.nyas.org/membership.

Journal Customer Services: For ordering information, claims, and any inquiry concerning your institutional subscription, please contact your nearest office:
UK: Email: customerservices@blackwellpublishing.com; Tel: +44 (0) 1865 778315; Fax +44 (0) 1865 471775
US: Email: customerservices@blackwellpublishing.com; Tel: +1 781 388 8599 or 1 800 835 6770 (Toll free in the USA); Fax: +1 781 388 8232
Asia: Email: customerservices@blackwellpublishing.com; Tel: +65 6511 8000; Fax: +61 3 8359 1120
Members: Claims and inquiries on member orders should be directed to the Academy at email: membership@nyas.org or Tel: +1 212 838 0230 (International) or 800-843-6927 (US only).

Printed in the USA.
Printed on acid-free paper.

Mailing: The *Annals of the New York Academy of Sciences* are mailed Standard Rate.
Postmaster: Send all address changes to *Annals of the New York Academy of Sciences*, Blackwell Publishing, Inc., Journals Subscription Department, 350 Main Street, Malden, MA 01248-5020. Mailing to rest of world by DHL Smart and Global Mail.

Copyright and Photocopying
© 2006 The New York Academy of Sciences. All rights reserved. No part of this publication may be reproduced, stored, or transmitted in any form or by any means without the prior permission in writing from the copyright holder. Authorization to photocopy items for internal and personal use is granted by the copyright holder for libraries and other users registered with their local Reproduction Rights Organization (RRO), e.g. Copyright Clearance Center (CCC), 222 Rosewood Drive, Danvers, MA 01923, USA (www.copyright.com), provided the appropriate fee is paid directly to the RRO. This consent does not extend to other kinds of copying such as copying for general distribution, for advertising or promotional purposes, for creating new collective works, or for resale. Special requests should be addressed to Blackwell Publishing at journalsrights@oxon.blackwellpublishing.com.

Disclaimer: The Publisher, the New York Academy of Sciences, and the Editors cannot be held responsible for errors or any consequences arising from the use of information contained in this publication; the views and opinions expressed do not necessarily reflect those of the Publisher, the New York Academy of Sciences, or the Editors.

Annals are available to subscribers online at the New York Academy of Sciences and also at Blackwell Synergy. Visit www.annalsnyas.org or www.blackwell-synergy.com to search the articles and register for table of contents e-mail alerts. Access to full text and PDF downloads of *Annals* articles are available to nonmembers and subscribers on a pay-per-view basis at www.annalsnyas.org.

The paper used in this publication meets the minimum requirements of the National Standard for Information Sciences Permanence of Paper for Printed Library Materials, ANSI Z39.48-1984.

ISSN: 0077-8923 (print); 1749-6632 (online)
ISBN-10: 1-57331-651-2 (paper); ISBN-13: 978-1-57331-651-4 (paper)

A catalogue record for this title is available from the British Library.

Digitization of the *Annals of the New York Academy of Sciences*

An agreement has recently been reached between Blackwell Publishing and the New York Academy of Sciences to digitize the entire run of the *Annals of the New York Academy of Sciences* back to volume one.

The back files, which have been defined as all of those issues published before 1997, will be sold to libraries as part of Blackwell Publishing's Legacy Sales Program and hosted on the Blackwell Synergy website.

Copyright of all material will remain with the rights holder. Contributors: Please contact Blackwell Publishing if you do not wish an article or picture from the *Annals of the New York Academy of Sciences* to be included in this digitization project.

In Memory of Horti and Larry Fairberg

ANNALS OF THE NEW YORK ACADEMY OF SCIENCES

Volume 1080
October 2006

INTERACTIVE AND INTEGRATIVE CARDIOLOGY

Editors
SAMUEL SIDEMAN, RAFAEL BEYAR, AND AMIR LANDESBERG

This volume is the result of a meeting entitled **Interactive and Integrative Cardiology: 4th Larry and Horti Fairberg Workshop,** held on April 23–27, 2006 in Charleston, South Carolina.

CONTENTS

Preface: The Challenge of Cardiac Modeling—Interaction and Integration. *By* SAMUEL SIDEMAN xi

Part I. Development and Genetics

Functional Studies of Individual Myosin Molecules. *By* JODY A. DANTZIG, TIM Y. LIU, AND YALE E. GOLDMAN 1

Recruitment of New Cells into the Postnatal Heart: Potential Modification of Phenotype by Periostin. *By* RICHARD P. VISCONTI AND ROGER R. MARKWALD 19

Cell-Based Approaches for Cardiac Repair. *By* MICHAEL RUBART AND LOREN J. FIELD 34

The Unstoppable Connexin43 Carboxyl-Terminus: New Roles in Gap Junction Organization and Wound Healing. *By* ROBERT G. GOURDIE, GAUTAM S. GHATNEKAR, MICHAEL O'QUINN, MATTHEW J. RHETT, RALPH J. BARKER, CHING ZHU, JANE JOURDAN, AND ANDREW W. HUNTER 49

The Developing Cardiac Myocyte: Maturation of Excitability and Excitation–Contraction Coupling. *By* ELIZABETH A. SCHRODER, YIDONG WEI, AND JONATHAN SATIN 63

Dynamic Interactions between Myocytes, Fibroblasts, and Extracellular Matrix. *By* INDRONEAL BANERJEE, KRISHNA YEKKALA, THOMAS K. BORG, AND TROY A. BAUDINO 76

Embryonic Heart Induction. *By* ANN C. FOLEY, RUCHIKA W. GUPTA, ROSA M. GUZZO, OKSANA KOROL, AND MARK MERCOLA 85

The Role of Basic Leucine Zipper Protein-Mediated Transcription in Physiological and Pathological Myocardial Hypertrophy. *By* IZHAK KEHAT, TAL HASIN, AND AMI ARONHEIM 97

Part II. Mechanochemical Interactions

Hypertrophy and Atrophy of the Heart: The Other Side of Remodeling. *By* PETER RAZEGHI AND HEINRICH TAEGTMEYER 110

Role of Cellular Compartmentation in the Metabolic Response to Stress: Mechanistic Insights from Computational Models. *By* LUFANG ZHOU, XIN YU, MARCO E. CABRERA, AND WILLIAM C. STANLEY 120

Maintenance of the Metabolic Homeostasis of the Heart: Developing a Systems Analysis Approach. *By* ROBERT S. BALABAN 140

Part III. Electrochemical Interactions

Diversity of Ca^{2+} Signaling in Developing Cardiac Cells. *By* EINSLEY JANOWSKI, LARS CLEEMANN, PHILIPP SASSE, AND MARTIN MORAD 154

Regulation of Ca^{2+} and Na^+ in Normal and Failing Cardiac Myocytes. *By* DONALD M. BERS, SANDA DESPA, AND JULIE BOSSUYT 165

The Integration of Spontaneous Intracellular Ca^{2+} Cycling and Surface Membrane Ion Channel Activation Entrains Normal Automaticity in Cells of the Heart's Pacemaker. *By* EDWARD G. LAKATTA, TATIANA VINOGRADOVA, ALEXEY LYASHKOV, SYEVDA SIRENKO, WEIZONG ZHU, ABDUL RUKNUDIN, AND VICTOR MALTSEV 178

Calcium Handling in Embryonic Stem Cell–Derived Cardiac Myocytes: Of Mice and Men. *By* ILANIT ITZHAKI, JACKIE SCHILLER, RAFAEL BEYAR, JONATHAN SATIN, AND LIOR GEPSTEIN 207

Cellular Alternans: A Mechanism Linking Calcium Cycling Proteins to Cardiac Arrhythmogenesis. *By* LANCE D. WILSON, XIAOPING WAN, AND DAVID S. ROSENBAUM 216

Part IV. Electromechanical Interactions

The Mechanoelectric Feedback: A Novel "Calcium Clamp" Method, using Tetanic Contraction, for Testing the Role of the Intracellular Free Calcium. *By* YAEL YANIV, CARMIT LEVY, AND AMIR LANDESBERG 235

Role of Sarcomere Mechanics and Ca^{2+} Overload in Ca^{2+} Waves and Arrhythmias in Rat Cardiac Muscle. *By* HENK E.D.J. TER KEURS, YUJI WAKAYAMA, YOSHINAO SUGAI, GUY PRICE, YUTAKA KAGAYA, PENELOPE A. BOYDEN, MASAHITO MIURA, AND BRUNO D.M. STUYVERS ... 248

Cellular Basis for the Repolarization Waves of the ECG. *By* CHARLES ANTZELEVITCH 268

Mechanosensitive-Mediated Interaction, Integration, and Cardiac Control. *By* MAX J. LAB 282

Three-Dimensional Models of Individual Cardiac Histoanatomy: Tools and Challenges. *By* REBECCA A.B. BURTON, GERNOT PLANK, JÜRGEN E. SCHNEIDER, VICENTE GRAU, HELMUT AHAMMER, STEPHEN L. KEELING, JACK LEE, NICOLAS P. SMITH, DAVID GAVAGHAN, NATALIA TRAYANOVA, AND PETER KOHL 301

Cardiac Defibrillation and the Role of Mechanoelectric Feedback in Postshock Arrhythmogenesis. *By* VIATCHESLAV GUREV, MARY M. MALECKAR, AND NATALIA A. TRAYANOVA 320

Part V. Integrated Models and Analysis

Modeling Cardiac Electrical Activity at the Cell and Tissue Levels. *By* TRAVIS M. AUSTIN, DARREN A. HOOKS, PETER J. HUNTER, DAVID P. NICKERSON, ANDREW J. PULLAN, GREGORY B. SANDS, BRUCE H. SMAILL, AND MARK L. TREW 334

Cardiac β-Adrenergic Signaling: From Subcellular Microdomains to Heart Failure. *By* JEFFREY J. SAUCERMAN AND ANDREW D. MCCULLOCH 348

Multiscale Modeling of Calcium Signaling in the Cardiac Dyad. *By* RAIMOND L. WINSLOW, ANTTI TANSKANEN, MINDAO CHEN, AND JOSEPH L. GREENSTEIN 362

Nonlinear Dynamics of Paced Cardiac Cells. *By* YOHANNES SHIFERAW, ZHILIN QU, ALAN GARFINKEL, ALAIN KARMA, AND JAMES N. WEISS 376

Modeling Cardiac Ischemia. *By* BLANCA RODRÍGUEZ, NATALIA TRAYANOVA, AND DENIS NOBLE 395

Part VI. Novel Therapeutics

Cardiovascular Therapeutic Aspects of Cell Therapy and Stem Cells. *By* LIOR GEPSTEIN 415

Adenylyl Cyclase Gene Transfer in Heart Failure. *By* H. KIRK HAMMOND 426

Genetic Engineering and Therapy for Inherited and Acquired Cardiomyopathies. *By* SHARLENE DAY, JENNIFER DAVIS, MARGARET WESTFALL, AND JOSEPH METZGER 437

Nanomedicine Opportunities in Cardiology. *By* GREGORY LANZA, PATRICK WINTER, TILLMANN CYRUS, SHELTON CARUTHERS, JON MARSH, MICHAEL HUGHES, AND SAMUEL WICKLINE 451

Effects of Synchronized Cardiac Assist Device on Cardiac Energetics. *By* AMIR LANDESBERG, AVSHALOM SHENHAV, RONA SHOFTY, EUGENE KONYUKHOV, CARMIT LEVY, OSCAR LICHTENSTEIN, RAFAEL BEYAR, HENK EDJ TER KEURS, GIORA LANDESBERG, MARCO CABRERA, WILLIAM STANLEY, AND GERALD M. SAIDEL 466

Index of Contributors 479

Financial assistance was received from:

- The Cardiac Muscle Society, USA
- Technion, Israel Institute of Technology, Haifa, Israel
- The Larry and Horti Fairberg Fund, ATS, New York, NY, USA

> The New York Academy of Sciences believes it has a responsibility to provide an open forum for discussion of scientific questions. The positions taken by the participants in the reported conferences are their own and not necessarily those of the Academy. The Academy has no intent to influence legislation by providing such forums.

Preface

The Challenge of Cardiac Modeling—Interaction and Integration

SAMUEL SIDEMAN

Faculty of Biomedical Engineering, Technion, Israel Institute of Technology, Haifa 32000, Israel

> ABSTRACT: The goal of clinical cardiology is to obtain an integrated picture of the interacting parameters of muscle and vessel mechanics, blood circulation and myocardial perfusion, oxygen consumption and energy metabolism, and electrical activation and heart rate, thus relating to the true physiological and pathophysiological characteristics of the heart. Scientific insight into the cardiac physiology and performance is achieved by utilizing life sciences, for example, molecular biology, genetics and related intra- and intercellular phenomena, as well as the exact sciences, for example, mathematics, computer science, and related imaging and visualization techniques. The tools to achieve these goals are based on the intimate interactions between engineering science and medicine and the developments of modern, medically oriented technology. Most significant is the beneficiary effect of the globalization of science, the Internet, and the unprecedented international interaction and scientific cooperation in facing difficult multidisciplined challenges. This meeting aims to explore some important interactions in the cardiac system and relate to the integration of spatial and temporal interacting system parameters, so as to gain better insight into the structure and function of the cardiac system, thus leading to better therapeutic modalities.
>
> KEYWORDS: multifunctional; multiscalar; biological; mathematical; systems analysis; cardiome; physiome

INTRODUCTION

Biochemical, electrical, and mechanical interactions, and the consequent physiological integrations of the interacting parameters, sustain and control the function of the heart in steady or unsteady conditions of health and disease. These include the cardiac response to sudden or gradual changes imposed

---

Address for correspondence: Sam Sideman, D.Sc., D.Sc.Hon., Faculty of Biomedical Engineering, Technion, Israel Institute of Technology, Haifa 32000, Israel. Voice: 972-4-829-4139; fax: 972-4-829-4599.
 e-mail: sam@bm.technion.ac.il

by environmental changes, for example, pathology, drugs, and aging. Insight into these phenomena in the cardiac system or in any living entity requires analysis based on a close interaction between physiology (i.e., biology, biophysics, biochemistry, and biomechanics), mathematics, and computational techniques. Last, but not least, we note the need for close interaction between scientists from all over the world. Effective integration of the contributions of multidisciplinary cardiac scientists is of great importance to the understanding of the cardiovascular system, its interactions with renal, respiratory, and other systems, and leads to improved therapies.

LIFE SCIENCES AND THE EXACT SCIENCES

Life sciences and the exact sciences owe much of their outstanding developments in the last century to the fast growth of technology. Most relevant is the huge effect that modern technology, associated with new macro- and microimaging together with molecular scale diagnostic techniques, had on expanding the frontiers of medical sciences, and cardiology in particular. These have had most significant effects on the health and longevity of mankind in the last century, and catalyzed the transformation from classical studies of measured parameters in the macro world of organisms and organs to the micro and nanoworld of genes and cells. Cardiac research, for example, has moved from physiology and rheology to molecular biology, and cellular and genetic engineering. Consequently, we can now focus on the causes rather than on the symptoms and on preventing undesired phenomena by controlling molecular scale phenomena and manipulating the cells to repair the ailing organs.

An important step in this new art of knowledge-based therapeutics is the utilization of sophisticated mathematics to gain insight into the multiparameter and multifunctional complexity of the heart.

Synergetic Effects between Physics and Mathematics

Mathematics has made enormous strides in the second half of the last century, and it is instructive to reflect on the synergetic effects of the interactions between mathematics and physics.[1] Most noticeable are the inventions of calculus by Isaac Newton and Gottfried W. Leibniz in the late 17th century, which were stimulated by physical problems, such as planetary orbits and optical calculations.

Mathematical analyses, including the differential and integral calculus of Newton and Leibniz, as well as the probability theory, allow better insight into, and a clearer understanding of, the biological world. Mathematical analysis represents the acknowledged watershed between ancient and modern scientific thinking. Needless to say that it is impossible to grasp much of modern science and technology without resort to the concepts of mathematical analysis. Closely related to the development of medical know-how and physiological insight are the recent advances in imaging techniques and image processing, which have been enhanced by new theoretical efforts of mathematics and engineering. This marriage of mathematics and computer vision, better known as computational vision, has yielded highly effective image processing capabilities that benefit medical imaging.

Biology and Mathematics

William Harvey's 1628 discovery of the blood circulatory system illustrates the advantages of combining simple mathematics with careful observation and common sense. Harvey, who studied medicine in Padua while Galileo was there, realized the existence of peripheral and ventricular one-way valves. Having measured the ventricular volume, the heartbeats, and the average human heart blood content, he inferred the existence of invisible small vessels between the arteries and the veins and postulated that the blood circulates in the body. Harvey's analysis is perhaps the pivotal event in modern interaction between mathematics and biology.[1]

Challenges from the biological world have enriched mathematics by provoking novel ideas. Cohen[1] lists some 18 examples of mathematical innovations triggered by biological reality, beginning with the social population studies of Euler in 1760 through van Newman's game theory in 1953, which rested on Francis Galton's work of 1889, to Kingman's 1982 coalescent genealogy of populations. The living world has at least a thousand times the diversity of the nonliving world as there are probably up to 100 million biological species on the Earth, generated from a small fraction of the naturally occurring elements.[1] Fundamental understanding of biology should thus stimulate the creation of entirely new realms of mathematics, because the living world is significantly more heterogeneous than the nonanimate one. The complexity of the cell-based function and the multiscaled cell-to-organ biological systems, with their intra- and intercellular signaling and interactions, presents an enormous challenge to any attempt to understand and quantify the multifunctional phenomena involved. Coping with the hyperdiversity of life with its spatial and temporal, multiscale organization requires sophisticated mathematics and, possibly, some novel fundamental conceptual advances in mathematics.[1]

Biology and mathematics thus seem destined to enrich and extend each other in the coming decades, stimulating the creation of qualitatively new realms of science. Present and future interactions with mathematics can help biologists in grasping very big (biosphere) or very small (molecular) structures, as well as very slow (macrocirculation) or very fast (picoseconds) phenomena (photosynthesis, molecular motors). New mathematics will be required to cope with unilevel ensemble properties and with the heterogeneity of the biological units that compose ensembles at each level.

The discovery of the microscope in the late 17th century stimulated a revolution in biology by revealing otherwise invisible and previously unsuspected worlds. The impact of mathematics on the life sciences could be even more pronounced. Charles Darwin noted that people with an understanding "of the great leading principles of mathematics... seem to have an extra sense." Indeed, mathematics can help interpret data and reveal invisible worlds in all levels of life. In this sense, "mathematics is biology's next microscope, only better."[1] Furthermore, mathematical analysis, which allows better insight into the physiological phenomena, is also of great practical value as a predictive and responsive tool to micro- and macroenvironmental changes. New developments in computer hardware are beginning to allow heart researchers to test their hunches on computer models, replacing years of experimenting on tissue, live hearts, and multiple rounds of human trials. Eventually, one could compute the effectiveness of a treatment as well as the side effects in a multitude of different heart types.

Mathematics and Genetics

Mathematics was crucial in the original discovery of genes by Mendel and in the development of Darwin's theory of evolution. Mathematics was, and continues to be, the principal means of integrating evolution and genetics since the classic work of R.A. Fisher, J.B.S. Haldane, and S. Wright in the first half of the 20th century.[2] The recently completed human genome sequence will further enhance the development of novel therapeutic agents in a variety of diseases. Functional genomics, a collection of disciplines that are used to identify the function of genes in a specific context, is a challenging new way to address a complex disease on a molecular level. A deeper understanding of molecular events within the tissue cells will provide not only a better understanding of pathogenesis mechanisms and the function of genes and proteins involved in disease initiation and progression, but will also stimulate new diagnostic markers and cellular targets for therapeutic intervention. This innovative technology represents a challenging approach complementing the classical research in disease-relevant genes. Large-scale functional genomics opens up new means to characterize genetic regulatory networks. This will include new unidentified players in disease-relevant intracellular signaling cascades. However, major challenges must be overcome in order to properly utilize the potential of this technology.

Classical Modeling of the Multifunctional Cardiac System

Understanding cardiac performance and its deviations from its normal function requires quantitative knowledge of the interactions between the many variables involved in maintaining the beating heart. Since many of these are difficult or impossible to measure we must rely on logical conceptual models that serve to analyze global or local performance under diverse operating conditions. The results of the analyses must then be verified against measurable properties.

Physiological models usually begin as logical "flow diagrams," linking known variables and then, following learning of the kinetics and the mechanisms of interactions, evolve to become mathematical models describing, often with several assumptions, the quantitative static, or dynamic, relationships between sets of variables in a system. Many models have been proposed to describe physiological phenomena and have been "validated" to a limited extent, in that the measured data have been fitted by model solutions.

Practically all these models are single scaled, in the sense that they relate to a relatively small and limited range of interest in a certain physiological element, say cell, organelle, tissue, or ventricle. Hence, relatively few parameters are considered, and it is assumed that all the other system parameters are either constants or negligible. However, in spite of their narrowness of focus, such studies have provided important stepping stones for better understanding of the cardiac system and further serve as elements in more integrated models. The success of some classical multifunctional single-scale models with a limited number of parameters, for example, the Hodgkin–Huxley model of the action potential in a membrane or Suga's elastance model[3] of the contracting heart, to describe and explain important physiological phenomena is most probably due to the fact that they capture the essence of the phenomenon under normal physiological circumstances.

It is interesting to note at this point that large multiparameter biological or/and man-made systems must be robust enough to cope with transient "local," "regional" disturbances. The alternative is a deterioration of the whole system due to relatively small local deviations from its ideal normal function. This notion has already been advanced by Claude Bernard's[4] suggestion in the 1870s that there are overriding features of human physiology that dominate over local events and result in relative stability or "homeostatic du milieu interieure." For example,[5] hemodynamics, wherein the stability of plasma electrolyte and substrates composition are due to the interactions of large numbers of ongoing processes. Transient or constant irregularities in one or two elements in the blood are compensated to assure continued steady-state performance. An interesting consequence of the interplay between the large system's robustness and local insensitivity is evident by the well-known fact that many given physiological phenomena can be described by a number of different models. This implies that a reasonable model, which is based on a limited number of parameters and some logical assumptions, may never be an exact representation of the real subsystem under consideration.

Returning to Suga's experimentally based elastance model, we can clearly identify a number of important ambiguities as, for instance, its inability to explain Starling's Law, Fenn's Effect,[6] and Suga's own observation of the linearity between muscle's power production and energy generation. As stated by Gibbs,[7] there is no linear relation between the force–length (FL) areas in the FL plane in Suga's Elastance theory, because too much extra energy is liberated when the muscles shorten. Similarly, the ingenious microscale chemomechanical model of Huxley[8] fails to predict the linearity between ATP consumption and the manifestation of the pressure–volume (PV) or force–length (FL) potential energy.[9] It required the application of the four-state tropomyosin model of Landesberg and Sideman[10,11] and the identification of two important intracellular feedback mechanisms[12] to overcome the limitations of Suga's model. Obviously, single-scale models have inherent limitations and must be expanded if a better and more accurate understanding of the physiological system under consideration is desired.

The application of a bidomain mathematical model to explore the mechanisms of transvenous cardiac defibrillation so as to improve clinical efficiency and efficacy, recently reported (http://www.ima.umn.edu/industrial/98_99/fishler/tsld024.htm) by M.G. Fishler of Jude Medical Inc., demonstrates the need to upgrade the mathematical arsenal when addressing a real complex biological system. Thus, clinically applicable insights must represent a high degree of the true complexity of the living organ and a realistic model must address a three-dimensional domain with heterogeneous nonuniform local electric fields with different wave fronts and wave tails in a heterogeneous tissue structure involving variations in myocyte shapes and sizes.

INTEGRATED MULTIFUNCTIONAL AND MULTISCALE MODELING

It is obvious that mathematical and computational approaches are needed for better understanding of complex biological entities. Biological mechanisms are not uniform in structure, operate in a nonlinear manner, and are by definition dynamic and temporal, continuously changing with time. Understanding these mechanisms requires physiological insight, sophisticated mathematical/computer modeling as well as proper technological capabilities; for example, magnetic resonance imaging and high-powered microscopes for minute measurements and verification.

Quantitative approaches to unraveling biological function are well established in physiology,[13] which bring together elements of molecular and cellular biology, biophysics, and biochemistry to study cell and tissue function in the context of the organism. Physiological modeling[14] combines these elements using explicit representations of biophysical processes and integrating the components involved in a large-scale modeling framework.

The genotype-to-phenotype relationship is now recognized to be one that lends itself to determining mechanisms, rather than an associative one.[5]

Consequently, systems biology[15,16] now studies the organism level with greater interest in the mechanistic aspects of the components. This is evident in Guyton's integrated analyses in physiology[17] and his pioneering application of engineering principles and large-scale systems analyses in the cardiovascular arena preceded and catalyzed the birth and growth of bioengineering and biomedical engineering approaches in the last quarter of the last century.

Sideman and Beyar initiated in 1982 an integrated engineering approach to the understanding of the cardiovascular system. Their early efforts to comprehend the cardiac system aimed at an integrated model of the interrelated multifunctional macroscale parameters of hemodynamics, coronary circulation, cardiac mechanics, cardiac metabolism, electrocardiography, imaging techniques, and other related parameters. Their three-dimensional imaging techniques and analytic quantitative cardiology allowed relating structure and function to mechanical, electrical, and hemodynamical parameters in the macroscale, followed by relating the ventricular function to the microcellular characteristics. A powerful tool toward integration was the initiation of a series of multidisciplinary international cardiac workshops, which stimulated scientific cooperation and enhanced the concept of system analysis and interaction.

The Goldberg/Fairberg Cardiac Workshops

The present Fairberg Cardiac Workshop continues to pursue the goals of the Henry Goldberg Cardiac Workshops, initiated in 1984, manifesting the need for scientific interaction in the development of cardiac science. The goals of these past and present cardiac workshops are to (*a*) foster interdisciplinary interaction, so as to identify missing knowledge and catalyze new research ideas; (*b*) relate basic microscale, molecular, and subcellular phenomena to the global clinically manifested cardiac performance; (*c*) apply conceptual modeling and quantitative analysis to better explore, describe, and understand cardiac physiology; (*d*) interpret available clinical data and design new revealing experiments; and (*e*) enhance international cooperation in the endless search for better understanding of the various interacting variables that govern the heart's functions and their implications in cardiac pathophysiology. The past Henry Goldberg and present Fairberg's series of annual conferences have pursued analytical quantitative insight into the cardiac system in a series of multidisciplinary workshops attended by leading cardiac scientists and practitioners of the clinical art. New analytical procedures were highlighted in the context of modern physiology and the practical clinical picture. These workshops emphasized the interaction between the micro- and macroparameters affecting the cardiac performance. The focal points in these workshops varied with time, going from the overall organ performance to the functions of the basic cellular elements of the cardiac system. A short overview of the focal points of these workshops is given in TABLE 1.

TABLE 1. Focal points of the Goldberg/Fairberg Cardiac Workshop

Year	Location	Focal points	Ref
1984	Haifa, Israel	Interaction of mechanics, electrical activation, and perfusion clinical imaging	18
1985	Haifa, Israel	Mechanics, electrical activation, circulation, and control	19
1986	Rutgers, NJ, USA	Micro to macro activation, energy metabolism, and mechanics	20
1987	Tiberias, Israel	Interacting parameters and cardiac performance; ischemia	21
1988	Cambridge, UK	Effect nonhomogeneity on cardiac performance	22
1989	Eilat, Israel	Imaging techniques and cardiac performance	23
1991	Gwatt, Switzerland	Microphenomena, electrical activation, and performance	24
1992	Bethesda, MD, USA	Application of cardiac research to clinical practice	25
1994	Haifa, Israel	Molecular and subcellular aspects of cardiac performance	26
1996	Haifa, Israel	Analytical and quantitative cardiology: genetics and function	27
2002	Antalya, Turkey	Engineering and clinical data by imaging and visualization	28
2003	Erice, Sicily	Combining analytical and engineering principles with molecular genetics: cellular control mechanism	29
2005	Sintra, Portugal	Intra- and intercellular signaling and cardiac communications	30
2006	Charleston, SC, USA	Multifunctional and multiscale interactions and integration in the cardiac system	31

The present, 4th Fairberg Workshop[31] seeks insight into cardiac function by relating to the various functional interactions in the cardiac system and exploring the analytical approaches to the integration of the functional single- and multiscale phenomena, which sustains the viability of the cardiac system.

The Challenge: The Cardiome

James Bassingthwaighte[32] put the cardiac system research efforts into a better perspective in 1995 by introducing the all-inclusive Cardiome concept. The Cardiome is a one-organ component of the Physiome, and the term is used to represent the multidimensional complexity of the cardiac system and the various parameters that affect the cardiac function. The major elements of interest of the whole *organ* can be grouped[32] by *structure* (fibers, directionalities, physical properties, composition, etc.), *state* (contraction, relaxation, pathophysiology, etc.), *kinetics* (rates of deformations, ejection, outputs, excitation, pressures, volumes, etc.), and *functions* (activation, contraction, relaxation, etc.). The next level of interest brings us to the *tissues*, again defined by *structure, state, kinetics*, and *function*. Going a level "deeper," we face the *cells* and then the *organelles*, and finally the *molecular* level, each defined by its *structure, state, kinetics*, and *function*. Clearly, an awesome array of interacting parameters! The inherent complexity of the Cardiome was thus established as a multiscale multiparameter description of the cardiac system.

Computation and Limitations

Integrated multifunctional, multiscale modeling, which encompasses genomics, molecular biology, cells, tissues, and organs, characterizes systems behavior. The lowest levels concern biophysical and biochemical events. The higher levels of organization in tissues, organs, and organism are complex, representing the dynamically varying behavior of billions of cells interacting together. The integrative systems approach to multiscale modeling relates to four complementary areas of research: (*a*) cardiovascular physiology and medicine; (*b*) systems optimization and parameterization; (*c*) signal analysis and control; and (*d*) molecular biology, cellular biophysics, and mathematics. These can be applied to formulate computationally feasible multiscale system descriptions, allowing adaptation to interventions or to changing environmental driving forces.

Effective comprehensible computational procedures require assumptions and simplifications, and models integrating cellular events into tissue and organ behavior are presently forced to resort to simplifications in order to minimize computation, consequently reducing the model's ability to respond correctly to dynamic changes in external conditions. Adjustments at protein and gene regulatory levels shortchange the simplified higher level representations. Bassingthwaighte[33] has recently suggested a cell primitive composed of a set of subcellular modules, each defining an intracellular function (action potential, trichloroacetic acid cycle, oxidative phosphorylation, glycolysis, calcium cycling, contraction, etc.), providing a so-called "eternal cell," which assumes that there is neither proteolysis nor protein synthesis. Cellular subregions are considered as stirred tanks, linked by diffusional or transporter-mediated exchange. This basic model uses ordinary differential equations rather than stochastic or partial differential equations, and is regarded as a primitive upon which to build models encompassing gene regulation, signaling, and long-term adaptations in structure and function. Simpler forms of the model can be used, when possible, to reduce computation, but more complex and detailed modules and elements need to be employed to improve model realism. Some potential computational approaches are reviewed by Bassingthwaighte.[33]

Models providing clinically applicable insights must represent a high degree of the true complexity of the living organ. A possible mechanism for handling this complexity is to adopt a modular and hierarchical approach to modeling, whereby mathematical representations of biological components are brought together and tuned appropriately to produce a model of a specific cell or tissue type. Perhaps the most desired way of achieving this is to retain biophysical detail at each level in a modeling hierarchy, which also provides an obvious mechanism for revision or improvement of selected parts of a large-scale simulation as new data are collected.[33]

THE PHYSIOME

The Physiome is a natural extension of the Cardiome, expressing the desire to integrate physiological information of a given species, and particularly the human species, in one large framework. The Physiome project, which was officially launched by the International Union of Physiology Scientists (IUPS) in 1997,[34] aims to obtain quantitative description and understanding of the human physiology in various states, from embryogenesis to ripe old age, and to place all the physiological information known about the human body into one database, and then utilize that data in specific models of cells, tissues, organs and, ultimately, the entire human system. The project was championed by a worldwide group of physiologists and bioengineers from Auckland, Oxford, Johns Hopkins, MIT, Washington, and the University of California, and is presently attracting scientists from all over the world. Physiome projects now in progress include the heart, lung, gut, and the musculoskeletal system.

The Physiome is the most challenging multiscale, multifunctional physiological model in creation today, and the databases needed are considered to be larger than those of the genome. The program combines computer science, physiology, and engineering to create digital simulations of biological systems. The project was significantly inspired by the success of Peter Hunter and Bruce Smaill in Auckland to develop clear and detailed images of the three-dimensional heart, lung, and later the skeleton.[35,36] Hunter's heart model, for example, can show any level of detail, down to the multicellular level, of how the heart functions. Utilizing detailed measurements in all regions of interest in the heart, their model is close to making the virtual heart almost real. A typical significant application of the virtual heart, developed by Denis Noble, involves rapid pharmaceutical target selection to explore the effects of known and new potential drugs on one or more targets in the cells and the consequent effect on the whole heart. Most important is the anticipated ability to predict the real heart's behavior by model simulation.

Obviously, all the computational multiscale limitations concerning the Cardiome are applicable to the far more complicated Physiome model. Interaction is one of the biggest challenges. Not only must this model account for the relationships within the organs, starting from their subcellular structures through to their whole organ function, it must also account for the way organs relate to one another within the whole body. Thus, compatible models of other organs are necessary for a complete picture, and this is the ultimate goal of the Physiome.

SUMMARY

The Cardiome is typically characterized by a wide range of spatial scales (from molecular to the tissue/organ level) and temporal scales (from picoseconds biochemical reactions and molecular motor actions to progression of disease over days, months, years, and slow aging). The challenge is to understand and actually describe the complex interactions by constructing "single" and multiscale models that relate to each other and can be integrated "horizontally" by function as well as "vertically" by scale to provide insight into all the levels in the complex physiological systems that sustain the heart's functions. Moreover, the desired Cardiome model should allow prediction of the system's response to any parametric change and deviation from normal function at all levels. Integration of simulation and experimental data is critical to the quantitative understanding of the complex Cardiome! Obviously, this task demands interaction of and integration of the worldwide know-how of the cardiac system and the international scientific cooperation in turning a virtual heart to a useful practical reality.

ACKNOWLEDGMENTS

We gratefully thank all those who helped transform this workshop from vision to reality. First and foremost, we salute the workshop participants whose excellence made the meeting an exciting meaningful affair, with particular kudos to Prof. Jim Bassingwaighte who actively encouraged and wisely contributed to *all* these Goldberg/Fairberg Cardiac Workshops. Next, we heartily thank the International Program Committee and the members of the Organizing Committee for endless suggestions and continuous vigilance. Special thanks go to Prof. Martin Morad, who helped set the meeting in The Inn Place, and old plantation in Charleston, SC, and to our local host, Prof. Roger Markwald, who helped make our meeting a most enjoyable experience. Their efforts made the workshop a great success. Thanks are also due to our secretary, Mrs. Betty Kazin, for devotion and care. Finally, we thank our sponsors, The Technion, Israel Institute of Technology, The Medical University of South Carolina, Charleston, SC, and the Cardiac Muscle Society, USA. Most sincerely, we gratefully remember our departed friends, Mr. Jack G. George of Los Angeles, CA for some financial support, and Horti and Larry Fairberg of the American Technion Society, New York, USA, whose endowment facilitated this important international event.

REFERENCES

1. COHEN, J.E. 2004. Mathematics is biology's next microscope, only better; biology is mathematics' next physics, only better. PLoS Biol. **2:** 2017–2023; e439.
2. PROVINE, W.B. 2001. The Origins of Theoretical Population Genetics, 2nd ed. University of Chicago Press. Chicago.
3. SUGA, H. 1990. Ventricular energetics. Physiol. Rev. **70:** 247–277.
4. BERNARD, C. 1878. Lectures on the Phenomena of Life Common to Animals and Plants. Translation by Hebbel E. Hoff, Roger Guillemin and Lucienne Guillemin. J. Libraire. Paris.
5. BASSINGTHWAIGHTE, J.B., H.S. CHIZECK, L.E. ATLAS & H. QIAN. 2005. Multiscale modeling of cardiac cellular energetics. Ann. N. Y. Acad. Sci. **1047:** 395–424.
6. FENN, W.O. 1923. A quantitative comparison between the energy liberated and the work performed by the isolated sartonius muscle of the frog. J. Physiol. **58:** 175–203.
7. GIBBS, C.L. 2003. Muscle mechanics and energetics: a comparative view cardiac energetics: sense and nonsense. Clin. Exp. Pharm. Physiol. **30:** 598–603.
8. HUXLEY, A.F. 1957. Muscle structure and theories of contraction. Prog. Biophys. Chem. **7:** 255–318.
9. GIBBS, C.L. & J.B. CHAPMAN. 1985. Cardiac mechanisms and energetics: chemomechanical transduction in cardiac muscle. Am. J. Physiol. **249:** H199–H206.
10. LANDESBERG, A. & S. SIDEMAN. 1994. Coupling calcium binding to Troponin-C and Xb cycling kinetics in skinned cardiac cells. Am. J. Physiol. **266** (Heart Circ Physiol. **35**): H1261–H1271.
11. LANDESBERG, A. & S. SIDEMAN. 1994. Mechanical regulation in the cardiac muscle by coupling calcium binding to troponin-C and Xb cycling. A dynamic model. Am. J. Physiol. **267** (Heart Cir. Physiol. **36**): H779–H795.
12. LANDESBERG, A., C. LEVY, Y. YANIV, & S. SIDEMAN. 2004. The adaptive intracellular control of cardiac muscle function. Ann. N. Y. Acad. Sci. **1015:** 71–83.
13. BOYD, C.A.R. & D. NOBLE. 1993. The Logic of Life: the Challenge of Integrative Physiology. Oxford University Press. New York.
14. NICHOLAS, P., et al. 2004. Modeling cellular and tissue function. Prog. Biophys. Mol. Biol. **85:** 117–119.
15. KITANO, H. 2002. Systems biology: a brief overview. Science **295:** 1662–1664.
16. NOBLE, D. 2002. Modeling the heart—from genes to cells to the whole organ. Science **295:** 1678–1682.
17. GUYTON, A.C., T.G. COLMAN & H.J. GRANGER. 1972. Circulation: overall regulation. Annu. Rev. Physiol. **34:** 13–46.
18. SIDEMAN, S. & R. BEYAR, Eds. 1985. Simulation and imaging of the cardiac system—state of the heart. Proc. 1st Henry Goldberg Workshop, Technion, Haifa, 1984. Martinus Nijhoff. Dordrecht, Boston.
19. SIDEMAN, S. & R. BEYAR, Eds. 1987. Simulation and control of the cardiac system. Parts I, II, III, Proc. 2nd Henry Goldberg Workshop, Haifa, 1985. CRC Press. Boca Raton, FL.
20. SIDEMAN, S. & R. BEYAR, Eds. 1987. Activation, metabolism and perfusion of the heart. Simulation and experimental models. Proc. 3rd Henry Goldberg Workshop, Rutgers Univ, USA, 1986. Martinus Nijhoff. Dordrecht, Boston.
21. SIDEMAN, S. & R. BEYAR, Eds. 1989. Analysis and simulation of the cardiac system—Ischemia. Proc. 4th Henry Goldberg Workshop, Tiberias, May 1987 (3 vols). CRC Press. Boca Raton, FL.

22. SIDEMAN, S. & R. BEYAR, Eds. 1990. Imaging, analysis and simulation of the cardiac system. Proc. 5th Henry Goldberg Workshop, Cambridge, UK, 1988. Freund Publishers. London.
23. SIDEMAN, S. & R. BEYAR, Eds. 1991. Imaging, measurements and analysis of the heart. Proc. 6th Henry Goldberg Workshop, Eilat, Dec. 1989. Hemisphere Publishers. New York.
24. SIDEMAN, S., R. BEYAR & A. KLEBER, Eds. 1991. Cardiac electrophysiology, circulation and transport. Proc. 7th Henry Goldberg Workshop, Gwatt, Switzerland, 1991. Kluwer. New York.
25. SIDEMAN, S. & R. BEYAR, Eds. 1993. Interactive phenomena in the cardiac system. Proc. of the 8th Henry Goldberg Workshop, Bethesda, MD, 1992. Plenum. New York.
26. SIDEMAN, S. & R. BEYAR, Eds. 1995. Molecular and subcellular cardiology: effects on structure and function. Proc. of the 9th Henry Goldberg Workshop, Haifa, Israel, 1994. Plenum. New York.
27. SIDEMAN, S. & R. BEYAR, Eds. 1997. Analytical and quantitative cardiology: from genetics to function. Proc. of the 10th Henry Goldberg Workshop, Haifa, Israel. Plenum. New York.
28. SIDEMAN, S. & A. LANDESBERG, Eds. 2002. Visualization and imaging in transport phenomena. Proc. of the 1st Larry and Horti Fairberg Workshop, Antalya, Turkey, Annals of the New York Academy Sciences./New York. Vol. 972.
29. SIDEMAN, S. & R. BEYAR, Eds. 2004. Cardiac engineering: from genes and cells to structure and function. Proc. of the 2nd Larry and Horti Fairberg Workshop, Erice, Sicily. Annals of the New York Academy of Sciences/New York, Vol. **1015**.
30. SIDEMAN, S., R. BEYAR & A. LANDESBERG. 2005. The communicative cardiac cell. Proc. of 3rd Larry & Horti Fairberg Workshop, Sintra, Portugal. Annals of the New York Academy of Sciences. New York Vol. 1047.
31. SIDEMAN, S., R. BEYAR & A. LANDESBERG, Eds. 2006. Interactive and Integrative cardiology. Proc. 4th Larry & Horti Fairberg Workshop, Charleston, SC, USA. Annals of the New York Academy of Sciences. New York vol 1080.
32. BASSINGTHWAIGHTE, J.B.. 1995. Toward modeling in human physiome. *In* Molecular and Subcellular Cardiology. S. Sideman & R. Beyar, Eds.: Adv Exp Med and Biol, Vol. 382. Plenum, New York.
33. BASSINGTHWAIGHTE, J.B. & K.C. VINNAKOTA. 2004. The computational integrated myocyte. A view into the virtual heart. Ann. N.Y. Acad. Sci. **1015:** 391–405.
34. BASSINGTHWAIGHTE, J.B. 2000. Strategies for the physiome project. Ann. Biomed. Eng. **28:** 1043–1058.
35. HUNTER, P.J. & B.H. SMAILL. 1989. The analysis of cardiac function: a continuum approach. Prog. Biophys. Mol. Biol. **52:** 101–164.
36. HUNTER, P.J., *et al*. 1992. An anatomical heart model with applications to myocardial activation and ventricular mechanics. Crit. Rev. Biomed. Eng. **20:** 403–427.

Functional Studies of Individual Myosin Molecules

JODY A. DANTZIG, TIM Y. LIU, AND YALE E. GOLDMAN

University of Pennsylvania School of Medicine, Pennsylvania Muscle Institute, Philadelphia, Pennsylvania 19104-6083, USA

> ABSTRACT: The "conventional" isoform of myosin that polymerizes into filaments (myosin II) is the molecular motor powering contraction in all three types of muscle. Considerable attention has been paid to the developmental progression, isoform distribution, and mutations that affect myocardial development, function, and adaptation. Optical trap (laser tweezer) experiments and various types of high-resolution fluorescence microscopy, capable of interrogating individual protein motors, are revealing novel and detailed information about their functionally relevant nanometer motions and pico-Newton forces. Single-molecule laser tweezer studies of cardiac myosin isoforms and their mutants have helped to elucidate the pathogenesis of familial hypertrophic cardiomyopathies. Surprisingly, some disease mutations seem to enhance myosin function. More broadly, the myosin superfamily includes more than 20 nonfilamentous members with myriad cellular functions, including targeted organelle transport, endocytosis, chemotaxis, cytokinesis, modulation of sensory systems, and signal transduction. Widely varying genetic, developmental and functional disorders of the nervous, pigmentation, and immune systems have been described in accordance with these many roles. Compared to the collective nature of myosin II, some myosin family members operate with only a few partners or even alone. Individual myosin V and VI molecules can carry cellular vesicular cargos much farther distances than their own size. Laser tweezer mechanics, single-molecule fluorescence polarization, and imaging with nanometer precision have elucidated the very different mechano-chemical properties of these isoforms. Critical contributions of nonsarcomeric myosins to myocardial development and adaptation are likely to be discovered in future studies, so these techniques and concepts may become important in cardiovascular research.
>
> KEYWORDS: myosin; molecular motors; laser tweezers; optical trap; TIRF microscopy; single molecule; cardiac

---

Address for correspondence: Yale E. Goldman, M.D., Ph.D., University of Pennsylvania School of Medicine, Pennsylvania Muscle Institute, 3700 Hamilton Walk, D700 Richards Building, Philadelphia, PA 19104-6083. Voice: 215-898-4247; fax: 215-898-2653.
  e-mail: goldmany@mail.med.upenn.edu

INTRODUCTION

In this article, we briefly describe several powerful techniques for studying macromolecules one at a time. Single-molecule biophysical studies are contributing to the understanding of sarcomeric myosins, including cardiac mutants that cause familial hypertrophic cardiomyopathy (FHC), and unconventional myosins that carry out essential functions in many cell types. Optical traps (laser tweezers), single-molecule fluorescence microscopy, single-molecule fluorescence polarization, and fluorescence imaging with one nanometer accuracy (FIONA) reveal the individual mechanical trajectories and structural dynamics of these molecular motors that are concealed by the averaging inherent in classical experiments on protein ensembles.[1-5] Applications relevant to the cardiovascular system are briefly described.

LASER TWEEZERS

Ashkin and Dziedzic[6] made the striking observation that a tightly focused laser beam would capture small refractile objects and prevent them from diffusing away. Since that initial finding, the technique of manipulating objects and measurement of their mechanical properties by focused light, often called *optical trap* or *laser tweezers*, has become a powerful and broadly applied tool in molecular biophysics. Optical traps are capable of detecting the nanometer motions and pico-Newton forces produced by macromolecules, such as molecular motors. Many dramatic discoveries have been made about molecular motors, nucleic acid processing enzymes, and membrane receptors using this kind of nanotechnology.[7,8]

The operating mechanism of the laser tweezers can be understood by considering the refraction or scattering of light rays by a small object, such as a 1-μm diameter plastic bead (FIG. 1).[9] A high numerical aperture microscope objective lens brings a collimated infrared laser beam ($\lambda = 1064$ nm) to an intense, diffraction-limited spot at its focal plane. If the bead is not centered within this spot, the intensity of light is higher toward the center of the trap (bright ray in FIG. 1 A). The bead acts as a tiny lens, refracting the infrared light at an angle, to the left in FIGURE 1 A, and the momentum of the photons, is altered (arrow Δ in the inset). In accordance with the conservation of momentum, the leftward mechanical impulse exerted by the bead on the photons is accompanied by a rightward force by the photons on the bead. This "optical trapping force" tends to cause the bead to migrate toward the center of the trap and thus be retained. Similar reasoning can be applied in the *z*-axis (optical axis), FIGURE 1 B, so the focused laser beam traps the bead in all three dimensions. Using sensitive detectors and appropriate calibration, the position and force on the bead are detectable at the resolutions required to study molecular events.[9,10]

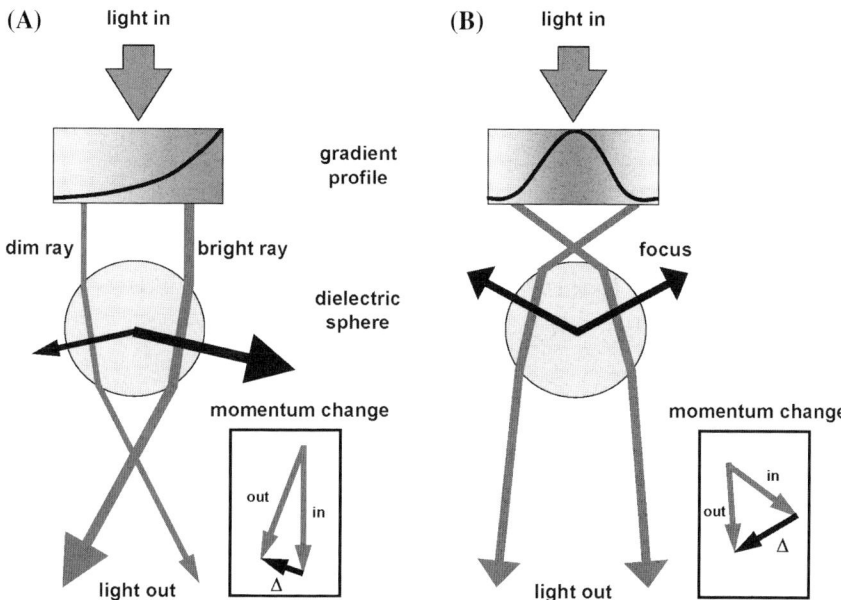

FIGURE 1. Ray optics diagram of the gradient forces on a transparent particle in an optical trap. The gradient profiles in the diagram show the intensity of an infrared laser beam ($\lambda = 1064$ nm). (**A**) Bead positioned leftward from the brightest spot, so the intensity is higher toward the right (thicker ray). Scattering (refraction) of the rays alters the momentum of the photons (Δ in the inset) causing an equal and opposite force on the bead (black arrows on bead). The net result is movement of the bead toward the highest intensity at the center of the beam. (**B**) Bead positioned below the focal spot. Refraction of the converging rays changes the photon momentum downward (Δ in the inset), leading to an upward trapping force on the bead, toward the focal plane. Thus the optical trapping force is toward the highest intensity in all three dimensions. "Photon pressure" causes the bead to settle slightly farther from the objective lens. Modified and reprinted, with permission, from the *Annu. Rev. Biophys. Biomolec. Struct.*, Volume 23, © 1994 by Annual Reviews www.annualreviews.org.

There are several ways to use the optical traps to study single-molecule mechanics. Measuring the force and displacement at the single-molecule level with the optical trap provides a molecular indication of the mechanical end point of energy transduction by actomyosin. A typical geometry for studying actomyosin is the *three-bead assay* (FIG. 2).[11,12] An actin filament is suspended securely between two beads which are held in dual optical traps. A third bead is attached to the substrate and sparsely coated with myosin. Positioning the actin near the myosin in a medium containing appropriate ionic constituents, including magnesium adenosine triphosphate (MgATP), allows the myosin to attach transiently to actin and deflect both beads from their central positions (FIG. 3, arrowheads).[13] These interactions are the individual displacement (panels A

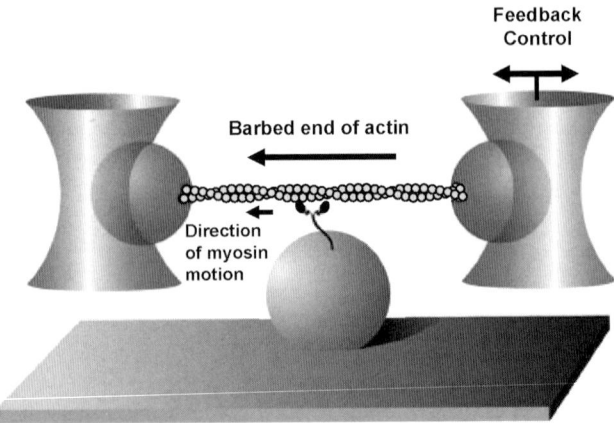

FIGURE 2. Three-bead geometry of an optical trap[11] originally described by Finer et al.[10] Polystyrene or ceramic beads sparsely coated with myosin (or fragments of myosin) are attached to a cover slip to raise the myosin above the surface. An actin filament is secured to two smaller latex beads captured in two optical traps. When the actin is brought close to the myosin, active interactions deflect the positions of the trapped beads. Feedback control of the bead positions enables measurement of force. Copyright 2001 National Academy of Sciences, USA.

and B) and force events (C and D) indicating transduction of the energy liberated from splitting of ATP into mechanical work. Individual muscle myosin II molecules produce a force of ~10 pN and a displacement of 5–10 nm, thus producing ~50 × 10^{-21} J of mechanical work from the ~100 × 10^{-21} J of free energy liberated from ATP hydrolysis.[14] In muscle and myocardium, these molecular events are amplified by the series/parallel filamentous structure of the sarcomeres to cause contraction. Work in our laboratory in this area has produced an enhancement of the three-bead assay to control and modulate the effective stiffness of the actin[14] and to study the mechanics of messenger RNA in ribosomes synthesizing proteins.[15]

APPLICATION TO FHC

Single-molecule techniques have recently been added to the tools used to study the pathology of cardiac disorders. FHC is an autosomal dominant inherited abnormality with variable penetrance leading to cardiomyocyte disarray, fibrosis, and hypertrophy in most cases. It has been linked to more than 100 individual missense mutations in several sarcomeric proteins including the β-myosin heavy chain (MHC), myosin regulatory and essential light chains, troponin, myosin binding protein C, actin, and titin.[16] One of the mutations causing disease with high penetration and sudden death is a point mutation at

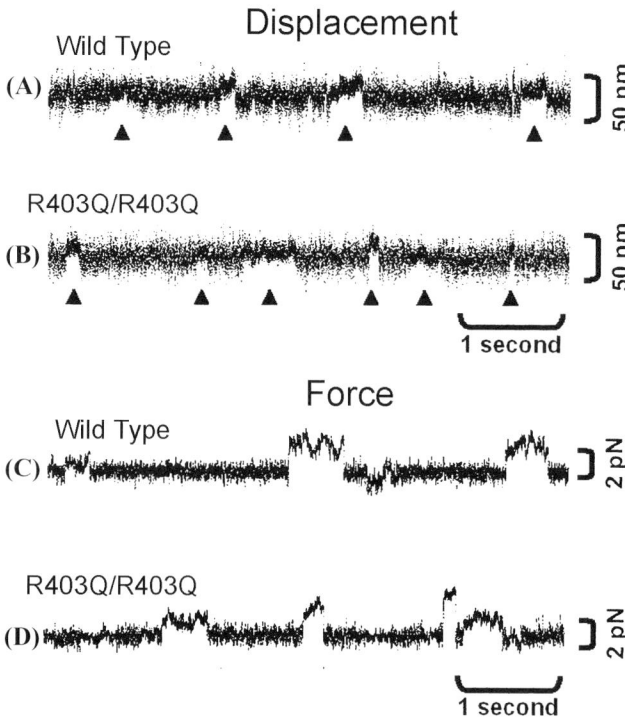

FIGURE 3. Single-molecule mechanical measurements of unitary displacement and force for mouse cardiac myosin. (**A**) and (**B**) Unitary displacement data from purified normal and R403Q/R403Q α-myosin heavy chain (α-MHC) using the three-bead assay described in FIGURE 2. (**C**) and (**D**) Unitary force measurements for normal and R403Q/R403Q α-MHC obtained by monitoring the force on the bead *via* a feedback circuit. Modified and reprinted with permission, Tyska, M.J. *et al.* 2000. *Circ. Res.* **86:** 737–744.

residue 403 of the MHC from the native arginine amino acid to glutamine (mutation R403Q). Arg^{403} is located in a peptide loop at the actin-binding interface of myosin, leading to its designation as the myopathy loop.[17,18] Myosins with mutations at the corresponding residue have been expressed in a number of backgrounds, such as cardiac α-MHC, smooth muscle, and the myosin II of the slime mold, *Dictyostelium discoideum*. The mutated myosins can be isolated from biopsies of human myocardium, soleus, and other slow skeletal muscles expressing the same β-MHC. Many studies found depressed function of the mutant myosin, such as ATPase rate, affinity for actin, and velocity of actin translocation by myosin with an *in vitro* gliding filament assay.[19–23] Experiments on whole slow muscles, skinned muscle fiber preparations, and transgenic mouse hearts also found the anticipated depressed force and diastolic dysfunction.[24–27] The power output deficit was consistent with the hypothesis that the hypertrophy was a compensatory mechanism to recover cardiac output. Interpretation of these early results was complicated by many factors especially the heterozygous expression of the mutant myosin and inability to purify the mutant from the normal myosin.

Recent studies using carefully purified myosin from transgenic mice and human biopsies have shown, instead, a moderate enhancement of function in R403Q MHC as well as other FHC mutations.[13,27–29] These studies found increased velocity for *in vitro* gliding, increased ATPase activity, and increased muscle fiber force production.[30] Using single molecules, optical trap recordings from the three-bead assay with purified wild-type α-MHC and R403Q mutant α-MHC from a transgenic mouse (FIG. 3)[13] show that the unitary displacement values (averaging 7 nm, upward deflections in FIG. 3 A, B) and unitary force events (averaging 1 pN, upward deflections in FIG. 3 C for wild-type and FIG. 3 D for R403Q α-MHC) are not appreciably different. A subsequent optical trap study of myosin purified from cardiac punch biopsies of heterozygotic R403Q and L908V patients found an enhanced detachment rate of individual actomyosin interactions in the FHC samples, consistent with the ~30% increased *in vitro* gliding velocity.[27]

Many factors may explain the discrepancy between these studies and the earlier ones, including differences in sources of myosin and conditions of experimentation. It is notable, however, that the study by Keller *et al*.[28] on R403W cardiac myosin from a human heart homozygous in this mutant, obtained following successful cardiac transplantation, avoided complications of heterozygous expression and unnatural background isoform. If we assume that the studies showing enhanced myosin function represent the actual performance because experimental problems, such as degradation during purification, are more likely to depress function than to improve it, a puzzling question arises: Why does a gain of function lead to hypertrophy and attendant mechanical and electrical dysfunction? Several hypotheses have been advanced, but the answer is not yet apparent.[27,30–32] Increased ATPase activity could lead to decreased efficiency and depressed energetic reserve. Force above the optimum design setting could disrupt attachments and alignment between myocardiocytes, causing disarray. Faster enzymatic cycling with a nearly constant actomyosin attachment time might lead to a higher-than-normal proportion of cross-bridge attachment time, slowed relaxation, and depressed diastolic filling. A reduced actomyosin interaction time at constant unitary force, would depress the average force during an enzymatic cycle. The release of adenosine diphosphate (ADP) from actomyosin may be the cross-bridge biochemical step that is regulated by the afterload during contraction,[33] but ADP release is not discriminated clearly for cardiac myosin in the optical trap. Thus the mechanochemical regulation of cycling, such as strain-dependent ADP dissociation, may be altered in FHC. That would allow premature detachment of force-generating cross-bridges and decreased force or excess ATP hydrolysis. The optical trap studies were conducted with unregulated actin filaments, but performance might be altered at submaximal Ca^{2+} activation, as exists during normal heartbeats. It is also possible that the mutations trigger hypertrophic signaling events by molecular interactions that are distinct from force production, which is probably the case for FHC mutations that mainly alter myofibril assembly.[34] The pathogenesis of FHC in individuals with mutations in other sarcomeric proteins is similarly baffling. Distinguishing among the possible mechanisms that link the genetic alterations to their phenotypes will require further studies of single molecules, cardiomyocytes, and whole hearts from additional animal models and human myocardial and slow skeletal muscle specimens.

UNCONVENTIONAL MYOSINS

At least 20 classes of myosin have been identified, 12 of which are expressed in humans (FIG. 4)[35,36] from the nearly 40 identified myosin genes detected in the human genome. Myosin molecules are involved in myriad cell developmental, functional, and maintenance roles including targeted organelle transport, endocytosis, chemotaxis, cytokinesis, modulation of sensory systems, and signal transduction. The "conventional" isoform of myosin that

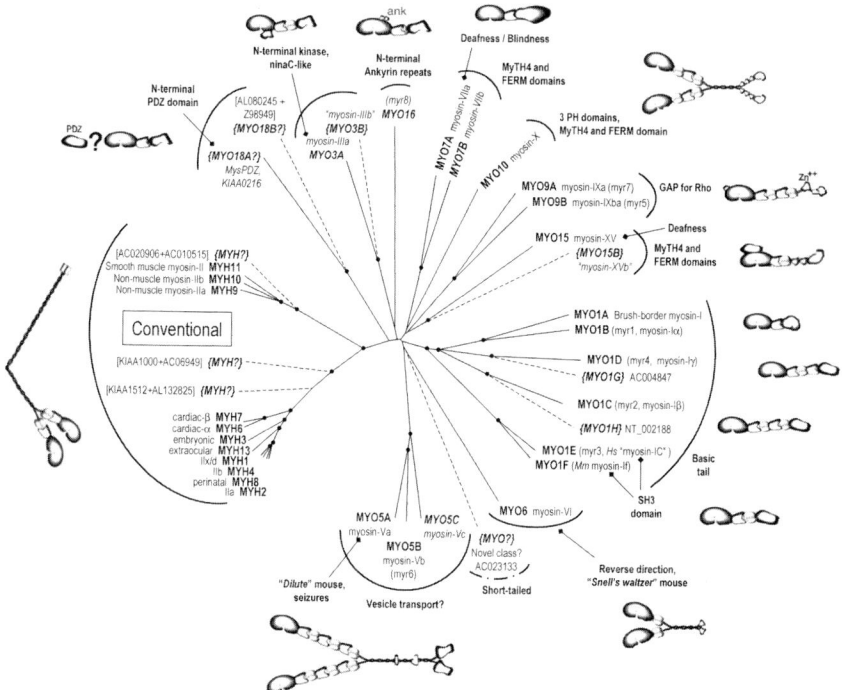

FIGURE 4. Phylogenetic tree of 35 human myosins with corresponding cartoon representations of the structures of each major class. Reprinted from *Mol. Biol. Cell* 2001 **12:** 780-794 with the permission of The American Society for Cell Biology. Cartoon representations of the myosin molecules are reprinted from *J. Cell Sci.* 2000 **113:** 3353-3354 with permission of Company of Biologists Ltd.

polymerizes into filaments and powers contraction in all three types of muscle was originally designated myosin II because it contains two globular heads containing the actin-binding ATPase motor domains. Besides powering muscle contraction myosin II also pinches the two daughter cells apart at the end of cell division[37] and causes cortical contraction at the trailing zone of locomoting leucocytes.[38]

The other myosin isoforms do not polymerize into filaments and many are single-headed. The diversity of the motor, regulatory, and cargo-binding tail domains of the myosin molecules allow them to perform many varied roles within the cell (FIG. 5).[39] In humans, eight single-headed isoforms of myosin I are responsible for linking the cytoskeleton to lipid membranes (FIG. 5 Bi), many membrane trafficking events,[40] and sensory-neural adaptation.[41] The three human myosin V genes express double-headed isoforms that power short range transport of vesicles and have a role in mRNA localization.

There is only one isoform of myosin VI found in humans, and its monomer/dimer transition may be under cellular regulation.[42,43] Myosin VI moves toward the minus ("pointed") end of actin,[44] opposite to the direction of other myosins, and it serves a role in endocytosis (FIG. 5 Be–g) as well as retrograde movement of vesicles toward the center of the cell (FIG. 5 Bg). Its unusual mechanism of motility has been the subject of many structural and single-molecule studies.[11,45–47]

The two isoforms of myosin VII are differentially expressed in many tissues and participate in cell adhesion, the structural organization of the actin cytoskeleton, as well as phagocytosis (FIG. 5 Bb). There is one widely expressed double-headed myosin X found in humans that is involved in nuclear positioning, filopodial extension (FIG. 5 Af), and pseudopod extension during phagocytosis (FIG. 5Ba). The varied functions of these and the other myosin isoforms are regulated by expression, phosphorylation, and other signaling mechanisms, providing the cell with a bustling and well-organized economy of motion.

Expression profiles of myosin isoforms among human tissues are shown in TABLE 1, obtained using the UniGene database (www.ncbi.nlm.nih.gov/UniGene)[48,49] to analyze the human transcriptome. The +, −, and 0 symbols indicate relative abundance of expressed sequence tags (ESTs), which are partial unique cDNA clones of mRNA transcripts in libraries from each tissue. There are caveats to inferring protein expression from this type of data, including errors of normalization, sequencing, reading direction, chimeras, contamination, and internal priming,[49–52] but general features of the expression levels emerge. Certain myosin isoforms (myosin I, II, VI), powering contraction, cell shape, and membrane trafficking, are expressed ubiquitously. Other isoforms (III and VII) are tissue-specific. Not surprisingly, mRNA transcripts for conventional myosin are present in high abundance in heart muscle. Many of the unconventional myosins (I, V, VI, IX, X, and XVIII) are also expressed in the myocardium.

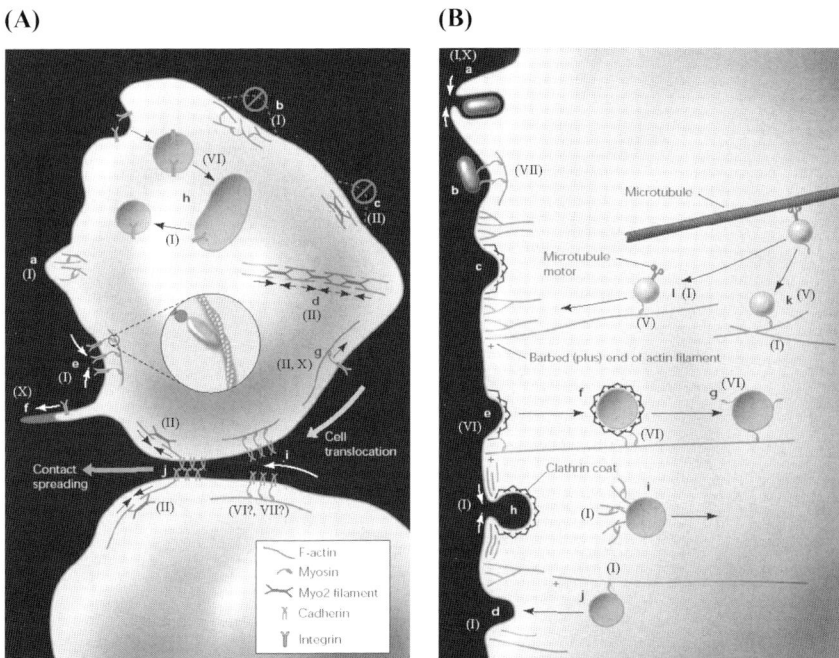

FIGURE 5. Functions of nonsarcomeric myosin isoforms. (**A**) Roles of myosin in cell motility and adhesion. (*a*) myosin I activation and nucleation of the actin related protein (ARP) 2/3 complex for lamellipodial protrusion. (*b*) myosin I limitation of lateral lamellipodial extension by regulation of cortical tension. (*c*) myosin II limitation of lateral extension driven by contractility. (*d*) myosin II retraction of the cell posterior. (*e*) clustering of the cell-substrate adhesion receptors. (*f*) myosin X transport of integrins or Wiscott–Aldrich syndrome proteins to the filopodial tip. (*g*) myosins II and X acting as a clutch coupling cell–substrate adhesion to forward movement of the cell. (*h*) cell adhesion receptor endocytosis and recycling. (*i*) clustering of cell–cell adhesion receptors. (*j*) myosin II-mediated zippering of cell–cell junctions. (**B**) Roles of myosin in membrane trafficking. (*a*) myosins I and X extending pseudopods for phagocytosis. (*b*) myosin VII-dependent cell adhesion of particles for phagocytosis. (*c*) reorganization of cortical actin for invagination of a clathrin-coated pit. (*d*) myosin I-mediated transport of an exocytic vesicle toward the plasma membrane. (*e*) myosin VI minus-end-directed deformation of the plasma membrane for clathrin pit formation and retrograde transportation of clathrin-coated vesicles (*f*) and uncoated vesicles (*g*). (*h*) membrane scission. (*i*) vesicle movement via myosin I-dependent ARP2/3 activation and actin polymerization. (*j*) myosin I movement of vesicles to the cell periphery. (*k*) switching between microtubule and myosin V actin-based transport with vesicle capture and anchoring. (*l*) short-range transport of actin filaments for relocation. The myosin isoform numbers are indicated by the Roman numerals within parentheses. Modified and reprinted from *Physiology (Bethesda)* **20**: 239–251, 2005, with permission of the American Physiological Society.

TABLE 1. Myosin classes expressed in humans

Myosin isoform	Blood	Bone	Brain	Heart	Liver Lung	Muscle	Skin	Testis Uterus	Vascular	Functions
I	++	++	+	++	++	++	++	++	++	Membrane trafficking, signal-transduction
II	+++	++	++	+++	++	+++	++	++	+++	Power muscle contraction, cell shape/polarity
III	+	0	±	0	±	±	+	+	+	Visual and auditory sensory cell functions
V	+	+	++	+	+	++	++	+	0	Short-range vesicle transport, mRNA localization
VI	+	+	+	+	+	++	+	+	+	Endocytosis, membrane trafficking, actin cytoskeleton
VII	+	+	±	0	+	+	0	+	0	Cell adhesion, phagocytosis, actin cytoskeleton
IX	++	+	+	+	+	+	++	+	+	Regulation of signaling
X	0	+	++	+	+	+	++	+	+	Links phosphoinositide signaling to phagocytosis, nuclear positioning
XV	++	+	+	0	±	+	0	+	0	Formation of actin-rich structures
XVIII	++	+	+	+	+	+	+	+	0	Unknown

NOTE: Expression of myosin classes in human tissues, based on analysis of the human transcriptome using the UniGene database (www.ncbi.nlm.nih.gov/UniGene) of relative abundance of ESTs. The symbols represent numbers of specific transcripts per million (TPM) total ESTs in each tissue: $0 = 0$, $\pm = 1$–10, $+ = 11$–100, $++ = 101$–549, and $+++ = \geq 550$ TPM.

SINGLE-MOLECULE STRUCTURAL DYNAMICS OF MYOSIN V

Biophysical experiments on individual molecules have been crucial to the basic understanding of several classes of unconventional myosins. Myosin V is interesting for single-molecule studies because it exhibits a very large step displacement (36 nm) and it undergoes dozens of mechanical steps per diffusional encounter with actin, a property termed processivity. These characteristics make it amenable to detailed mechanical experiments using optical traps as well as structural dynamics studies by single-molecule fluorescence microscopy. FIONA (FIG. 6 A),[5] a technological advance made by Selvin and colleagues,[5,53] localizes the position of individual fluorescent probes at a much higher precision than the ∼250 nm resolution limit usually ascribed to conventional optical microscopy. The fluorescent-labeled molecules of interest are applied to a very clean sample chamber in a total internal reflection fluorescence (TIRF) microscope and detected by a sensitive charge-coupled device camera.

If only one molecule is contributing fluorescence to a particular small region of the magnified image in the TIRF microscope, fitting the intensity distribution (termed the point spread function), with an appropriate theoretical curve, such as a two-dimensional Gaussian function, enables location of the probe at a much higher precision than the width of the distribution (FIG. 6 A). Steps produced in this assay by myosin V, translocating processively along actin, and several other molecular motors (myosin VI and kinesin),[54,55] showed that they walk along actin with a hand-over-hand mechanism (FIG. 6 B). This enables them to progress a much greater distance than their own size without losing contact with actin and to navigate through the dense cytoplasm carrying relatively huge cargoes, such as membrane-bound vesicles.[56–59]

Using polarized light to detect the spatial orientation of the fluorescent probe also showed that the light chain domain (containing calmodulins in myosin V) tilts forward or backward each time the motor takes a step,[60,61] also compatible with hand-over-hand motility. Theoretical considerations have made tilting of myosin the likely cause of filament sliding in skeletal, smooth and cardiac muscle, dating from the discovery of sliding filaments 50 years ago.[62–68] Tilting of the light chain region also explains the motions of unconventional myosins and the dependence of their step size on the number of light chains in their lever arm.[69] However, direct evidence for tilting of the light chain region was lacking until the development of these single-molecule techniques. The demonstration of light chain tilting in muscle is not as direct.[70]

NONSARCOMERIC AND DEVELOPMENTAL MOLECULAR MOTORS IN THE MYOCARDIUM

Given the essential roles ascribed to all three families of molecular motors, kinesins, dyneins and myosins, and the microtubule and actin cytoskeletal

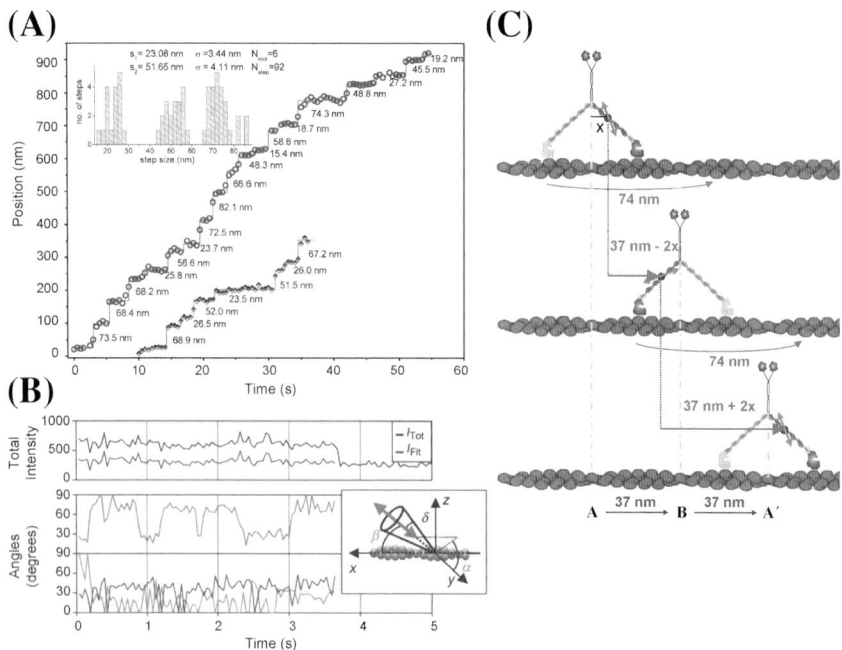

FIGURE 6. FIONA and single-molecule polarized fluorescence measurements on actomyosin V. (**A**) Stepping traces from two bifunctional rhodamine-labeled myosin V molecules with alternating step sizes. The data from several myosin V molecules, representing 92 steps, are compiled in the histograms. The majority of the steps alternates between 52 nm and 23 nm. Some longer steps are observed due to two smaller steps unresolved at the 0.5 s time resolution. (**B**) Single-molecule polarized fluorescence data for myosin V moving along an actin filament. The timed traces are records of the total light intensity (I_{Tot}, black), weighted total fitted intensity (I_{Fit}, blue), angular orientations of the probe labeling the myosin (β, red: α, green), and the extent of slow wobble (δ, blue) as defined in the inset. (**C**) Hand-over-hand model of myosin V. A single-labeled calmodulin subunit (blue dot with red arrow representing the fluorescent dipole) is incorporated into the myosin molecule. The rear head moves 74 nm toward the barbed end of actin while the lead head remains stationery. The coiled-coil neck domain moves 37 nm while the labeled calmodulin takes alternating $37 \pm 2x$ nm steps, where x is the distance from the probe to the center of mass of the molecule. Panels A and B are reprinted from Yildiz, A. *et al.*, (*Science* **300:** 2061-2065, 2003) with permission. Panel C is reprinted from Forkey, J.N. *et al.* (*Nature* **422:** 399-404, 2003) with permission.

systems in general cell and developmental biology,[71–74] it is surprising to us how few reports have specifically identified these responsibilities in the heart. A search of MedLine or Google Scholar identifies thousands of papers published on molecular motors in brain and sensory neural organs. This may be a fertile research direction for cardiovascular scientists, as well. Kinesins and dyneins, driving ciliary motion, partly determine sidedness during development,[72] a crucial facet of myocardial development.[75,76] Although many of the genes for hypertrophic cardiomyopathy and glycogenopathies have been identified, the causes of several of the dilated and restrictive cardiomyopathies, and arrhythmogenic right ventricular dysplasia are unknown.[34]

Defects in unconventional myosins have recently been correlated with a few cardiac diseases. In heart myosin Ic is essential for the translocation of the GLUT4 glucose transporter. In the resting heart, a majority of cellular energy is derived from lipid sources, but during exercise or in certain pathological situations, glucose metabolism can predominate. If the functionality of the myosin Ic is altered, the energy supply may be compromised.[77]

Myosin VI is also expressed in the heart, but its function and cellular localization are not known.[78] It may be associated with the Golgi complex, clathrin-coated vesicles, or play a role in cell migration and morphogenesis. Mohiddin *et al.*[79] identified a hereditary multisystem disorder having a genetic linkage of cardiac and auditory dysfunction with a mutation of the myosin VI gene in all affected members of a kindred. A missense mutation at a highly conserved location in the motor domain (His^{246}) causes an autosomal dominant sensorineural hearing loss[80] that co-segregates with mild FHC and long QT interval. The penetrance of both of these deficits is age-related, suggesting that manifestation of symptoms requires prolonged abnormal function of myosin VI.[79]

A mutation in the actin-binding domain of perinatal myosin II, found in both skeletal and cardiac muscle (MYH8), has been implicated as the primary cause of trismus-pseudocamptodactyly syndrome (TPC), a rare muscle disorder causing contractures of the jaw and hand muscles.[81] Patients with the same mutation also present with a mild variant of Carney complex (CNC), a multiple neoplasia syndrome including cardiac myxomas. Mutations in protein kinase A have also been implicated in Carney complex. Proliferation of myofibroblasts can occur, leading to tumorigenesis after injury, remodeling, or ischemia.

Complimentary cell biological, genetic, and single-molecule biophysical studies are making rapid progress toward elucidating the functions and mechanisms of these interesting cellular nano-machines. Their involvement in pathogenesis of human disease is becoming more apparent as specific examples are identified.[82,83]

SUMMARY AND FUTURE DIRECTIONS

Molecular motor research is impacting on progress in developmental biology, understanding of muscle and myocardial function, and human diseases. Further interrogation of biophysical mechanisms of conventional myosin may help to resolve the many uncertainties in heart disease. Inasmuch as unconventional myosins are expressed broadly in the cardiovascular system, their roles will be elucidated when they are studied in myocardium and the vasculature. Get to know unconventional myosins and stay ahead of the cardiology research curve!

REFERENCES

1. BARBARA, P.F. 2005. Single-molecule spectroscopy. Acc. Chem. Res. **38**: 503.
2. ROSENBERG, S.A., M.E. QUINLAN, J.N. FORKEY & Y.E. GOLDMAN. 2005. Rotational motions of macro-molecules by single-molecule fluorescence microscopy. Acc. Chem. Res. **38**: 583–593.
3. BOKINSKY, G. & X. ZHUANG. 2005. Single-molecule RNA folding. Acc. Chem. Res. **38**: 566–573.
4. RASNIK, I., S.A. MCKINNEY & T. HA. 2005. Surfaces and orientations: much to FRET about? Acc. Chem. Res. **38**: 542–548.
5. YILDIZ, A. & P.R. SELVIN. 2005. Fluorescence imaging with one nanometer accuracy: application to molecular motors. Acc. Chem. Res. **38**: 574–582.
6. ASHKIN, A. & J.M. DZIEDZIC. 1987. Optical trapping and manipulation of viruses and bacteria. Science **235**: 1517–1520.
7. KUO, S.C. 2001. Using optics to measure biological forces and mechanics. Traffic **2**: 757–763.
8. KNIGHT, A.E., G. MASHANOV & J.E. MOLLOY. 2005. Single molecule measurements and biological motors. Eur. Biophys. J. **35**: 89.
9. SVOBODA, K. & S.M. BLOCK. 1994. Biological applications of optical forces. Annu. Rev. Biophys. Biomol. Struct. **23**: 247–285.
10. SHEETZ, M.P. 1998. Laser Tweezers in Cell Biology, Vol. 55. Academic Press. San Diego, CA.
11. ROCK, R.S., S.E. RICE, A.L. WELLS, *et al*. 2001. Myosin VI is a processive motor with a large step size. Proc. Natl. Acad. Sci. USA **98**: 13655–13659.
12. FINER, J.T., R.M. SIMMONS & J.A. SPUDICH. 1994. Single myosin molecule mechanics: piconewton forces and nanometre steps. Nature **368**: 113–119.
13. TYSKA, M.J., E. HAYES, M. GIEWAT, *et al*. 2000. Single-molecule mechanics of R403Q cardiac myosin isolated from the mouse model of familial hypertrophic cardiomyopathy. Circ. Res. **86**: 737–744.
14. TAKAGI, Y., E.E. HOMSHER, Y.E. GOLDMAN, *et al*. 2006. Force generation in single conventional actomyosin complexes under high dynamic load. Biophys. J. **90**: 1295–1307.
15. VANZI, F., Y. TAKAGI, H. SHUMAN, *et al*. 2005. Mechanical studies of single ribosome/mRNA complexes. Biophys. J. **89**: 1909–1919.
16. SEIDMAN J.G. & C. SEIDMAN. 2001. The genetic basis for cardiomyopathy: from mutation identification to mechanistic paradigms. Cell **104**: 557–567.
17. GEISTERFER-LOWRANCE, A.A.T., S. KASS, G. TANIGAWA, *et al*. 1990. A molecular basis for familial hypertrophic cardiomyopathy: a β cardiac myosin heavy chain gene missense mutation. Cell **62**: 999–1006.
18. BEMENT, W.M. & M.S. MOOSEKER. 1995. TEDS rule: a molecular rationale for differential regulation of myosins by phosphorylation of the heavy chain head. Cell Motil. Cytoskel. **31**: 87–92.
19. CUDA, G., L. FANANAPAZIR, W.S. ZHU, *et al*. 1993. Skeletal muscle expression and abnormal function of β-myosin in hypertrophic cardiomyopathy. J. Clin. Invest. **91**: 2861–2865.
20. CUDA, G., L. FANANAPAZIR, N.D. EPSTEIN, *et al*. 1997. The in vitro motility activity of β-cardiac myosin depends on the nature of the β-myosin heavy chain

gene mutation in hypertrophic cardiomyopathy. J. Musc. Res. Cell Motil. **18:** 275–283.
21. SWEENEY, H.L., A.J. STRACESKI, L.A. LEINWAND, *et al.* 1994. Heterologous expression of a cardiomyopathic myosin that is defective in its actin interaction. J. Biol. Chem. **269:** 1603–1605.
22. SATA, M. & M. IKEBE. 1996. Functional analysis of the mutations in the human cardiac β-myosin that are responsible for familial hypertrophic cardiomyopathy. Implication for the clinical outcome. J. Clin. Invest. **98:** 2866–2873.
23. ROOPNARINE, O. & L.A. LEINWAND. 1998. Functional analysis of myosin mutations that cause familial hypertrophic cardiomyopathy. Biophys. J. **75:** 3023–3030.
24. THOMPSON, C.H., G.J. KEMP, D.J. TAYLOR, *et al.* 1997. Abnormal skeletal muscle bioenergetics in familial hypertrophic cardiomyopathy. Heart **78:** 177–181.
25. BLANCHARD, E., C. SEIDMAN, J.G. SEIDMAN, *et al.* 1999. Altered crossbridge kinetics in the $\alpha MHC^{403/+}$ mouse model of familial hypertrophic cardiomyopathy. Circ. Res. **84:** 475–483.
26. LANKFORD, E.B., N.D. EPSTEIN, L. FANANAPAZIR, *et al.* 1995. Abnormal contractile properties of muscle fibers expressing β-myosin heavy chain gene mutations in patients with hypertrophic cardiomyopathy. J. Clin. Invest. **95:** 1409–1414.
27. PALMITER, K.A., M.J. TYSKA, J.R. HAEBERLE, *et al.* 2000. R403Q and L908V mutant β-cardiac myosin from patients with familial hypertrophic cardiomyopathy exhibit enhanced mechanical performance at the single molecule level. J Musc. Res. Cell Motil. **21:** 609–620.
28. KELLER, D.I., C. COIRAULT, T. RAU, *et al.* 2004. Human homozygous R403W mutant cardiac myosin presents disproportionate enhancement of mechanical and enzymatic properties. J. Mol. Cell Cardiol. **36:** 355–362.
29. ALPERT, N.R., S.A. MOHIDDIN, D. TRIPODI, *et al.* 2005. Molecular and phenotypic effects of heterozygous, homozygous, and compound heterozygote myosin heavy-chain mutations. Am. J. Physiol. Heart Circ. Physiol. **288:** H1097–H1102.
30. KÖHLER J., G. WINKLER, I. SCHULTE, *et al.* 2002. Mutation of the myosin converter domain alters cross-bridge elasticity. Proc. Natl. Acad. Sci. USA **99:** 3557–3562.
31. MOSS, R.L. & J.S.A. PERIERA. 2000. Enhanced myosin function due to a point mutation causing a familial hypertrophic cardiomyopathy. Circ. Res. **86:** 720–722.
32. INGWALL, J.S. & R.G. WEISS. 2004. Is the failing heart energy starved? On using chemical energy to support cardiac function. Circ. Res. **95:** 135–145.
33. NYITRAI M. & M.A. GEEVES. 2004. Adenosine diphosphate and strain sensitivity in myosin motors. Phil. Trans. R. Soc. B. **359:** 1867–1877.
34. AHMAD, F., J.G. SEIDMAN & C.E. SEIDMAN. 2005. The genetic basis for cardiac remodeling. Annu. Rev. Genomics Hum. Genet. **6:** 185–216.
35. BERG, J.S., B.C. POWELL & R.E. CHENEY. 2001. A millennial myosin census. Mol. Biol. Cell **12:** 780–794.
36. HODGE, T. & M.J.T.V. COPE. 2000. A myosin family tree. J. Cell Sci. **113:** 3353–3354.
37. SANGER, J.M., B. MITTAL, J.S. DOME, *et al.* 1989. Analysis of cell division using fluorescently labeled actin and myosin in living PtK2 cells. Cell Motil. Cytoskel. **14:** 201–219.
38. DEVREOTES, P. & C. JANETOPOULOS. 2003. Eukaryotic chemotaxis: distinctions between directional sensing and polarization. J. Biol. Chem. **278:** 20445–20448.
39. KRENDEL, M. & M. MOOSEKER. 2005. Myosins: tails (and heads) of functional diversity. Physiology (Bethesda) **20:** 239–251.

40. DE LA CRUZ, E.M. & E.M. OSTAP. 2004. Relating biochemistry and function in the myosin superfamily. Curr. Opin. Cell Biol. **16:** 61–67.
41. GILLESPIE, P.G. & J.L. CYR. 2004. Myosin-1c, the hair cell's adaptation motor. Annu. Rev. Physiol. **66:** 521–545.
42. LISTER I., S. SCHMITZ, M. WALKER, et al. 2004. A monomeric myosin VI with a large working stroke. EMBO J. **23:** 1729–1738.
43. PARK, H., B. RAMAMURTHY, M. TRAVAGLIA, et al. 2006. Full-length myosin VI dimerizes and moves processively along actin filaments upon monomer clustering. Mol. Cell. **21:** 331–336.
44. WELLS, A.L., A.W. LIN, L.-Q. CHEN, et al. 1999. Myosin VI is an actin-based motor that moves backwards. Nature **401:** 505–508.
45. ALTMAN, D., H.L. SWEENEY & J.A. SPUDICH. 2004. The mechanism of myosin VI translocation and its load-induced anchoring. Cell **116:** 737–749.
46. MÉNÉTREY, J., A. BAHLOUL, A.L. WELLS, et al. 2005. The structure of the myosin VI motor reveals the mechanism of directionality reversal. Nature **435:** 779–785.
47. SUN, Y., H.W. SCHROEDER, J.F. BEAUSANG, et al. 2005. Single molecule fluorescence polarization of calmodulin in myosin VI. Biophys. J. **90:** 431a.
48. SCHULER, G.D., M.S. BOGUSKI, E.A. STEWART, et al. 1996. A gene map of the human genome. Science **274:** 540–546.
49. PONTIUS, J.U., L. WAGNER & G.D. SCHULER. 2003. UniGene: a unified view of the transcriptome. In The NCBI Handbook. National Center for Biotechnology Information. Bethesda, MD. (www.ncbi.nlm.nih.gov/UniGene).
50. BOUCK, J., W. YU, R. GIBBS & K. WORLEY. 1999. Comparison of gene indexing databases. Trends Gen. **15:** 159–162.
51. BURKE, J., H. WANG, W. HIDE, et al. 1998. Alternative gene form discovery and candidate gene selection from gene indexing projects. Genome Res. **8:** 276–290.
52. PANDEY, A. & F. LEWITTER. 1999. Nucleotide sequence databases: a gold mine for biologists. Trends Biochem. Sci. **24:** 276–280.
53. YILDIZ, A., J.N. FORKEY, S.A. MCKINNEY, et al. 2003. Myosin V walks hand-over-hand: single fluorophore imaging with 1.5-nm localization. Science **300:** 2061–2065.
54. YILDIZ, A., M. TOMISHIGE, R.D. VALE, et al. 2004. Kinesin walks hand-over-hand. Science **303:** 676–678.
55. YILDIZ, A., H. PARK, D. SAFER, et al. 2004. Myosin VI steps via a hand-over-hand mechanism with its lever arm undergoing fluctuations when attached to actin. J. Biol. Chem. **279:** 37223–37226.
56. HEUSER, J.E. & M.W. KIRSCHNER. 1980. Filament organization revealed in platinum replicas of freeze-dried cytoskeletons. J. Cell Biol. **86:** 212–234.
57. MEDALIA, O., I. WEBER, A.S. FRANGAKIS, et al. 2002. Macromolecular architecture in eukaryotic cells visualized by cryoelectron tomography. Science **298:** 1209–1213.
58. LANGFORD, G.M. 2002. Myosin-V, a versatile motor for short-range vesicle transport. Traffic **3:** 859–865.
59. FRANK, D.J., T. NOGUCHI & K.G. MILLER. 2004. Myosin VI: a structural role in actin organization important for protein and organelle localization and trafficking. Curr. Opin. Cell Biol. **16:** 189–194.
60. FORKEY, J.N., M.E. QUINLAN, M.A. SHAW, et al. 2003. Three-dimensional structural dynamics of myosin V by single-molecule fluorescence polarization. Nature **422:** 399–404.

61. QUINLAN, M.E., J.N. FORKEY & Y.E. GOLDMAN. 2005. Orientation of the myosin light chain region by single molecule total internal reflection fluorescence polarization microscopy. Biophys. J. **89:** 1132–1142.
62. HUXLEY, A.F. & R. NIEDERGERKE. 1954. Structural changes in muscle during contraction; interference microscopy of living muscle fibres. Nature **173:** 971–973.
63. HUXLEY, H. & J. HANSON. 1954. Changes in the cross-striations of muscle during contraction and stretch and their structural interpretation. Nature **173:** 973–976.
64. HANSON, J. & H.E. HUXLEY. 1955. The structural basis of contraction in striated muscle. Symp. Soc. Exp. Biol. **9:** 228–264.
65. HUXLEY, A.F. 1957. Muscle structure and theories of contraction. Prog. Biophys. Biophys. Chem. **7:** 255–318.
66. HUXLEY, H.E. 1969. The mechanism of muscular contraction. Science **164:** 1356–1366.
67. HUXLEY, A.F. & R.M. SIMMONS. 1971. Proposed mechanism of force generation in striated muscle. Nature **233:** 533–538.
68. RAYMENT, I., H.M. HOLDEN, M. WHITTAKER, *et al.* 1993. Structure of the actin-myosin complex and its implications for muscle contraction. Science **261:** 58–65.
69. WARSHAW, D.M. 2004. Lever arms and necks: a common mechanistic theme across the myosin superfamily. J. Musc. Res. Cell Motil. **25:** 467–474.
70. HOPKINS, S.C., C. SABIDO-DAVID, J.E.T. CORRIE, *et al.* 1998. Fluorescence polarization transients from rhodamine isomers on the myosin regulatory light chain in skeletal muscle fibers. Biophys. J. **74:** 3093–3110.
71. POLLARD, T.D. & W.C. EARNSHAW. 2002. Cell Biology. Chaps: 35–42. Saunders. Philadelphia, PA.
72. HIROKAWA, N. & R. TAKEMURA. 2004. Kinesin superfamily proteins and their various functions and dynamics. Exp. Cell Res. **301:** 50–59.
73. HOLZBAUR, E.L.F. 2004. Motor neurons rely on motor proteins. Trends Cell Biol. **14:** 233–240.
74. BROWN, M.E. & P.C. BRIDGMAN. 2003. Myosin function in nervous and sensory systems. J. Neurobiol. **58:** 118–130.
75. LEVIN, M. 2004. The embryonic origins of left-right asymmetry. Crit. Rev. Oral. Biol. Med. **15:** 197–206.
76. QIU, D., S.M. CHENG, L. WOZNIAK, *et al.* 2005. Localization and loss-of-function implicates ciliary proteins in early, cytoplasmic roles in left-right asymmetry. Dev. Dyn. **234:** 176–189.
77. ABEL, E.D., H.C. KAULBACH, R. TIAN, *et al.* 1999. Cardiac hypertrophy with preserved contractile function after selective deletion of GLUT4 from the heart. J. Clin. Invest. **104:** 1703–1714.
78. AVRAHAM, K.B., T. HASSON, T. SOBE, *et al.* 1997. Characterization of unconventional MYO6, the human homologue of the gene responsible for deafness in Snell's waltzer mice. Hum. Mol. Genet. **6:** 1225–1231.
79. MOHIDDIN, S.A., Z.M. AHMED, A.J. GRIFFITH, *et al.* 2004. Novel association of hypertrophic cardiomyopathy, sensorineural deafness, and a mutation in unconventional myosin VI (MYO6). J. Med. Genet. **41:** 309–314.
80. MELCHIONDA, S., N. AHITUV, L. BISCEGLIA, *et al.* 2001. *MYO6,* the human homologue of the gene responsible for deafness in *Snell's Waltzer* mice, is mutated in autosomal dominant nonsyndromic hearing loss. Am. J. Hum. Genet. **69:** 635–640.

81. VEUGELERS, M., M. BRESSAN, D.A. MCDERMOTT, *et al*. 2004. Mutation of perinatal myosin heavy chain with a Carney complex variant. N. Engl. J. Med. **351:** 460–469.
82. POLLARD, T.D. 2003. The cytoskeleton, cellular motility and the reductionist agenda. Nature **422:** 741–745.
83. SCHLIWA, M. & G. WOEHLKE. 2003. Molecular motors. Nature **422:** 759–765.

Recruitment of New Cells into the Postnatal Heart

Potential Modification of Phenotype by Periostin

RICHARD P. VISCONTI AND ROGER R. MARKWALD

Department of Cell Biology and Anatomy and the Cardiovascular Developmental Biology Center, Medical University of South Carolina, South Carolina 29425, USA

ABSTRACT: Establishment of the circulatory system occurs very early in development to support the rapid growth of the embryo. Therefore, the heart is the first functional organ to be formed during both avian and mammalian development. Historically, cardiac development has been considered to occur only during embryogenesis from cell sources located within the primordial structures that generate the myocardium and associated coronary vascular endothelium and smooth muscle and cardiac fibroblasts. Recently, however, contribution to the cardiac structures has been demonstrated to occur during embryonic development from extracardiac sources, like the anterior heart field, raising questions as to whether cardiogenesis may be an ongoing process that extends into adult life. In this brief article, we describe the contribution of circulating adult bone marrow hematopoietic stem cells to the cardiac cell populations and the potential regulation of their differentiation by the extracellular matrix protein, periostin.

KEYWORDS: cardiac development; fibroblast; cardiomyocyte; periostin; stem cell; plasticity

INTRODUCTION

Regenerative medicine is defined as the repair and replacement of diseased tissues and organs. In the instance of the heart, there have been two general approaches to replacing diseased tissues by adding new cells. The first utilizes an external approach, for example, the engineering of cellular or tissue

Address for correspondence: Roger R. Markwald, Ph.D., Department of Cell Biology and Anatomy, Medical University of South Carolina, 173 Ashley Avenue, CRI605 Charleston, SC 29425. Voice: 843-792-5880; fax: 843-792-0664.
  e-mail: markwald@musc.edu

constructs that can be surgically implanted, inserted with a catheter, or directly injected as with different types of adult stem cells.[1–6] In the second approach, the effort is directed toward promoting cell renewal from within. This raises the question as to whether new autologous cells are really being added to the heart by natural mechanisms in adult life. If this is indeed the case, this represents a continuation of developmental processes postnatally. Heart development is a dynamic process with new cells continuously being added to the embryonic and fetal heart during development.[7–13] As recently reviewed, they are recruited at both the venous and arteriole poles from secondary heart fields as well as from migratory cell populations including neural crest cells and epicardially derived cells.[14] Importantly, cells are also recruited from the embryonic circulation and added to the myocardium.[15] Such recruitment is in addition to proliferation that occurs intrinsically to establish the compact myocardium.[16,17] That cells extrinsic to the heart are recruited for the cardiac lineages in the embryo raises questions as to whether cells from outside the heart may contribute to cardiac tissues in the adult. The objective of this brief article is to discuss whether new cells are added to the heart, and if so what is their source, their phenotype, and the potential regulation of their differentiation.

EMBRYONIC CARDIAC MORPHOGENESIS

The onset of formation of a functional beating heart occurs very early during murine and avian embryogenesis since blood circulation is crucial to the development of the rapidly growing embryo. Cardiac morphogenesis begins at the onset of gastrulation when the embryo still exhibits a relatively simple planar organization composed of the three primary germ layers. At this stage of development, the myocardial progenitors are located at the anterior half of the embryo within two bilaterally distributed regions of the mesoderm referred to as the primary heart fields or precardiac mesoderm.[18,19] As cardiogenesis proceeds, the lateral mesoderm separates into distinct dorsal and ventral layers and the cardiac progenitors segregate into the ventral splanchnic mesoderm.[20,21] The bilateral heart-forming fields subsequently move anteriorly toward the ventral midline and begin to merge to form the three-dimensional primary heart tube.[22,23] As these morphogenetic events take place, cells within the heart fields begin to display a cardiac phenotype. Expression of cardiac cytoskeletal proteins is detected during the early stages of heart field fusion.[24–30] Beating of the primitive heart tube begins shortly thereafter, concomitant with the appearance of striated muscle.

After the onset of beating, the heart-forming fields continue to fuse at the posterior pole of the primary heart tube to form the atrioventricular (AV) canal and the atrial pole of the heart.[31] The final cardiac segment, the outflow tract, is added to the anterior pole of the primitive heart by recruitment of mesodermal tissue located anterior to the newly formed heart tube.[7–9] This represents a distinct origin for the myocardium of the conotruncus. The anterior mesodermal field that gives rise to this outflow tract myocardium is referred to as the anterior or secondary heart field.[7,8] Formation of the outflow tract from the anterior heart field marks the completion of the earliest stage of heart formation. However, cardiac morphogenesis does not end at this point. To meet the needs of the growing embryo and subsequent adult life, the primitive heart tube must undergo substantial growth and remodeling.

As the primitive embryonic heart tube is remodeled into a four-chambered heart that is capable of supporting extra-uterine life, a number of extracardiac cells contribute to populations within the cardiac lineages. For example, subsequent growth and remodeling of the embryonic heart include muscularization of the septae and the venous pole of the heart.[10–13] During this process, additional cardiomyocytes are produced by the proliferation of existing myocardium and also recruitment of new cardiomyocytes from intracardiac and extracardiac mesenchyme adjacent to the expanding myocardium.[10–13] In addition to expansion of the cardiomyocyte population, other cardiac cell types are added to the developing heart. For example, the epicardial anlage serves as another extrinsic source of cells for the developing embryonic heart. The epicardial anlage appears as an outcropping proximal to the embryonic liver. Shortly after looping of the primitive heart tube, cells from this pro-epicardial structure migrate over the surface of the embryonic myocardium and flatten to form an epithelium. Cells of this epithelial sheet undergo epithelial-to-mesenchymal transformation and invade the subepicardial space and the myocardium. An intriguing property of these cells is their ability to differentiate into specific cell types based on positional information. A number of elegant studies employing lineage-tracing reagents have demonstrated that these cells give rise to coronary vessel endothelium[32–35] and smooth muscle cells[32,35,36] as well as interstitial fibroblasts.[32,35,36] These cells provide structural integrity and requisite perfusion to the heart. Other investigators have demonstrated that cells derived from the epicardial anlagen also contribute to the AV valve interstitial cell population.[32] Valve interstitial cells exhibit an array of phenotypes ranging from fibroblastic[37–39] and myofibroblastic[40,41] to smooth muscle cell-like.[38,39,42] In addition to being derived from the embryonic epicardium,[32,36,43] there is also contribution to this lineage by the epicardially derived mesenchymal cells that populate primitive embryonic valves/endocardial cushions.[44]

Collectively, these studies demonstrate that cardiac morphogenesis is a dynamic process involving not only expansion of intrinsic cardiac cell populations but also contribution from a variety of extracardiac sources. This contribution of extrinsic cells to the heart raises questions as to whether cardiac development is indeed a lifelong process, wherein cells of extracardiac origin are continuously added to the cardiac tissues.

CONTRIBUTION BY CIRCULATING CELLS TO THE ADULT CARDIAC TISSUES

A number of groups have reported adult stem cell contribution to cardiac cell populations in response to injury.[6,45–49] These reports raise exciting possibilities for the application of stem cells and tissue engineering technologies to regeneration of the diseased or damaged heart. Further, the contribution of stem cells to postinjury tissue repair and remodeling raises the question of whether there is contribution of circulating cells to the adult heart during normal tissue homeostasis.

To investigate this possibility, we have developed a protocol that permits the potential of a single hematopoietic stem cell (HSC) to be evaluated *in vivo*. This strategy employs congenic clonal HSC transplantation[50] wherein the bone marrow (BM) of lethally irradiated recipient mice is repopulated with a small population of cells derived from a single lineage-marked (enhanced green fluorescence protein [EGFP])[51] HSC. To accomplish this (FIG. 1), BM cells are collected from the femurs and tibiae of EGFP$^+$/Ly5.2 mice, pooled and the mononuclear cells isolated by gradient separation. Lineage negative (Lin$^-$) cells are prepared by negative immunomagnetic selection using antibodies to

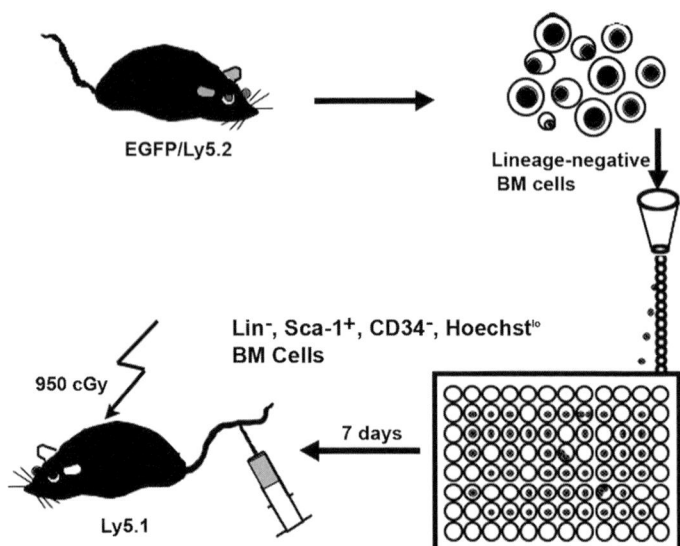

FIGURE 1. Enrichment and identification of candidate BM HSCs for clonal BM reconstitution. Donor BM cells are isolated from EGFP$^+$/Ly5.2 mice. Lin$^-$ cells are isolated by immunomagnetic selection. Next, HSCs are enriched by FACS for CD34$^-$ cells followed by FACS for Hoechst^{lo}, c-kit 1$^+$, Sca-1$^+$ cells (SP 'tip' cells). These cells are plated at clonal density in HSC-specific medium. After 7 days, candidate HSCs are selected for clonal transplantation into lethally irradiated congenic (Ly5.1) recipient mice.

Mac-1, B220, Gr-1, CD4, CD8, and TER-119. Lin$^-$ CD34$^-$ cells are subsequently isolated by fluorescence-activated cell sorting (FACS). Finally, the HSCs are further enriched in the Lin$^-$ CD34$^-$ population based on the ability of HSCs to efficiently exclude dyes, such as rhodamine 123 and Hoechst 33342.[52] Goodell et al.[52,53] demonstrated that a population of BM cells defined by two-color sorting with Hoechst 33342 dye, the side population (SP), is highly enriched for HSCs. The highest degree of HSC enrichment, however, appears to be achieved through FACS using both surface markers and dye exclusion. As reported by Matsuzaki et al.,[54] a high incidence of Lin$^-$ c-kit$^+$ Sca-1$^+$ CD34$^-$ HSCs were present in the "tip" portion of the SP of cells. Therefore, we isolate the Lin$^-$ c-kit$^+$ Sca-1$^+$ CD34$^-$ SP "tip" cells from EGFP mice fraction of BM mononuclear cells and deposit individual cells into wells of U-bottom 96-well culture plates.

These populations are maintained in culture for 1 week in fortified medium that supports HSC survival during the culture period. Based on their growth characteristics during this period, we select candidate HSC clones for transplantation into lethally irradiated non-EGFP/Ly5.1 mice by tail vein injection. Successful transplantation of HSCs is demonstrated by evidence of long-term multilineage hematopoietic reconstitution. If donor cells do not include an HSC, irradiated recipient mice do not exhibit repopulation at the BM and die due to postirradiative impairment of hematopoiesis. We have been able to achieve high levels of HSC engraftment using these techniques.[55-59] When EGFP$^+$ donor cells, derived from a single HSC, are transplanted into lethally irradiated congenic EGFP$^-$ recipient mice, the progeny of donor adult BM HSCs (EGFP$^+$ cells) can be identified as they repopulate the BM, enter the peripheral circulation, and engraft into other tissues. To control for the effects of cell culture on HSC potential, a separate cohort of mice receives 100 noncultured Lin$^-$ c-kit$^+$ Sca-1$^+$ CD34$^-$ SP "tip" cells from EGFP$^+$/LY5.2 mice. Mice from both transplant groups are assayed at 60 days posttransplantation for high levels of hematopoietic chimerism and multilineage hemtopoietic reconstitution. Using this system, we have previously demonstrated an HSC origin of microglial cells in the brain,[56] kidney glomerular mesangial cells,[55] and interstitial and perivascular cells in the tumor stroma and capsule.[58] As our transplantation strategy demonstrated that adult BM HSC-derived cells are able to engraft into a number of other organs and respond to cues provided by the extracellular milieu, we sought to identify contribution of these unequivocally HSC-derived cells to the cardiac lineages under normal (nonpathological) conditions.

When the cardiac tissues from engrafted mice were examined at periods ranging from 3 to 12 months posttransplantation, EFGP$^+$ cells were detected in a number of defined tissues in all recipient mice. In the ventricles, EGFP$^+$ cells were observed intercalated between cardiomyocytes, subadjacent to both the epicardium and the endocardium, and in the vascular connective tissue.

Further, examination of the cardiac valves revealed engraftment of HSC-derived (EGFP$^+$) cells in the leaflets of the AV and outflow valves of every engrafted mouse.

A subpopulation of cells that were intercalated between ventricular cardiomyocytes exhibited a fibroblastic morphology and HSC-derived cells that had engrafted into the valve interstitium were morphologically indistinguishable from recipient valve interstitial cells.[59] Therefore, we sought to investigate whether HSCs might contribute to the cardiac fibroblast population. To distinguish these cells as other than differentiated cells of the hematopoietic (blood) lineages, we performed a number of protein and RNA analyses to define their fibroblastic phenotype. Immunolabeling analysis of HSC-derived cells revealed that cells with fibroblastic/interstitial cell morphology were immunoreactive with antibodies to the discoidin domain type 2 receptor (FIG. 2 A), a collagen type 1 receptor tyrosine kinase that has been shown to be expressed exclusively by fibroblasts in the cardiac tissues.[60] Further, ultrastructural analysis demonstrated that EGFP$^+$ (HSC-derived) cells exhibit large prominent nuclei, lack of basal lamina, and close association with cardiomyocytes (FIG. 2 B): all characteristics of cardiac fibroblasts. RNA analysis revealed expression of collagen type I message,[59] demonstrating that HSC-derived cells have integrated into the cardiac tissues where they exhibit tissue-specific gene expression normally associated with cardiac fibroblastic cells. In support of our *in vivo* findings, we have also demonstrated HSC contribution to the fibroblast lineages *in vitro*. When BM mononuclear cells from mice that have been engrafted with a clonal population derived from a single EGFP$^+$ HSC are plated onto RetroNectin, they form fibroblast colony-forming units. Further, when peripheral blood mononuclear cells from these mice are cultured on fibronectin in selective culture medium, they adopt a fibroblastic morphology and express fibroblast-specific genes.[57]

Contribution of HSC-derived cells to the cardiac fibroblast population represents an entirely new paradigm for contribution to this lineage. As described

FIGURE 2. HSC contribution to the cardiac interstitial cell population. (**A**) EGFP$^+$ HSC-derived cells (green) in the myocardium are labeled with antibody to the discoidin domain-2 receptor (red), which is expressed only by fibroblasts in the cardiac tissues. (**B**) Transmission electron microscopic analysis of immunogold labeling shows that cells with fibroblastic morphology are labeled with anti-GFP. The fibroblastic cell depicted here is located in the infarcted myocardium in close association with a dying cardiomyocyte (∗). (**C**) z-Projection of laser scanning confocal analysis over the surface of an infarcted heart reveals that the infarcted portion of the myocardium (green) is densely populated with HSC-derived (EGFP$^+$) cells compared to the viable myocardium (purple). The red and blue wavelengths have been artificially amplified to assist in viewing the noninfarcted tissue. (**D**) Sectional analysis of the infarcted myocardium reveals HSC-derived (EGFP$^+$) cells with a fibroblastic morphology throughout the infarct zone. (**E**) HSC-derived (EGFP$^+$) cells (green) are surrounded by periostin (red) in the infarcted myocardium.

VISCONTI & MARKWALD: CELL RECRUITMENT TO THE POSTNATAL HEART 25

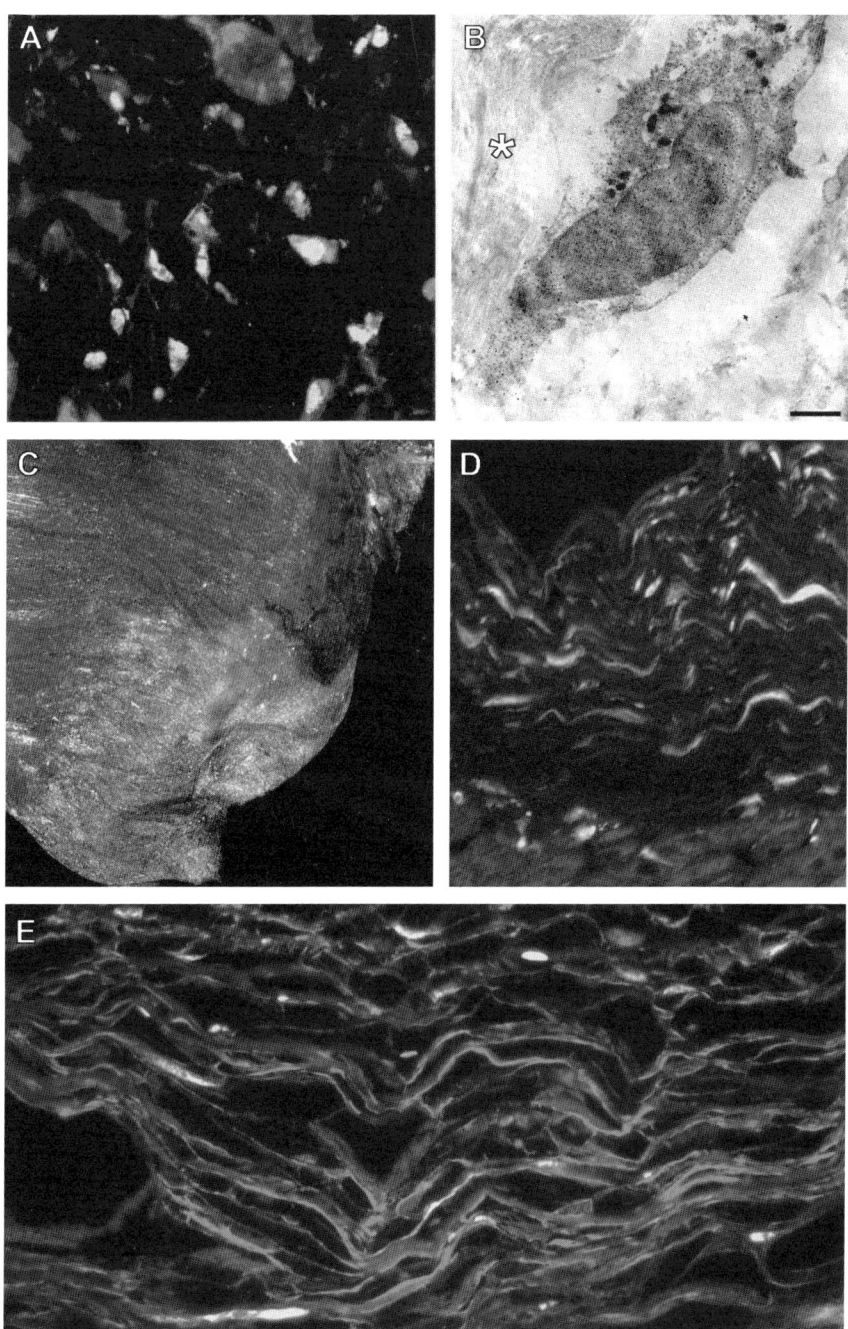

above, cardiac fibroblasts are considered to be derived from embryonic sources during early cardiac morphogenesis. Like the cardiomyocytes of the postnatal heart, the cardiac interstitial cell population has long been considered to be a static population that exhibits very limited turnover due to observed low levels of cell division. This is especially striking with respect to valve interstitial fibroblasts, which exhibit a very high level of extracellular matrix (ECM) synthesis but very low levels of cell division.[61] Our observation of contribution of circulating cells derived from the BM to the cardiac tissues suggests that cardiac development is a lifelong process wherein circulating cells of BM HSC origin contribute to the specialized fibroblasts of the myocardial and valve interstitium.

RESPONSE OF CIRCULATING CELLS TO INJURY

Our demonstration of the contribution of BM HSC-derived cells to the cardiac tissues during normal cardiac tissue homeostasis led us to explore what would be the response of these cells to cardiac injury. A number of groups have reported differing but promising results with regard to the ability of stem cells to regenerate the damaged myocardium.[6,45–49] A unique aspect of our system is that it permits us to observe the physiological response of adult BM HSCs to myocardial injury. Since we replace host BM with EGFP$^+$ cells derived from a single unequivocal HSC, we can easily and reproducibly observe the response of endogenous BM cells to experimentally induced injury. To accomplish this, we subjected clonal EGFP$^+$ HSC-engrafted mice to infarction by permanent occlusion of the left anterior descending coronary artery.[62] Examination of infarcted tissue during the acute stage of postinfarction remodeling revealed that cells of hematopoietic origin had infiltrated the infarct zone. Further, examination of infarcted hearts at 30 days postinfarction, a point at which the inflammatory response is resolved,[63,64] revealed that the infarcted region of the myocardium is still densely populated by EGFP$^+$ (HSC-derived) cells (FIG. 2 C). Strikingly, a population of EGFP$^+$ cells with a clearly fibroblastic/myofibroblastic morphology was observed in the infarct zone (FIG. 2 D) surrounded by a periostin-rich ECM (FIG. 2 E) (discussed below). RNA analysis revealed that these cells express a message for collagen type I, a function not normally associated with the hematopoietic lineage, strongly supporting our contention that BM HSCs contribute to the fibroblast population and that these HSC-derived cells participate in the elaboration of the postinfarction scar. That HSC-derived cells are so highly responsive to myocardial infarction raises exciting possibilities for treatment of postinfarction pathological remodeling. Use of autologous BM to carry modulators of postinfarction pathological remodeling, whether pharmacological or genetic, would be much more cost- and time-effective and less risky than more invasive procedures using cells from allogenic sources.

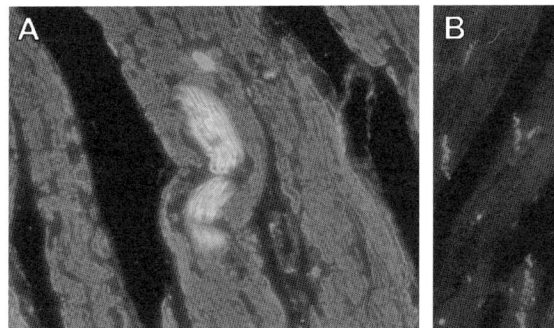 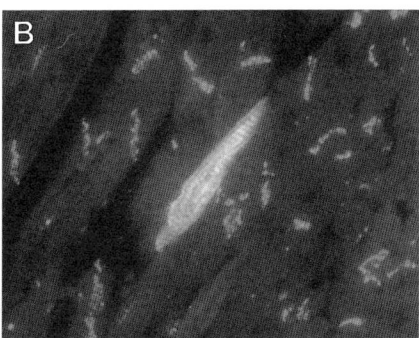

FIGURE 3. HSC contribution to the cardiomyocyte population. (**A**) HSC-derived cardiomyocytes (green) are immunoreactive with antibody to sarcomeric actin (red) and (**B**) express connexin 43 (red) where they contact adjacent host cardiomyocytes.

Additionally, we detect rare and isolated HSC-derived cardiomyocytes in the ventricles of transplanted mice. These myocytes, derived from clonally transplanted unequivocal HSCs, are detected both in control mice and mice subjected to infarction, with no significant difference in occurrence between these two groups. Further, we do not detect HSC-derived cardiomyocytes within the infarct zone. EGFP+ myocytes are localized within the infarct border zone and the viable myocardium. These HSC-derived cells express cardiomyocyte-specific markers and, at the light microscopic level of resolution, appear to be connected to host cardiomyocytes by gap-junctional complexes (FIG. 3). While these cells clearly demonstrate that circulating BM HSCs do indeed possess the plasticity to contribute both to the cardiac fibroblast and cardiomyocyte populations, it also suggests these cells are not capable of differentiating into cardiomyocytes when they are exposed to the cytokine signaling and transitional matrix of the infarcted region of the ventricle.

ECM IN STEM CELL DIFFERENTIATION

ECM and cytokines are potent effectors of a number of cell behaviors including cell migration and chemotaxis, proliferation and apoptosis, and differentiation and maintenance of phenotype. HSCs, the archetypal stem cell, have been shown to be dependent upon maintenance of ECM[65,66] and adhesion molecule-specific ligation[67,68] for maintenance of normal hematopoiesis. The question is what components of the ECM might be directing or sustaining HSC differentiation into fibroblastic lineages when they engraft into the heart (and elsewhere). One candidate ECM protein is periostin which increases 8- to 40-fold in myocardial remodeling diseases.[69,70] Periostin is expressed only by fibroblasts or by mesenchymal cells that differentiate into fibroblasts as in the embryonic heart during valvulogenesis.[71,72] Periostin is a unique, secreted ECM protein that is related to the *Drosophila fasciclin* gene family. It is a highly conserved protein (mouse and human are 90% identical) that has four fasciclin domains that are capable of forming multimers or binding to integrin receptors (alpha$_v$, beta$_3$ or alpha$_v$, beta$_1$) and to other ECM scaffold proteins (collagen, fibronectin).[73] Periostin signaling through integrin receptors and Akt pathways promotes cell migration and expression of growth factor receptors.[74–76] Based on studies in MC3T3 cells, a preosteogenic cell line, we have proposed a "periostin hypothesis," which proposes that periostin promotes and sustains differentiation into a fibroblastic phenotype and/or inhibits differentiation into other mesodermal lineages,[74–76] for example, bone or cartilage. The phenotype of periostin null hearts supports this hypothesis in two ways. Although deleting periostin is not lethal, periostin null mice are 25% smaller than wild type and their hearts have a marked increase in the ratio of ventricular wall thickness to the lumen, which is similar to adult myocardial hypertrophy.[77] Second, the presence of ectopic myocardial cells and undifferentiated mesenchyme in the valve leaflets and the cardiac fibrous skeleton indicates that some cardiac progenitor cells have failed to normally differentiate.[78] Because periostin is expressed only in fibroblastic tissue and its expression is increased up to 40-fold during adult remodeling diseases (see FIG. 2 E), it would suggest that undifferentiated HSCs that engraft into ECM of the heart would most likely be directed to differentiate into fibrous tissue (and not myocardium). To initially test this hypothesis, we made periostin full-length sense and antisense cDNA adenoviral vectors that were used to infect isolated embryonic cardiac cushion mesenchyme. Cushion cells normally differentiate into valvular fibroblasts, but when infected with 500 multiplicity of infection (MOI) viral vectors (FIG. 4), antisense vectors

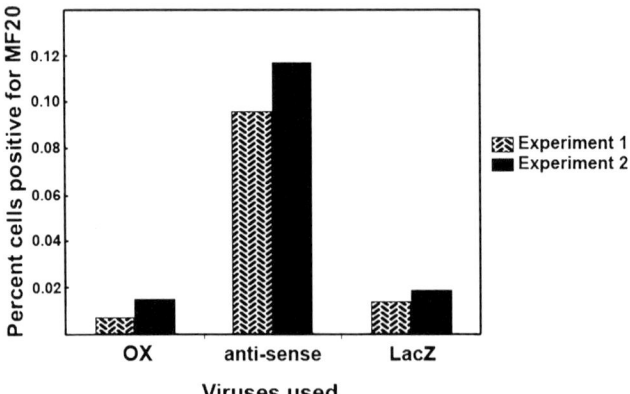

FIGURE 4. MF20 expression in cultured valve cells. Valve mesenchymal stem cells are isolated by enzymatic digestion and subsequently infected with full-length antisense periostin cDNA (or LacZ control vectors) using an adenoviral vector. Infected cells are permitted to form aggregates. Aggregates are then placed onto collagen gels and cultured for 72 h. Aggregates are harvested and assayed for expression of MF20 by FACS.

increased differentiation into cardiomyocytes nearly fourfold compared to sense and LacZ control vectors.

SUMMARY

While the degree to which embryonic developmental processes are recapitulated in response to injury is largely unknown, these preliminary data do strongly support that one role of periostin may be to direct pathological scar formation by HSC rather than myocardial regeneration. One future therapeutic approach might be to infect clonal HSCs with periostin antisense vectors to assess whether the ability to alter the composition of the postinfarction ECM or the signaling cascades that are activated in the progenitor cells can tip the balance between pathological remodeling and tissue regeneration.[73] A more complete understanding of the commonalities shared by developmental and injury response will be tremendously useful for application to tissue engineering and regenerative medicine.

REFERENCES

1. ASSMUS, B. *et al.* 2002. Transplantation of progenitor cells and regeneration enhancement in acute myocardial infarction (TOPCARE-AMI). Circulation **106:** 3009–3017.
2. STRAUER, B.E. *et al.* 2005. Regeneration of human infarcted heart muscle by intracoronary autologous bone marrow cell transplantation in chronic coronary artery disease: the IACT Study. J. Am. Coll. Cardiol. **46:** 1651–1658.
3. STRAUER, B.E. *et al.* 2002. Repair of infarcted myocardium by autologous intracoronary mononuclear bone marrow cell transplantation in humans. Circulation **106:** 1913–1918.
4. SCHACHINGER, V. *et al.* 2004. Transplantation of progenitor cells and regeneration enhancement in acute myocardial infarction: final one-year results of the TOPCARE-AMI Trial. J. Am. Coll. Cardiol. **44:** 1690–1699.
5. GALINANES, M. *et al.* 2004. Autotransplantation of unmanipulated bone marrow into scarred myocardium is safe and enhances cardiac function in humans. Cell Transplant. **13:** 7–13.
6. ORLIC, D. *et al.* 2001. Transplanted adult bone marrow cells repair myocardial infarcts in mice. Ann. N. Y. Acad. Sci. **938:** 221–229; discussion 229–230.
7. KELLY, R.G. & M.E. BUCKINGHAM. 2002. The anterior heart-forming field: voyage to the arterial pole of the heart. Trends Genet. **18:** 210–216.
8. MJAATVEDT, C.H. *et al.* 2001. The outflow tract of the heart is recruited from a novel heart-forming field. Dev. Biol. **238:** 97–109.
9. WALDO, K.L. *et al.* 2001. Conotruncal myocardium arises from a secondary heart field. Development **128:** 3179–3188.
10. KRUITHOF, B.P. *et al.* 2003. Recruitment of intra- and extracardiac cells into the myocardial lineage during mouse development. Anat. Rec. A Discov. Mol. Cell Evol. Biol. **271:** 303–314.

11. KRUITHOF, B.P. *et al.* 2003. Cardiac muscle cell formation after development of the linear heart tube. Dev. Dyn. **227:** 1–13.
12. VAN DEN HOFF, M.J. *et al.* 2001. Formation of myocardium after the initial development of the linear heart tube. Dev. Biol. **240:** 61–76.
13. VAN DEN HOFF, M.J. *et al.* 1999. Myocardialization of the cardiac outflow tract. Dev. Biol. **212:** 477–490.
14. EISENBERG, L.M. & R.R. MARKWALD. 2004. Cellular recruitment and the development of the myocardium. Dev. Biol. **274:** 225–232.
15. ZHANG, N. *et al.* 2006. Blood-borne stem cells differentiate into vascular and cardiac lineages during normal development. Stem Cells Dev. **15:** 17–28.
16. SEDMERA, D. *et al.* 2002. Cellular changes in experimental left heart hypoplasia. Anat. Rec. **267:** 137–145.
17. SEDMERA, D. *et al.* 2003. Spatiotemporal pattern of commitment to slowed proliferation in the embryonic mouse heart indicates progressive differentiation of the cardiac conduction system. Anat. Rec. A Discov. Mol. Cell Evol. Biol. **274:** 773–777.
18. REDKAR, A., M. MONTGOMERY & J. LITVIN. 2001. Fate map of early avian cardiac progenitor cells. Development **128:** 2269–2279.
19. STALSBERG, H. & R.L. DEHAAN. 1969. The precardiac areas and formation of the tubular heart in the chick embryo. Dev. Biol. **19:** 128–159.
20. DEHAAN, R.L. 1963. Regional organization of pre-pacemaker cells in the cardiac primordia of the early chick embryo. J. Embryol. Exp. Morphol. **11:** 65–76.
21. LINASK, K.K. 1992. N-cadherin localization in early heart development and polar expression of Na+,K(+)-ATPase, and integrin during pericardial coelom formation and epithelialization of the differentiating myocardium. Dev. Biol. **151:** 213–224.
22. DEHAAN, R.L. 1965. Morphogenesis of the vertebrate heart. *In* Organogenesis. R.L. Dehaan, H. Upsprung, Eds.: 377–419. Holt, Rinehart and Winston. New York.
23. EISENBERG, L.M. & EISENBERG, C.A. 2002. Onset of a cardiac phenotype in the early embryo. *In* Cardiovascular Molecular Morphogenesis: Myofibrillogenesis. D.K. Dube, Ed.: 181–205. Springer Verlag. New York.
24. BISAHA, J.G. & D. BADER. 1991. Identification and characterization of a ventricular-specific avian myosin heavy chain, VMHC1: expression in differentiating cardiac and skeletal muscle. Dev. Biol. **148:** 355–364.
25. COLAS, J.F., A. LAWSON & G.C. Schoenwolf. 2000. Evidence that translation of smooth muscle alpha-actin mRNA is delayed in the chick promyocardium until fusion of the bilateral heart-forming regions. Dev. Dyn. **218:** 316–330.
26. DE JONG, F. *et al.* 1990. Isomyosin expression pattern during formation of the tubular chicken heart: a three-dimensional immunohistochemical analysis. Anat. Rec. **226:** 213–227.
27. HAN, Y. *et al.* 1992. Expression of sarcomeric myosin in the presumptive myocardium of chicken embryos occurs within six hours of myocyte commitment. Dev. Dyn. **193:** 257–265.
28. RUZICKA, D.L. & R.J. SCHWARTZ. 1988. Sequential activation of alpha-actin genes during avian cardiogenesis: vascular smooth muscle alpha-actin gene transcripts mark the onset of cardiomyocyte differentiation. J. Cell Biol. **107:** 2575–2586.
29. TOKUYASU, K.T. & P.A. MAHER. 1987. Immunocytochemical studies of cardiac myofibrillogenesis in early chick embryos. I. Presence of immunofluorescent titin spots in premyofibril stages. J. Cell Biol. **105:** 2781–2793.

30. TOKUYASU, K.T. & P.A. MAHER. 1987. Immunocytochemical studies of cardiac myofibrillogenesis in early chick embryos. II. Generation of alpha-actinin dots within titin spots at the time of the first myofibril formation. J. Cell Biol. **105:** 2795–2801.
31. DE LA CRUZ, M.V. & R.R. MARKWALD. 1998. Living morphogenesis of the heart. *In* Cardiovascular Molecular Morphogenesis. R.R. Markwald, Ed.: 131–156. Birkhauser/Springer-Verlag. Boston, New York.
32. GITTENBERGER-DE GROOT, A.C. *et al*. 1998. Epicardium-derived cells contribute a novel population to the myocardial wall and the atrioventricular cushions. Circ. Res. **82:** 1043–1052.
33. PEREZ-POMARES, J.M. *et al*. 2002. Origin of coronary endothelial cells from epicardial mesothelium in avian embryos. Int. J. Dev. Biol. **46:** 1005–1013.
34. POELMANN, R.E., H. LIE-VENEMA & A.C. GITTENBERGER-DE GROOT. 2002. The role of the epicardium and neural crest as extracardiac contributors to coronary vascular development. Tex. Heart Inst. J. **29:** 255–261.
35. VRANCKEN PEETERS, M.P. *et al*. 1999. Smooth muscle cells and fibroblasts of the coronary arteries derive from epithelial-mesenchymal transformation of the epicardium. Anat. Embryol. (Berl.) **199:** 367–378.
36. DETTMAN, R.W. *et al*. 1998. Common epicardial origin of coronary vascular smooth muscle, perivascular fibroblasts, and intermyocardial fibroblasts in the avian heart. Dev. Biol. **193:** 169–181.
37. LESTER, W. *et al*. 1988. Porcine mitral valve interstitial cells in culture. Lab. Invest. **59:** 710–719.
38. ICARDO, J.M. & E. COLVEE. 1995. Atrioventricular valves of the mouse: II. Light and transmission electron microscopy. Anat. Rec. **241:** 391–400.
39. MARRON, K. *et al*. 1996. Innervation of human atrioventricular and arterial valves. Circulation **94:** 368–375.
40. TAYLOR, P.M., S.P. ALLEN & M.H. YACOUB. 2000. Phenotypic and functional characterization of interstitial cells from human heart valves, pericardium and skin. J. Heart Valve Dis. **9:** 150–158.
41. MAISH, M.S. *et al*. 2003. Tricuspid valve biopsy: a potential source of cardiac myofibroblast cells for tissue-engineered cardiac valves. J. Heart Valve Dis. **12:** 264–269.
42. FILIP, D.A., A. RADU & M. SIMIONESCU. 1986. Interstitial cells of the heart valves possess characteristics similar to smooth muscle cells. Circ. Res. **59:** 310–320.
43. GITTENBERGER-DE GROOT, A.C. *et al*. 2000. Epicardial outgrowth inhibition leads to compensatory mesothelial outflow tract collar and abnormal cardiac septation and coronary formation. Circ. Res. **87:** 969–971.
44. WESSELS, A. & J.M. PEREZ-POMARES. 2004. The epicardium and epicardially derived cells (EPDCs) as cardiac stem cells. Anat. Rec. **276A:** 43–57.
45. YEH, E.T. *et al*. 2003. Transdifferentiation of human peripheral blood CD34+-enriched cell population into cardiomyocytes, endothelial cells, and smooth muscle cells in vivo. Circulation **108:** 2070–2073.
46. JIANG, Y. *et al*. 2002. Pluripotency of mesenchymal stem cells derived from adult marrow. Nature **418:** 41–49.
47. JACKSON, K.A. *et al*. 2001. Regeneration of ischemic cardiac muscle and vascular endothelium by adult stem cells. J. Clin. Invest. **107:** 1395–1402.
48. KOCHER, A.A. *et al*. 2001. Neovascularization of ischemic myocardium by human bone-marrow-derived angioblasts prevents cardiomyocyte apoptosis, reduces remodeling and improves cardiac function. Nat. Med. **7:** 430–436.

49. ORLIC, D. *et al*. 2001. Mobilized bone marrow cells repair the infarcted heart, improving function and survival. Proc. Natl. Acad. Sci. USA **98:** 10344–10349.
50. OSAWA, M. *et al*. 1996. Long-term lymphohematopoietic reconstitution by a single CD34-low/negative hematopoietic stem cell. Science **273:** 242–245.
51. OKABE, M. *et al*. 1997. 'Green mice' as a source of ubiquitous green cells. FEBS Lett. **407:** 313–319.
52. GOODELL, M.A. *et al*. 1996. Isolation and functional properties of murine hematopoietic stem cells that are replicating *in vivo*. J. Exp. Med. **183:** 1797–1806.
53. GOODELL, M.A. *et al*. 1997. Dye efflux studies suggest that hematopoietic stem cells expressing low or undetectable levels of CD34 antigen exist in multiple species. Nat. Med. **3:** 1337–1345.
54. MATSUZAKI, Y. *et al*. 2004. Unexpectedly efficient homing capacity of purified murine hematopoietic stem cells. Immunity **20:** 87–93.
55. MASUYA, M. *et al*. 2003. Hematopoietic origin of glomerular mesangial cells. Blood **101:** 2215–2218.
56. HESS, D.C. *et al*. 2004. Hematopoietic origin of microglial and perivascular cells in brain. Exp. Neurol. **186:** 134–144.
57. EBIHARA, Y. *et al*. 2006. Hematopoietic origins of fibroblasts: II. *In vitro* studies of fibroblasts, CFU-F, and fibrocytes. Exp. Hematol. **34:** 219–229.
58. LARUE, A.C. *et al*. 2006. Hematopoietic origins of fibroblasts: I. In vivo studies of fibroblasts associated with solid tumors. Exp. Hematol. **34:** 208–218.
59. VISCONTI, R.P. *et al*. 2006. An in vivo analysis of hematopoietic stem cell potential: hematopoietic origin of cardiac valve interstitial cells. Circ. Res. **98:** 690–696.
60. GOLDSMITH, E.C. *et al*. 2004. Organization of fibroblasts in the heart. Dev. Dyn. **230:** 787–794.
61. DECK, J.D. *et al*. 1988. Structure, stress, and tissue repair in aortic valve leaflets. Cardiovasc. Res. **22:** 7–16.
62. TARNAVSKI, O. *et al*. 2004. Mouse cardiac surgery: comprehensive techniques for the generation of mouse models of human diseases and their application for genomic studies. Physiol. Genomics **16:** 349–360.
63. DEWALD, O. *et al*. 2004. Of mice and dogs: species-specific differences in the inflammatory response following myocardial infarction. Am. J. Pathol. **164:** 665–677.
64. YANG, F. *et al*. 2002. Myocardial infarction and cardiac remodelling in mice. Exp. Physiol. **87:** 547–555.
65. JANOWSKA-WIECZOREK, A., A. MATSUZAKI & L.A. MARQUEZ 2000. The hematopoietic microenvironment: matrix metalloproteinases in the hematopoietic microenvironment. Hematology **4:** 515–527.
66. KLEIN, G. 1995. The extracellular matrix of the hematopoietic microenvironment. Experientia **51:** 914–926.
67. COULOMBEL, L. *et al*. 1997. Expression and function of integrins on hematopoietic progenitor cells. Acta Haematol. **97:** 13–21.
68. SIMMONS, P.J., J.P. LEVESQUE & A.C. ZANNETTINO. 1997. Adhesion molecules in haemopoiesis. Baillieres Clin. Haematol. **10:** 485–505.
69. KATSURAGI, N. *et al*. 2004. Periostin as a novel factor responsible for ventricular dilation. Circulation **110:** 1806–1813.
70. WANG, D. *et al*. 2003. Effects of pressure overload on extracellular matrix expression in the heart of the atrial natriuretic peptide-null mouse. Hypertension **42:** 88–95.

71. KRUZYNSKA-FREJTAG, A. *et al.* 2001. Periostin (an osteoblast-specific factor) is expressed within the embryonic mouse heart during valve formation. Mech. Dev. **103:** 183–188.
72. NORRIS, R.A. *et al.* 2004. Identification and detection of the periostin gene in cardiac development. Anat. Rec. A Discov. Mol. Cell Evol. Biol. **281:** 1227–1233.
73. LITVIN, J. *et al.* 2005. Periostin family of proteins: therapeutic targets for heart disease. Anat. Rec. A Discov. Mol. Cell Evol. Biol. **287:** 1205–1212.
74. BAO, S. *et al.* 2004. Periostin potently promotes metastatic growth of colon cancer by augmenting cell survival via the Akt/PKB pathway. Cancer Cell **5:** 329–339.
75. GILLAN, L. *et al.* 2002. Periostin secreted by epithelial ovarian carcinoma is a ligand for alpha(V)beta(3) and alpha(V)beta(5) integrins and promotes cell motility. Cancer Res. **62:** 5358–5364.
76. KIM, C.J. *et al.* 2005. Periostin is down-regulated in high grade human bladder cancers and suppresses in vitro cell invasiveness and in vivo metastasis of cancer cells. Int. J. Cancer **117:** 51–58.
77. RIOS, H. *et al.* 2005. Periostin null mice exhibit dwarfism, incisor enamel defects, and an early-onset periodontal disease-like phenotype. Mol. Cell Biol. **25:** 11131–11144.
78. GAUSSIN, V. *et al.* 2005. Alk3/Bmpr1a receptor is required for development of the atrioventricular canal into valves and annulus fibrosus. Circ. Res. **97:** 219–226.

Cell-Based Approaches for Cardiac Repair

MICHAEL RUBART AND LOREN J. FIELD

Herman B Wells Center for Pediatric Research and Krannert Institute of Cardiology, Indiana University School of Medicine, Indianapolis, Indiana 46202, USA

ABSTRACT: Many forms of cardiovascular disease are associated with cardiomyocyte loss via necrosis and/or apoptosis. The cumulative loss of contractile cells ultimately results in diminished cardiac function. Numerous approaches have been employed to reduce the rate of cardiomyocyte loss, or alternatively, to repopulate the heart with new cardiomyocytes. Strategies aimed at repopulating the heart include cardiomyocyte cell therapy, myogenic stem cell therapy, and cell cycle activation therapy. All three approaches are based on the assumption that the *de novo* cardiomyocytes will participate in a functional syncytium with the surviving myocardium. This review will discuss the current status of interventions aimed at repopulating the heart with functional cardiomyocytes.

KEYWORDS: myocardial regeneration; stem cells; cardiomyocyte proliferation; apoptosis

INTRODUCTION

During development, increases in cardiac mass are largely due to the differentiation and subsequent proliferation of cardiomyocytes. After birth, the level of cardiomyocyte cell cycle activity is dramatically reduced and subsequent increases in cardiac mass occur predominantly from hypertrophic cardiomyocyte growth. The intrinsic proliferative capacity of terminally differentiated adult cardiomyocytes appears to be rather limited, as evidenced by the very low rates of DNA synthesis using radioisotope incorporation assays.[1–3] Although a number of studies have suggested that cardiomyogenic stem cells are present in adult hearts, the ability of these cells to reconstitute significant amounts of myocardial tissue in the absence of exogenous inducers also appears to be quite limited.[4] Consequently, myocardial injury typically resolves with scar formation as opposed to regenerative muscle growth. A number of approaches

Address for correspondence: Prof. Loren J. Field, Ph.D., Herman B Wells Center for Pediatric Research, Indiana University School of Medicine, 1044 West Walnut Street, RM W376, Indianapolis, IN 46202, USA. Voice: 317-274-5225; fax: 317-274-8679.
  e-mail: ljfield@iupui.edu

have emerged to lessen the degree of myocyte loss following injury, as well as to promote repopulation of damaged areas with functional cardiomyocytes. This review will focus on interventions aimed at repopulating damaged hearts with functional cardiomyocytes. Initial efforts aimed at the transplantation of cardiomyocytes as well as myogenic stem cells will be discussed. More recent studies suggesting that stem cell mobilization can be employed to promote cardiomyocyte repopulation in adult hearts are also discussed. This is followed by a review of interventions aimed at inducing cell cycle activity in cardiomyocytes surviving myocardial injury.

Cardiomyocyte Cell Therapy

The notion of direct transplantation of donor cardiomyocytes as a mechanism to promote repopulation in normal or injured myocardium dates to the early 1990s. Fetal or neonatal cardiomyocytes would *a priori* appear to be the ideal donor cell, as they express all of the molecular and physiologic attributes necessary for functional integration with the host myocardium. Proof of concept studies used donor fetal cardiomyocyte from transgenic mice expressing a cardiomyocyte-restricted, nuclear localized beta-galactosidase reporter transgene. After transplantation into the hearts of nontransgenic host mice, donor cells were readily identified based on the presence of nuclear beta-galactosidase activity.[5] Subsequent ultrastructure studies confirmed the presence of gap junctions between donor and host cardiomyocytes,[6] and numerous studies demonstrated that fetal cardiomyocytes could be transplanted into normal or injured hearts. Moreover, delivery of cardiomyocytes into injured hearts was frequently shown to have a positive impact on myocardial function, suggesting a potential therapeutic value (the reader is referred to the recent review by Dowell *et al.*[7]).

Despite these promising results, direct demonstration of physiologic coupling between donor and host cardiomyocytes required the development of imaging systems capable of monitoring intracellular calcium transients in individual cells within intact hearts;[8] these studies demonstrated that the donor cardiomyocytes could participate in a functional syncytium with the host myocardium.

Given that embryonic stem (ES) cells can give rise to highly differentiated cardiomyocytes *in vitro*,[9] additional studies were performed to assess the suitability of ES-derived cardiomyocytes as donor cells for transplantation experiments. Initial studies used a relatively simple antibiotic selection protocol to generate pure cultures of ES-derived cardiomyocytes; these cells were able to form stable grafts following transplantation into recipient hearts.[10] Subsequent studies demonstrated that this selection protocol was easily scalable to bioreactor vessels, and yields as high as 10^9 cardiomyocytes per 2 L volume were obtained.[11,12] The use of ES-derived cells for the treatment of injured hearts has recently been reviewed.[13]

Myogenic Stem Cell Therapy

In addition to differentiated cardiomyocytes, therapies aimed at transplanting myogenic, or preferably cardiomyogenic, stem cells have been initiated. The first efforts focused on the use of skeletal myoblasts (SMBs). SMBs can be isolated from relatively small tissue biopsies, and can be amplified to large numbers *in vitro*. When cultured under appropriate conditions, SMBs will differentiate into nascent skeletal myotubes. The first demonstration that transplanted SMBs differentiated into myotubes and formed stable grafts following intracardiac delivery used C2C12 cell lines, and relied on differential expression of myofiber contractile protein isoforms to distinguish donor and host myocytes.[14] Light and ultrastructure analyses suggested that the nascent myotubes were structurally uncoupled from the host myocardium. Subsequent studies demonstrated that SMBs could readily engraft infarcted myocardium,[15] and furthermore could result in functional improvement following engraftment.[16] Although several groups suggested that nascent myotubes reconstituted "functioning muscle,"[16-18] subsequent studies demonstrated that the donor-derived cells were electrically isolated from the host myocardium[19,20] (with the exception of extremely rare fusion events which occurred between donor SMBs and host cardiomyocytes at the graft/myocardium border).[20] The improvement in cardiac function observed following SMB transplantation more likely resulted from a beneficial impact on postinfarction ventricular remodeling.[21] Nonetheless, the observation that SMB transplantation could promote some degree of functional recovery promoted several phase I clinical trials to test the feasibility and safety of the approach;[22-24] the current status of these trials was recently reviewed.[25]

A number of studies suggested the existence of extracardiac stem cells with cardiomyogenic potential. For example, transplantation of wild-type male hematopoietic stem cells (HSCs) into lethally irradiated female mdx mice resulted in the presence of a low number of dystrophin-positive cardiomyocytes that appeared to contain a Y-chromosome.[26] Similarly, transplantation of HSCs from mice carrying a ubiquitously expressed beta-galactosidase reporter gene into irradiated recipients gave rise to beta-galactosidase expressing cardiomyocytes.[27] These observations suggested that marrow-derived cells could contribute to the adult myocardium, albeit at very low frequencies. This view was supported indirectly by pathologic analysis of female human hearts, which had been transplanted into male recipients: cardiomyocytes harboring a Y-chromosome could be detected. However, the frequency of this phenomenon varied tremendously from lab to lab, ranging from as high as 14% of the cardiomyocytes in one study[28] to very few or none of the cardiomyocytes in other studies.[29-31] Subsequent demonstration of heterokaryon formation between HSCs and resident cardiomyocytes strongly argued that fusion events gave rise to "cardiomyocyte formation" in the basic and clinical studies described above.[32,33]

The early suggestion that HSC marrow reconstitution might result in the formation of cardiomyocytes prompted several groups to directly transplant these cells into injured hearts. One study reported very high rates of "transdifferentiation" of HSCs into cardiomyocytes, resulting in a remarkable reconstitution of muscle mass and concomitant functional improvement.[34] In contrast, several other studies using both lineage-restricted and cell fate reporter trangenes demonstrated that HSCs failed to differentiate into cardiomyocytes following transplantation into injured hearts.[35–37] It was suggested that differences in the rigor of the assays used to monitor cardiomyogenic differentiation likely contributed to these markedly differing results.[38]

Other marrow-derived cells have been reported to exhibit cardiomyogenic activity, and/or can improve function following transplantation into injured hearts.[39–43] Of particular interest, Dzau and colleagues suggested that mesenchymal stem cells (MSCs) differentiated into cardiomyocytes with a concomitant marked improvement in cardiac function following transplantation into infarcted hearts.[44] However, subsequent studies from this group revealed that the observed functional improvement resulted from an antiapoptotic paracrine effect of the donor cells on at-risk cardiomyocytes as opposed to regenerative growth of the myocardium;[45] a similar mechanism could very well account for the functional improvement seen in the initial HSC transplantation experiments.[34] Indeed, marrow-derived cells have previously been implicated in neovascularization events.[46] Those observations prompted a number of phase I clinical trials, enthusiasm for which was bolstered somewhat by the initial suggestion of transdifferentiation activity.[47–53] Although a slight to moderate improvement in cardiac function was noted following delivery of marrow- or peripheral blood-derived progenitor cells in most instances, the functional assays employed were unable to distinguish between an indirect effect (e.g., angiogenesis) imparted upon the surviving myocardium and a direct contribution of functional *de novo* cardiomyocytes. The current status of clinical trials using stem cells from the marrow or the peripheral circulation was recently reviewed.[25]

It has also been reported that treatment with cytokines, which mobilize marrow-derived HSCs, resulted in marked regeneration of infarcted hearts in mice.[54] Given that the same cytokines are routinely and effectively used clinically for HSCs' transplantation in cancer patients, several clinical trials were rapidly initiated to test their impact on postinfarction function in humans. The absence of any improvement (or deterioration) in cardiac function in a large, randomized clinical trial[55] suggests that this treatment lacks the ability to induce cardiomyogenic differentiation. In support of this, subsequent reports in mice using more rigorous experimental readouts failed to see regenerative growth in infarcted animals, despite a similar degree of HSC mobilization as reported in the earlier study.[37,56] Cytokine treatment may have beneficial albeit indirect effects on postinfarction remodeling;[57] however, value of this activity must be weighed against potentially deleterious vascular effects in patients with

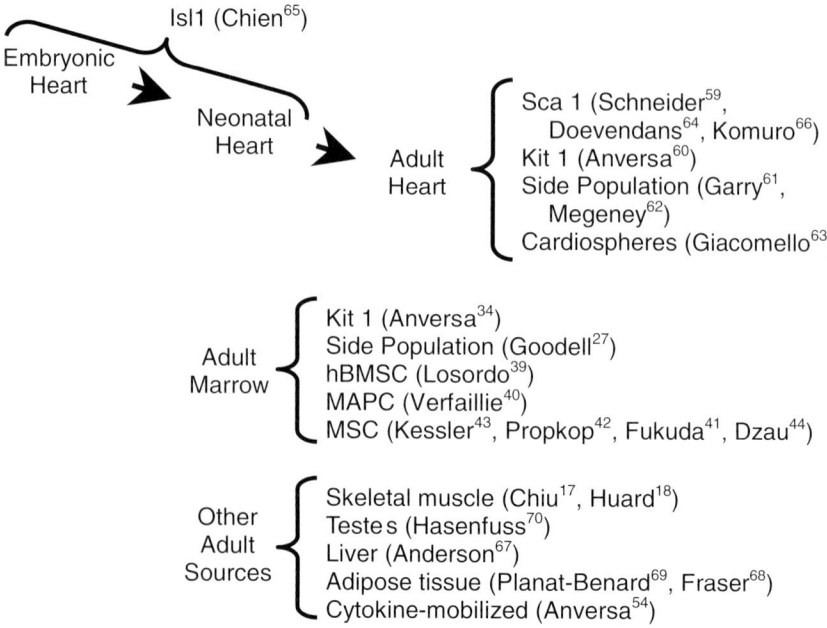

FIGURE 1. Representative studies suggesting that neonatal or adult-derived stem cells possess cardiomyogenic activity (names in parentheses indicate the senior author of the studies, and superscript numbers indicate the citations).

coronary artery disease, as exemplified by the perhaps predictable observation that cytokine treatment accelerated in-stent coronary artery restenosis.[58] Finally, cardiac-resident stem cells have also been recently described in the neonatal and adult heart.[59–64] Several studies indicated that these cells can be transplanted in or mobilized to injured myocardium, with apparent cardiomyogenic differentiation. Of particular interest are the Isl-1 cells described by Chien and coworkers[65] and the Sca-1 cells described by Komuro and colleagues,[66] as they appear to be able to undergo bona fide cardiomyogenic differentiation *in vitro*. Cells with apparent cardiomyogenic potential have also been reported in the liver,[67] adipose tissue,[68,69] and testes.[70]

FIGURE 1 lists representative studies suggesting that neonatal- or adult-derived stem cells possess cardiomyogenic activity. While it is exciting to anticipate the potential impact such cells might have on repopulating injured myocardium, it is important to keep in mind that injured hearts typically exhibit little regenerative capacity.[1,3] Moreover, deregulation of intracellular signaling pathways typically leads to neoplastic growth in organ systems with robust stem cell activity; in contrast, neoplastic growth of the myocardium is virtually nonexistent.[71] These observations indicate that under normal circumstances, cardiomyogenic stem cell activity in adult mammals is quite limited. While it is possible that *ex vivo* growth of stem cells might enhance their ability to repopulate the heart (as was suggested for mesenchymal adult progenitor cells),[40] considerable manipulation *in vitro* and/or *in vivo* might be required to obtain effective repopulation in injured hearts with these cells.

Cell Cycle Activation Therapy

Cell cycle activation constitutes an alternative approach with which to repopulate damaged cardiac tissue with functional cardiomyocytes. As indicated above, cardiomyocytes withdraw from the cell cycle shortly after birth, and increases in cardiac mass during postnatal life are due predominantly to hypertrophic growth. Cardiac injury typically has only a modest impact on cardiomyocyte cell cycle activity. Using a lineage-restricted transgenic reporter system, only 0.008% of the cardiomyocytes at the infarct border zone exhibit cell cycle activity 1 week following permanent coronary artery occlusion, with even lower levels of cell cycle activity in the remote myocardium.[72] While it is likely that both species and strain differences can impact on the absolute rate of cardiomyocyte proliferation (the previous experiments were performed in a DBA/2J genetic background), a survey of the literature confirms that the proliferative response following myocardial injury is limited.[73]

Given the potential utility of cell cycle activation as an approach to repopulate injured hearts, considerable effort has been invested to elucidate factors and gene products that regulate cardiomyocyte proliferation.[74] These efforts have been greatly aided by the use of transgenic animals (which overexpress a specific gene product) or gene-targeted animals (which either do not express a specific gene product or express an altered form of a gene product). These systems effectively permit gain-of-function, loss-of-function, and change-of-function genetic modifications of virtually any gene product, and combinatorial effects can readily be studied by simple interbreeding genetically modified animals.

The first animal models which exhibited altered cardiomyocyte cell cycle activity relied on targeted expression of the SV40 Large T Antigen oncoprotein to cardiomyocytes in transgenic mice.[75–77] These animals developed tumors comprised of differentiated, proliferating cardiomyocytes, and thus demonstrated that cardiomyocyte cell cycle activity can be readily modulated genetically. Subsequent studies identified a multitude of gene products which, when misexpressed in genetically modified animals, resulted in marked deregulation of cardiomyocyte cell cycle activity (the reader is referred to several recent reviews).[74,78] In most instances, the effect on cardiomyocyte cell cycle activity was observed to occur in embryonic hearts; this skew in temporal distribution reflects in part the fact that many of the genetic alterations resulted in embryonic or neonatal lethality (thereby precluding the ability to ascertain the effect of the alteration at later stages of development). Nonetheless, a number of models also had altered cardiomyocyte cell cycle activity in neonatal and adult hearts.

Cell cycle progression is regulated by a number of checkpoints which rely on protein kinase signaling cascades.[79] A key regulatory node is the restriction point, transit through which commits the cell to a new round of DNA synthesis and cell division. Restriction point transit relies on the activation of cyclin-dependent kinase (CDK) 4 and 6. CDK activity in turn is dependent upon the induction of their obligate activating partners, the D-type cyclins. Factors which positively regulate cell cycle progression (i.e., sufficient nutrients, presence of growth factors, etc.) activate signal transduction pathways, which induce transcription of the D-type cyclins. Newly synthesized D-type cyclins bind to and activate CDKs, which then phoshorylate members of the retinoblastoma gene family. Phosphorylation of retinoblastoma proteins results in the release of active E2F transcription factors and the subsequent transcription of genes required for DNA synthesis. Conversely, factors that negatively regulate cell cycle progression (inhibitory cytokines, intrinsic transduction pathways, etc.) act predominantly by suppressing CDK activity either directly or indirectly.

The majority of genes that have been shown to impact cardiomyocyte cell cycle activity in adult genetically modified mice are involved in some aspect of restriction point transit (FIG. 2). For example, an approximate 5-fold increase in cardiac IGF-1 expression led to a 16-fold increase in the number of DNA synthesizing cardiomyocytes in adult mice as compared to their nontransgenic littermates.[80] Similarly, induction of c-myc activity in conditional transgenic mice resulted in cardiac hypertrophy which was accompanied by reactivation of cardiomyocyte DNA synthesis and the formation of multinucleated cardiomyocytes.[81] In other studies, inhibition of p38 mitogen-activated protein (MAP) kinase activity (either pharmacologically in cultured cells or *in vivo* using cardiomyocyte-restricted gene targeting) resulted in cardiomyocyte DNA synthesis and proliferation.[82] Thus, modulation of positive or negative signal transduction regulatory pathways which act upstream of the restriction point is sufficient to drive cardiomyocyte cell cycle activity in adult hearts.

Other experiments have manipulated the activities of molecules that directly regulate restriction point transit. Indeed, SV40 large T antigen regulates cell cycle activity by binding to and inhibiting the activity of retinoblastoma family members;[83] thus cardiomyocyte cell cycle induction in transgenic mice expressing this protein[75–77] resulted from direct manipulation of restriction point regulatory proteins. In agreement with this, a recent study has shown that combinatorial deletion of retinoblastoma protein and its closely related family member p130 resulted in a 135-fold increase in DNA synthesizing cells as compared to control animals.[84] A similar effect was observed when D-type cyclin expression was targeted to cardiomyocytes. Adult mice expressing either cyclin D1, D2, or D3 show a remarkable 200-fold increase in DNA synthesizing cardiomyocytes as compared to their nontransgenic littermates.[85,86] Finally, overexpression of CDK-2, which acts downstream of CDKs 4 and 6, had a similar impact on cardiomyocyte DNA synthesis (approximately 100-fold increase as compared to nontransgenic littermates).[87] Thus, manipulation

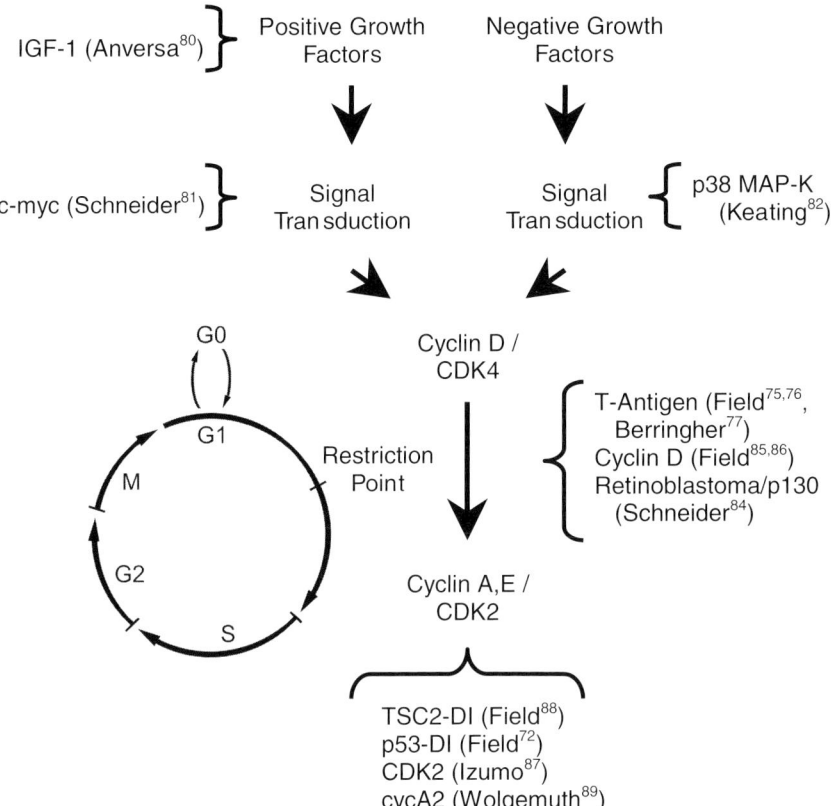

FIGURE 2. A schematic diagram of the cell cycle highlighted with studies wherein genetic manipulation resulted in cardiomyocyte cell cycle activity in adult hearts (names in parentheses indicate the senior author of the studies, and superscript numbers indicate the citations).

of molecules that directly regulate the restriction point is sufficient to drive cardiomyocyte DNA synthesis in adult hearts.

The activity of regulatory proteins, which act between the restriction point and the G1/S phase boundary of the cell cycle, has also been modulated in cardiomyocytes of genetically modified animals. For example, expression of either dominant interfering p53[72] or dominant interfering TSC2[88] was sufficient to promote cardiomyocyte DNA synthesis in adult hearts following myocardial injury. Both p53 and TSC2 are positive regulators of p27 (which is a negative regulator of CDK2); hence expression of dominant interfering p53 or TSC2 would interfere with p27-mediated cell cycle inhibition. Similarly, overexpression of cyclin A2, which acts at the G1/S boundary, also resulted in a slight increase in cardiomyocyte DNA synthesis levels as compared to nontransgenic littermates.[89] Finally, overexpression of either dominant interfering p193[72] or wild-type Bcl-2[90] resulted in enhanced levels of cardiomyocyte DNA synthesis in adult hearts; both molecules have been shown to inhibit apoptosis, but the mechanism by which their expression modulated cardiomyocyte cell cycle activity remains elusive.

An important caveat in many of the transgenic and gene targeting experiments described above is that alteration of gene expression often occurred prior to cardiomyocyte terminal differentiation. As such, modulation of these proteins in terminally differentiated cardiomyocytes might yield a different result. In the case of the dominant interfering TSC2, p53, and p193 models, cardiomyocyte DNA synthesis was not observed under baseline conditions in adult hearts, but was only observed following myocardial injury. Thus it is likely that much, if not all, of the terminal differentiation program was enacted prior to cell cycle induction in these mice. Although transgene expression of cyclin D preceded cardiomyocyte terminal differentiation, a similar effect on cell cycle activity was observed following adenoviral delivery of cyclin D1 (containing a nuclear localization motif) and CDK4.[91] In the case of conditional myc expression and pharmacologic p38 inhibition, these manipulations were also performed after cardiomyocyte terminal differentiation (although in the case of p38 inhibition, the potential impact culturing the cardiomyocytes might constitute a confounding issue). Nonetheless, these data all strongly support the notion that with appropriate manipulation adult cardiomyocytes can reenter the cell cycle.

Although many of the experiments described above used cardiomyocyte DNA synthesis as an assay for cell cycle induction, it is clear that the cardiomyocytes must progress through the cell cycle and divide, and furthermore, that the *de novo* formed cardiomyocytes must participate in a functional syncytium with the remainder of the heart if the activity is to be of any therapeutic value. Modulation of IGF-1, p38 MAP kinase, retinoblastoma/p130, cyclin D, and CDK2 activity was associated with increased cardiomyocyte cell number and/or immune-histologic evidence of cell cycle progression. In the case of IGF-1, transgene expression was associated with improved cardiac function following injury; however, it was not clear if this resulted from cardiomyocyte cell cycle activity, or from the well-established antiapoptotic activity of this molecule.[92] In contrast, cardiomyocyte cell cycle induction in mice expressing cyclin D2 resulted in regeneration of muscle mass following permanent coronary artery occlusion in mice.[86] Improvement in cardiac structure in these animals was accompanied by a marked restoration in cardiac function, as measured by intraventricular pressure–volume recordings.[93] Paradoxically, myocardial injury in mice expressing CDK2 (which exhibited a similar increase in cardiomyocyte cell cycle activity as was seen in the cyclin D mice) resulted in a maladaptive hypertrophic response and marked deterioration in cardiac function.[87] The mechanistic basis for these different responses to injury is currently not clear.

SUMMARY

The studies described above demonstrate that ability to repopulate the heart in experimental animals using cell-based approaches is now well established. In some instances, cardiomyocyte repopulation was directly associated with improved cardiac function following injury. Clearly, many challenges must be overcome for successful clinical application of these approaches. For example, it may prove to be impossible to modulate some of the pathways in an organ- or cell-type-specific manner, thus rendering them unsuitable for therapeutic use. It is also likely that some of the interventions described will be species specific (and thus not translatable to humans), or alternatively will simply not be reproducible by other groups. Nonetheless, the scope and sheer number of interventions which appear to have a positive impact on the heart, is unprecedented. Thus, the potential for successful restoration of cardiac structure and function following injury is greater now than at any previous time. Concerted efforts on research in this area will hopefully turn this dream to reality.

ACKNOWLEDGMENT

We thank the National Heart, Lung, and Blood Institute for support.

REFERENCES

1. RUMIANTSEV, P.P. 1991. Growth and hyperplasia of cardiac muscle cells. Harwood Academic Publishers. London; New York, N.Y.
2. SOONPAA, M.H. & L.J. FIELD. 1994. Assessment of cardiomyocyte DNA synthesis during hypertrophy in adult mice. Am. J. Physiol. **266:** H1439–H1445.
3. SOONPAA, M.H. & L.J. FIELD. 1997. Assessment of cardiomyocyte DNA synthesis in normal and injured adult mouse hearts. Am. J. Physiol. **272:** H220–H226.
4. DIMMELER, S., A.M. ZEIHER & M.D. SCHNEIDER. 2005. Unchain my heart: the scientific foundations of cardiac repair. J. Clin. Invest. **115:** 572–583.
5. SOONPAA, M.H. *et al.* 1994. Formation of nascent intercalated disks between grafted fetal cardiomyocytes and host myocardium. Science **264:** 98–101.
6. KOH, G.Y. *et al.* 1995. Stable fetal cardiomyocyte grafts in the hearts of dystrophic mice and dogs. J. Clin. Invest. **96:** 2034–2042.
7. DOWELL, J.D. *et al.* 2003. Myocyte and myogenic stem cell transplantation in the heart. Cardiovasc. Res. **58:** 336–350.
8. RUBART, M. *et al.* 2003. Physiological coupling of donor and host cardiomyocytes after cellular transplantation. Circ. Res. **92:** 1217–1224.
9. DOETSCHMAN, T.C. *et al.* 1985. The *in vitro* development of blastocyst-derived embryonic stem cell lines: formation of visceral yolk sac, blood islands and myocardium. J. Embryol. Exp. Morphol. **87:** 27–45.
10. KLUG, M.G. *et al.* 1996. Genetically selected cardiomyocytes from differentiating embryonic stem cells form stable intracardiac grafts. J. Clin. Invest. **98:** 216–224.

11. SCHROEDER, M. et al. 2005. Differentiation and lineage selection of mouse embryonic stem cells in a stirred bench scale bioreactor with automated process control. Biotechnol. Bioeng. **92:** 920–933.
12. ZANDSTRA, P.W. et al. 2003. Scalable production of embryonic stem cell-derived cardiomyocytes. Tissue Eng. **9:** 767–778.
13. RUBART, M. & L.J. FIELD. 2006. Cardiac repair by embryonic stem-derived cells. Handb. Exp. Pharmaco. 73–100.
14. KOH, G.Y. et al. 1993. Differentiation and long-term survival of C2C12 myoblast grafts in heart. J. Clin. Invest. **92:** 1548–1554.
15. MURRY, C.E. et al. 1996. Muscle differentiation during repair of myocardial necrosis in rats via gene transfer with MyoD. J. Clin. Invest. **98:** 2209–2217.
16. TAYLOR, D.A. et al. 1998. Regenerating functional myocardium: improved performance after skeletal myoblast transplantation. Nat. Med. **4:** 929–933.
17. CHIU, R.C., A. ZIBAITIS & R.L. KAO. 1995. Cellular cardiomyoplasty: myocardial regeneration with satellite cell implantation. Ann. Thorac. Surg. **60:** 12–18.
18. OSHIMA, H. et al. 2005. Differential myocardial infarct repair with muscle stem cells compared to myoblasts. Mol. Ther. **12:** 1130–1141.
19. LEOBON, B. et al. 2003. Myoblasts transplanted into rat infarcted myocardium are functionally isolated from their host. Proc. Natl. Acad. Sci. USA **100:** 7808–7811.
20. RUBART, M. et al. 2004. Spontaneous and evoked intracellular calcium transients in donor-derived myocytes following intracardiac myoblast transplantation. J. Clin. Invest. **114:** 775–783.
21. REINLIB, L. & L. FIELD. 2000. Cell transplantation as future therapy for cardiovascular disease?: a workshop of the National Heart, Lung, and Blood Institute. Circulation **101:** E182–E187.
22. MENASCHE, P. et al. 2003. Autologous skeletal myoblast transplantation for severe postinfarction left ventricular dysfunction. J. Am. Coll. Cardiol. **41:** 1078–1083.
23. PAGANI, F.D. et al. 2003. Autologous skeletal myoblasts transplanted to ischemia-damaged myocardium in humans. Histological analysis of cell survival and differentiation. J. Am. Coll. Cardiol. **41:** 879–888.
24. SIMINIAK, T. et al. 2005. Percutaneous trans-coronary-venous transplantation of autologous skeletal myoblasts in the treatment of post-infarction myocardial contractility impairment: the POZNAN trial. Eur. Heart J. **26:** 1188–1195.
25. MURRY, C.E., L.J. FIELD & P. MENASCHE. 2005. Cell-based cardiac repair: reflections at the 10-year point. Circulation **112:** 3174–3183.
26. BITTNER, R.E. et al. 1999. Recruitment of bone-marrow-derived cells by skeletal and cardiac muscle in adult dystrophic mdx mice. Anat. Embryol. (Berl.) **199:** 391–396.
27. JACKSON, K.A. et al. 2001. Regeneration of ischemic cardiac muscle and vascular endothelium by adult stem cells. J. Clin. Invest. **107:** 1395–1402.
28. QUAINI, F. et al. 2002. Chimerism of the transplanted heart. N. Engl. J. Med. **346:** 5–15.
29. LAFLAMME, M.A. et al. 2002. Evidence for cardiomyocyte repopulation by extra-cardiac progenitors in transplanted human hearts. Circ. Res. **90:** 634–640.
30. HRUBAN, R.H. et al. 1993. Fluorescence in situ hybridization for the Y-chromosome can be used to detect cells of recipient origin in allografted hearts following cardiac transplantation. Am. J. Pathol. **142:** 975–980.
31. GLASER, R. et al. 2002. Smooth muscle cells, but not myocytes, of host origin in transplanted human hearts. Circulation **106:** 17–19.

32. ALVAREZ-DOLADO, M. *et al.* 2003. Fusion of bone-marrow-derived cells with Purkinje neurons, cardiomyocytes and hepatocytes. Nature **425:** 968–973.
33. WAGERS, A.J. *et al.* 2002. Little evidence for developmental plasticity of adult hematopoietic stem cells. Science **297:** 2256–2259.
34. ORLIC, D. *et al.* 2001. Bone marrow cells regenerate infarcted myocardium. Nature **410:** 701–705.
35. MURRY, C.E. *et al.* 2004. Haematopoietic stem cells do not transdifferentiate into cardiac myocytes in myocardial infarcts. Nature **428:** 664–668.
36. BALSAM, L.B. *et al.* 2004. Haematopoietic stem cells adopt mature haematopoietic fates in ischaemic myocardium. Nature **428:** 668–673.
37. NYGREN, J.M. *et al.* 2004. Bone marrow-derived hematopoietic cells generate cardiomyocytes at a low frequency through cell fusion, but not transdifferentiation. Nat. Med. **10:** 494–501.
38. CHIEN, K.R. 2004. Stem cells: lost in translation. Nature **428:** 607–608.
39. YOON, Y.S. *et al.* 2005. Clonally expanded novel multipotent stem cells from human bone marrow regenerate myocardium after myocardial infarction. J. Clin. Invest. **115:** 326–338.
40. JIANG, Y. *et al.* 2002. Pluripotency of mesenchymal stem cells derived from adult marrow. Nature. **418:** 41–49.
41. KAWADA, H. *et al.* 2004. Nonhematopoietic mesenchymal stem cells can be mobilized and differentiate into cardiomyocytes after myocardial infarction. Blood **104:** 3581–3587.
42. POCHAMPALLY, R.R. *et al.* 2004. Rat adult stem cells (marrow stromal cells) engraft and differentiate in chick embryos without evidence of cell fusion. Proc. Natl. Acad. Sci. USA **101:** 9282–9285.
43. TOMA, C. *et al.* 2002. Human mesenchymal stem cells differentiate to a cardiomyocyte phenotype in the adult murine heart. Circulation **105:** 93–98.
44. MANGI, A.A. *et al.* 2003. Mesenchymal stem cells modified with Akt prevent remodeling and restore performance of infarcted hearts. Nat. Med. **9:** 1195–1201.
45. GNECCHI, M. *et al.* 2005. Paracrine action accounts for marked protection of ischemic heart by Akt-modified mesenchymal stem cells. Nat. Med. **11:** 367–368.
46. LOSORDO, D.W. & S. DIMMELER. 2004. Therapeutic angiogenesis and vasculogenesis for ischemic disease: part II: cell-based therapies. Circulation **109:** 2692–2697.
47. PERIN, E.C. *et al.* 2003. Transendocardial, autologous bone marrow cell transplantation for severe, chronic ischemic heart failure. Circulation **107:** 2294–2302.
48. FUCHS, S. *et al.* 2003. Catheter-based autologous bone marrow myocardial injection in no-option patients with advanced coronary artery disease: a feasibility study. J. Am. Coll. Cardiol. **41:** 1721–1724.
49. STRAUER, B.E. *et al.* 2002. Repair of infarcted myocardium by autologous intracoronary mononuclear bone marrow cell transplantation in humans. Circulation **106:** 1913–1918.
50. TSE, H.F. *et al.* 2003. Angiogenesis in ischaemic myocardium by intramyocardial autologous bone marrow mononuclear cell implantation. Lancet **361:** 47–49.
51. ASSMUS, B. *et al.* 2002. Transplantation of progenitor cells and regeneration enhancement in acute myocardial infarction (TOPCARE-AMI). Circulation **106:** 3009–3017.

52. WOLLERT, K.C. *et al.* 2004. Intracoronary autologous bone-marrow cell transfer after myocardial infarction: the BOOST randomised controlled clinical trial. Lancet **364:** 141–148.
53. CHEN, S.L. *et al.* 2004. Effect on left ventricular function of intracoronary transplantation of autologous bone marrow mesenchymal stem cell in patients with acute myocardial infarction. Am. J. Cardiol. **94:** 92–95.
54. ORLIC, D. *et al.* 2001. Mobilized bone marrow cells repair the infarcted heart, improving function and survival. Proc. Natl. Acad. Sci. USA **98:** 10344–10349.
55. ZOHLNHOFER, D. *et al.* 2006. Stem cell mobilization by granulocyte colony-stimulating factor in patients with acute myocardial infarction: a randomized controlled trial. JAMA **295:** 1003–1010.
56. DETEN, A. *et al.* 2005. Hematopoietic stem cells do not repair the infarcted mouse heart. Cardiovasc. Res. **65:** 52–63.
57. HASEGAWA, H. *et al.* 2006. Cardioprotective effects of granulocyte colony-stimulating factor in swine with chronic myocardial ischemia. J. Am. Coll. Cardiol. **47:** 842–849.
58. KANG, H.J. *et al.* 2004. Effects of intracoronary infusion of peripheral blood stem-cells mobilised with granulocyte-colony stimulating factor on left ventricular systolic function and restenosis after coronary stenting in myocardial infarction: the MAGIC cell randomised clinical trial. Lancet **363:** 751–756.
59. OH, H. *et al.* 2003. Cardiac progenitor cells from adult myocardium: homing, differentiation, and fusion after infarction. Proc. Natl. Acad. Sci. USA **100:** 12313–12318.
60. BELTRAMI, A.P. *et al.* 2003. Adult cardiac stem cells are multipotent and support myocardial regeneration. Cell **114:** 763–776.
61. MARTIN, C.M. *et al.* 2004. Persistent expression of the ATP-binding cassette transporter, Abcg2, identifies cardiac SP cells in the developing and adult heart. Dev. Biol. **265:** 262–275.
62. HIERLIHY, A.M. *et al.* 2002. The post-natal heart contains a myocardial stem cell population. FEBS Lett. **530:** 239–243.
63. MESSINA, E. *et al.* 2004. Isolation and expansion of adult cardiac stem cells from human and murine heart. Circ. Res. **95:** 911–921.
64. GOUMANS, M. *et al.* 2005. Human cardiac progenitor cells are able to differentiate into cardiomyocytes *In Vitro.* American Heart Association 2005 Scientific Sessions [Abstract No. 337]. Dallas, TX.
65. LAUGWITZ, K.L. *et al.* 2005. Postnatal isl1+ cardioblasts enter fully differentiated cardiomyocyte lineages. Nature **433:** 647–653.
66. MATSUURA, K. *et al.* 2004. Adult cardiac Sca-1-positive cells differentiate into beating cardiomyocytes. J. Biol. Chem. **279:** 11384–11391.
67. MALOUF, N.N. *et al.* 2001. Adult-derived stem cells from the liver become myocytes in the heart *in vivo.* Am. J. Pathol. **158:** 1929–1935.
68. STREM, B.M. *et al.* 2005. Expression of cardiomyocytic markers on adipose tissue-derived cells in a murine model of acute myocardial injury. Cytotherapy **7:** 282–291.
69. PLANAT-BENARD, V. *et al.* 2004. Spontaneous cardiomyocyte differentiation from adipose tissue stroma cells. Circ. Res. **94:** 223–229.
70. GUAN, K. *et al.* 2006. Pluripotency of spermatogonial stem cells from adult mouse testis. Nature **440:** 1199–1203.
71. BUTANY, J. *et al.* 2005. Cardiac tumours: diagnosis and management. Lancet Oncol. **6:** 219–228.

72. NAKAJIMA, H. *et al.* 2004. Expression of mutant p193 and p53 permits cardiomyocyte cell cycle reentry after myocardial infarction in transgenic mice. Circ. Res. **94:** 1606–1614.
73. SOONPAA, M.H. & L.J. FIELD. 1998. Survey of studies examining mammalian cardiomyocyte DNA synthesis. Circ. Res. **83:** 15–26.
74. PASUMARTHI, K.B. & L.J. FIELD. 2002. Cardiomyocyte enrichment in differentiating ES cell cultures: strategies and applications. Methods Mol. Biol. **185:** 157–168.
75. FIELD, L.J. 1988. Atrial natriuretic factor-SV40 T antigen transgenes produce tumors and cardiac arrhythmias in mice. Science **239:** 1029–1033.
76. BEHRINGER, R.R. *et al.* 1988. Heart and bone tumors in transgenic mice. Proc. Natl. Acad. Sci. USA **85:** 2648–2652.
77. KATZ, E.B. *et al.* 1992. Cardiomyocyte proliferation in mice expressing alpha-cardiac myosin heavy chain-SV40 T-antigen transgenes. Am. J. Physiol. **262:** H1867–H1876.
78. FIELD, L.J. 2004. Modulation of the cardiomyocyte cell cycle in genetically altered animals. Ann. N. Y. Acad. Sci. **1015:** 160–170.
79. SCHANG, L.M. 2003. The cell cycle, cyclin-dependent kinases, and viral infections: new horizons and unexpected connections. Prog. Cell Cycle Res. **5:** 103–124.
80. REISS, K. *et al.* 1996. Overexpression of insulin-like growth factor-1 in the heart is coupled with myocyte proliferation in transgenic mice. Proc. Natl. Acad. Sci. USA **93:** 8630–8635.
81. XIAO, G. *et al.* 2001. Inducible activation of c-Myc in adult myocardium *in vivo* provokes cardiac myocyte hypertrophy and reactivation of DNA synthesis. Circ. Res. **89:** 1122–1129.
82. ENGEL, F.B. *et al.* 2005. p38 MAP kinase inhibition enables proliferation of adult mammalian cardiomyocytes. Genes Dev. **19:** 1175–1187.
83. DECAPRIO, J.A. *et al.* 1988. SV40 large tumor antigen forms a specific complex with the product of the retinoblastoma susceptibility gene. Cell **54:** 275–283.
84. MACLELLAN, W.R. *et al.* 2005. Overlapping roles of pocket proteins in the myocardium are unmasked by germ line deletion of p130 plus heart-specific deletion of Rb. Mol. Cell Biol. **25:** 2486–2497.
85. SOONPAA, M.H. *et al.* 1997. Cyclin D1 overexpression promotes cardiomyocyte DNA synthesis and multinucleation in transgenic mice. J. Clin. Invest. **99:** 2644–2654.
86. PASUMARTHI, K.B. *et al.* 2005. Targeted expression of cyclin D2 results in cardiomyocyte DNA synthesis and infarct regression in transgenic mice. Circ. Res. **96:** 110–118.
87. LIAO, H.S. *et al.* 2001. Cardiac-specific overexpression of cyclin-dependent kinase 2 increases smaller mononuclear cardiomyocytes. Circ. Res. **88:** 443–450.
88. PASUMARTHI, K.B. *et al.* 2000. Enhanced cardiomyocyte DNA synthesis during myocardial hypertrophy in mice expressing a modified TSC2 transgene. Circ. Res. **86:** 1069–1077.
89. CHAUDHRY, H.W. *et al.* 2004. Cyclin A2 mediates cardiomyocyte mitosis in the postmitotic myocardium. J. Biol. Chem. **279:** 35858–35866.
90. LIMANA, F. *et al.* 2002. bcl-2 overexpression promotes myocyte proliferation. Proc. Natl. Acad. Sci. Usa **99:** 6257–6262.
91. TAMAMORI-ADACHI, M. *et al.* 2003. Critical role of cyclin D1 nuclear import in cardiomyocyte proliferation. Circ. Res. **92:** e12–e19.

92. LI, Q. *et al.* 1997. Overexpression of insulin-like growth factor-1 in mice protects from myocyte death after infarction, attenuating ventricular dilation, wall stress, and cardiac hypertrophy. J. Clin. Invest. **100:** 1991–1999.
93. HASSINK, R.J. *et al.* Cardiomyocyte cell cycle activation improves cardiac function after myocardial infarction. Submitted.

The Unstoppable Connexin43 Carboxyl-Terminus

New Roles in Gap Junction Organization and Wound Healing

ROBERT G. GOURDIE,[a,b] GAUTAM S. GHATNEKAR,[a] MICHAEL O'QUINN,[a] MATTHEW J. RHETT,[a] RALPH J. BARKER,[a] CHING ZHU,[a] JANE JOURDAN,[a] AND ANDREW W. HUNTER[a]

[a]*Department of Cell Biology and Anatomy, Center for Cardiovascular Development Biology, Medical University of South Carolina, Charleston, South Carolina 29425, USA*
[b]*Department of Bioengineering, Clemson University, Clemson, South Carolina 29634, USA*

> ABSTRACT: Intercellular connectivity mediated by gap junctions (GJs) composed of connexin43 ($C \times 43$) is critical to the function of excitable tissues such as the heart and brain. Disruptions to $C \times 43$ GJ organization are thought to be a factor in cardiac arrhythmias and are also implicated in epilepsy. This article is based on a presentation to the 4th Larry and Horti Fairberg Workshop on Interactive and Integrative Cardiology and summarizes the work of Gourdie and his lab on $C \times 43$ GJs in the heart. Background and perspective of recently published studies on the function of $C \times 43$-interacting protein zonula occludens-(ZO)-1 in determining the organization of GJ plaques are provided. In addition how a peptide containing a PDZ-binding sequence of $C \times 43$, developed as part of the work on cardiac GJ organization is also described, which has led to evidence for novel and unexpected roles for $C \times 43$ in modulating healing following tissue injury.
>
> KEYWORDS: gap junctions; connexin; electrical coupling; conduction; wound healing

INTRODUCTION

The gap junction (GJ) plaque is an aggregate of intercellular channels that provides for exchange of nutrients, messengers, and ions between the cytoplasms of neighboring cells.[1–3] The channels comprising the GJ are made up

Address for correspondence: Robert Gourdie, Ph.D., Department of Cell Biology and Anatomy, Medical University of South Carolina, Charleston, SC 29425. Fax: 843-792-0664.
e-mail: gourdier@musc.edu

of proteins encoded by the connexin gene family.[4] Assembly of GJs from connexins is understood to proceed in multiple steps.[5] Following translation, six connexins oligomerize into a connexin hemichannel, which is then trafficked to the cell membrane. The hemichannel docks with a second hemichannel from the apposed membrane of an adjacent cell to form an intercellular channel. In a process that may occur in association with the docking step, intercellular channels aggregate to form the GJ plaque. Phosphorylation is a posttranslational modification that appears to be of particular significance to the function and life cycle of connexins.[6,7]

In the heart and other excitable tissues, electrotonic couplings mediated by GJ aggregates contribute to uniform propagation of electrical activation.[8-13] Disruptions to GJ organization are thought to be a factor in cardiac arrhythmias[8-16] and have been implicated in a form of epilepsy.[17] As cellular circuits defined by GJs are recognized as important in health and disease, the mechanisms determining the size and positioning of GJs between cells are attracting increasing attention by researchers. Moreover, the prospect that the connexin subunits of GJs may have functions that are independent of intercellular communication is arousing interest and debate.[18-21]

Here, we review our work on the main GJ protein in the mammalian heart $\alpha 1$ connexin43 ($C \times 43$), with particular focus on its interaction with zonula occludens (ZO)-1, a protein directly interacting with the carboxyl terminus of $C \times 43$. Among other information, a perspective is given on our studies of how ZO-1 interaction with $C \times 43$ may determine GJ organizational patterns and we also outline evidence for a novel and unexpected role for peptide fragments derived from the $C \times 43$ carboxyl terminal (Ct) in wound healing.

CARDIAC GJs SHOW HIGHLY REGULAR PATTERNS OF SPATIAL ORGANIZATION

The main GJ proteins in the mammalian heart are Cx40, $C \times 43$, and Cx45.[8-16,20-31] $C \times 43$ is expressed in atrial myocardium and parts of the conduction system, but is found most prominently in the ventricle where numerous GJs composed of $C \times 43$ couple working ventricular myocytes together. Cx40 and Cx45 are also expressed in atrial myocardium and comprise GJs within tissues of the pacemaking and conduction system. There is evidence for conservation of Cx40 and Cx45 in the hearts of nonmammalian vertebrates.[28,32,33] However, mammals appear to be unique among the chordates in expressing $C \times 43$ in cardiac muscle.[33] This phylogenetic oddity is made even more curious by the high abundance at which $C \times 43$ is expressed in hearts of all mammalian species relative to the near undetectable levels of connexin of any type present in the working myocardium of adult nonmammals (reviewed in Ref. 9)

The large numbers of $C \times 43$ GJs in the working ventricular myocardium of the adult mammal display characteristic and highly regular patterns of spatial

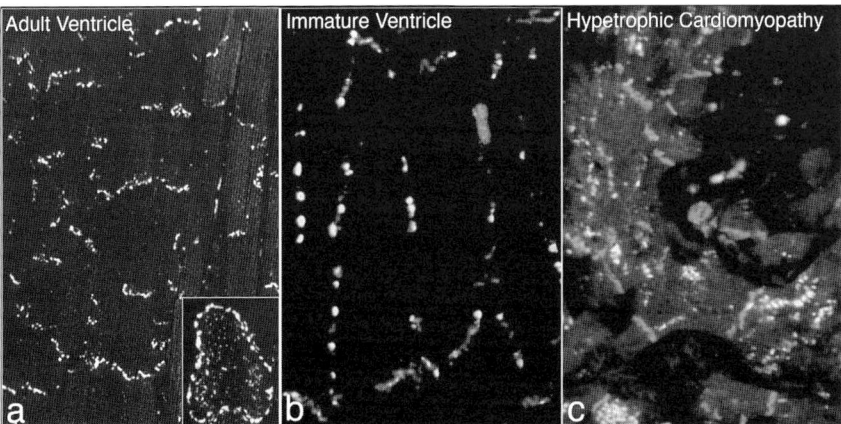

FIGURE 1. C×43 GJ organization in the adult, immature, and diseased mammalian ventricular myocardium. (**A**) Immunolabeled C×43 GJs are largely polarized at myocyte intercalated disks in the normal adult mammalian ventricle.[25] Inset (A) Large C×43 GJs form prominent rings encircling the intercalated disk. (**B**) C×43 GJs (green) are distributed along lateral membranes and dissociated from the heaviest concentrations of intercellular adhesion junctions (as delineated by red desmoplakin-labeled desmosomes) at intercalated disks in the immature mammalian ventricle.[40] (**C**) C×43 GJs (green) are dissociated from desmoplakin-labeled (red) intercalated disks in a zone of myofiber disarray in a human patient with hypertrophic cardiomyopathy (HCM).[44] The dissociation in electrical and mechanical intercellular junction distribution in HCM is reminiscent of the pattern seen during developmental remodeling of C×43 GJs from lateral distributions to intercalated disks (i.e., as in FIG. 1 B). Shown in color in the online version.

organization.[9,10,15,16,25,26,33–40] The polarized localization of GJs at intercalated disks is perhaps the most widely appreciated of these characteristics (FIG. 1 A). Further evidence of the regulated order of GJs in the ventricle can be recognized at the scale of the intercalated disk. Confocal imaging reveals ring-like arrangements of large GJs encircling the perimeter of disks[25,35] (inset FIG. 1 A). An even finer substructure has been discriminated within the plaque of individual GJs. Ultrarapid freezing has shown GJs at the intercalated disk to be irregularly packed structures comprising small rafts of uniformly aggregated channels separated by narrow particle-free aisles.[36]

POSTNATAL REMODELING OF LATERAL Cx43 GJs INTO INTERCALATED DISKS

Characterization of the developmental processes accounting for the spatial order of C×43 GJs in ventricular myocardium has been a long-term focus of the lab. The first descriptions of how C×43 GJs change from lateral distributions at side-by-side appositions between myocytes to become polarized at intercalated disks over postnatal growth of the rat heart were provided by Gourdie and co-workers[26,37]—a phenomenon later confirmed by others in mice[38] and humans.[39] Subsequently, we showed that postnatal remodeling of GJs was preceded by striking increases in intercellular adhesion junctions at intercalated disks and proposed that this transient dissociation in the distribution of electrical and mechanical junctions (e.g., FIG. 1 B) was key to understanding how GJs progressively assume mature organizational patterns in ventricular myocardium following birth.[40] Our proposal was that GJs are maintained within the intercalated disk (and conversely lost from lateral membranes over postnatal development) owing to a stabilizing proximity of disk-localized GJs to adherens junctions and desmosomes in the mechanically active tissue.

The concept that intercellular mechanical junctions are critical for GJ stability has received support from studies by other workers. First, it has been demonstrated that the components of the adherens junction and $C \times 43$ GJ form a multiprotein complex in NIH-3T3 cells.[41] Second, a hierarchical interdependence between maintenance of GJs and calcium-dependent adhesion junctions has been shown in Drosophila embryos.[42] Third, elegant transgenic work from Radice and co-workers have demonstrated that cardiac-specific knockout of N-cadherin in postnatal mice results in dissolution of intercalated disk structure, loss of membrane localization of $C \times 43$ GJs, and progressive lethality from ventricular arrhythmia.[43] Finally, evidence for interdependence of the stability of electrical and desmosomal intercellular junctions have come from studies of human patients with hypertrophic cardiomyopathy and inherited diseases of the myocardium (FIG. 1 C).[44,45]

INTERACTION OF THE ACTIN-BINDING MAGUK PROTEIN ZO-1 WITH Cx43

In addition to describing processes giving rise to the characteristic organizational patterns of GJs in the mammalian heart, we are also interested in the intracellular machinery governing the generation of this spatial order. The actin-binding protein ZO-1 has been proposed as a candidate for regulating cardiac GJ organization at the molecular level[46,47] and has been a major focus of our research of the last 5 years. Originally discovered in association with the tight junction, ZO-1 is a member of the membrane-associated guanylate kinase (MAGUK) family of proteins that function in targeting, signal transduction, and determination of cell polarity.[48] In immunoprecipitation studies in cultured cells, and in yeast-two hybrid analyses, it was shown that $C \times 43$ interacts with the second PDZ domain of ZO-1 via a short PDZ-binding motif at extreme carboxyl terminus of $C \times 43$.[46,47]

Initially, it was assumed that the function of ZO-1 interaction with $C \times 43$ was analogous to the presumed role of ZO-1 as a scaffolding protein at the tight junction. Namely, ZO-1 was thought to stabilize GJs at the plasma membrane by linkage to the actin cytoskeleton. However, subsequent reports have indicated that protein–protein interactions between connexins and ZO-1 encompass other, more dynamic functions. In particular, changes in ZO-1–C×43 interactions have been noted during remodeling of the organization and subcellular distribution of C×43 GJs in various cell types.[49–54]

Interaction between C×43 and ZO-1 during Remodeling of GJ Organization

Based on reports that ZO-1 interacts with C×43,[46,47] we investigated ZO-1 and C×43 association in the rat ventricular myocardium *in vivo*.[52] Our initial goal was to probe whether ZO-1 served within an actin scaffold, stabilizing GJs at the intercalated disk by direct interaction with C×43. However, results from immunofluorescence, immunoelectron microscopic, and immunoprecipitation studies did not seem to fit well with this proposal. First, we found that levels of co-localization between C×43 and ZO-1 in the ventricle *in vivo* were relatively modest. Second, it was determined that enzymatic dissociation of myocytes, a treatment causing loss of GJs from the sarcolemmal membrane,[55] increased C×43-ZO-1 association levels. Subsequently, other workers have confirmed that GJ-localized connexins and ZO-1 show modest levels of co-localization *in vivo*.[56,57] Moreover, others have confirmed increased association between C×43 and ZO-1 following induction of GJ re-distribution from the membrane to the cytoplasm.[54]

Fusion of GFP to the C×43 Carboxyl Terminus Yields a Connexin Molecule That Is Incompetent to Interact with ZO-1 and a Loss of GJ Size Control

We next attempted to observe the dynamics of C×43 and ZO-1 interaction directly in living cells.[58,59] To achieve this goal, we generated HeLa cell lines stably expressing C×43-GFP (Fig. 2). However, it was found that GJ plaques formed by C×43-GFP excluded ZO-1.[59] We later realized that this loss of ZO-1 co-localization was consistent with previous results from Giepmans and co-workers.[60] In pull-down studies, this group had shown that Ct tagging of C×43 with GFP, as well as other sequences, resulted in loss of function of the C×43 PDZ-binding domain. Although a setback, as outlined in Hunter *et al.*,[58] we soon appreciated that the loss of competence of the C×43-GFP mutant protein in interacting with ZO-1 provided a useful opportunity.

As is illustrated in Figure 2, the GJs formed by C×43-GFP molecules are abnormally large, relative to GJs formed by wild-type C×43 in HeLa cells (e.g., Fig. 2 B) and also in comparison with C×43 GJs observed *in vivo* (e.g., Fig. 1). To determine whether the organization of the large C×43-GFP GJs

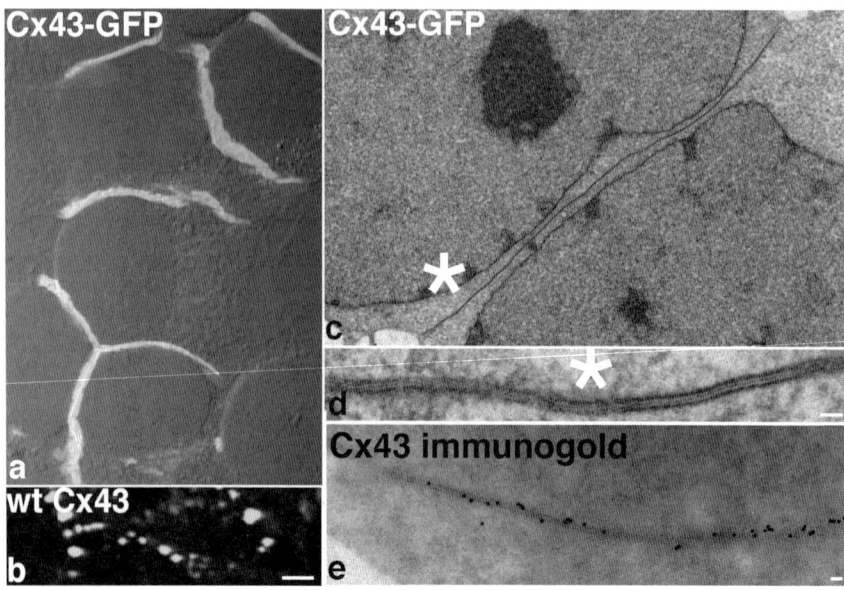

FIGURE 2. A C×43-GFP construct that is incompetent to interact with ZO-1 (see Refs. 58 and 59). (**A**) HeLa cells stably expressing the C×43-GFP construct form large, sheet-like GJs. White-gray signal at cell borders is GFP fluorescence. Darker gray background is a differential interference contrast image of the HeLa cells. (**B**) Normally sized and distributed punctate GJs in HeLa cells stably expressing wild-type (wt) C×43 as immunolabeled by anti-C×43 antibodies. (**C**) Transmission electron micrograph of an ultrathin section showing a large GJ between two C×43-GFP expressing HeLa cells. Note that the GJ spans the entire width of the interface between the two cells. Asterisk marks the region of GJ shown at higher resolution in (**D**). (**E**) anti-C×43 immunogold labeling electron micrograph of a GJ between two HeLa-C×43-GFP cells. Scale: A, B = 1 μm; D, F = 40 nm.

could be altered or rescued to be more *in vivo*-like, we expressed wild-type C×43 at varying levels in the HeLa cell line.[58] As relative amounts of wild-type C×43 increased, GJs in the C×43-GFP expressing cell line assumed regular size distributions and organizations. Pulse chase labeling studies with [^{35}S]-methionine established that there was little difference in half-life between C×43-GFP and wild-type C×43 when expressed singly or together, suggesting that C×43-GFP GJs did not get larger as a result of slowed turn-over of the mutant protein.[58] In experiments using immunoprecipitation of metabolically labeled connexins, we determined that an average stoichiometry of 1 C×43-GFP to 5.4 wild-type C×43 molecules was required for normalization of GJ organization.[58] This result suggested that it was necessary for each six-subunit hemichannel aggregated within a GJ needed to be mostly composed of wild-type C×43 for size control to be recovered for the GJ as a whole.

Binding of ZO-1 Regulates the Rate of Accretion of C×43 Hemichannels to the GJ

In Zhu et al.,[61] we reported high-resolution analyses of ZO-1 localization patterns at C×43 GJs in cultured monolayers of neonatal myocytes. These studies revealed a preferential association of ZO-1 with the perimeter of the C×43 GJ plaque. Subsequently, in Hunter et al.,[58] we determined that the rescue of size control in C×43-GFP expressing HeLa cells by expression of wild-type C×43 was associated with the re-establishment of localization of ZO-1 to the GJ periphery. In earlier work, Ellisman and co-workers[62] identified the GJ periphery as a site of assembly for new junctional membrane. Based on our data, we hypothesized that ZO-1 may be regulating GJ size via governing the rate of recruitment of C×43 hemichannels at the plaque periphery.

Our next step was to develop a strategy for inhibiting ZO-1 binding in situ at already established GJs between C×43-expressing cells. To achieve this goal, we synthesized a short peptide comprised of an antennapedia internalization sequence linked to the PDZ-binding domain of C×43[58] (FIG. 3 A). This rationally designed inhibitor of ZO-1 interaction with C×43 was shown to specifically interact with the PDZ2 domain of ZO-1 and inhibited PDZ2 interaction with normal full-length C×43 in vivo (FIG. 3 B). Importantly, we demonstrated that the inhibitor measurably reduced levels of ZO-1 localization at the GJ plaque edge in vivo (FIG. 3 C) and increased GJ size in neonatal myocytes and in HeLa cells expressing wild-type C×43 (FIG. 3 C).

Consistent with the concept that ZO-1-C×43 binding influences GJ size via affecting recruitment of C×43, changes in GJ size and ZO-1 co-localization induced by the peptide were similar, albeit less pronounced, to those observed in the C×43-GFP expressing HeLa cells. Western blotting indicated that this increase in GJ size was not associated with an increase in C×43 abundance.[58] These results were interpreted as indicating that the peptide caused redistribution between different parts of the cellular pool C×43—i.e., as opposed to increasing bulk levels of the protein. To probe this hypothesis, detergent fractionation was used to segregate the cellular pool of C×43 into junctional and nonjunctional components.[58] Consistent with the increase in GJ size observed in response to the peptide, fractionation of C×43 in this assay indicated a shift in C×43 from nonjunctional to junctional pools following peptide treatment.

Based on the microscopic and biochemical evidence, we concluded that ZO-1 limits C×43 GJ size via influencing rate of accretion of channels to the GJ. This rate-affecting mechanism is probably most active at the periphery of the GJ, where assembly of new junctional membrane proceeds. As such, ZO-1 may be conceived as somewhat like a "gate keeper" regulating, though not inhibiting, admission of hemichannels to the GJ channel aggregate. An interesting possibility is that regulation of ZO-1 interaction level provides a mechanism for altering C×43 hemichannel density in the plasma membrane. In such a scenario, dynamic adjustment to ZO-1 levels at the plaque edge might

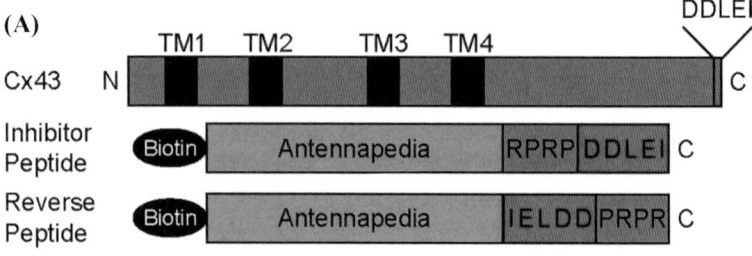
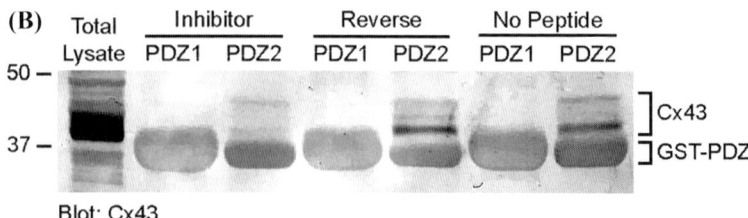
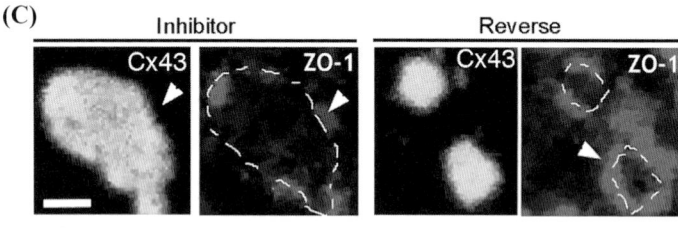

FIGURE 3. A peptide that specifically binds ZO-1 and blocks interaction with C×43.[60] (**A**) C×43, inhibitory peptide and reverse control peptide. (**B**) Blot showing that C×43 pulled down from HeLa lysates by GST-PDZ2 beads was reduced by inhibitor peptide. (**C**) In HeLa cells the peptide reduces C×43 GJ size and ZO-1 localization at the GJ perimeter as compared to reverse peptide treated cells. Two channel views of C×43 and ZO-1 signals are shown from a double immunolabeling. The perimeter of GJ plaques is indicated on the ZO-1 channel by dotted lines. Scale: C = 1 μm.

prompt conversion of dispersed connexons into GJ aggregates, reducing the numbers of hemichannel available for opening in response to an appropriate prompt.

ROLE OF PEPTIDE CONTAINING Cx43 PDZ DOMAIN IN WOUND HEALING

Intercellular communication between cells is a key aspect of tissue repair following injury.[63] While specific mechanisms remain to be characterized,

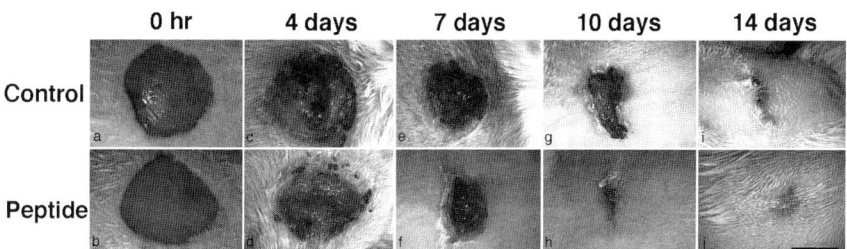

FIGURE 4. The inhibitory peptide improves healing of a excisional skin injury in adult mice. Anesthetized adult mice had 8-mm wide excisional skin injuries made by scalpel down to the underlying muscle in the dorsal mid line between the shoulder blades [i.e., as shown in (**A**) and (**B**)]. Hundred microliters of a solution of 30% pluronic gel containing either no (control) or dissolved peptide (FIG. 3 A) at a concentration of 100 μM was then applied to the injuries. Control or peptide containing gel was applied again subsequently 24 h. The peptide-treated excisional injury (B, D, F, H, I) was less inflamed, healed faster, and had better appearance than the control injury (A, C, E, G, J) over the 14-day time course. Note that images of the same injury on the same animal are shown at the different time points during the healing time course. Scale = 4 mm.

connexins appear to have functions in coordinating inflammatory response, wound repair, and scar tissue formation following injury.[63–66] Of particular note, downregulation of C×43 mRNA by antisense targeting has been shown to accelerate healing and reduce scar differentiation in a wound model of mouse skin.[64] Moreover, ZO-1 localization patterns in migrating fibroblasts in corneal injury have recently led Taliana and co-workers to propose roles for ZO-1 in coordination of cell migration and adhesion during wound healing.[67]

Based on the literature and experiments on cell migration from "scratch wounds" of NIH-3T3 fibroblast monolayers, we undertook studies of the effects of the PDZ-targeting peptide (as shown in FIG. 3 A) on skin wound healing in a mouse model *in vivo*.[68] The data indicated that relative to controls, the peptide increased the healing rate of excisional wounds and promoted the generation of skin with more normal-looking histology following closure of the injury (FIG. 4). Additionally, strength testing of 90-day-old healed wounds indicated peptide treatment resulted in significantly improved mechanical properties compared to controls. The effects of the peptide on wound healing were in some respects not similar to those reported for C×43 antisense treatment,[64] and it is unclear whether the C×43 antisense or the peptide designed to target ZO-1 act via related mechanisms.

CONCLUDING REMARKS

Can results obtained from skin be applied to a cryo-injury model of the heart? A further interesting question is whether our synthetic peptide is enhancing an endogenous response of mammalian tissues to injury involving the C×43 carboxyl terminus. This issue brings us to a point raised at the outset of this review. It is widely accepted that orderly C×43-based coupling between cardiac muscle cells is required for the stability of the heartbeat. However, it is remains unclear why mammals express C×43 in the heart at such abundance, or indeed at all. Efficient electrical coupling is achieved between heart muscle cells in nonmammalian chordates from tunicates to birds in the absence of C×43, and with only a tiny fraction of the intercellular channels that are apparently required in mammals.[9] Cardiac-specific gene knockout of C×43 in mice, while eventually causing lethal arrhythmia during postnatal life, is in fact consistent with regular propagation of cardiac activation up to the point that these transgenics succumb to conduction instability.[69] Could it be that C×43 is required for both the stability of the heartbeat and cardiac injury response in mammals? C×43 is also expressed at high levels in mammalian skin,[63–66] as well as other tissues, especially in embryonic development.[70] Apart from perfunctory assumptions about the importance of communication to cell and tissue homeostasis, the actual requirement for abundant C×43 expression in tissues like the skin, as in the heart, is not that well understood. In our ongoing work, we seek to determine whether C×43 has a generic role in mediating response to injury in mammals. Also, it will be of great interest to determine whether the peptide based on the PDZ-binding domain of C×43 shifts the balance during healing from fibrotic scar tissue to regeneration of cardiac muscle in the injured heart.

ACKNOWLEDGMENTS

The work reviewed here was supported by grants to A.W.H. and M.J.R. (NIH, HL07260), M.O. (AHA Pre-Doctoral Fellowship), and R.G.G. (NIH, HL56728, HL36059, HD39946). Many thanks to Dr. Robert Price and Mr. Jeff Davis (USC Medical School) for electron microscopy.

REFERENCES

1. HARRIS, A.L. 2001. Emerging issues of connexin channels: biophysics fills the gap. Q. Rev. Biophys. **34:** 325–472.
2. EVANS, W.H. & P.E. MARTIN. 2002. Gap junctions: structure and function. Mol. Membr. Biol. **19:** 121–136.
3. GOODENOUGH, D.A. & D.L. PAUL. 2003. Beyond the gap: functions of unpaired connexon channels. Nat. Rev. Mol. Cell. Biol. **4:** 285–294.
4. WILLECKE, K. et al. 2002. Structural and functional diversity of connexin genes in the mouse and human genome. Biol. Chem. **383:** 725–737.
5. MUSIL, L.S. & D.A. GOODENOUGH. 1993. Multisubunit assembly of an integral plasma membrane channel protein, gap junction connexin43, occurs after exit from the ER. Cell **74:** 1065–1077.

6. LAMPE, P.D. & A.F. LAU. 2004. The effects of connexin phosphorylation on gap junctional communication. Int. J. Biochem. Cell Biol. **36:** 1171–1186.
7. LAIRD, D.W. 2005. Connexin phosphorylation as a regulatory event linked to gap junction internalization and degradation. Biochim. Biophys. Acta **1711:** 172–182.
8. WEI, C.J. *et al.* 2004. Connexins and cell signaling in development and disease. Annu. Rev. Cell Dev. Biol. **20:** 811–838.
9. BARKER, R.J. & GOURDIE R.G. 2002. JNK bond regulation: why do mammalian hearts invest in connexin43? Circ. Res. **91:** 556–558.
10. SEVERS, N.J. *et al.* 2004. Gap junction alterations in human cardiac disease. Cardiovasc. Res. **62:** 368–377.
11. SPACH, M.S. 2003. Transition from a continuous to discontinuous understanding of cardiac conduction. Circ. Res. **92:** 125–126.
12. COTTRELL, G.T. & J.M. BURT. 2005. Functional consequences of heterogeneous gap junction channel formation and its influence in health and disease. Biochim. Biophys. Acta **1711:** 126–141.
13. SAFFITZ, J.E. & A.G. KLEBER. 2004. Effects of mechanical forces and mediators of hypertrophy on remodeling of gap junctions in the heart. Circ. Res. **94:** 585–591.
14. SHAH, M. *et al.* 2005. Molecular basis of arrhythmias. Circulation **112:** 2517–2529.
15. POELZING, S. & D.S. ROSENBAUM. 2004. Nature, significance, and mechanisms of **280:** 1010–1017.
16. PETERS, N.S. & A.L. WIT. 2000. Gap junction remodeling in infarction: Does it play a role in arrhythmogenesis? J. Cardiovasc. Electrophysiol. **11:** 488–490.
17. FONSECA, C.G., C.R. GREEN & L.F. NICHOLSON. 2002. Upregulation in astrocytic connexin 43 gap junction levels may exacerbate generalized seizures in mesial temporal lobe epilepsy. Brain Res. **929:** 105–116.
18. STOUT, C. *et al.* 2004. Connexins: functions without junctions. Curr. Opin. Cell Biol. **16:** 507–512.
19. KARDAMI, E. *et al.* 2003. PKC-dependent phosphorylation may regulate the ability of connexin43 to inhibit DNA synthesis. Cell Commun. Adhes. **10:** 293–297.
20. BOENGLER, K. *et al.* 2005. Connexin 43 in cardiomyocyte mitochondria and its increase by ischemic preconditioning. Cardiovasc. Res. 67: 234–244.
21. SALAMEH, A. & S. DHEIN. 2005. Pharmacology of gap junctions. New pharmacological targets for treatment of arrhythmia, seizure and cancer? Biochim. Biophys. Acta. **1719:** 36–58.
22. MANJUNATH, C., G. GOINGS & E. PAGE. 1984. Cytoplasmic surface and intramembrane components of rat heart gap junctional proteins. Am. J. Physiol. **246:** H865-H875.
23. BEYER, E.C. *et al.* 1987. Connexin43: a protein from rat heart homologous to a gap junction protein from liver. J. Cell Biol. **105:** 2621–2629.
24. DELMAR, M. *et al.* 2004. Structural bases for the chemical regulation of Connexin43 channels. Cardiovasc. Res. **62:** 268–275.
25. GOURDIE, R.G. *et al.* 1991. Gap junction distribution in adult mammalian myocardium revealed by an anti-peptide antibody and laser scanning confocal microscopy. J. Cell Sci. **99:** 41–55.
26. GOURDIE, R.G. *et al.* 1992. Immunolabelling patterns of gap junction connexins in the developing and mature rat heart. Anat. Embryol. **185:** 363–378.
27. GOURDIE, R.G. *et al.* 1993a. The spatial distribution and relative abundance of gap junctional connexin40 and connexin43 correlate to functional properties of the components of the cardiac AV conduction system. J. Cell Sci. **105:** 985–991.

28. GOURDIE, R.G. *et al.* 1993b. Evidence for a distinct gap-junctional phenotype in conduction tissues of the developing and mature avian heart. Circ. Res. **72:** 278–289.
29. KANTER, H.L. *et al.* 1993. Distinct patterns of connexin expression in canine Purkinje fibers and ventricular muscle. Circ. Res. **72:** 1124–1131.
30. GROS, D.B. & H.J. JONGSMA. 1996. Connexins in mammalian heart function. Bioessays **18:** 719–730.
31. COPPEN, S.R. *et al.* 1999. Connexin45 (alpha 6) expression delineates an extended conduction system in the embryonic and mature rodent heart. Dev. Genet. **24:** 82–90.
32. BEYER, E.C. 1990. Molecular cloning and developmental expression of two chick embryo gap junction proteins. J Biol Chem. **265:** 14439–14443; Christie, T.L., et al. 2004. Molecular cloning, functional analysis, and RNA expression analysis of connexin45.6: A zebrafish cardiovascular connexin. Am. J. Physiol. Heart Circ. Physiol. **286**: H1623–H1633.
33. BECKER, D.L. *et al.* 1998. Expression of major gap junction connexin types in the working myocardium of eight chordates. Cell Biol. Int. **22:** 527–543.
34. GOURDIE, R.G. & C.W. LO. 2000. C×43 gap junctions in cardiac development and disease. *In* Current Topics in Cell Biology. Vol. 49, Gap Junctions. C. Perrachia, Ed.: 581–602. Academic Press. New York.
35. GOURDIE, R.G. *et al.* 1990. Cardiac gap junctions in rat ventricle: Localization using site-directed antibodies and laser scanning confocal microscopy. Cardioscience **1:** 75–82.
36. GREEN, C.R. & N.J. SEVERS. 1984. Gap junction connexon configuration in rapidly frozen myocardium and isolated intercalated disks. J. Cell Biol. **99:** 453–463.
37. GOURDIE, R.G. *et al.* 1990. Three-dimensional reconstruction of gap junction arrangement in developing and adult rat hearts. Transact. Royal Microsc. Soc. **1:** 417–420.
38. FROMAGET, C. *et al.* 1992. Distribution pattern of connexin43, a gap-junctional protein, during the differentiation of mouse heart myocytes. Differentiation **51:** 9–20.
39. PETERS, N.S. *et al.* 1994. Spatiotemporal relation between gap junctions and fascia adherens junctions during postnatal development of human ventricular myocardium. Circulation **90:** 713–725.
40. ANGST, B.D. *et al.* 1997. Dissociated spatial patterning of gap junctions and cell adhesion junctions during postnatal differentiation of ventricular myocardium. Circ. Res. **80:** 88–94.
41. WEI, C.J. *et al.* 2005. Connexin43 associated with an N-cadherin-containing multiprotein complex is required for gap junction formation in NIH3T3 cells. J. Biol. Chem. **280:** 19925–19936.
42. BAUER, R. *et al.* 2004. Gap junction channel protein innexin 2 is essential for epithelial morphogenesis in the Drosophila embryo. Mol. Biol. Cell **15:** 2992–3004.
43. LI, J. *et al.* 2005. Cardiac-specific loss of N-cadherin leads to alteration in connexins with conduction slowing and arrhythmogenesis. Circ. Res. **97:** 474–481.
44. SEPP, R. *et al.*1996. Altered patterns of cardiac intercellular junction distribution in hypertrophic cardiomyopathy. Heart **76:** 412–417.
45. SAFFITZ, J.E. 2005. Dependence of electrical coupling on mechanical coupling in cardiac myocytes: insights gained from cardiomyopathies caused by defects in cell–cell connections. Ann. N. Y. Acad. Sci. **1047:** 336–344.

46. GIEPMANS, B.N. & W.H. MOOLENAAR. 1998. The gap junction protein connexin43 interacts with the second PDZ domain of the zona occludens-1 protein. Curr. Biol. **8:** 931–934.
47. TOYOFUKU, T.M. *et al.* 1998. Direct association of the gap junction protein connexin-43 with ZO-1 in cardiac myocytes. J. Biol. Chem. **273:** 12725–12731.
48. STEVENSON, B.R. *et al.* 1986. Identification of ZO-1: a high molecular weight polypeptide associated with the tight junction (zonula occludens) in a variety of epithelia. J. Cell Biol. **103:** 755–766.
49. TOYOFUKU, T.Y. *et al.* 2001. c-Src regulates the interaction between connexin-43 and ZO-1 in cardiac myocytes. J. Biol. Chem. **276:** 1780–1788.
50. DEFAMIE, N.B. *et al.* 2001. Disruption of gap junctional intercellular communication by lindane is associated with aberrant localization of connexin43 and zonula occludens-1 in 42GPA9 Sertoli cells Y. Carcinogenesis **22:** 1537–1542.
51. BARKER, R.J. *et al.* 2001. Increased co-localization of connexin43 and ZO-1 in dissociated adult myocytes. Cell Commun. Adhes. **8:** 205–208.
52. BARKER, R.J. *et al.* 2002. Increased association of ZO-1 with connexin43 during remodeling of cardiac gap junctions. Circ. Res. **22**;90:317–324.
53. BARKER, R.J. & R.G. GOURDIE. 2003. Connexin interacting proteins. *In* Heart Cell Coupling and Impulse Propagation in Health and Disease. W.C. De Mello & M.J. Janse, Eds.: 25–50. Kluwer. Boston.
54. SEGRETAIN, D. *et al.* 2004. A proposed role for ZO-1 in targeting connexin 43 gap junctions to the endocytic pathway. Biochimie **86:** 241–244.
55. SEVERS, N.J. *et al.* 1989. Fate of gap junctions in isolated adult mammalian cardiomyocytes. Circ. Res. **65:** 22–42.
56. NIELSEN, P.A. *et al.* 2002. Molecular cloning, functional expression, and tissue distribution of a novel human gap junction-forming protein, connexin-31.9. Interaction with zona occludens protein-1. J. Biol. Chem. **277:** 38272–38283.
57. DUFFY, H.S. *et al.* 2004. Regulation of connexin43 protein complexes by intracellular acidification. Circ. Res. **94:** 215–222.
58. HUNTER, A.W. *et al.* 2005. ZO-1 alters connexin43 gap junction size and organization by influencing channel accretion. Mol. Biol. Cell **16:** 5686–5698.
59. HUNTER, A.W. *et al.* 2003. Fusion of GFP to the carboxyl terminus of connexin43 increases gap junction size in HeLa cells. Cell Commun. Adhes. **10:** 211–214.
60. GIEPMANS, B.N. *et al.* 2001. Connexin-43 interactions with ZO-1 and alpha- and beta-tubulin. Cell Commun. Adhes. **8:** 219–223.
61. ZHU, C. *et al.* 2005. Quantitative analysis of ZO-1 colocalization with C×43 gap junction plaques in cultures of rat neonatal cardiomyocytes. Microsc. Microanal. **11:** 244–248.
62. GAIETTA, G. *et al.* 2002. Multicolor and electron microscopic imaging of connexin trafficking. Science **296:** 503–507.
63. CHANSON, M. *et al.* 2004. Gap junctional communication in tissue inflammation and repair. Biochim. Biophys. Acta **1711:** 197–207.
64. QIU, C. *et al.* 2003.Targeting connexin43 expression accelerates the rate of wound repair. Curr. Biol. **13:** 1697–1703.
65. SAITOH, M., M. OYAMADA, Y. OYAMADA, *et al.* 1997. Changes in the expression of gap junction proteins (connexins) in hamster tongue epithelium during wound healing and carcinogenesis. Carcinogenesis **18:** 1319–1328.
66. COUTINHO, P., C. QIU, S. FRANK, *et al.* 2003. Dynamic changes in connexin expression correlate with key events in the wound healing process. Cell Biol. Int. **27:** 525–541.

67. TALIANA, L. *et al*. 2005. M. ZO-1: Lamellipodial localization in a corneal fibroblast wound model. Invest. Ophthalmol. Vis. Sci. **46:** 96–103.
68. GHATNEKAR, G.S., J.L. JOURDAN & R.G. GOURDIE. 2006. Novel connexin based peptides accelerate wound closure and reduce inflammation and scarring in cutaneous wounds [abstract]. Wound Repair Regen., in press.
69. GUTSTEIN, D.E *et al*. 2001. Conduction slowing and sudden arrhythmic death in mice with cardiac-restricted inactivation of connexin43 Circ. Res. **88:** 333–339.
70. RUANGVORAVAT, C.P. & C.W. LO. 1992. Connexin43 expression in the mouse embryo: Localization of transcripts within developmentally significant domains Dev. Dyn. **194:** 261–281.

The Developing Cardiac Myocyte

Maturation of Excitability and Excitation–Contraction Coupling

ELIZABETH A. SCHRODER, YIDONG WEI, AND JONATHAN SATIN

Department of Physiology, University of Kentucky College of Medicine, Lexington, Kentucky 40536-0298, USA

ABSTRACT: The study of cardiac myocyte (CM) differentiation, development, and maturation is of interest for several compelling reasons. First, mechanisms of development are of fundamental biological interest. Second, congenital malformation of the heart may be related to CM dysfunction during embryonic/fetal development. Third, adult myocardium in a variety of diseased states re-expresses a fetal-like gene program. Fourth, the mature heart cannot readily regenerate itself. Thus, cell replacement therapy is an emerging treatment paradigm. Among the obstacles for the realization of cell replacement therapy is our incomplete understanding of the function during CM maturation. This is crucial in the potential use of embryonic stem (ES) cell-derived CMs as a cell source. Although much progress has been realized with mouse ES-CMs, our understanding of human counterparts is scant. Here we discuss key molecular underpinnings of excitability and excitation–contraction coupling in developing mouse heart. We focus on the Ca channel multimeric complex and Ca handling. We compare mouse embryonic physiology to that previously described in mouse ES-CMs and draw parallels and highlight distinctions to human ES-CMs. During mouse embryonic and fetal maturation, the L-type Ca channel current ($I_{Ca,L}$) predominates, but embryonic/fetal $I_{Ca,L}$ has distinct properties from mature $I_{Ca,L}$. In addition T-type Ca current ($I_{Ca,T}$) present in the fetus is not present in the adult. It is neither ethical nor practical to experiment with live human embryonic/fetal CMs for I_{Ca} and Ca handling studies, but we can draw inferences from human heart cell function based on studies of human ES-CMs, using the parallels noted between mouse embryonic heart cells and mouse ES-CMs.

KEYWORDS: ion channel; calcium channel; heart development; voltage-gated ion channel; cardiac electrophysiology

Address for correspondence: Jonathan Satin, Ph.D., Department of Physiology, MS-508, University of Kentucky College of Medicine, Lexington, KY 40536-0298. Voice: 859-323-5356; fax: 859-323-1070.
  e-mail: jsatin1@uky.edu

INTRODUCTION

The embryonic myocardium undergoes simultaneous maturation of structure and function at the tissue, cell, and subcellular levels. During development cardiac muscle progresses from a thin layer of myocardium surrounding a thick layer of cardiac jelly with a thin internal layer of endocardium to a highly organized myofibrillar structure optimized for efficient function. Simultaneously, myocardial cells proceed toward an efficient mechanism for Ca cycling and muscle contraction (excitation–contraction [EC] coupling). In this article, we discuss novel aspects of murine cardiac myocyte (CM) Ca channels in embryonic development.

EMBRYONIC HEART MODEL SYSTEMS

Ideally we would prefer to study human heart cells to understand human heart development. This, of course, is ethically challenged, and thus we must rely on a combination of model systems. Perhaps the best-studied animal model of late is the mouse. The main advantage of the mouse heart is the ability to manipulate gene expression, and as a result we have gained a great deal of insight, despite the well-established CM physiological differences between mouse and humans. Of central interest to our focus is the fact that EC coupling in mouse cells utilizes significantly more sarcoplasmic reticulum (SR) than plasma membrane (PM) Ca flux, exhibits dramatically faster heart rates, and exhibits a significantly more sympathetic tone than in human cells. Nonetheless, each of these factors is reduced in native developing mouse heart. For example, there is relatively more PM Ca influx, slower heart rate, and likely less sympathetic tone. Of central importance is the question, "what molecular components mediate these developmental distinctions?" Whether features of mouse heart development applies to human CMs as well requires knowledge of human embryonic stem (ES)-CMs, comparisons with mouse ES-CMs. We can draw inferences regarding native human development based on parallels between murine ES-CM and murine native heart cell development. These relationships are demonstrated in FIGURE 1.

EMBRYONIC PHYSIOLOGICAL DEVELOPMENT

In mature myocardium PM Ca channels permit Ca entry that initiates SR release, a process commonly referred to as Ca-induced Ca release (CICR). Ca entry via the PM is not sufficient to elicit contraction. PM Ca entry stimulates approximately a 10-fold more release of SR Ca via ryanodine receptors (RyRs). Localization of PM L-type Ca channels in the T tubules and junctional SR RyRs in dyadic junctions facilitate CICR in the adult myocardium. SR Ca release is

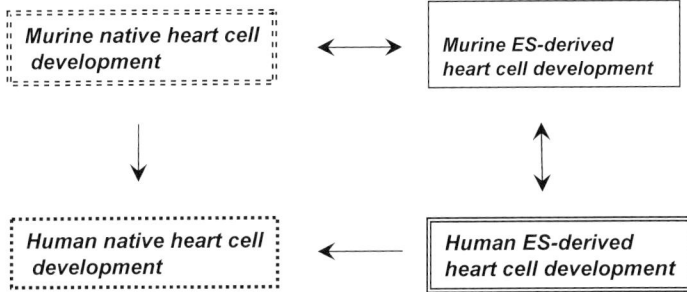

FIGURE 1. Native, live human heart cell development is inaccessible for study, but the human ES-CMs serve as a useful model system. Murine heart development, in some respects, is captured by murine ES-CMs *in vitro* maturation. Therefore, studying both human and mouse ES-CM differentiation and maturation allows us to make inferences regarding human heart development.

graded as a function of L-type Ca currents.[1] Although L-type Ca channels are most commonly thought of as the "trigger" for SR Ca release, Ca influx from T-type channels[2] and the Na–Ca exchanger[3] may also play a role under certain conditions.

In contrast, embryonic ventricular myocytes (EVM) have a poorly developed SR, and the embryonic and fetal heart is more dependent on trans-PM Ca^{2+} influx, rather than Ca^{2+} released from the SR.[4] In addition, mature components like L-type channels, the main trigger for SR release, and the Na–Ca exchanger appear to be both present and functioning before birth. T tubules are not present in many species until weeks to months after birth. This lack of physical/functional coupling at the dyadic junction may account for the lack of a phenotypically mature CICR in the late fetal and neonatal stages of development. Recently, embryonic lethality between E10.5–11.5 of mice carrying a gene inactivation of the ryanodine receptor 2 (RyR2) was described.[5] While the hearts of $RyR2^{-/-}$ mutant mice started to spontaneously contract at E9.5, severe morphological changes of the SR and the mitochondria were detected. RyR2 may not be required for EC coupling in EVM but may play a crucial role in Ca homeostasis. Thus, PM Ca entry pathways such as voltage-gated Ca channels may be critical contributors to EVM excitability and Ca handling.

The molecular characterization of embryonic heart function is important for several reasons. First, the mature heart in disease states often re-expresses an embryonic phenotype. Elucidation of the molecular basis for excitability in the developing heart offers a glimpse of mechanisms underlying heart cell function in pathology. Second, cells hoped to be useful for regenerative cell therapies are often derived from ES cells. For the mouse, ES cell function during development has been partially characterized. Unfortunately, there is a paucity of native developmental data that precludes definitive interpretation of ES cell function as mirroring native development. Therefore, it is imperative to describe the molecular basis for the function of the developing native heart. Trans-PM Ca handling is an early step that ultimately controls contractility. However, the Ca channels that mediate Ca flux in EVM are poorly defined. EVM express multiple voltage-gated Ca channel types. $Ca_V1.2$ knockout mice are embryonic lethal,[6] and $Ca_V1.3$ may substitute for $Ca_V1.2$ in early embryonic development.[7] T-type Ca channels ($Ca_V3.1$) are also expressed in murine EVM.[8] $Ca_V1.3$ and $Ca_V3.1$ share the functional property that they conduct Ca at relatively hyperpolarized potentials compared to $Ca_V1.2$.[7,9] Moreover, cloning and heterologous expression of $Ca_V3.1$ reveals that this channel type may contribute to cytosolic Ca entry in steady state at potentials corresponding to diastole in the heart. In the potential range from ~ -70 to -45 mV, $Ca_V3.1$ does not fully inactivate, but does exhibit a small open probability.[10] It has been widely suggested that Ca entry via T-type Ca channels may serve as a current injector to initiate depolarization.

The literature describing excitability and Ca handling in the developing heart is better developed from ES cell studies than that from native heart. At the extreme, ES cells early in the pathway to cardiac differentiation do not even require external Ca for activity.[11] Maturation of Ca handling has been inferred by ES-cell-derived cardiac precursor cell physiology from mouse[12] and most recently human origins.[13,14] Functional expression of L-type Ca channels is a hallmark of cardiomyogenesis in ES-derived cardiomyocytes, although RyR-sensitive stores are delayed.[12] Neonatal heart cells utilize a phosphatidylinositol 3-kinase(PI_3K)–IP_3-IP_3R pathway for generating spontaneous Ca oscillations.[15]

RESULTS AND DISCUSSION

Role of PM Ca Channels in Spontaneous Activity

A major functional distinction of EVM to mature ventricular myocytes is that EVM exhibit spontaneous electrical and contractile activity. The lack of a well-defined T-tubule network and incompletely developed SR suggests that EVM has an increased emphasis on PM Ca handling for EC coupling. To dissect the role of PM Ca channels and internal stores in spontaneous electrical and contractile activity, we used functional assays in concert with pharmacological profiles to evaluate contributions by at least three different PM Ca current components. The mature cardiac Ca channel, $Ca_V1.2$, is blocked by dihydropyridines, such as nifedipine. FIGURE 2 A shows representative cytosolic Ca transients in Ca-containing and Ca-free bath solution in a mouse day 10 EVM. In contrast to early mouse ES-CMs, removal of bath Ca^{2+} eliminates Ca transients (FIG. 2 B). One micromolar nifedipine blocks adult cardiac $Ca_V1.2$ Ca^{2+} current but has little effect on EVM Ca^{2+} transients (FIG. 2 C), and 10 μM nifedipine partially inhibits spontaneous Ca transients (FIG. 2 D). Ten micromolar nifedipine significantly reduced the amplitude and slowed the

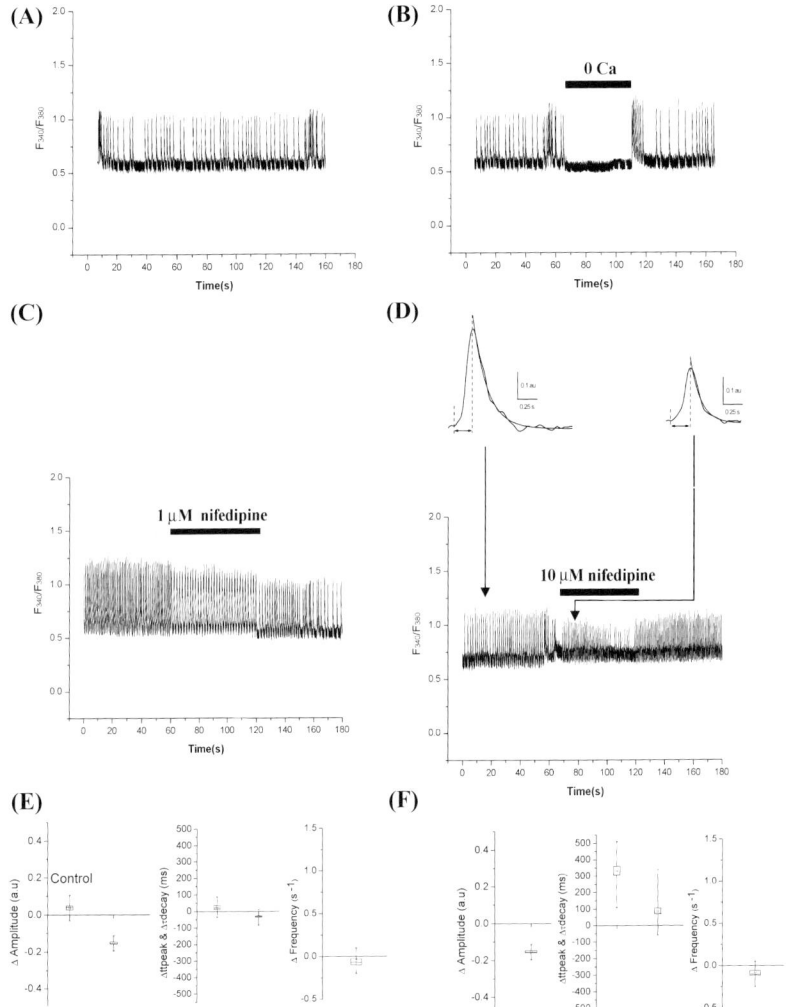

FIGURE 2. External Ca and a relatively nifedipine-resistant Ca entry pathway are required for spontaneous activity in ED16 EVM. Representative spontaneous fura-2 transients. (**A**) Control conditions and (**B**) upon removal of external Ca. (**C**) One micromolar nifedipine does not inhibit spontaneous activity. The trend for a slight slow rate was not statistically significant. (**D**) Ten micromolar nifedipine reversibly inhibits spontaneous activity with a lag. Note the decrease of amplitude. Inset, single transients shown on an expanded timescale to illustrate measurement of summary data as follows. (**E, F**) Pooled data for response to 1 μM (**E**) and 10 μM nifedipine (**F**). Δ refers to the difference before and after drug addition for a given recording. The box in the summary plot shows the median 75% of the data and the lines extending from the boxes show the range of all data. Amplitude is from baseline to peak; ttp (time to peak) is the duration from the upstroke to peak. The decay is a single exponential fit of the decay of the transient and Δfrequency is the beat rate difference. Note that 10 μM nifedipine significantly reduced Δamplitude and slowed the kinetics without a change in frequency.

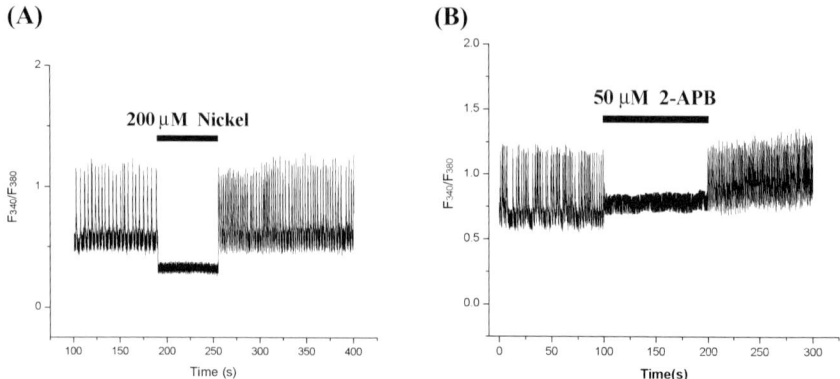

FIGURE 3. (**A**) Ni^{2+} blocks spontaneous activity and reduces resting cytosolic Ca. Two hundred micromolar Ni^{2+} applied at indicated time. In addition to blockade of spontaneous activity, the resting Ca level was inhibited. Washout of Ni^{2+} coincides with elevation of diastolic Ca and resumption of automaticity. (**B**) Spontaneous activity, but not resting Ca is sensitive to 2-APB. Fifty micromolar 2-APB applied during time indicated. Note that frequency and diastolic Ca were elevated with 2-APB washout.

kinetics of the Ca transients (FIG. 2 F). These findings are consistent with reduced PM Ca entry via the relatively nifedipine-insensitive $Ca_V1.3$ channel. Requirements for spontaneous activity and requirements for heart development, function, or survival are clearly independent of one another, as illustrated by the absence of sub-μM nifedipine effects on spontaneous Ca transients (FIG. 1 B), but of $Ca_V1.2$ expression is required for viable heart development past ED14 in the mouse.[6]

Nickel was used to further determine PM Ca channel contribution to EC coupling. Ni at sub-mM concentrations blocks Ca_V1 and Ca_V3 channels,[16,17] including $Ca_V3.1$ type expressed by embryonic mouse heart,[8] but has no effect on NCX. Two hundred micromolar Ni^{2+} rapidly and reversibly inhibits spontaneous Ca transients (FIG. 3 A). Also, there was a reversible decrease of diastolic Ca during the application of Ni^{2+}. This suggests that Ca_V3 or Ni-sensitive Ca_V1 channels are critical for Ca entry.

Internal Ca Stores Are Not Required, but Can Modulate Spontaneous Activity

To test for RyR2 involvement in spontaneous activity, we either blocked RyR with ruthenium red or used caffeine to release RyR-store Ca. In contrast to mature cardiomyocyte Ca^{2+} handling, 10 μM ruthenium red, an inhibitor of RyR had no effect on spontaneous Ca transients. However, the RyR2 agonist, caffeine, causes an increase of rate and an increase of diastolic Ca in EVM (FIG. 4 A). The caffeine effect on individual transients was restricted to a change in beat frequency; there was no significant effect on the Ca transient amplitude or kinetics. Although RyR2 function is not required for spontaneous activity,

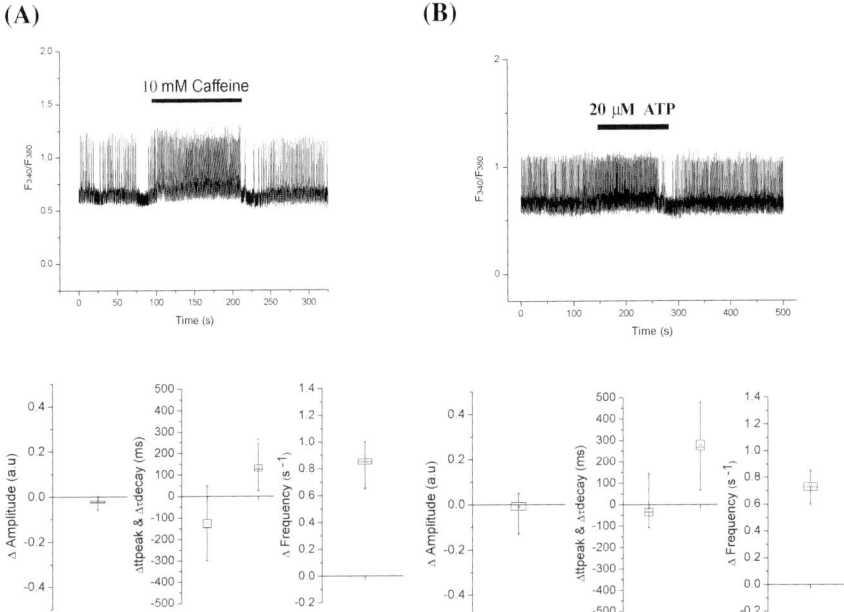

FIGURE 4. Internal Ca stores modulate, but are not required for spontaneous activity. Ryanodine receptor release pathway. (**A**) Ten millimolar caffeine significantly increases the spontaneous frequency. (**B**) Twenty micromolar ATP significantly increases rate. This suggests that the IP_3R pathway may not contribute to basal automaticity, but stimulation of the IP_3R pathway can release sufficient Ca to modulate Ca cycling. Summary plots are as described in FIGURE 2.

caffeine-releasable Ca pools can modulate the beat rate. Moreover, these effects on individual transients are distinct from slower transient kinetics induced by partial PM Ca channel block by nifedipine.

Studies of embryonic heart cells and immature heart cells derived from stem cells suggest that internal store Ca^{2+} release via IP_3R is a major pathway of cytosolic Ca^{2+} entry. To evaluate IP_3R involvement, we stimulated IP_3R-releasable Ca with the purinergic receptor agonist, adenosine 5′-triphosphate (ATP). ATP reversibly speeded the spontaneous Ca transient frequency (FIG. 4 B). ATP-purinergic receptor signaling in neonatal heart is mediated via a PI_3Kinase pathway to increase cytosolic IP_3 formation.[15] Wortmannin inhibits this PI_3K- and ATP-induced formation of IP_3. Given that IP_3-releasable Ca may be important for EVM activity, we tested the ability of wortmannin to inhibit transients. Wortmannin had no effect suggesting the absence of basal purinergic receptor tone.

The principal antagonistic effect of 2-aminoethyl diphenylborate (2-APB) is on cytosolic Ca entry. However, the molecular target for 2-APB is unclear. Numerous early studies with 2-APB claim that it is an efficacious inhibitor of IP_3R-mediated store Ca release, including ventricular myocytes.[18] In adult heart cells, 2 μM 2-APB is sufficient for attenuating IP_3R-mediated cytosolic Ca entry.[19] In EVM, however, 2 μM 2-APB has no effect on spontaneous activity. The 2-APB concentration dependence was steep with no effect seen for eight of eight trials using <30 μM, but six of six trials with 50 μM 2-APB resulted in reversible cessation of spontaneous activity, but without a reduction of diastolic Ca (FIG. 3 B). This suggests a different molecular target for 2-APB versus Ni^{2+}. Collectively, these data show that EVM does not utilize the same major components of CICR as adult myocytes; rather, our pharmacological evidence suggests that PM Ca^{2+} flux and IP_3R may be required.

More recent studies have shown, however, that 2-APB also inhibits Ca pumps and has a slowly reversible action on store-operated Ca entry channels in mature atrial myocytes.[20] 2-APB blocks electrically stimulated Ca transients in atrial rat myocytes in the same concentration range as we observed in 2-APB inhibition of EVM spontaneous Ca transients. As noted above, Ni^{2+} decreased resting Ca, whereas 2-APB increased diastolic Ca. This could be explained by a 2-APB inhibition of Ca pump.[21,22] Thus, three mutually exclusive possibilities can explain 2-APB effects on spontaneous Ca transients: block of IP_3R release, block of SERCA, or block of $Ca_V1.3$, and to a lesser extent $Ca_V3.1$ channels. Indirect evidence against a pure effect on SERCA is the reversibility of 2-APB (FIG. 2 B). In past studies, higher concentrations of 2-APB were necessary to show accumulation of cytosolic Ca, and these effects were irreversible[23] as expected for action on an intracellular target. However, our data clearly show that upon 2-APB washout, spontaneous Ca activity instantly resumes. This said, we consistently noted a slight rise of diastolic Ca, which is a finding that is consistent with cytosolic Ca overload. It is probable that 2-APB blocks Ca transients via multiple targets including SERCA, $Ca_V1.3$, and $Ca_V3.1$ channels but not necessarily via IP_3R release alone.

Ca Current Expressed by EVM Are Distinct from Mature Ventricle

The reliance of PM Ca flux for spontaneous activity prompted us to explore the voltage-dependent Ca current in EVM. We compared mature ventricular myocyte whole-cell Ca current to that expressed by EVM. In mature cells, Ca current (L-type) was not dependent on holding potential difference between −80 and −40 mV. In contrast, EVM shows a >50% decrease of current following V_{hold} −40 compared to −80 mV (FIG. 5 A). In addition, EVM I_{Ca} voltage dependence was different than mature I_{Ca}. The peak current was slightly more hyperpolarized and an additional low-voltage-activated component was manifested as a −40 mV V_{hold}-sensitive current (FIG. 5 B). Fifty micromolar 2-APB-blocked spontaneous Ca transients and also blocked all components of EVM I_{Ca}. In contrast, this same concentration of 2-APB had no effect on mature ventricular myocyte I_{Ca}. It is well known that mature heart cells express predominantly $Ca_V1.2$. In contrast, the differing voltage dependence

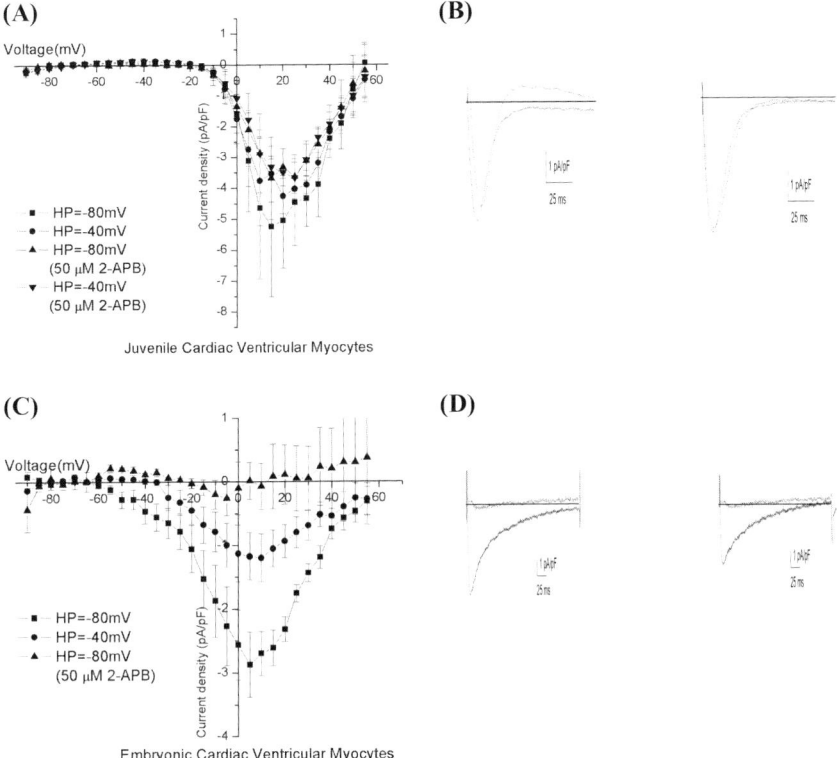

FIGURE 5. EVM and mature ventricle express distinct Ca current signatures. (**A**) Whole-cell Ca current–voltage curves recorded from single cells from mature mouse ventricle. In control, bath solution V_{hold} −80 (squares) versus −40 mV (circles) had negligible effects on measured Ca current. Fifty micromolars 2-APB (triangles) had no effect on I_{Ca} from mature myocytes. (**B**) Left: Representative ionic current for V_{test} 0 mV, V_{hold} −80 or −40 mV superimposed. Right: Same voltage steps in the presence of 50 μM 2-APB. (**C**) Embryonic ventricular myocyte I_{Ca} is sensitive to V_{hold} in range from −80 to −40 mV. Current–voltage curve shows that V_{hold} −40 mV reduces available current to ∼60% of that measured for V_{hold} −80 mV. Fifty micromolar 2-APB completely blocks EVM I_{Ca}. (**D**) Representative current traces for EVM as described in panel B.

and pharmacological sensitivity of embryonic compared to mature I_{Ca} is consistent with differential Ca channel α-subunit expression (not shown). The low-voltage activation range suggests functional expression of $Ca_V 1.3$ and/or $Ca_V 3.1$.

2-APB Blocks $Ca_V 1.3 > Ca_V 3.1$ but Has No Effect on $Ca_V 1.2$

Although 2-APB is often used to evaluate SOC-IP_3R Ca^{2+} fluxes,[23] we next tested the straightforward possibility that 2-APB blocked $Ca_V 3.1$ or $Ca_V 1.3$

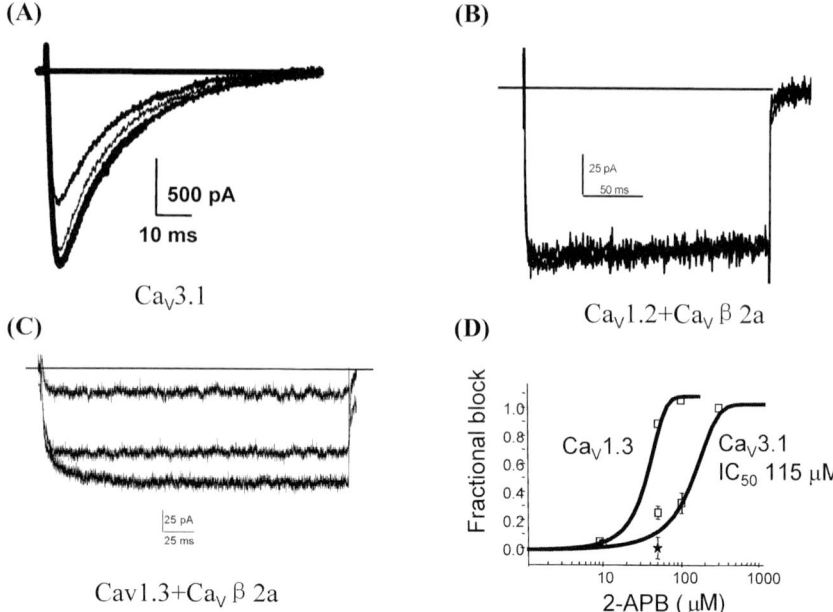

FIGURE 6. $Ca_V1.3$ and $Ca_V3.1$ are sensitive to 2-APB block in the same range as 2-APB block of spontaneous activity. (**A**) $Ca_V3.1$, (**B**) $Ca_V1.2$, or (**C**) $Ca_V1.3$ were heterologously expressed by HEK 293 cells. (A–C) V_{hold} −80 mV, V_{test} 0 mV for control, 50 μM 2-APB, and washout superimposed. (**D**) Dose–response curve. Smooth lines are single-site inhibition curves for $Ca_V3.1$ and $Ca_V1.3$. No curve is shown for $Ca_V1.2$ because no block was observed (solid star).

ionic current. For these experiments, we measured the efficacy of 2-APB blockade of current through Ca channels expressed in HEK 293 cells. 2-APB is an inhibitor of $Ca_V3.1$ (FIG. 6 A) with partial current block at 50 μM and an EC_{50} of 115 μM (FIG. 6 D). 2-APB does not alter current kinetics or voltage dependence of activation or inactivation. Moreover, pulse trains showed no use dependence (data not shown). Thus, 2-APB block is neither voltage nor channel state dependent. Given the unforeseen block of $Ca_V3.1$ by 2-APB, we also tested 2-APB block of $Ca_V1.2$. $Ca_V1.2$ is the predominant mature cardiac Ca current. Thirty micromolar 2-APB has no effect on $Ca_V1.2$, and for 300 μM 2-APB only partial block was observed (FIG. 4 B). $Ca_V1.3$ was potently inhibited by 2-APB with 50 μM causing 80% current block. Taken together, these results are consistent with $Ca_V1.3$ and $Ca_V3.1$, 2-APB-sensitive pathways for Ca^{2+} entry that underlie spontaneous beating in the developing heart.

SUMMARY AND CONCLUSIONS

In this study we focused on the role of multiple PM Ca channel types in the maintenance of spontaneous activity in the developing murine ventricle.

Spontaneous activity distinguishes embryonic from mature ventricular myocytes, and the present work shows that $Ca_V1.3$ and possibly $Ca_V3.1$ are major contributors to PM Ca flux. Although intracellular Ca stores can modulate Ca transient frequency, store Ca may not be required for spontaneous activity in the developing heart. Finally, we now show that 2-APB blocks $Ca_V1.3$ current within the same concentration range of its block of spontaneous activity. This suggests 2-APB is a useful drug to dissect $Ca_V1.2$ versus $Ca_V1.3$ currents in heart cells.

The present study shows that EVM Ca current is sensitive to V_{hold} -80 versus -40 mV. This is sharply contrasted in mature mouse heart where the same V_{hold} range has negligible effects on Ca current properties (FIG. 6). Most previous studies of murine EVM I_{Ca} only consider the current elicited by relatively depolarized V_{hold}.[6,7,24–26] Also, most of these studies used elevated bath Ba concentration; in contrast we used physiological Ca level (2 mM). Nonetheless, in the one study using 2 mM Ba the current density recorded from E18-derived cells was similar to that which we reported.[24] Davies et al.[26] showed no holding potential in the range of -90 to -50 for EVM I_{Ca}. The higher divalent cation concentration used in that study should contribute to a depolarizing shift of the inactivation voltage dependence, thus masking the effect of physiological V_{hold} dependence on Ca current amplitude. Such a divalent cation dependence for voltage gating of $Ca_V1.3$ channels has been elegantly documented.[27] We therefore suggest that given the 2-APB pharmacology and the V_{hold} dependence of current that $Ca_V1.3$ may be a major PM Ca pathway for EVM.

Mouse ES-CMs and native mouse ventricular myocytes tend to have similar functional properties.[28] This contention is based on broad measures and requires more refined testing. For example, it is not established which Ca channel subtypes underlie I_{Ca} in mouse ES-CMs. We cannot access primary human embryonic heart cells, but have initiated physiological studies of human ES-CMs. The major similarity of electrical properties between human and mouse ES-CMs is the absence of Kir (inward rectifier K-current) in relatively early developmental stages. Relatively early refers to species-specific gestational age adjusted. Beyond this simple correlation, there are few commonalities between mouse and human ES-CM excitability. Human ES-CMs contain a different mixture of ion channels[13] and exhibit markedly different Ca handling properties in comparison to mouse counterparts (Izhaki et al., unpublished). Recognition of the uniqueness of human cells should spur additional human ES-CM studies. Though the mouse is an important model, the study of human ES-CMs presents an exciting and unique opportunity to elaborate human physiological heart cell development in living cells.

ACKNOWLEDGMENTS

This work was supported by NIH-HL074091, and JS is an Established Investigator of the AHA.

REFERENCES

1. BERS, D.M. 2001. Excitation–Contraction Coupling and Cardiac Contractile Force, 2nd ed. Kluwer Academic Publishers. Dordrecht.
2. SHOROFSKY, S.R. & C.T. JANUARY. 1992. L-type and T-type Ca^{2+} channels in canine cardiac Purkinje cells—single-channel demonstration of L-type Ca^{2+} window current. Circ. Res. **70:** 456–464.
3. VORNANEN, M., N. SHEPHERD & G. ISENBERG. 1994. Tension-voltage relations of single myocytes reflect Ca release triggered by Na/Ca exchange at 35 degrees C but not 23 degrees C. Am. J. Physiol. **267:** C623–C632.
4. KLITZNER, T.S. & W.F. FRIEDMAN. 1989. A diminished role for the sarcoplasmic reticulum in newborn myocardial contraction: effects of ryanodine. Pediatr. Res. **26:** 98–101.
5. TAKESHIMA, H., S. KOMAZAKI, et al. 1998. Embryonic lethality and abnormal cardiac myocytes in mice lacking ryanodine receptor type 2. EMBO J. **17:** 3309–3316.
6. SEISENBERGER, C., V. SPECHT, et al. 2000. Functional embryonic cardiomyocytes after disruption of the L-type α1C (Cav1.2) calcium channel gene in the mouse. J. Biol. Chem. **275:** 39193–39199.
7. XU, M., A. WELLING, S. PAPARISTO, et al. 2003. Enhanced expression of L-type Cav1.3 calcium channels in murine embryonic hearts from Cav1.2-deficient mice. J. Biol. Chem. **278:** 40837–40841.
8. CRIBBS, L.L., B.L. MARTIN, E.A. SCHRODER, et al. 2001. Identification of the T-type calcium channel (CaV3.1d) in developing mouse heart. Circ. Res. **88:** 403–407.
9. SATIN, J. & L.L. CRIBBS. 2000. Identification of a T-type calcium channel isoform in murine atrial myocytes (AT-1). Circ. Res. **86:** 636–642.
10. SATIN, J. & L.A. BURNS. 2001. Steady-state calcium flux through T-type calcium channels require active Ca-calmodulin kinase. Circulation **104:** II-251.
11. VIATCHENKO-KARPINSKI, S., et al. 1999. Intracellular Ca^{2+} oscillations drive spontaneous contractions in cardiomyocytes during early development. Proc. Natl. Acad. Sci. USA **96:** 8259–8264.
12. KOLOSSOV, E., B.K. FLEISCHMANN, Q. LIU, et al. 1998. Functional characteristics of ES cell-derived cardiac precursor cells identified by tissue-specific expression of the green fluorescent protein. J. Cell Biol. **143:** 2045–2056.
13. SATIN, J., I. KEHAT, O. CASPI, et al. 2004. Mechanism of spontaneous excitability in human embryonic stem cell derived cardiomyocytes. J. Physiol. **559:** 479–496.
14. SAUER, H., T. THEBEN, J. HESCHELER, et al. 2001. Characteristics of calcium sparks in cardiomyocytes derived from embryonic stem cells. Am. J. Physiol. Heart Circ. Physiol. **281:** H411–H421.
15. BONY, C., S. ROCHE, U. SHUICHI, et al. 2001. A specific role of phosphatidylinositol 3-kinase {gamma}: a regulation of autonomic Ca^{2+} oscillations in cardiac cells. J. Cell Biol. **152:** 717–728.
16. LEE, J.-H., J.C. GOMORA, L.L. CRIBBS & E. PEREZ-REYES. 1999. Nickel block of three cloned T-type calcium channels: low concentrations selectively block α1H. Biophys. J. **77:** 3034–3042.
17. ZAMPONI, G.W., E. BOURINET & T.P. SNUTCH. 1996. Nickel block of a family of neuronal calcium channels: subtype and subunit-dependent action at multiple sites. J. Membr. Biol. **151:** 77–90.

18. GYSEMBERGH, A., S. LEMAIRE, et al. 1999. Pharmacological manipulation of Ins(1,4,5)P3 signaling mimics preconditioning in rabbit heart. Am. J. Physiol. Heart Circ. Physiol. **277:** H2458–H2469.
19. MACKENZIE, L., M.D. BOOTMAN, et al. 2002. The role of inositol 1,4,5-trisphosphate receptors in Ca^{2+} signalling and the generation of arrhythmias in rat atrial myocytes. J. Physiol. (Lond.) **541:** 395–409.
20. PEPPIATT, C.M., T.J. COLLINS, et al. 2003. 2-Aminoethoxydiphenyl borate (2-APB) antagonises inositol 1,4,5-trisphosphate-induced calcium release, inhibits calcium pumps and has a use-dependent and slowly reversible action on store-operated calcium entry channels. Cell Calcium **34:** 97–108.
21. MISSIAEN, L., G. CALLEWAERT, H. DE SMEDT & J.B. PARYS. 2001. 2-Aminoethoxydiphenyl borate affects the inositol 1,4,5-trisphosphate receptor, the intracellular Ca^{2+} pump and the non-specific Ca^{2+} leak from the non-mitochondrial Ca^{2+} stores in permeabilized A7r5 cells. Cell Calcium **29:** 111–116.
22. MARUYAMA, T., T. KANAJI, S. NAKADE, et al. 1997. 2-Aminoethoxydiphenyl borate, a membrane-penetrable modulator of Ins(1,4,5)P3-induced Ca^{2+} release. J. Biochem. (Tokyo) **122:** 498–505.
23. BOOTMAN, M.D., T.J. COLLINS, et al. 2002. 2-Aminoethoxydiphenyl borate (2-APB) is a reliable blocker of store-operated Ca^{2+} entry but an inconsistent inhibitor of InsP3-induced Ca^{2+} release. FASEB J. **16:** 1145–1150.
24. LIU, W., K. YASUI, T. OPTHOF, et al. 2002. Developmental changes of Ca^{2+} handling in mouse ventricular cells from early embryo to adulthood. Life Sci. **71:** 1279–1292.
25. AN, R.H., M.P. DAVIES, et al. 1996. Developmental changes in beta-adrenergic modulation of L-type Ca^{2+} channels in embryonic mouse heart. Circ. Res. **78:** 371–378.
26. DAVIES, M.P., R.H. AN, et al. 1996. Developmental changes in ionic channel activity in the embryonic murine heart. Circ. Res. **78:** 15–25.
27. XU, W. & D. LIPSCOMBE. 2001. Neuronal $Ca_V1.3$ L-type channels activate at relatively hyperpolarized membrane potentials and are incompletely inhibited by dihydropyridines. J. Neurosci. **21:** 5944–5951.
28. FIJNVANDRAAT, A.C., A.C. VAN GINNEKEN, et al. 2003. Cardiomyocytes derived from embryonic stem cells resemble cardiomyocytes of the embryonic heart tube. Cardiovasc. Res. **58:** 399–409.

Dynamic Interactions between Myocytes, Fibroblasts, and Extracellular Matrix

INDRONEAL BANERJEE, KRISHNA YEKKALA, THOMAS K. BORG, AND TROY A. BAUDINO

Department of Cell and Developmental Biology and Anatomy, University of South Carolina, School of Medicine, Columbia, South Carolina 29208 USA

ABSTRACT: Cardiac function is determined by the coordinated and dynamic interaction of several cell types together with components of the extracellular matrix (ECM). This interaction is regulated by mechanical, chemical, and electrical signals between the cellular and noncellular components of the heart. Recent studies using fluorescence-activated cell sorting indicate that the number of myocytes remains relatively constant during development and disease, whereas the number of fibroblasts and other cell types can change dramatically. Cardiac fibroblasts appear to have different origins at different stages of development and fluctuate in response to a variety of physiological signals. Fibroblasts form a network of cells that are connected to each other via specific cadherins and connexins, to the ECM via integrins, and to myocytes by a variety of receptors, including connexins. Examples of the integration of signals include the role of angiotensin II (Ang II), which stimulates mechanical contraction of fibroblasts, as well as cytokine signaling. Cytokine signaling alters connexin and K^+ channel activation, which in turn is regulated by Ang II, essentially forming a feedback loop. Quantitative changes in mechanical, chemical, and electrical signals that can alter the overall cardiac form and function will be discussed here.

KEYWORDS: myocytes; fibroblasts; extracellular matrix; connexins; cadherins

INTRODUCTION

The function of any organ is dependent upon the interaction of all the cellular components that comprise the particular tissue. These interactions result in a dynamic interplay of mechanical, electrical, and chemical signals as well as a communication between inter- and intracellular signals. In the heart, the cellular components primarily consist of myocytes, fibroblasts, and the vascular system. In addition, transient cells, such as mast cells, macrophages, and

Address for correspondence: Thomas K. Borg, Cell and Developmental Biology and Anatomy, University of South Carolina, School of Medicine, Columbia, SC 29208. Voice: 803-733-1562; fax: 803-733-3115.
e-mail: borg@med.sc.edu

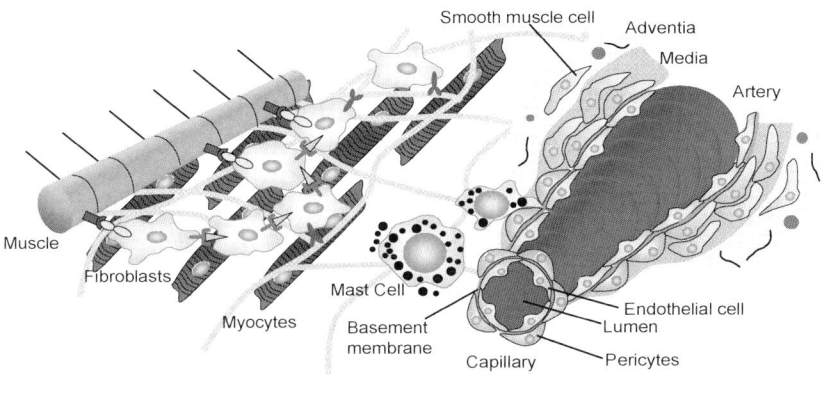

FIGURE 1. Model of interactions between cells and extracellular matrix in the heart.

lymphocytes, can be found under certain conditions, such as in response to pathophysiological stimuli (FIG. 1).[1]

Most evaluations on the number and type of cells in the heart have been by arbitrary methods to produce qualitative descriptions under a variety of conditions.[2] Initial investigations by earlier investigators simply separated cells into two populations: myocyte or myosin positive cells and nonmyocyte (myosin negative) populations. These initial studies determined that the ratio of fibroblasts to myocytes was approximately 70:30.[3] As has been pointed out in numerous studies, myocytes make up the largest volume of the heart, but little quantitative information has been done on both myocytes and other cell types.

Analysis by flow-assisted cell sorting (FACS) has revealed that the number and type of cells in the heart vary greatly depending on the developmental stage, as well as with potential pathophysiological conditions (FIG. 2 A, B). While the number of myocytes appears to be fairly constant, the other cell types vary with the physiological condition of the heart. Clearly the numbers of fibroblasts are variable, as are smooth muscle cells. These data indicate that cell sorting can be used to determine both cell number and type during various physiological conditions. FACS can also be used to determine the rate of cellular proliferation and apoptosis of individual populations (data not shown).

Distribution of Fibroblasts in the Heart

Few studies have attempted to document differences in fibroblast distribution in the heart, yet thorough examination of the data shows that fibroblasts are not

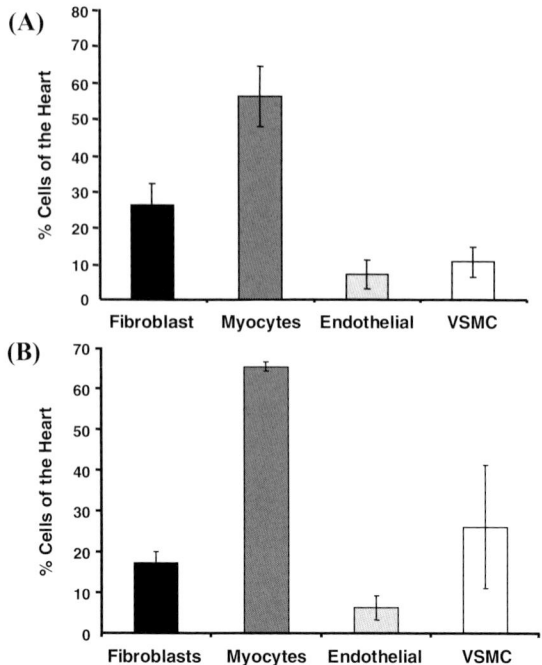

FIGURE 2. Cellular populations of the heart. Percentages of fibroblasts, myocytes, endothelial cells (EC), or vascular smooth muscle cells (VSMC) in the adult murine heart (**A**) or in an E18.5 murine heart as determined by FACS analyses.

distributed equally throughout the heart.[4,5] For example, studies by Kohl and colleagues have examined fibroblasts in the sino-atrial node, where fibroblasts outnumber the myocytes.[4,5] Other investigations have demonstrated that the number of fibroblasts appear to vary with physiological condition.[6,7] In hypertrophy, an abundance of fibroblasts are apparent in the ventricular free wall; however, comparative studies documenting the number of fibroblasts in other areas, such as the septum or right ventricle are lacking. Moreover, the number of fibroblasts appears to dramatically increase in relation to remodeling and repair of different regions of the heart. For example, in myocardial infarctions, abundant fibroblasts can be found within and surrounding the scar.[8] Yet the physiological function of the fibroblasts as a function of number is still poorly understood.

FIBROBLAST–MYOCYTE–ECM INTERACTION

Histological examination of the heart shows that myocytes are arranged in laminae, 2–5 layers in thickness.[9,10] These laminae are surrounded by a weave network of endomysial collagen. Recent studies have demonstrated that fibroblasts lie within this endomysial network.[6,7] The fibroblasts in the endomysial collagen display three types of connections: (*a*) fibroblast–fibroblast contacts via long filapodia; (*b*) cell–extracellular matrix (ECM) interactions, principally with surrounding collagen, and (*c*) fibroblast–myocyte interactions.[1,11]

Fibroblast–fibroblast connections are presumed to be regulated by a variety of molecules including connexins and cadherins, as well as unknown proteins.[12,13] Connexins have primarily been studied in myocytes and display varied distribution.[6,14] In most cases, their function(s) appear to be related arrhythmias and other electrical events. Furthermore, recent studies have shown that connexin43 (Cx43) may be regulated via heparin binding-epidermal growth factor (EGF).[15] These findings, which were performed in myocytes, demonstrate that signals within the microenvironment can be critical in regulating cellular hypertrophy. Extending these studies to include cardiac fibroblasts and myocytes will likely show that they also play an essential role in the three-dimensional signaling. Understanding the dynamic signaling by the various connexins in both fibroblasts and myocytes will be essential in understanding basic processes, such as ECM turnover, growth regulation, and remodeling in response to physiological signals.

Cadherins are also present in the heart on both fibroblasts and myocytes. Principally, N-cadherin is expressed by cardiac myocytes but also appears to be present in cell–cell contacts between fibroblasts.[16] Cadherin-11 or OB-cadherin is a specific marker of fibroblasts whose function is not well understood.[17] In other mesenchymal cells, cadherin-11 expression is closely linked to the expression of vascular endothelial growth factor-D (VEGF-D) and preliminary studies with cardiac fibroblasts indicate that the same relationship is also true in the heart (FIG. 3).[18] This association of cadherin-11 and VEGF-D may be important for the angiogenic process.

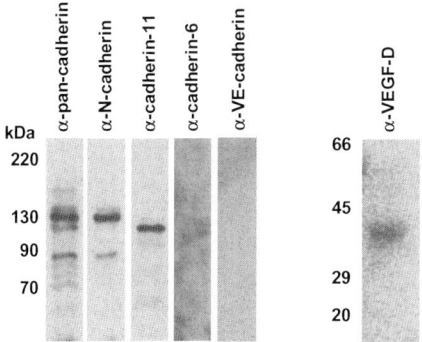

FIGURE 3. Cadherin and VEGF-D expression in cardiac fibroblasts. Western blot analyses of cardiac fibroblasts showing expression of N-cadherin, cadherin-11, cadherin-6, VE-cadherin, and VEGF-D.

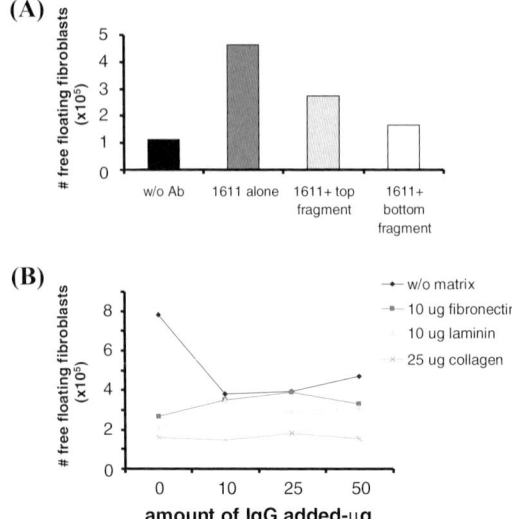

FIGURE 4. Inhibition of fibroblast–myocyte interactions. (**A**) Fibroblast–myocyte interactions were blocked through the addition of 50 g of antibody 1611 (antibody against the entire fibroblast membrane fraction), antibody against the upper (100 kDa and above) or lower (100 kDa and below) membrane fractions. As a control we used IgG or pre-immune serum. (**B**) Effect of antibody 1611 on fibroblast–ECM interactions. Fibroblast–ECM interactions were unaffected by addition of antibody 1611.

Recent studies in our laboratory show that antibodies made against the detergent soluble membrane fraction of cardiac fibroblasts have the ability to block myocyte–fibroblast interactions (FIG. 4 A). In these assays, neonatal myocytes were allowed to establish a rod-like phenotype on aligned collagen and fibroblasts were subsequently added to these cells. In this adhesion assay, the antibodies were not effective in blocking fibroblast–ECM interactions (FIG. 4 B), but did block fibroblast–myocyte interactions (FIG. 4 A).

In addition to the cell adhesion studies to determine fibroblast–myocyte interaction, cell aggregation assays can also be used to quantitatively examine the cellular interactions. These assays have been used as models of heart differentiation and tissue interaction.[19,20] Using an aggregation assay, fibroblasts were placed in rotational culture alone or with neonatal myocytes. Over a 24-h period, specific cell–cell interactions produced large cellular aggregates. Antibodies against the fibroblast membrane fraction dramatically reduced the size of the aggregates by apparently blocking cell–cell interactions (FIG. 5). From these two different assays, it is apparent that the antibodies against the fibroblast membrane proteins block cell–cell adhesion, but the nature of these proteins are not yet known. Clearly low molecular weight dyes can pass between fibroblasts and myocyte, but the physiological nature of these signals is not known.

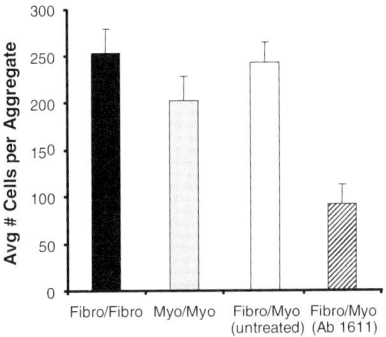

FIGURE 5. Aggregate cultures of cardiac fibroblasts and myocytes. Cardiac fibroblasts or myocytes were incubated alone (6×10^6 cells/10 mL) or together in the presence or absence of antibody in BSA-coated 50 mL Erlenmeyer flasks ON with shaking at 37° individual aggregates were isolated, disrupted, and cells were counted using a Nikon T$100 inverted microscope (Melville, NY). Results are presented as the average number of cells/aggregate ± SD from five individual aggregates in each culture.

What Are the Fibroblasts Telling the Myocytes?

The fact that fibroblasts are in direct contact with each other and with myocytes, does not imply that physiological signals are being sent or received between them. Previous *in vitro* studies with fibroblasts in collagen gels have demonstrated that the fibroblasts, which are in contact with each other, contract the collagen via mechanical force.[21] Inhibition of fibroblast interactions can block the contraction, as can a wide variety of reagents including connexins, cadherins, integrins, and matrix metalloproteinases (MMPs).[22] The arrangement of fibroblasts *in vivo*, with the fibroblasts in contact with each other in the endomyosial collagen, is analogous to their behavior observed in collagen gels.[11] However, the exact nature of these cellular signals is not currently known.

To determine if cell–cell interactions between fibroblasts or fibroblasts and myocytes actually potentiate signals between each other, cells were loaded with fluorescent dyes that could be transferred across the membrane.[20] In studies using fibroblasts associated with myocytes on aligned collagen gels, the low molecular weight component CMFDA was transferred from the fibroblast to the myocyte, whereas large molecular weight components, such as fluorescent dextran, did not pass across the cell membrane (data not shown). The same pattern of dye transfer was also observed (data not shown) in cell aggregate studies.

The aggregation and adhesion studies demonstrate that low molecular weight material can be passed across the cell membrane (via gap junctions?) but these experiments do not give information about autocrine and/or paracrine

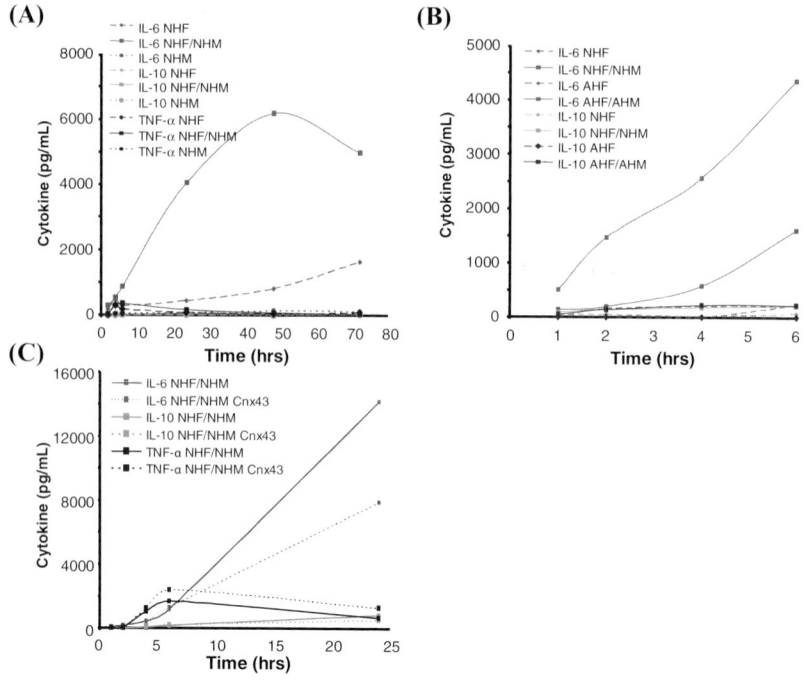

FIGURE 6. BioPlex measurements of various cytokines in cardiac cells. (**A**) Expression of IL-6, IL-10, and TNF-α in neonatal heart fibroblasts (NHF), neonatal heart myocytes (NHM), or NHFs and NHMs in co-culture. (**B**) Expression of IL-6 and IL-10 in adult heart fibroblasts (AHF), adult heart myocytes (AHM), or AHFs and AHMs in co-culture. (**C**) Effect of blocking Cx43 on cytokine expression in neonatal fibroblasts and myocytes.

signaling. Short range signals are likely to be components, such as cytokines and growth factors.[23,24] Using a BioRad Bioplex assay, the expression of interleukin-1 (IL-1), IL-6, IL-10, and tumor necrosis factor-α (TNF-α) were analyzed under a variety of experimental conditions. Interactions between myocytes and fibroblasts resulted in changes of expression of IL-6 and IL-10 (FIG. 6 A). We have also obtained similar results to those measured by extraction of adult hearts (FIG. 6 B). Interestingly, the addition of antibodies against Cx43 and/or fibroblast membranes caused a significant reduction in the expression of the various cytokines (FIG. 6 C and data not shown). These data suggest that direct cell–cell interactions are required for proper gene expression and proper cardiac function *in vivo*.

Electrophysiological Implications

Previous studies examining fibroblast–myocyte interactions have indicated that there are potentially important changes in ion channels that result in electrophysiological patterns.[25] Indeed, addition of adult myocytes to cardiac fibroblasts results in an activation of fibroblast-specific K^+ channels.[25] Moreover, various reports have demonstrated that the addition of growth factors and/or hormones can also affect the expression of these ion channels.[26] This regulation of various ion channels can affect a variety of cellular functions and it is important to understand how these various physiological signals are integrated at the molecular, cellular, and organ level.

SUMMARY

The organization of fibroblasts in the heart indicates that, in addition to the production of ECM components, these cells are critical in a variety of physiological functions. Fibroblasts can respond to a variety of mechanical, electrical, and chemical signals that are critical in the dynamics of proper cardiac function. Understanding the integration of these chemical, electrical, and mechanical signals under different physiological conditions is essential to understanding normal heart development as well as its response to disease.

ACKNOWLEDGMENTS

The research was supported in part by funds from NIH P20RR 1643401 (COBRE), HL-68038, and P20RR 16461 (INBRE).

REFERENCES

1. BAUDINO, T.A., W. CARVER, W. GILLES & T.K. BORG. 2005. Cardiac fibroblasts: friend or Foe? Am. J. Physiol. Epub ahead of print.
2. BUGAISKY, L., R. ZAK. 1979. Cellular growth of cardiac muscle after birth. Tex. Rep. Biol. Med. **39:** 123–138.
3. NAG, A. 1980. Study of non-muscle cells of the adult mammalian heart. A fine structural analysis & distribution. Cytobios **28:** 41–61.
4. CAMELLITI, P., C.R. GREEN, I. LEGRICE & P. KOHL. 2004. Fibroblast network in rabbit sino-atrial node: structural and functional identification of homo-and heterologous cell coupling. Circ. Res. **94:** 828–835.
5. KOHL, P. 2004. Cardiac cellular heterogeneity and remodelling. Cardiovasc. Res. **64:** 195–197.
6. GOLDSMITH, E.C., HOFFMAN, et al. 2004. Organization of fibroblasts in the heart. Dev. Dyn. **230:** 787–794.
7. MORALES, M.O., R.L. PRICE & E.C. GOLDSMITH. 2005. Expression of discoidin domain receptor 2 (DDR2) in the developing heart. Microsc. Microanal. **11:** 260–267.
8. HOLMES, J.W., T.K. BORG & J.W. COVELL. 2005. Structure and mechanics of healing myocardial infarcts. Annu. Rev. Biomed. Eng. **7:** 223–253.

9. YOUNG, A.A., I.J. LEGRICE, M.A. YOUNG & B.H. SMAILL. 1998. Extended confocal microscopy of myocardial laminae and collagen network. J. Microsc. **192:** 139–150.
10. BORG, T.K. & J.B. CAULFIELD. 1981. The collagen matrix of the heart. Fed. Proc. **40:** 2037–2041.
11. CAMELLITI, P., T.K. BORG & P. KOHL. 2005. Structural and functional characterization of cardiac fibroblasts. Cardiovasc. Res. **65:** 40–51.
12. LAIRD, D.W. 2006. Life cycle of connexins in health and disease. Biochem. J. **394:** 527–543
13. GUMBINER, B.M. 2005. Regulation of cadherin-mediated adhesion in morphogenesis. Nat. Rev. Mol. Cell. Biol. **6:** 622–634
14. CAMELLITI, P., G.P. DEVLIN, et al. 2004. Spatially and temporally distinct expression of fibroblast connexins after sheep ventricular infarction. Cardiovasc. Res. **62:** 415–425,
15. OSHIOKA, J., R.N. PRINCE, et al. 2005. Cardiomyocyte hypertrophy and degradation of connexin 43 through spatially restricted autocrine/paracrine heparin-binding EGF. PNAS **102:** 10622–10627.
16. LI, J., V.V. PATEL, I. KOSTETSKII, et al. 2005. Cardiac-specific loss of N-cadherin leads to alteration in connexins with conduction slowing and arrhythmogenesis. Circ. Res. **97:** 474–481.
17. VALENCIA, X., J.M. HIGGINS, et al. 2004. Cadherin-11 provides specific cellular adhesion between fibroblast-like synoviocytes. J. Exp. Med. **200:** 1673–1679.
18. ORLANDINI, M. & S. OLIVIERO. 2001. In fibroblasts VEGF-D expression is induced by cell-cell contact mediated by cadherin-11. J. Biol. Chem. **276:** 6576–6581.
19. KELM, J.M. & M. FUSSENEGGER. 2004. Microscale tissue engineering using gravity-enforced cell assembly. Trends Biotech. **22:** 195–202.
20. KELM, J.M., E. EHLER, L.K. NIELSEN, et al 2004. Design of artificial myocardial microtissues. Tissue Eng. **10:** 201–214.
21. GRINNELL, F. 2003. Fibroblast biology in three-dimensional collagen matrices. Trends Cell. Biol. **13:** 264–269.
22. GRINNELL, F., L.B. ROCHA, et al. 2006. Nested collagen matrices: a new model to study migration of human fibroblast populations in three dimensions. Exp. Cell. Res. **312:** 86–94.
23. PRABHU, S. 2004. Cytokine-induced modulation of cardiac function. Circ. Res. **95:** 1140–1153
24. TOMANEK, R.J., W. ZHENG & X. YUE. 2004. Growth factor activation in myocardial vascularization: therapeutic implications. Mol. Cell. Biochem. **264:** 3–11.
25. SHIBUKAWA, Y., E.L. CHILTON, K.A. MACCANNELL, et al. 2005. K+ currents activated by depolarization in cardiac fibroblasts. Biophys. J. **88:** 3924–3935.
26. DELPON, E., R. CABALLERO, R. GOMEZ, et al. 2005. Angiotensin II, angiotensin II antagonists and spironolactone and their modulation of cardiac repolarization. Trends Pharmacol. Sci. **26:** 155–161.

Embryonic Heart Induction

ANN C. FOLEY, RUCHIKA W. GUPTA, ROSA M. GUZZO,
OKSANA KOROL, AND MARK MERCOLA

Burnham Institute for Medical Research, La Jolla, California 92037, USA

ABSTRACT: We have characterized two signaling pathways that induce heart tissue during embryonic development. The first is initiated by the Wnt antagonist Dickkopf1 (Dkk1) and involves the homeodomain transcription factor Hex. Other Wnt antagonists are less effective and the potency of Dkk1 might be due to synergy between Wnt antagonizing and another, novel activity emanating from its amino terminal cysteine-rich domain. The second signal is initiated by Nodal and its co-receptor Cripto. Importantly, both the Dkk1/Wnt antagonism and Nodal pathways act on the endoderm that underlies the future heart to control secretion of diffusible factors that induce cardiogenesis in adjacent mesoderm. In this article, we summarize data that Dkk1 induces cardiogenic differentiation cell non-autonomously through the action of the homeodomain transcription factor Hex. We also discuss recent data showing that Nodal also acts indirectly through stimulation of the secreted protein Cerberus, which is a member of the differential-screening selected aberrant in neuroblastoma (DAN) family of secreted proteins. Finally, we present the model that signaling from Dkk1 regulates novel activities, in addition to Wnt antagonism, which are essential for progression beyond initiation of cardiogenesis to control later stages of cardiomyocyte differentiation and myocardial tissue organization.

KEYWORDS: cardiogenesis; heart; *Xenopus*; Wnt; Dickkopf1; Nodal

INTRODUCTION

Classical experiments beginning in the 1920s using amphibians, chicks, and later mice, mapped the regions of the mesoderm that give rise to the heart. Prospective heart-forming regions, when removed from the embryo prior to specification and placed in culture, do not form heart tissue unless grafted to other tissues that provide the necessary inductive stimuli. Such recombination assays using amphibian heart primordia eventually led to the identification of dorsal midline mesoderm that gives rise to the notochord and head mesoderm,[1,2] and anterior endoderm[2-4] as potent sources of heart-inducing substances (FIG. 1). Amphibian dorsal midline mesoderm is known as

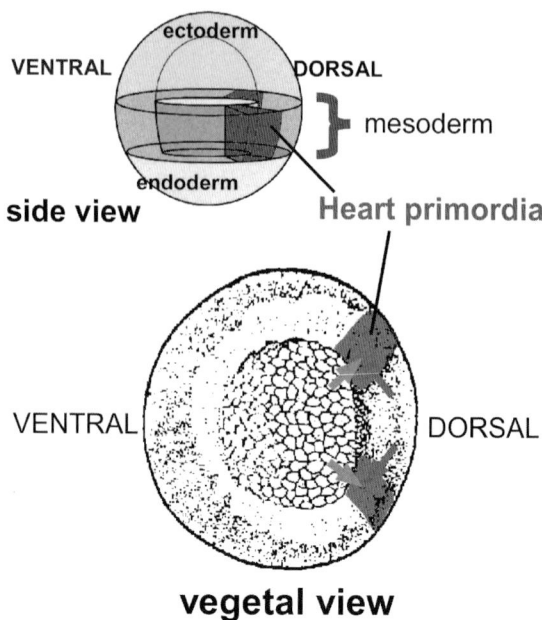

FIGURE 1. Heart-inducing tissues in *Xenopus*. Heart mesoderm is induced at the onset of gastrulation by signals from the deep endoderm and Speman's Organizer (dorsal midline mesoderm).[31]

Spemann's Organizer and shares the ability to induce an ectopic body axis with Hensen's node in the chick, the node in mouse, and the shield in zebrafish. In chicks, extraembryonic cells of the anterior hypoblast[5] and anterior definitive endoderm[6,7] both induce heart. Initiating signals in mice originate from the anterior visceral and definitive endoderm,[8] which is extraembryonic and has signaling properties in common with both the hypoblast in chicks and the deep endoderm in *Xenopus*.

Proteins that are essential for heart induction have been reviewed[9,10] and include Wnt antagonists, the transforming growth factor-β (TGF-β) family member Nodal, and bone morphogenetic proteins (BMPs). Dickkopf1 (Dkk1) and Crescent block signaling from secreted Wnt proteins and induce hearts in non-heart mesoderm.[11,12] Wnt antagonists must inhibit canonical Wnt->β-catenin signaling in order to induce heart. Dkk1 is particularly potent whereas Crescent is a weak inducer of ectopic hearts in the *Xenopus* assay, while other Wnt antagonists do not induce cardiomyocytes. The reason for varying potency is not clear but might reflect affinity for particular Wnts and possibly novel activities of Dkk1.

In addition to inhibition of the canonical Wnt/β-catenin signal transduction pathway, cardiogenesis is enhanced by activation of non-canonical Wnt signaling. The first of these activates Jun-N-terminal kinase (JNK) and the small GTPase RhoA, whereas the second involves intracellular calcium release and activation of phospholipase C (PLC) and protein kinase C (PKC).[13,14] In mESCs, cardiomyogenesis depends on the upregulation of PKC isoforms ζ and ϵ.[15] The intracellular protein dishevelled modulates both canonical and non-canonical pathways and Strabismus, Naked Cuticle, together with PKC and Calmodulin kinase II (also a target of the Wnt/Ca^{++} pathway), inhibit canonical β-catenin signaling[16–19]; thus, teasing apart the relative influences of activation of non-canonical signaling from inhibition of canonical signaling on cardiogenesis has not been completely resolved.

Additionally, the TGF-β-family member Nodal and its essential, membrane-bound co-receptor Cripto are important in heart induction in embryos and in embryonic stem cells (ESCs). Cripto$^{-/-}$ mESCs form mesoderm but do not undergo cardiogenesis.[20] Cripto$^{-/-}$ embryos also form mesoderm, but lack anteroposterior axial development and do not form cardiomyocytes.[21,22] Comparison of the phenotypes of Cripto$^{-/-}$ and Nodal$^{-/-}$ embryos indicates that Cripto is essential for Nodal to signal in both the epiblast and the anterior visceral endoderm (AVE) that overlies the epiblast. Considerable evidence shows that the AVE is essential for induction of the heart[8] and other anterior structures;[23] thus, Nodal is likely to be involved in heart induction.

BMPs also promote cardiogenesis in embryos, and synergize with fibroblast growth factor (FGF) isoforms to extend the cardiogenic region posteriorly.[24–26] Embryological studies in *Xenopus* suggest BMPs function after Wnt antagonism or Nodal and are required to sustain cardiogenesis from the Nkx2.5 positive state.[27] BMPs also stimulate ESC cardiogenesis,[28,29] and are required for cardiomyocyte differentiation of Sca1$^+$ cells obtained from the adult heart.[30]

WNT ANTAGONISM CAN INITIATE CARDIOGENESIS

Our earlier studies showed that whereas both the dorsal midline mesoderm (Spemann's Organizer, which forms head mesoderm and notochord) are required together to induce heart tissue, neither alone can function in this capacity[31,32] (FIG. 1). Two Wnt antagonists secreted by dorsal midline mesoderm, Dkk1 and Crescent, are sufficient to induce ectopic hearts and ectopic Wnt was found to block normal heart formation in both *Xenopus*[11] and chick[12] embryonic tissues.

We pursued the mechanism of induction by asking if Wnt antagonism is required in the cells that form heart tissue or if it operates on nearby cells to control production of a diffusible inducer.[33] We performed a mosaic analysis in which the cell-autonomous Wnt/β-catenin pathway antagonists dnTCF3 and GSK3β were each coinjected with a Texas Red-lysinated dextran (10,000MW) as a lineage label to track the progeny of the injected cells (FIG. 2 A). The injections were targeted to the non-cardiogenic mesendoderm of the ventroposterior marginal zone (VMZ). Cardiac markers were induced at a distance from the

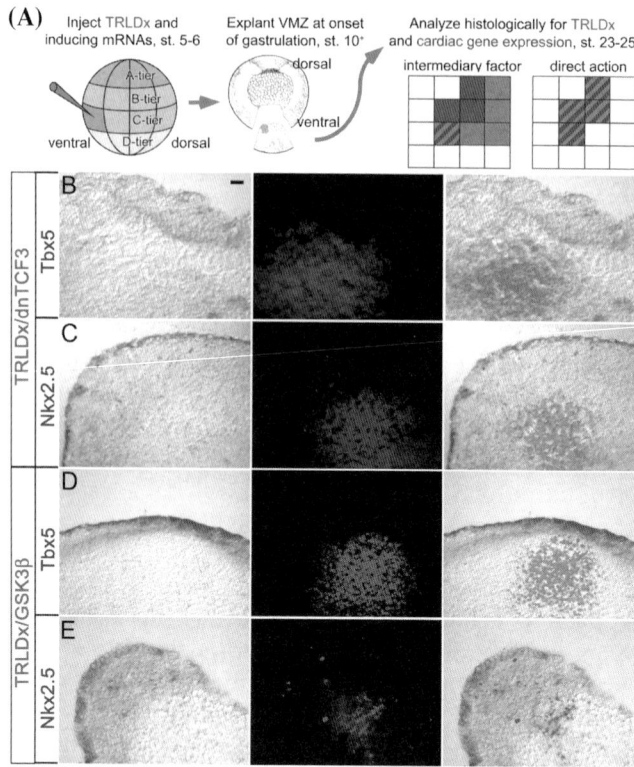

FIGURE 2. Wnt antagonism induces cardiogenesis cell non-autonomously. (**A**) Single cells in the non-cardiac VMZ mesendoderm were injected to express either dnTCF3 or GSK3β, and these regions were then explanted, cultured, and evaluated at later stages for expression of Tbx5 or Nkx2.5. (**B-E**) Cardiac mRNAs (colorimetric *in situ* hybridization signal) induced at a distance from the progeny of the injected cells (tracked by presence of the fluorescent Texas Red-lysinated dextran, TRLDx). Left panels, *in situ* hybridization signal; middle, fluorescent lineage label; right, merge. This figure is reproduced from the original color version[33] with permission.

progeny of the injected cells, revealing that inhibition of canonical Wnt/β-catenin signaling controls production of a diffusible heart-inducing factor (FIG. 2 B–E). Targeting the injections to deliver mRNA to endoderm was necessary for efficacious induction of heart markers. Cardiac tissue was induced more superficially as would be expected for mesoderm.

This microinjection assay for ectopic heart induction was used to screen cRNAs to identify novel heart-inducing molecules, some of which we hoped would act downstream of Wnt antagonism. One active cRNA encoded the divergent homeodomain protein Hex (FIG. 3), which was previously implicated in hematopoietic development. Key evidence that Hex acts downstream of

(A) *Hex mRNA is expressed by anterior endoderm*

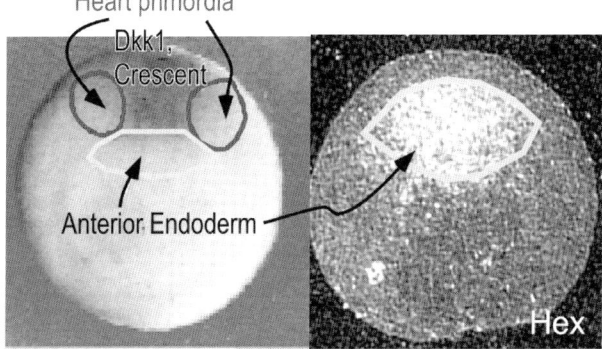

(B) *Hex induces Nkx2.5 and Tbx5 non-cell autonomously*

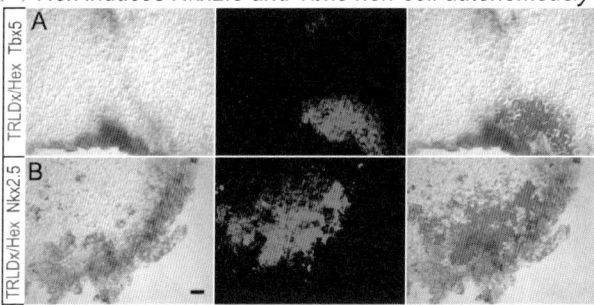

FIGURE 3. Involvement of the homeodomain transcriptional repressor Hex in heart induction. (**A**) Hex is expressed in endoderm adjacent to heart primordial and Dkk1 (and Crescent) expression in organizer (ventral views of st. 10 embryos; left, Dkk1 colorimetric *in situ* hybridization, Crescent has same pattern; right, Hex^{35}S *in situ* hybridization, viewed by darkfield illumination). (**B**) Injection of Hex mRNA induces ectopic cardiac markers in adjacent tissue. Experiment in panel B is of same design as in FIGURE 2A. (Panel B. reprinted from the color original[33] with permission from Cold Spring Harbor Laboratory Press.)

Dkk1 to regulate a heart-inducing factor includes:[33] (*a*) Hex mRNA is normally present in dorsoanterior endoderm (FIG. 3 A), (*b*) Dkk1 induces Hex mRNA, (*c*) Hex morpholinos block heart induction by Dkk1, (*d*) a constitutively active HexVP16 fusion protein also blocks, indicating that it is the transcriptional repressing function of Hex that is essential for heart induction, and, most importantly, (*e*) Hex injection also initiates ectopic heart formation (FIG. 3 B). Because it is the repressive function of Hex that is important, Hex might either (*a*) suppress a repressor of a diffusible heart-inducer or (*b*) repress a diffusible heart-suppressor. Thus it appears that Dkk-1 promotes cardiomyogenesis indirectly by inducing Hex expression in the underlying endoderm.

Bogue et al.[34] used homologous recombination to create transgenic mice that lack Hex. These mice develop a number of congenital cardiac abnormalities, including hypolasia of the right ventricle, ventricular septal defects, outflow tract anomalies, atrioventricular valve dysplasia, and aberrant development of the myocardial compact layer. We do not yet know the extent to which these defects arise from early errors in cardiogenesis, as discussed above, or are consequences of the systemic loss of Hex in these embryos that is known to cause vascular problems, which could affect heart development secondarily. Nonetheless, the involvement of Hex is an important finding that offers a means of identifying downstream proteins that directly initiate cardiogenesis in competent mesoderm.

CERBERUS MEDIATES INDUCTIVE SIGNALING FROM NODAL

Signaling from the TGF-β family member Nodal was also found to induce cardiac differentiation in the ectopic heart-induction assay. Although cardiogenesis in response to Nodal and its Cripto co-receptor has been known from previous work in ESCs (see above), the mechanism of action and the identity of downstream factors have never been investigated. Using the mosaic assay, our recent data, to be published elsewhere, revealed that heart tissue was induced at a distance from the cells in which Nodal signaling was activated, indicating that a diffusible molecule functions downstream of Nodal. The same result was obtained either by coinjection of Nodal (XNr-1) and Cripto or by injection of caAlk4 mRNAs.

Since we had found the spatiotemporal domain of Cerberus mRNA to correspond precisely to the region of endoderm needed for cardiogenesis[34] and Nodal/Cripto or Alk4 injection-induced Cerberus directly (not shown; see Refs. 35 and 36), we went on to position Cerberus as an essential component of the Nodal/Cripto pathway for heart induction. Like other DAN proteins, *Xenopus* Cerberus is a BMP antagonist; however, it also inhibits Wnt and Nodal activities.[36,37] Prior studies had shown that *Xenopus* Cerberus or mouse Cerberus-like is capable of inducing early cardiac markers in animal cap ectoderm.[37-40] When misexpressed in non-cardiogenic *Xenopus* mesendoderm, we found that non-cardiogenic Cerberus induced Nkx2.5 and Tbx5. To determine if it is involved in native or ectopic heart induction, we then injected specific antisense morpholino oligonucleotides to attenuate Cerberus expression. Analyses of histological sections, to be published elsewhere, revealed that specific morpholino knockdown blocked heart induction in response to Nodal signaling. Since Cerberus was also induced by Nodal/Cripto or caAlk4 injection, we conclude that Cerberus functions downstream of Nodal.

Importantly, Cerberus morpholinos did not block heart induction by Dkk1 and Nodal/Cripto signaling does not induce Hex; thus, the Dkk1 and Nodal

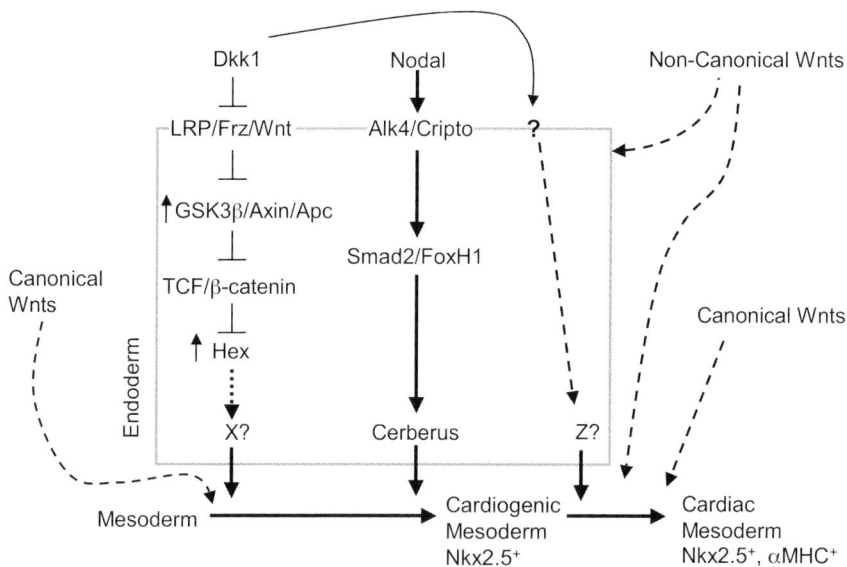

FIGURE 4. Nodal and Dkk1 signal transduction pathways in dorsoanterior endoderm. Our mosaic analyses (as in FIG. 2) indicate that the Dkk1 and Nodal/Cripto/Alk4 pathways function within endoderm. Based on morpholino knockdown data,[33] the suppressive function of Hex is required for cardiogenesis and is illustrated here as indirectly regulating an inducer (labeled X?). Hex is not induced by Nodal (not shown). Conversely, specific morpholino knockdown of Cerberus implicate it in Nodal, but not the Dkk1 pathway; thus, the cardiogenic function of these two pathways appears to be distinct at the levels of Hex and Cerberus. Non-canonical Wnt signal transduction promotes cardiogenesis,[14] but whether this pathway acts via endoderm or directly on cardiogenic mesoderm has not been resolved. Last, canonical Wnt signal transduction is likely to be important for cardiomyogenesis based on experiments using P19 embryonal carcinoma cells[42] and murine ESCs (Michael Schneider, Baylor, *personal communication*). Whether it is involved in differentiation of Nkx2.5$^+$ cardiac mesoderm and/or for production of competent mesoderm is under investigation, as is the question of whether it acts directly on cardiogenic mesoderm.

pathways appear distinct at least at the level of Cerberus and Hex (diagrammed in FIG. 4). The existence of parallel pathways indicates a potential redundancy that might complicate interpretation of knockout phenotypes, such as Hex$^{-/-}$ embryos discussed above, by providing a means for cardiac development to continue even following attenuation of one pathway.

Our studies support the model that heart induction in mesoderm is initiated by signals from foregut endoderm. Production of endodermally derived heart-inducing factors is controlled by Dkk1 and other antagonists of canonical Wnt/β-catenin signaling, at least in part through regulation by the homeodomain transcriptional repressor Hex (FIG. 4). Similarly, signaling from Nodal and its co-receptor Cripto functions within the endoderm to control production of Cerberus, which in turn induces cardiogenesis in mesoderm.

DKK1 MIGHT HARBOR A NOVEL INDUCTIVE ACTIVITY

Understanding the signaling pathways that control myocardial organization after initial induction is a fascinating problem that has not been explored at the molecular genetic level. An intriguing finding from our heart induction studies was that Dkk1 is remarkably efficient at inducing intact, rhythmically beating myocardial tubes (Ref. 11 60% of explants, FIG. 5). In contrast, Hex, although required for Dkk1 to induce hearts, on its own induced only expression of early heart markers, such as Nkx2.5 and Tbx5, but never contractile protein gene expression.[33] Experimental activation of intermediate points in the pathway between Dkk1 and Hex caused correspondingly intermediate levels of heart morphogenesis (FIG. 5). This suggests that signaling pathways that branch from the canonical Dkk1/Wnt antagonist/Hex pathway induce other signals needed for progression from initial induction, to cardiomyocyte differentiation, to acquisition of rhythmic beating, and, finally, to tube formation. The nature of the molecules that mediate progression from cardiogenic mesoderm to cardiomyogenesis remains to be elucidated.

It is striking that Dkk1 is unique among Wnt antagonists in inducing robustly beating heart tubes. Crescent, in comparison, induces about 4–5× fewer beating structures and other Wnt antagonists, such as WIF1 and FrzB induce only early (e.g., Nkx2.5, Tbx5, GATA4) but not late (e.g., contractile protein gene expression) cardiac marker gene expression.[33] Thus, we favor the view that Dkk1 harbors a novel signaling capacity relevant for later differentiation of cardiac mesoderm and tissue morphogenesis distinct from its ability to inhibit canonical Wnt/β-catenin signal transduction. The Wnt inhibitory activity of Dkk1 is localized to its carboxyl-terminal cysteine-rich domain (CRD) that, by binding to low-density lipoprotein-related protein (LRP) on the cell surface, disrupts the interaction between the Frizzled receptor, LRP5/6, and Wnt protein that transduces the Wnt signal into the cell.[41] Our recent results (Gupta & Mercola, submitted elsewhere for publication) indicate that the amino-terminal CRD possesses a novel activity related to cell migration and we speculate that this might mediate a novel signal that complements Wnt antagonism to promote progression to later stages of cardiomyocyte differentiation and/or tissue organization.

SUMMARY

Both Dkk1 and Nodal induce heart tissue indirectly by acting on adjacent foregut endoderm. Dkk1 induces Hex to regulate an unknown diffusible factor

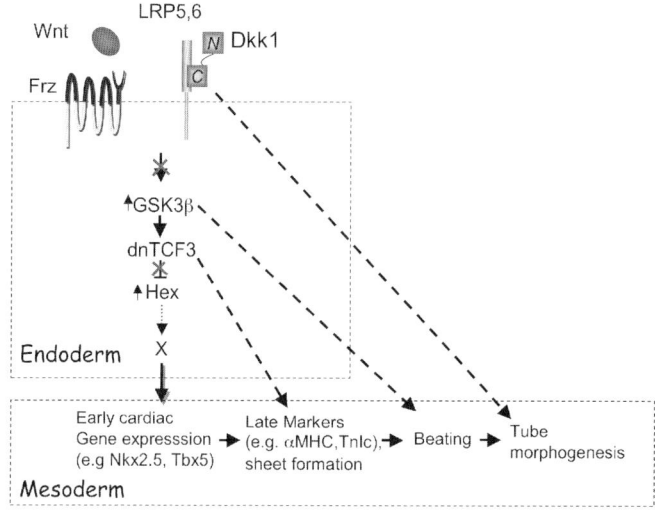

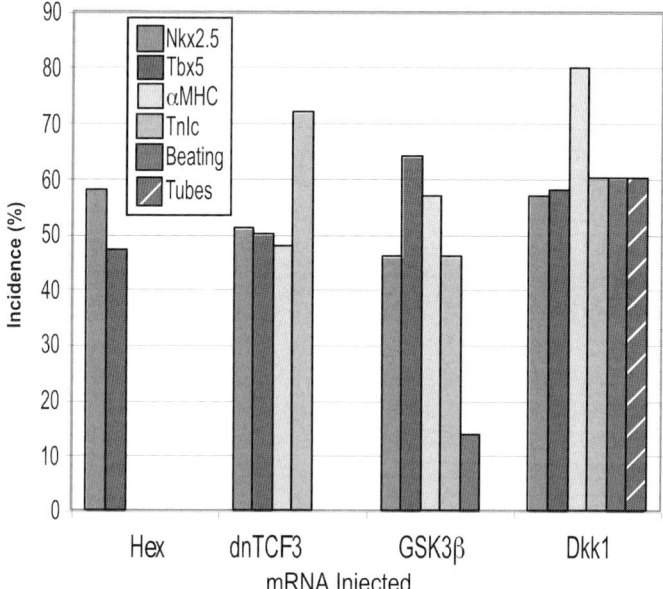

FIGURE 5. Divergent branches of the Dkk1 pathway stimulate later stages of cardiomyogenesis. The upper panel diagram components of the Dkk1 signal transduction pathway leading to heart induction. The lower panel shows incidence of explants expressing markers or exhibiting morphological characteristics of heart formation as a function of different proteins misexpressed in non-cardiogenic mesendoderm (VMZ) by mRNA microinjection as diagrammed in FIGURE 2.

involved in initiation of cardiogenesis. Nodal stimulates production of the secreted protein Cerberus, which also initiates cardiogenesis. Progression to later stages of cardiomocyte differentiation and heart tube morphogenesis involves additional pathways, possibly branching from the Dkk1/Wnt antagonism signaling cascade. Last, novel signaling from Dkk1 in addition to inhibition of Wnt/β-catenin signal transduction might account for promotion of later stages of myocardial differentiation.

ACKNOWLEDGMENTS

The authors thank Michael Oubré for editing the article and Ashley Lakoduk and Yessenia Ibarra for quantitative PCR analyses. The research cited in this article was supported by RO1 HL059502 to M.M. and an NIH NRSA postdoctoral fellowship to A.C.F.

REFERENCES

1. SATER, A.K. & A.G. JACOBSON. 1990. The role of the dorsal lip in the induction of heart mesoderm in Xenopus laevis. Development **108**: 461–470.
2. NASCONE, N. & M. MERCOLA. 1995. An inductive role for the endoderm in Xenopus cardiogenesis. Development **121**: 515–523.
3. JACOBSON, A.G. 1960. Influences of ectoderm and endoderm on heart differentiation in the newt. Dev. Biol. **2**: 138–154.
4. FULLILOVE, S.L. 1970. Heart induction: distribution of active factors in newt endoderm. J. Exp. Zool. **175**: 323–326.
5. YATSKIEVYCH, T.A., A.N. LADD & P.B. ANTIN. 1997. Induction of cardiac myogenesis in avian pregastrula epiblast: the role of the hypoblast and activin. Development **124**: 2561–2570.
6. SCHULTHEISS, T.M., S. XYDAS & A.B. LASSAR. 1995. Induction of avian cardiac myogenesis by anterior endoderm. Development **121**: 4203–4214.
7. SUGI, Y. & J. LOUGH. 1994. Anterior endoderm is a specific effector of terminal cardiac myocyte differentiation of cells from the embryonic heart forming region. Dev. Dyn. **200**: 155–162.
8. ARAI, A., K. YAMAMOTO & J. TOYAMA. 1997. Murine cardiac progenitor cells require visceral embryonic endoderm and primitive streak for terminal differentiation. Dev. Dyn. **210**: 344–353.
9. FOLEY, A. & M. MERCOLA. 2004. Heart induction: embryology to cardiomyocyte regeneration. Trends Cardiovasc. Med. **14**: 121–125.
10. SOLLOWAY, M.J. & R.P. HARVEY. 2003. Molecular pathways in myocardial development: a stem cell perspective. Cardiovasc. Res. **58**: 264–277.
11. SCHNEIDER, V.A. & M. MERCOLA. 2001. Wnt antagonism initiates cardiogenesis in *Xenopus laevis*. Genes Dev. **15**: 304–315.
12. MARVIN, M.J. *et al.* 2001. Inhibition of Wnt activity induces heart formation from posterior mesoderm. Genes Dev. **15**: 316–327.
13. SHELDAHL, L.C. *et al.* 2003. Dishevelled activates Ca2+ flux, PKC, and CamKII in vertebrate embryos. J. Cell. Biol. **161**: 769–777.

14. PANDUR, P. et al. 2002. Wnt-11 activation of a non-canonical Wnt signalling pathway is required for cardiogenesis. Nature **418:** 636–641.
15. ZHOU, X., E. QUANN & G.I. GALLICANO. 2003. Differentiation of nonbeating embryonic stem cells into beating cardiomyocytes is dependent on downregulation of PKC beta and zeta in concert with upregulation of PKC epsilon. Dev. Biol. **255:** 407–422.
16. ALVAREZ-BUYLLA, E.R. et al. 2000. MADS-box gene evolution beyond flowers: expression in pollen, endosperm, guard cells, roots and trichomes.[erratum appears in Plant J 2001 Mar;25(5):593]. Proc. Natl. Acad. Sci. USA **97:** 5328–5333.
17. KUHL, M. et al. 2001. Antagonistic regulation of convergent extension movements in Xenopus by Wnt/beta-catenin and Wnt/Ca2+ signaling. Mech. Dev. **106:** 61–76.
18. DARKEN, R.S. et al. 2002. The planar polarity gene strabismus regulates convergent extension movements in Xenopus. Embo. J. **21:** 976–985.
19. PARK, M. & R.T. MOON. 2002. The planar cell-polarity gene stbm regulates cell behaviour and cell fate in vertebrate embryos. Nat. Cell. Biol. **4:** 20–25.
20. XU, C. et al. 1998. Specific arrest of cardiogenesis in cultured embryonic stem cells lacking Cripto-1. Dev. Biol. **196:** 237–247.
21. DING, J. et al. 1998. Cripto is required for correct orientation of the anterior-posterior axis in the mouse embryo. Nature **395:** 702–707.
22. XU, C. et al. 1999. Abrogation of the Cripto gene in mouse leads to failure of postgastrulation morphogenesis and lack of differentiation of cardiomyocytes. Development **126:** 483–494.
23. BEDDINGTON, R.S. & E.J. ROBERTSON. 1999. Axis development and early asymmetry in mammals. Cell **96:** 195–209.
24. LOUGH, J. et al. 1996. Combined BMP-2 and FGF-4, but neither factor alone, induces cardiogenesis in non-precardiac embryonic mesoderm. Dev. Biol. **178:** 198–202.
25. SCHLANGE, T. et al. 2000. BMP2 is required for early heart development during a distinct time period. Mech. Dev. **91:** 259–270.
26. SCHULTHEISS, T.M., J.B. BURCH & A.B. LASSAR. 1997. A role for bone morphogenetic proteins in the induction of cardiac myogenesis. Genes Dev. **11:** 451–462.
27. SHI, Y. et al. 2000. BMP signaling is required for heart formation in vertebrates. Dev. Biol. **224:** 226–237.
28. BEHFAR, A. et al. 2002. Stem cell differentiation requires a paracrine pathway in the heart. FASEB J. **16:** 1558–1566.
29. KAWAI, T. et al. 2004. Efficient cardiomyogenic differentiation of embryonic stem cell by fibroblast growth factor 2 and bone morphogenetic protein 2. Circ. J. **68:** 691–702.
30. OH, H. et al. 2003. Cardiac progenitor cells from adult myocardium: homing, differentiation, and fusion after infarction. Proc. Natl. Acad. Sci. USA **100:** 12313–12318.
31. NASCONE, N. & M. MERCOLA. 1995. An inductive role for the endoderm in *Xenopus* cardiogenesis. Development **121:** 515–523.
32. SCHNEIDER, V.A. & M. MERCOLA. 1999. Spatially distinct head and heart inducers within the *Xenopus* organizer region. Curr. Biol. **9:** 800–809.
33. FOLEY, A.C. & M. MERCOLA. 2005. Heart induction by Wnt antagonists depends on the homeodomain transcription factor Hex. Genes Dev. **19:** 387–396.

34. BOGUE, C.W. et al. 2003. Impaired B cell development and function in mice with a targeted disruption of the homeobox gene Hex. Proc. Natl. Acad. Sci. USA **100**: 556–561.
35. OSADA, S.I. & C.V. WRIGHT. 1999. Xenopus nodal-related signaling is essential for mesendodermal patterning during early embryogenesis. Development **126**: 3229–3240.
36. PICCOLO, S. et al. 1999. The head inducer Cerberus is a multifunctional antagonist of Nodal, BMP and Wnt signals. Nature **397**: 707–710.
37. BOUWMEESTER, T. et al. 1996. Cerberus is a head-inducing secreted factor expressed in the anterior endoderm of Spemann's organizer. Nature **382**: 595–601.
38. LATINKIC, B.V., S. KOTECHA & T.J. MOHUN. 2003. Induction of cardiomyocytes by GATA4 in Xenopus ectodermal explants. Development **130**: 3865–3876.
39. BELO, J.A. et al. 1997. *Cerberus-like* is a secreted factor with neuralizing activity expressed in the anterior primitive endoderm of the mouse gastrula. Mech. Dev. **68**: 45–57.
40. BIBEN, C. et al. 1998. Murine cerberus homologue mCer-1: a candidate anterior patterning molecule. Dev. Biol. **194**: 135–151.
41. BROTT, B.K. & S.Y. SOKOL. 2002. Regulation of Wnt/LRP signaling by distinct domains of Dickkopf proteins. Mol. Cell. Biol. **22**: 6100–6110.
42. NAKAMURA, T. et al. 2003. A Wnt- and beta-catenin-dependent pathway for mammalian cardiac myogenesis. Proc. Natl. Acad. Sci. USA **100**: 5834–5839.

The Role of Basic Leucine Zipper Protein-Mediated Transcription in Physiological and Pathological Myocardial Hypertrophy

IZHAK KEHAT,[a,b] TAL HASIN,[a,b] AND AMI ARONHEIM[b]

[a]*Department of Cardiology, Rambam Medical Center, Haifa, Israel 31096*
[b]*Department of Molecular Genetics, The Rappaport Family Institute in the Medical Sciences, Technion, Israel Institute of Technology, Haifa, Israel 31096*

ABSTRACT: Accumulating evidence suggests that nuclear transcription factors from the basic leucine zipper (bZIP) family play an important role in cardiac development and function. This class includes the CREB/ATF family of transcription factors, namely CREB, cAMP response element modulator (CREM), ATF, and the related AP-1 and C/EBP families. An effort has been made to elucidate the role of specific bZIP members in the heart. Unfortunately, little insight could be gained from knockout experiments, either due to embryonic lethal phenotypes or functional compensation by other bZIP family members. Surprisingly, cardiac overexpression of several inhibitory transcription factors from the bZIP family, such as a nonphosphorylatable form of CREB (CREB$_{ser133}$), a nonfunctional isoform of CREM, or ATF3 resulted in massive atrial dilatation. In order to try and characterize this pathway we have expressed the potent bZIP inhibitory protein, Jun dimerization protein 2 (JDP2), specifically in the mouse heart in a temporally controlled manner. Expression of JDP2 resulted in massive biatrial dilatation; loss of connexin 40 (Cx40), connexin43 (C×43), and myosin light chain 2 (MLC2a) expression; atrioventricular defects in conduction; and a lethal phenotype. All these effects were independent of any developmental events acquired during adulthood, and were totally reversible upon abolishing the bZIP inhibition. The results of this article suggest that bZIP inhibition is sufficient to cause atrial dilation, that this dilatation is acquired postnatally, and that it is reversible upon the relief of inhibition. Thus, bZIP repressors may serve as novel drug targets for the prevention of atrial dilatation a major risk of atrial fibrillation (AF).

KEYWORDS: transcription factors; atrium; hypertrophy

Address for correspondence: Izhak Kehat, Technion, Israel Institute of Technology, Rappaport Family Institute in the Medical Sciences, the B. Rappaport Faculty of Medicine, Haifa, Israel 31096. Voice: 972-4-829-5226; fax: 972-4-829-5325.
  e-mail: ikehat@tx.technion.ac.il

INTRODUCTION

Myocardial hypertrophy is a leading predictor for the development of serious cardiac complications, such as the development of arrhythmias, sudden death, and heart failure.[1,2] Current medical treatments for the prevention of pathological hypertrophy rely on the pharmacological blockade of key membrane-bound receptors that respond to neuroendocrine stimuli, such as angiotensin II, aldosterone, and catecholamines. Yet, despite the capacity for a near-complete pharmacological blockade of the neurohumoral axis, the incidence of heart failure, with its associated morbidity and mortality are still on the rise.[3] Given these clinical observations, new therapeutic strategies, potentially directed at signaling pathways that transduce the neuroendocrine or the stretch-mediated signals are direly needed.

A growing number of intracellular signaling pathways have been characterized as important transducers of the membrane-bound and stretch-mediated signals including G proteins, small GTPase, protein kinase C, the mitogen-activated protein kinase (MAPK) pathways, and others. Of these, the MAPK cascades, have been postulated to function as one of the transducers, involved in the transition between compensated hypertrophy and the more serious disease sequelae, such as heart failure.[4] The above cascades, and others, usually result in phosphorylation, activation, and nuclear translocation of several transcription factors that are responsible for a shift in gene expression, the key process in the development of hypertrophy. This shift in gene expression is characterized by a coordinated pattern of expression, which includes an early transient expression of immediate-early genes, followed by a recapitulation of an embryonic pattern of genetic transcription, and an increase in contractile protein content.[5]

Basic leucine zipper (bZIP) transcription factors are exclusively eukaryotic proteins that bind to specific double-stranded DNA sequences as homodimers or heterodimers to either activate or repress gene transcription[6] (FIG. 1). Amino acid alignment of bZIP proteins allowed the identification of the bZIP motif, a long bipartite α-helix that is 60 to 80 amino acids long.[7] The N-terminal half contains two clusters of basic amino acids responsible for sequence-specific DNA binding, while the C-terminal half contains a protein sequence of variable length with a leucine residue at six amino acids interval. This sequence, termed the *leucine zipper*, mediates homo- and heterodimerization of the bZIP proteins. During the 1980s, several mammalian bZIP proteins were purified, and the genes encoding these proteins were cloned. Among the first cloned were the AP-1 (c-Fos and c-Jun) heterodimer, the CREB homodimer, and the C/EBP homodimer. These newly isolated genes were used as probes in low-stringency DNA hybridizations to identify new sequence-related bZIP proteins. Thus the different bZIP proteins were originally grouped to AP-1, CREB/ATF, and to the C/EBP families. More recently, when published DNA sequences of the human genome were examined, 53 genes that contain the bZIP motif were identified,

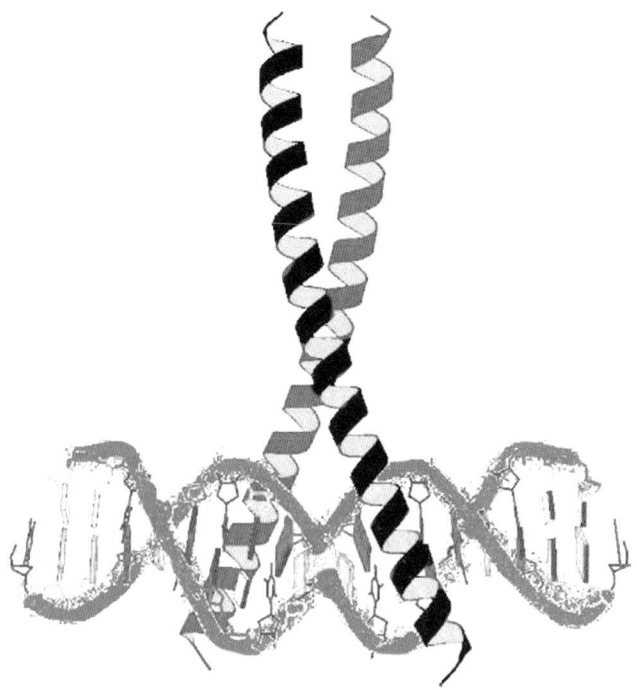

FIGURE 1. bZIP transcription factors are exclusively eukaryotic proteins that bind to specific double-stranded DNA sequences as homodimers or heterodimers. A schematic representation of a bZIP heterodimer bound to DNA is shown.

with the potential to form 2809 combinations of different dimers.[8] This creates the possibility for a tremendous range of transcriptional control. It is not surprising therefore, that the potential role of this transcriptional machinery in the heart is eagerly studied.

ACTIVATING PROTEIN 1 (AP-1) SIGNALING AND HYPERTROPHY

Several lines of evidence suggest that the transcription factor complex AP-1 plays a major role in myocardial hypertrophy. AP-1 is composed of dimeric combinatorial complex of members of the c-Jun homodimers (c-Jun, JunD, and JunB) or c-Jun heterodimer with Fos family members (c-Fos, Fos B, and Fra1, 2), and some members of the ATF and CREB protein families (reviewed in Ref. 9). Several models have shown that hypertrophy in the heart is accompanied by an increase in the expression of c-Fos and c-Jun transcription factor family members.[10,11] Some reports suggested that mechanical overload causes only a transient increase in c-Jun expression[10,12] in the myocardium.

However, several lines of evidence also indicated that this transcription factor might be important for the subsequent activation of genes that are characteristically expressed during cardiac hypertrophy, such as α-skeletal actin and atrial natriuretic factor.[12] In addition, sustained upregulation of AP-1 was also found in the chronic phase of left ventricular remodeling after myocardial infarction in rats and in failing human hearts.[13]

Several approaches were used to verify, *in vitro*, the causal role of AP-1 in the development of hypertrophy. Transfection of cultured cardiac myocytes with a dominant negative form of c-Jun has been shown to inhibit cardiac myocyte hypertrophy in response to phenylephrine and endothelin, suggesting that c-Jun might play an important causal role in the development of cardiac hypertrophy.[14] Studies on isolated adult ventricular myocytes have shown that both α- and β-adrenergic stimulation are associated with an increase in c-Jun and c-Fos. Blockade of this pathway by CRE decoy oligonucleotides was shown to prevent α- but not β-adrenergic-mediated hypertrophy.[15] Targeted disruption of c-Jun and JunB is embryonic lethal. c-Jun$^{-/-}$ fetuses had a malformation of the outflow tract of the heart, suggesting that this factor may also have an important developmental role.[16] Collectively, these *in vitro* data suggest that AP-1 may play a causal role in the development of myocardial hypertrophy and thus may serve as a potential drug target for the prevention of hypertrophy.

Yet, it is important to realize that many discrepancies exist between *in vitro* data and that obtained from animal models. For example, most reports that relied exclusive on culture-based models of cellular growth proposed a prohypertrophic regulatory role for JNK and p38 signaling. More recently, a number of studies in genetically modified animal models have challenged this view and suggest that *in vivo* these factors may actually serve as negative regulators of hypertrophy.[4] Given the reported conflicting data between *in vitro* and *in vivo* experiments it may be of paramount importance to assess the causal role of AP-1 in an animal model.

Disruption of the AP-1 Transcription Pathway

Since the AP-1 transcription factor is composed of dimeric combinatorial complex of several proteins, disruption of this pathway poses a special problem. Members of the AP-1 proteins share a high degree of homology, similar DNA binding specificity, and comparable transcription activation capacity. It remains unclear to what extent family members may share common biological roles. Although JunB was thought to be an antagonist of c-Jun, it was shown that JunB can largely substitute for c-Jun *in vivo*.[17] c-Jun knockout mice have arrested liver development and develop cardiac malformation.[16] Homozygous knockin mice with JunB expressed from the c-Jun locus develop to birth and show normal liver morphogenesis but still show a malformed cardiac outflow tract,[17] suggesting that JunB can compensate for c-Jun in the liver but not in the heart during development. The AP-1 member junD, although dispensable in development,[18] has been shown to be involved in muscle cell differentiation.[19] Interestingly, junD is specifically expressed in the developing heart and cardiovascular system.[18] Reduced junD expression has also been reported in human failing hearts.[20] Mice lacking junD develop less adaptive hypertrophy in heart after mechanical pressure overload, while cardiomyocyte-specific expression of junD in mice results in spontaneous ventricular dilation and decreased contractility.[21] There are conflicting data regarding fra-1 expression upon cardiac hypertrophic stimuli. One study demonstrated that fra-1 is not induced upon aortic banding,[10] whereas another study reported both repression and induction of fra-1 expression in cardiomyocytes *in vitro*, depending on the stimulation.[22] Interestingly, it has been reported that fra-1 seems to regulate the cardiac hypertrophy gene ANF.[23] Fra-1 overexpression resulted in dilatation and reduced cardiac contractility. Increased mortality was observed after TAC or isoproteranol infusion.[21] Thus a comprehensive assessment of the role of AP-1 may require the inactivation of several members, and the developmental role AP-1-mediated transcription should also be differentiated from the postnatal effects.

CRE Signaling and Hypertrophy

CREB is a 43-kD bZIP transcription factor that binds an octanucleotide sequence, called cyclic AMP response element (CRE), both as a homodimer and as a heterodimer in association with other members of the CREB/ATF and AP-1 families. CREB plays a critical role in regulating gene expression in response to a variety of extracellular signals. The transcriptional activity of CREB is positively regulated by phosphorylation of a Serine residue (Ser 133) located in the kinase-inducible domain.[24] Phosphorylation of CREB on Ser 133 facilitates its interaction with the 265-kD CREB-binding protein (CBP), which in turn is able to interact with, and activate the basal transcription complex.[25] A mutant CREB molecule, $CREB_{A133}$ containing a Serine 133 to Alanine substitution functions as a potent dominant negative repressor of CREB-dependent gene expression both *in vitro* and *in vivo*.[26] Previous studies have provided evidence suggesting that CREB might be an important regulator of cardiac myocyte gene expression. G-protein-coupled receptors, such as the β-adrenergic receptors are important regulators of the contractile state of cardiac myocytes. Such receptors mediate their effects by altering intracellular levels of cAMP, which, in turn, is an important regulator of CREB activity.[27] Mice with overexpression of the $CREB_{A133}$ displayed a phenotype that closely resembles the pathological, hemodynamic, and clinical features of the human of inherited dilated cardiomyopathy.[28]

ATRIAL HYPERTROPHY AND DILATATION

Atrial fibrillation (AF) is the most common sustained arrhythmia in clinical practice. Atrial dilatation is often associated with AF, but it appears to be both the cause and a consequence of the arrhythmia.[29] Several lines of evidence suggest that atrial enlargement predispose to AF. Prospective studies have showed that left atrial enlargement is an independent risk factor for the development of AF.[30,31] Acute atrial dilatation also increased the vulnerability to AF in langendorff-perfused rabbit.[29] It should be noted, however, that other studies suggested that AF itself can also cause atrial dilatation,[32] and restoration of sinus rhythm can reduce LA size. Thus it appears that atrial dilatation and AF may be mutually dependent and constitute a vicious circle.

Despite an intensive research directed at elucidating the pathways involved in ventricular hypertrophy, the mechanisms involved in atrial dilatation and hypertrophy remain largely unstudied. The chambers of the mammalian heart are specialized in order to handle differing physiological conditions, throughout embryonic and adult life. Therefore each chamber is composed of cells with unique functional, structural, metabolic, and electrophysiological characteristics. Moreover, each chamber has a different expression profile.[33] It is therefore possible that hypertrophy and hypertrophy pathways differ between the atria and ventricles.

Since the CRE and AP-1 DNA motifs appear in numerous promotors,[34] including those of many cardiac-specific genes, an effort has been made to elucidate the role of specific bZIP members in the heart. Unfortunately, little insight could be gained from knockout experiments due to either embryonic lethal phenotypes or to functional compensation by other bZIP family members.[16,35,36] Consequently, transgenic models with overexpression of native or mutant bZIP proteins were developed. Surprisingly, overexpression of several inhibitory bZIP proteins in the heart resulted in massive atrial dilatation and hypertrophy.

Cardiac overexpression of the dominant negative $CREB_{A133}$ in the mouse heart resulted in progressive four chamber cardiac dilatation, interstitial cardiac fibrosis with myocyte heterogeneity and vacuolization, intracardiac thrombi, and signs of severe chronic venous congestion.[28] The mice also demonstrated significantly depressed left ventricular systolic function and abnormal diastolic relaxation, and a significant increase in mortality. Detailed electrophysiological analysis showed that young transgenic mice developed abnormalities in atrioventricular nodal conduction. These mice developed abnormalities of infrahisian and interventricular conduction at older age. Since in this model, mice display four chambers hypertrophy, it is not clear whether or not atrial dilatation represented a primary phenomena or it was secondary to the ventricular disarrangement. Moreover, the molecular mechanism responsible for the atrial dilatation was not clear. There are at least three different mechanisms by which overexpression of $CREB_{A133}$ could dysregulate CREB-dependent transcription. First, because $CREB_{A133}$ can bind to DNA but fails to activate transcription, it has been shown to displace transcriptionally active CREB from CRE sites and thereby downregulate CREB-dependent transcription. Second, $CREB_{A133}$ protein may displace wild-type CREB from the appropriate CREB kinases. Third, overexpression of $CREB_{A133}$ might also squelch CREB/ATF-dependent transcription by altering the balance of different CREB/ATF dimers present in the cell. Atrial dilatation could result from any of these mechanisms. Moreover, it is possible that the ventricular dilatation results predominantly from one of the above suggested mechanism while the cause of atrial dilation differs.

To further study the CRE signaling in the heart, mice with overexpression of a nonfunctional isoform of CRE binding protein (CREB)/CRE modulator (CREM) were generated.[37] This isoform termed *CREM-IbΔC-X*, is composed of the basic and leucine zipper domain responsible for dimerization and CRE-specific DNA binding and act as suppressors of CRE-mediated transcriptional activation. Following overexpression of this isoform transgenic mice hearts developed considerable atrial dilatation, with absolute and relative atrial weights increased more than sixfold. At 7 weeks, transgenic mice displayed sinus rhythm combined with enlarged atria. AF began at 8 weeks, and AF was observed in all transgenic animals investigated at 16 weeks, suggesting that AF occurred as a consequence of atrial dilatation. Mean survival times were decreased in the transgenic lines as compared with wild-type controls. The ventricular phenotype of CREM-IbΔC-X transgenic mice was fundamentally different from the phenotypes of transgenic mice with $CREB_{A133}$ overexpression. While $CREB_{A133}$ mice displayed signs of heart failure with depressed LV function, hypertrophy of ventricles, and edema, the CREM-IbΔC-X displayed ventricular hypertrophy and increased LV performance. In this model, the atrial dilatation appears to be a primary phenomenon and cannot be ascribed to the ventricular phenotype, as invasive measurements did not show increased ventricular pressures. Nevertheless, phosphorylation of CREB was reduced, no compensatory increase in CREM-IbΔC-X transgenic hearts was observed. Thus the precise molecular mechanism responsible for the atrial dilatation cannot be ascertained.

Another inhibitory member of the CREB/ATF family of bZIP transcription factors that was studied in the heart is ATF3.[38] Evidence indicates that ATF3 is induced by a variety of stress signals in different cell types.[39] It was also demonstrated that the mRNA level of ATF3 greatly increases in the heart after myocardial ischemia, and ischemia coupled with ischemia reperfusion.[40] Mice with cardiac overexpression of ATF3 showed biatrial enlargement starting at 3 weeks of age. There was also a small but statistically significant increase in ventricular weight. An *in vitro* assay on isolated ventricular myocytes derived from these transgenic mice showed a reduction in percent cell shortening, suggesting decreased ventricular contractility. Similar to the $CREB_{A133}$ and the CREM-IbΔC-X mice, the ATF3 mice also showed disturbances in atrioventricular conduction.

Taken together these data suggest that inhibition of CRE-mediated transcription causes atrial dilatation. However, a difficulty in the interpretation of the atrial phenotype in the above-mentioned models stems from the use of the α-myosin heavy chain (α-MHC) promotor to direct the cardiac transgene expression.[28,37,38] The α-MHC promotor was reported to be active in the atria on embryonic day 10, whereas in the ventricles the promotor becomes active only 12 h before birth.[41] Hence, it was postulated that atrial dilatation actually resulted from the selective early expression of the transgene in the atria,[38] and thus represented a secondary developmental event.[28,38]

Overexpression of JDP2 in the Mouse Heart

To determine whether the bZIP inhibition of transcription is a primary event sufficient to cause atrial dilatation, we overexpressed another inhibitory bZIP transcription factor–Jun dimerization protein 2 (JDP2) in the mouse heart in a temporally controlled manner.[42] c-Jun dimerization protein 2 is a potent inhibitory bZIP protein that can form a stable homodimer as well as a heterodimer with Jun family members and ATF2; it binds DNA, and represses transcription by multiple mechanisms.[43,44] JDP2 exhibits a 47% identity overall with ATF3 and up to 90% similarity within the bZIP motif. However, unlike ATF3, which is an immediate early gene, JDP2 is constitutively expressed in all cell lines and tissues tested. In addition, whereas ATF3 is able to activate/repress transcription, depending on its dimerization state,[45–47] JDP2 represses transcription either as a homo- or heterodimer.[43,44]

Expression of JDP2 in the mouse heart resulted in massive biatrial dilatation with increased trabeculation, without apparent hypertrophy of chamber walls. Histological sections revealed hypertrophic cardiomyocytes in the atria with a significant increase in atrial, but not ventricular, myofibrillar cross-sectional diameter. Importantly, there was no evidence for elevated diastolic pressures. Thus, transcriptional inhibition by bZIP proteins is sufficient to cause atrial dilatation (Fig. 2).

Similar to all previous models, the JDP2 transgenics displayed increased mortality rate and atrioventricular conduction defects. Since conduction in the heart is dependent on the presence of the gap junction proteins, namely connexins, the expression of these proteins was analyzed. This analysis showed a markedly lower expression of the atrial isoform Cx40 and of $C\times43$ in the JDP2-transgenics atria. We also showed that both JDP2 and ATF3 are able to bind the CRE binding sequences located at the Cx40 promotor and inhibit its transcription.

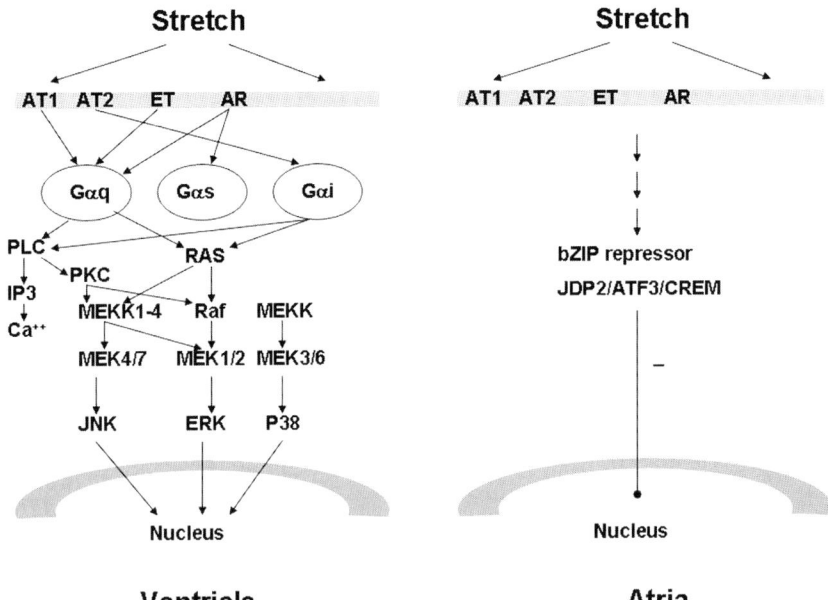

FIGURE 2. A schematic representation of some of the hypertrophy pathways known to be involved in ventricular hypertrophy (left), and atrial hypertrophy (right). The top bar depicts the cell membrane and the various receptors that initiate signaling through G-proteins. Stretch activates these upstream events as well as other less defined stress sensing mechanism to promote activation of MEKKs, which in turn activate the MAP kinase kinases, culminating in MAPK activation (JNK, ERK, and p38). These terminal kinases then proceed to phosphorylate transcription factors within the nucleus, as well as other regulatory proteins in the nucleus and cytoplasm. In the atria inhibitory bZIP proteins are sufficient to cause hypertrophy and dilatation. Abbreviations: Et, endothelin receptor; AT, angiotensin II receptor; AR, adrenergic receptor; PLC, phospholipase C; PKC, protein kinase C; PI3K, phosphoinositide 3′-OH kinase; IP3, inositol triphosphate.

Another target gene that was found to be significantly downregulated in the atria is the myosin light chain 2 (MLC2) atrial isoform. Similar to Cx40, this effect was reversible upon abolishing of JDP2 expression. Sarcomeric myosin provides the molecular motor for force production, and each myosin hexamer is composed of two heavy chains and four light chains, two essential MLC1/3 molecules, and two regulatory MLC2 molecules. The most striking mechanical effect of MLC2 is on the physiological speed of shortening of the actomyosin complex; removal of MLC2 significantly decreases the velocity of actin movement on skeletal myosin.[48] Two MLC2 isoforms are present in mammalian heart: MLC2V in the ventricles and MLC2A in the atrium. MLC2a disruption in mice is embryonically lethal as this is the major isoform in embryonic chamber; however, embryos display enlarged atria.[49] Overexpression of an interfering mutant, nonphosphorylatable MLC2v, in the mouse heart also caused marked biatrial hypertrophy and dilatation without appreciable effects in the ventricle.[50] A study of human atrial and ventricular strips showed similar results.[51] This study showed that α1-adrenergic receptors mediate a prominent increase in contractile force in human atria, but not in the human ventricle that is accompanied by an increase in MLC2a phosphorylation. Collectively, these data suggest that the reduced expression of MLC2a in JDP2-expressing mice may have a causal effect in the development of atrial dilatation. Thus pathways converging on MLC2a levels and phosphorylation state may have importance in mediating atrial size and function.

The α-MHC promotor was reported to be active in the atria on embryonic day 10, whereas in the ventricles the promotor becomes active shortly before birth.[41] To examine whether the pronounced atrial effect was due to developmental differences in the activity of the α-MHC promotor, we used the binary "tet-off" system and took advantage of the ability to regulate the binding activity of the tetracycline activator by the use of doxycycline. We could show an identical phenotype in animals in which JDP2 overexpression was allowed only after birth. Thus, the observed phenotype was independent of any developmental or early postnatal events. We could also demonstrate that the phenotype was totally reversible upon abolishing of bZIP inhibition.

Atrial and Ventricular Effects of bZIP Repressors

Although overexpression of repressing bZIP proteins resulted in strikingly similar massive atrial dilatation and hypertrophy, the ventricular effects were more variable. Overexpression of $CREB_{ser133}$[28] resulted in massive ventricular dilatation and an overt heart failure with edema. The overexpression of CREM-IbΔC-X resulted in a ventricular hypertrophy without increased pressures.[37] Overexpression of ATF3 resulted in only a small increase in ventricular weight, suggesting cardiac hypertrophy, without signs of heart failure.[38] JDP2 overexpression resulted in a slight (10%) increase in ventricular weight with no evidence of either systemic or pulmonary edema, strongly suggesting no increased cardiac pressures. Nevertheless, molecular markers for ventricular hypertrophy in the ventricles were observed. The almost identical atrial phenotype, along with the variable ventricular one in the different mouse models, strongly suggests that the atrial dilatation is a primary event, independent of the ventricles. It is possible that bZIP inhibition has a dominant effect in the atria resulting in dilatation, whereas other, yet to be determined, independent mechanisms account for the ventricular hypertrophy.

SUMMARY

Accumulating evidence suggests that nuclear transcription factors from the bZIP family play an important role in cardiac development and function.

Expression of inhibitory members of this family: JDP2, ATF3, and CREM, in transgenic animals induce massive atrial hypertrophy and dilatation. This hypertrophy is accompanied by the loss of Cx40, C×43, and MLC2 expression, atrioventricular defects in conduction, and the development of AF. In contrast, only mild ventricular hypertrophy is noted. These data suggest that atrial and ventricular hypertrophies are different entities, governed by different signaling pathways. Since atrial dilatation and hypertrophy is the harbinger of AF, further studies are necessary to dissect the atrial pathways of hypertrophy.

ACKNOWLEDGMENTS

This work was partially supported by the Israel Cancer Research Foundation Research Career Development Award to AA and The Israel Ministry of Health to AA and IK.

REFERENCES

1. Ho, K.K., J.L. Pinsky, W.B. Kannel & D. Levy. 1993. The epidemiology of heart failure: the Framingham Study. J. Am. Coll. Cardiol. **22:** 6A–13A.
2. Levy, D. et al. 2002. Long-term trends in the incidence of and survival with heart failure. N. Engl. J. Med. **347:** 1397–1402.
3. Klein, L. et al. 2003. Pharmacologic therapy for patients with chronic heart failure and reduced systolic function: review of trials and practical considerations. Am. J. Cardiol. **91:** 18F–40F.
4. Liang, Q. & J.D. Molkentin. 2003. Redefining the roles of p38 and JNK signaling in cardiac hypertrophy: dichotomy between cultured myocytes and animal models. J. Mol. Cell. Cardiol. **35:** 1385–1394.
5. Komuro, I. & Y. Yazaki. 1993. Control of cardiac gene expression by mechanical stress. Annu. Rev. Physiol. **55:** 55–75.
6. Hurst, H.C. 1995. Transcription factors 1: bZIP proteins. Protein Profile **2:** 101–168.
7. Vinson, C.R., P.B. Sigler & S.L. McKnight. 1989. Scissors-grip model for DNA recognition by a family of leucine zipper proteins. Science **246:** 911–916.
8. Vinson, C. et al. 2002. Classification of human B-ZIP proteins based on dimerization properties. Mol. Cell. Biol. **22:** 6321–6335.
9. Shaulian, E. & M. Karin. 2001. AP-1 in cell proliferation and survival. Oncogene **20:** 2390–2400.
10. Rockman, H.A. et al. 1991. Segregation of atrial-specific and inducible expression of an atrial natriuretic factor transgene in an in vivo murine model of cardiac hypertrophy. Proc. Natl. Acad. Sci. USA **88:** 8277–8281.
11. Nadruz, W. Jr., C.B. Kobarg, J. Kobarg & K.G. Franchini. 2004. c-Jun is regulated by combination of enhanced expression and phosphorylation in acute-overloaded rat heart. Am. J. Physiol. Heart Circ. Physiol. **286:** H760–H767.
12. Cornelius, T., S.R. Holmer, F.U. Muller, et al. 1997. Regulation of the rat atrial natriuretic peptide gene after acute imposition of left ventricular pressure overload. Hypertension **30:** 1348–1355.

13. FRANTZ, S. *et al*. 2003. Sustained activation of nuclear factor kappa B and activator protein 1 in chronic heart failure. Cardiovasc. Res. **57:** 749–756.
14. YOSHIDA, K. *et al*. 2001. Activation of mitogen-activated protein kinases in the non-ischemic myocardium of an acute myocardial infarction in rats. Jpn. Circ. J. **65:** 808–814.
15. TAIMOR, G., K.D. SCHLUTER, P. BEST, *et al*. 2004. Transcription activator protein 1 mediates alpha- but not beta-adrenergic hypertrophic growth responses in adult cardiomyocytes. Am. J. Physiol. Heart Circ. Physiol. **286:** H2369–H2375.
16. EFERL, R. *et al*. 1999. Functions of c-Jun in liver and heart development. J. Cell. Biol. **145:** 1049–1061.
17. PASSEGUE, E., W. JOCHUM, A. BEHRENS, *et al*. 2002. JunB can substitute for Jun in mouse development and cell proliferation. Nat. Genet. **30:** 158–166.
18. THEPOT, D. *et al*. 2000. Targeted disruption of the murine junD gene results in multiple defects in male reproductive function. Development **127:** 143–153.
19. ANDREUCCI, J.J. *et al*. 2002. Composition and function of AP-1 transcription complexes during muscle cell differentiation. J. Biol. Chem. **277:** 16426–16432.
20. POLLACK, P.S. *et al*. 1997. Differential expression of c-jun and junD in end-stage human cardiomyopathy. J. Cell. Biochem. **65:** 245–253.
21. RICCI, R. *et al*. 2005. Distinct functions of junD in cardiac hypertrophy and heart failure. Genes Dev. **19:** 208–213.
22. VAN WAMEL, A.J., C. RUWHOF, L.J. VAN DER VALK-KOKSHOORN, *et al*. 2000. Rapid effects of stretched myocardial and vascular cells on gene expression of neonatal rat cardiomyocytes with emphasis on autocrine and paracrine mechanisms. Arch. Biochem. Biophys. **381:** 67–73.
23. KOVACIC-MILIVOJEVIC, B. & D.G. GARDNER. 1995. Fra-1, a Fos gene family member that activates atrial natriuretic peptide gene transcription. Hypertension **25:** 679–682.
24. GONZALEZ, G.A. & M.R. MONTMINY. 1989. Cyclic AMP stimulates somatostatin gene transcription by phosphorylation of CREB at serine 133. Cell **59:** 675–680.
25. KWOK, R.P. *et al*. 1994. Nuclear protein CBP is a coactivator for the transcription factor CREB. Nature **370:** 223–226.
26. LAMPH, W.W., V.J. DWARKI, R. OFIR, *et al*. 1990. Negative and positive regulation by transcription factor cAMP response element-binding protein is modulated by phosphorylation. Proc. Natl. Acad. Sci. USA **87:** 4320–4324.
27. YAMAMOTO, K.K., G.A. GONZALEZ, W.H. BIGGS III & M.R. MONTMINY. 1988. Phosphorylation-induced binding and transcriptional efficacy of nuclear factor CREB. Nature **334:** 494–498.
28. FENTZKE, R.C., C.E. KORCARZ, R.M. LANG, *et al*. 1998. Dilated cardiomyopathy in transgenic mice expressing a dominant-negative CREB transcription factor in the heart. J. Clin. Invest. **101:** 2415–2426.
29. LIU, T., G.P. LI & L.J. LI. 2005. Atrial dilatation and atrial fibrillation: a vicious circle? Med. Hypotheses **65:** 410–411.
30. VAZIRI, S.M., M.G. LARSON, E.J. BENJAMIN & D. LEVY. 1994. Echocardiographic predictors of nonrheumatic atrial fibrillation. The Framingham Heart Study. Circulation **89:** 724–730.
31. PSATY, B.M. *et al*. 1997. Incidence of and risk factors for atrial fibrillation in older adults. Circulation **96:** 2455–2461.
32. DITTRICH, H.C. *et al*. 1999. Left atrial diameter in nonvalvular atrial fibrillation: an echocardiographic study. Stroke Prevention in Atrial Fibrillation Investigators. Am. Heart J. **137:** 494–499.

33. TABIBIAZAR, R., R.A. WAGNER, A. LIAO & T. QUERTERMOUS. 2003. Transcriptional profiling of the heart reveals chamber-specific gene expression patterns. Circ. Res. **93:** 1193–1201.
34. MAYR, B. & M. MONTMINY. 2001. Transcriptional regulation by the phosphorylation-dependent factor CREB. Nat. Rev. Mol. Cell. Biol. **2:** 599–609.
35. RUDOLPH, D. *et al*. 1998. Impaired fetal T cell development and perinatal lethality in mice lacking the cAMP response element binding protein. Proc. Natl. Acad. Sci. USA **95:** 4481–4486.
36. HUMMLER, E. *et al*. 1994. Targeted mutation of the CREB gene: compensation within the CREB/ATF family of transcription factors. Proc. Natl. Acad. Sci. USA **91:** 5647–5651.
37. MULLER, F.U. *et al*. 2005. Heart-directed expression of a human cardiac isoform of cAMP-response element modulator in transgenic mice. J. Biol. Chem. **280:** 6906–6914.
38. OKAMOTO, Y. *et al*. 2001. Transgenic mice with cardiac-specific expression of activating transcription factor 3, a stress-inducible gene, have conduction abnormalities and contractile dysfunction. Am. J. Pathol. **159:** 639–650.
39. HAI, T., C.D. WOLFGANG, D.K. MARSEE, *et al.*1999. ATF3 and stress responses. Gene Express. **7:** 321–335.
40. YIN, T. *et al*. 1997. Tissue-specific pattern of stress kinase activation in ischemic/reperfused heart and kidney. J. Biol. Chem. **272:** 19943–19950.
41. SUBRAMANIAM, A. *et al*. 1991. Tissue-specific regulation of the alpha-myosin heavy chain gene promotor in transgenic mice. J. Biol. Chem. **266:** 24613–24620.
42. KEHAT, I. *et al*. 2006. Inhibition of basic leucine zipper transcription is a major mediator of atrial dilatation. Cardiovasc. Res. **70:** 543–554.
43. JIN, C. *et al*. 2001. Identification of mouse Jun dimerization protein 2 as a novel repressor of ATF-2. FEBS Lett. **489:** 34–41.
44. ARONHEIM, A., E. ZANDI, H. HENNEMANN, *et al*. 1997. Isolation of an AP-1 repressor by a novel method for detecting protein-protein interactions. Mol. Cell. Biol. **17:** 3094–3102.
45. HAI, T.W., F. LIU, W.J. COUKOS & M.R. GREEN 1989. Transcription factor ATF cDNA clones: an extensive family of leucine zipper proteins able to selectively form DNA-binding heterodimers. Genes Dev. **3:** 2083–2090.
46. HSU, J.C., R. BRAVO & R. TAUB 1992. Interactions among LRF-1, JunB, c-Jun, and c-Fos define a regulatory program in the G1 phase of liver regeneration. Mol. Cell. Biol. **12:** 4654–4665.
47. LIANG, G., C.D. WOLFGANG, B.P. CHEN, *et al*. 1996. ATF3 gene. Genomic organization, promotor, and regulation. J. Biol. Chem. **271:** 1695–1701.
48. LOWEY, S., G.S. WALLER & K.M. TRYBUS. 1993. Skeletal muscle myosin light chains are essential for physiological speeds of shortening. Nature **365:** 454–456.
49. HUANG, C. *et al*. 2003. Embryonic atrial function is essential for mouse embryogenesis, cardiac morphogenesis and angiogenesis. Development **130:** 6111–6119.
50. SANBE, A. *et al*. 1999. Abnormal cardiac structure and function in mice expressing nonphosphorylatable cardiac regulatory myosin light chain 2. J. Biol. Chem. **274:** 21085–21094.
51. GRIMM, M. *et al*. 2005. Key role of myosin light chain (MLC) kinase-mediated MLC2a phosphorylation in the alpha 1-adrenergic positive inotropic effect in human atrium. Cardiovasc. Res. **65:** 211–220.

Hypertrophy and Atrophy of the Heart

The Other Side of Remodeling

PETER RAZEGHI AND HEINRICH TAEGTMEYER

Division of Cardiology, University of Texas Houston Medical School, Houston, Texas, 77030, USA

ABSTRACT: The size of a cardiomyocyte is determined by relative rates of protein synthesis and degradation. Signaling pathways regulating myocardial protein synthesis have been extensively investigated, not the least because in patients hypertrophy increases cardiovascular morbidity and mortality. Until now strategies to reverse hypertrophy have relied on the inhibition of prohypertrophic signaling pathways. Here we review signaling pathways of atrophy in the heart and we present evidence in support of the idea that activating proatrophic signaling pathways in the presence of prohypertrophic signaling may be an attractive strategy to reverse hypertrophy.

KEYWORDS: atrophy; ubiquitin; proteasome; remodeling

INTRODUCTION

Left ventricular hypertrophy (LVH) is a feature of the failing heart[1] and associated with increased cardiovascular morbidity and mortality.[2] There is strong evidence for LVH to be maladaptive because pharmacological or transgenic inhibition of pressure-induced hypertrophy does not compromise cardiac function.[3,4] In addition, regression of hypertrophy improves cardiac function even in the presence of a sustained prohypertrophic stimulus.[5] Until now the focus for treatment of heart failure has been on the prevention, or on early recognition and delay of LVH. Reversal of LVH through activation of atrophic signaling pathways has not been extensively considered.[6]

In broad terms, hypertrophy is the result of an increase in the ratio of protein synthesis to protein degradation.[7] Prohypertrophic signals increase protein synthesis by well-known mechanisms.[8] Their effects on protein degradation is not known.[8] Attempts to reverse hypertrophy by inhibiting prohypertrophic signaling[9] is often unsuccessful in decreasing cell size, because of the great

---

Address for correspondence: Heinrich Taegtmeyer, University of Texas Houston Medical School, 6431 Fannin, MSB 1.246, Houston, TX 77030. Voice: 713-500-6569; fax: 713-500-0637.
e-mail: Heinrich.Taegtmeyer@uth.tmc.edu

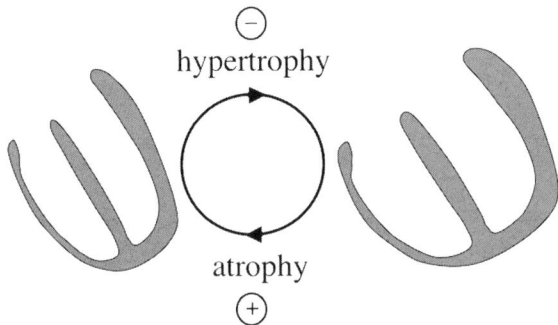

FIGURE 1. Cardiac hypertrophy can be reversed by inhibiting prohypertrophic or activating proatrophic signaling pathways.

redundancy of prohypertrophic signaling pathways. An alternative way to reverse hypertrophy is the activation of protein degradation. This mechanism would also rebalance the protein turnover, even in the presence of prohypertrophic signaling (FIG. 1). Such an approach does not depend on the inhibition of the key regulatory component of a complex signaling network, but rather on the activation of a single pathway. Such a strategy would make it necessary to understand the pathways regulating protein degradation in the heart. We will therefore discuss different models and signaling pathways of cardiac atrophy, and we will highlight potential targets for antihypertrophic therapy.

SIGNALING PATHWAYS REGULATING PROTEIN DEGRADATION

Like hypertrophy, atrophy can also be caused by a variety of different stimuli (e.g., disuse, cachexia, starvation, denervation). At present, relatively little is known about signaling pathways regulating atrophy in the heart. Most of our knowledge is derived from skeletal muscle where three major proteolytic systems have been identified: (*a*) the calcium-dependent calpain system, (*b*) the lysosomal protease system, and (*c*) the ubiquitin proteasome system (UPS) (FIG. 2).[10] Although we will mainly discuss the UPS, we will begin with the two other proteolytic systems.

(1) The calcium-dependent calpain system is part of the early process of proteolysis. Calpains exist in two forms, microcalpain and millicalpain.[11] The terms *microcalpain* and *millicalpain* refer to the micromolar calcium-requiring and the millimolar calcium-requiring proteases, respectively. Calpains are regulated by the intracellular calcium concentration, by their endogenous inhibitor calpastatin, and possibly by their

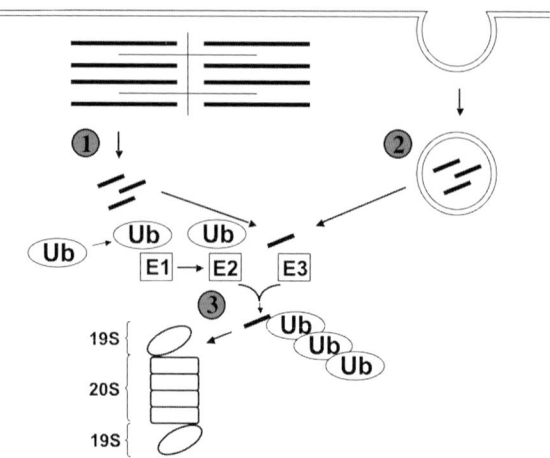

FIGURE 2. Protein degradation in muscle is regulated by three major pathways, which are connected with each other. (1) Calpains disintegrate myofibrillar proteins. (2) Lysosomes mainly degrade membranous and extracellular proteins. (3) The UPS is responsible for the major bulk of protein degradation during atrophy.

intracellular location.[11] Calpains disintegrate myofibrillar proteins and make them available for the UPS. Inhibition of calpains during skeletal muscle unloading attenuates muscle atrophy.[12] The calpain system exists in the heart and is involved in ischemia reperfusion-induced injury.[13] In an animal model of myocardial infarction pharmacological inhibition of the calpains reduces infarct size, but the role of calpains in physiologic protein turnover of the heart is not yet established.[14] Preliminary data suggest that the calpain system is activated during atrophic remodeling of the unloaded normal rat heart and the unloaded failing human heart (Razeghi and Taegtmeyer, unpublished results).

(2) Lysosomes are cell organelles that contain several acid proteases (e.g., cathepsins B, D, H, and L) and other hydrolases. Lysosomal proteolysis is involved in the degradation of membranous proteins (e.g., membrane receptors), but is not quantitatively important in the breakdown of muscle proteins in catabolic states.[15] Inhibition of lysosomal protein degradation does not significantly decrease myofibrillar proteolysis in the unloaded skeletal muscle.[16] Although lysosomal proteinases do not contribute to the bulk of myofibrillar protein degradation, they may contribute to the atrophy phenotype by degrading membrane-associated proteins. Alterations in the distribution of lysosomal enzyme activities from sedimented (intact lysosomes) to nonsedimented (fragmented lysosomes) seem to correlate with increased proteolysis in perfused rat heart,[17] and the total activity of Cathepsin D changes during thyrotoxic cardiac hypertrophy[18] and its regression.[19]

(3) The selective degradation of many short-lived proteins in eukaryotic cells is carried out by the UPS.[20] In this pathway, proteins are targeted for degradation by covalent ligation to ubiquitin, a highly conserved peptide. The ligation of ubiquitin was discovered as an "ATP dependent proteolysis factor" (APF1)[21] because it is energy dependent.[22] It involves the successive action of three types of enzymes (FIG. 2). Ubiquitin is activated by the ubiquitin-activating enzyme (E1) in an ATP-dependent reaction. Activated ubiquitin is transferred to an ubiquitin-conjugating enzyme (E2) and then linked to the lysine residue in proteins destined for degradation. This reaction is catalyzed by the ubiquitin ligases (E3). The same process is repeated to form an ubiquitin chain. The ubiquitin-conjugated proteins are recognized by the 19S subunit of the proteasome and subsequently degraded into peptides in the 20S core proteasome. The peptides are then released from the proteasome and degraded to amino acids by peptidases in the cytoplasma. Our recent work suggests that this pathway is prominent in cardiac atrophy *in vivo*.[23,24] Here, it needs to be emphasized that ubiquitination and degradation of proteins not only control cell size, but also cell function at many different levels, from transcriptional activity to enzyme activity.

PROTEIN TURNOVER IN CARDIAC ATROPHY

Cardiac atrophy can be induced by hormonal, nutritional, and mechanical interventions. Early studies examined cardiac atrophy after hypophysectomy and thyroidectomy.[25-27] Ablation of hormones from the pituitary gland and/or the thyroid gland suppresses protein synthesis and increases the activity of the lysosomal enzyme Cathepsin D, leading to a reduction in the cardiomyocyte cross-sectional area.[25-27] Consistent with the decrease in protein synthesis is the decrease in myocardial polysomes after hypophysectomy.[25] Interestingly the amount of ribosomal subunits increases in the same model, suggesting decreased efficiency in the polysome assembly.[25]

Similar to the atrophy models induced by hormonal ablation, nutrient deprivation also decreases heart size and delays physiologic cardiac growth.[28-30] Starvation downregulates proteins synthesis and increases fractional rates of protein degradation. Increased protein degradation is associated with increased activity of Cathepsin D, suggesting that this model also activates lysosomal proteolysis.[29]

The plasticity of the myocardium to respond to changes in load was first demonstrated in a model of unloading induced by severing the chordae tendineae of a single right ventricular papillary muscle.[31] Unloading induced a decrease in the cardiomyocyte cross-sectional area and mitochondrial density, while myofibrillar disarray increased.[31,32] In addition, large areas of cytoplasm became devoid of organelles. The plasticity of atrophic remodeling in the heart is given by the fact that reloading the papillary muscle by attaching its apex to the ventricular-free wall reversed unloading-induced changes in the cardiomyocyte.[31]

Another model used to study unloading-induced cardiac atrophy is the heterotopically transplanted heart. This model can be applied to the normal, ischemic, or hypertrophied heart resembling in many ways the failing human heart supported with a mechanical assist device.[33–36] In addition, the transplantation of hearts of genetically modified animals allows to study mechanisms of reverse remodeling. The heterotopically transplanted rat heart rapidly decreases in size within a few days after surgery, but continues to beat.[23] The decrease in heart size is mainly caused by a decrease in cell size rather than a loss of cells through apoptosis.[37] The reduction of heart size may be prevented by isovolumic loading and reloading the transplanted rat heart *ex vivo* reverses unloading-induced changes in metabolic gene expression.[33,38] These findings suggest that load, rather then denervation, regulates cardiac atrophy and metabolic gene expression in the heterotopically transplanted rat heart.

Unloading induced atrophy is associated with an increase in the expression of ubiquitin B, the ubiquitin-conjugating enzyme UbcH2, and polyubiquitinated proteins, suggesting that the UPS is activated in the heterotopically transplanted rat heart.[23,24] While a coherent concept of protein degradation seems to emerge, the effect of mechanical unloading on protein synthesis remains a controversial issue. The rate of total protein synthesis decreases in the heterotopically transplanted rat heart, while the fractional protein synthesis rate shows a nonsignificant increase in the same study.[39] Measuring specific radioactivity of sarcomeric polypeptides, others found a relative increase in polypeptide synthesis in the same model.[40] The latter finding is consistent with an increase in the activity of downstream effectors of the mammalian target of rapamycin (mTOR) in the unloaded rat heart.[23] MTOR is a central regulator of proteins synthesis and regulates the activity of p70S6k and 4EBP1, two critical regulators of protein synthesis. Consistent with the increase in mTOR activity in the unloaded rat heart, rapamycin augments unloading-induced cardiac atrophy.[23] One possible explanation for the activation of mTOR is the increase of insulin-like growth factor 1 (IGF-1) in the transplanted heart.[41] IGF-1 activates mTOR by Akt dependent and independent pathways.[42] Because Akt is not activated in the heterotopically transplanted rat heart, mTOR must be activated by Akt independent pathways in this model of cardiac atrophy.[41] Also consistent with the increase in protein synthesis in the unloaded rat heart is the increase of transcriptional regulators of ribosomal biogenesis and the activation of a hypertrophic gene program.[43] We have therefore proposed, that atrophic remodeling of the unloaded heart activates both protein synthesis and degradation.[44] Because atrophy decreases cell mass, protein degradation must outweigh protein synthesis. Interestingly, transcriptional regulators of the UPS also increase during hypertrophic remodeling of the heart, suggesting that protein degradation increases in the hypertrophied heart, albeit to a lesser degree than protein synthesis.[24] Therefore, load-induced changes in myocardial mass increase both protein synthesis and degradation. The relative balance of these two processes determines the trophic response.[44]

REGULATORS OF ATROPHY AS POTENTIAL TARGETS TO REVERSE HYPERTROPHY

The activation of proatrophic signaling pathways reverses cardiac hypertrophy. This approach may be more successful than inhibiting prohypertrophic signaling, because it allows to reverse hypertrophy in the presence of prohypertrophic signals and does not rely on the complete inhibition of a network of redundant pathways. In order to apply this novel strategy to reverse hypertrophy, it is necessary to identify key regulators of cardiac atrophy. Most attention has been paid to the two ubiquitin ligases: Muscle and atrophy F-box protein (Mafbx) and Atrogin-1 and Muscle and Ring Finger protein-1 (MuRF-1). Both ligases were discovered in models of skeletal muscle atrophy and were found to be essential for the atrophic response.[45,46] Transcriptional regulators of these ligases are the forkhead transcription factors of the FOXO subgroup (e.g., FOXO3a).[47] The nuclear translocation of these transcription factors is inhibited by phosphorylation through Akt.[47] Transfection of cardiomyocytes with FOXO3a or Mafbx/Atrogin-1 decreases cell size and reverses cardiac hypertrophy.[48-50] A possible mechanism for this effect is that Mafbx/Atrogin-1 targets the prohypertrophic phosphatase calcineurin for ubiquitin-mediated proteolysis.[49] In addition, MuRF-1 inhibits protein kinase C epsilon activation, suggesting that both ligases induce atrophy by inhibiting prohypertrophic signaling.[50]

Unexpectedly, the expression of Mafbx/Atrogin-1 and MuRF-1 decreases in the unloaded rat heart and increases with pressure overload (FIG. 3).[24] One explanation for the decrease of both ligases in the heterotopically transplanted rat heart is the increase in IGF-1 in the same model.[41] IGF-1 inhibits FOXO3a activation and therefore the transcription of both ligases.[48] The transcriptional increase of both ligases during pressure overload-induced hypertrophy maybe an adaptive response to prevent an excessive increase in myocardial mass, because transfection of Mafbx/Atrogin-1 in the same model reverses hypertrophy.[49] Because both ligases reverse hypertrophy by inhibiting prohypertrophic signaling, it will be important to investigate whether other proatrophic signaling pathways exist, which reverse hypertrophy independent of the inhibition of prohypertrophic signaling. Attractive targets are the calpain system (discussed above) and the NF-κB signaling pathway. Both systems are important regulators in skeletal muscle atrophy,[51,52] and preliminary data show that they

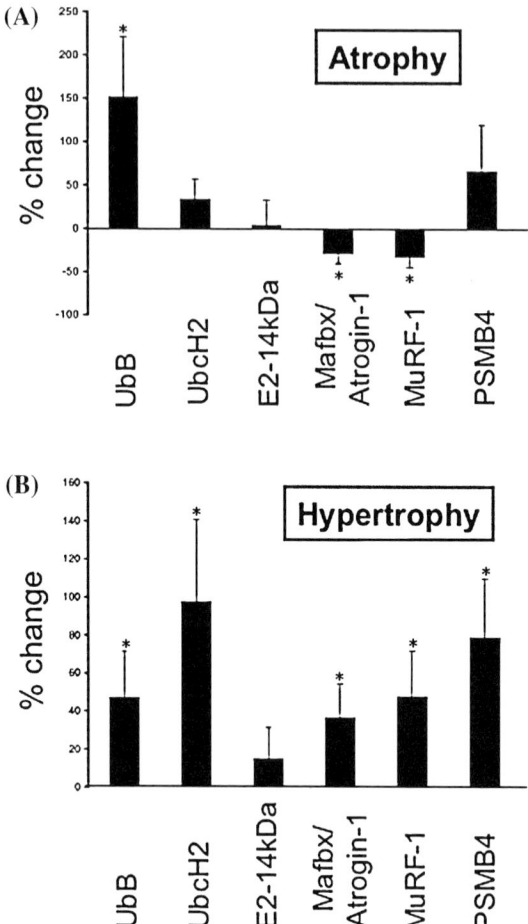

FIGURE 3. Myocardial transcript levels of regulators of the UPS are differentially expressed during (**A**) unloading-induced atrophy (*significant changes, $n = 7$) and (**B**) pressure-induced hypertrophy (*significant changes, $n = 5$).[24] (Reprinted with permission.)

are activated during atrophic remodeling of the unloaded rat heart (Razeghi & Taegtmeyer, unpublished results).

SUMMARY

The dynamic nature of protein turnover that was recognized already more than half a century ago[53] endows the heart with the plasticity to respond to multiple environmental stimuli (e.g., load, nutrients, or oxygen supply). Protein turnover is a function of protein synthesis and degradation. A refined understanding in the regulation of protein degradation in the heart seems to be essential for the development of strategies to rebuild the cardiomyocyte "from within."

ACKNOWLEDGMENTS

We thank Roxy Ann Tate for help with the preparation of the manuscript and past as well as present members of the laboratory for many discussions. Work in the laboratory is supported by a grant from the National Heart, Lung and Blood Institute (R01-HL-61483). P.R. is the recipient of a fellowship from the Roderick Duncan MacDonald Foundation of St. Luke's Episcopal Hospital, Houston, Texas.

REFERENCES

1. IZUMO, S. & H. AOKI. 1998. Calcineurin–the missing link in cardiac hypertrophy. Nat. Med. **4:** 661–662.
2. LEVY, D. et al. 1990. Prognostic implications of echocardiographically determined left ventricular mass in the Framingham Heart Study. N. Engl. J. Med. **322:** 1561–1566.
3. HILL, J.A. et al. 2000. Cardiac hypertrophy is not a required compensatory response to short-term pressure overload. Circulation **101:** 2863–2869.
4. ICHIHARA, S. et al. 2001. Angiotensin II type 2 receptor is essential for left ventricular hypertrophy and cardiac fibrosis in chronic angiotensin II-induced hypertension. Circulation **104:** 346–351.
5. ESPOSITO, G. et al. 2002. Genetic alterations that inhibit in vivo pressure-overload hypertrophy prevent cardiac dysfunction despite increased wall stress. Circulation **105:** 85–92.
6. PATTERSON, C. & D. CYR. 2002. Welcome to the machine: a cardiologist's introduction to protein folding and degradation. Circulation **106:** 2741–2746.
7. MEERSON, F.Z. 1983. The Failing Heart: adaptation and Deadaptation. pp.1–5. Raven Press. New York.
8. MORGAN, H.E. et al. 1987. Biochemical mechanisms of cardiac hypertrophy. Annu. Rev. Physiol. **49:** 533–543.
9. FREY, N. et al. 2004. Hypertrophy of the heart: a new therapeutic target? Circulation **109:** 1580–1589.
10. JACKMAN, R.W. & S.C. KANDARIAN. 2004. The molecular basis of skeletal muscle atrophy. Am. J. Physiol. Cell. Physiol. **287:** C834–C843.
11. GOLL, D.E. et al. 2003. The calpain system. Physiol. Rev. **83:** 731–801.
12. TIDBALL, J.G. & M.J. SPENCER. 2002. Expression of a calpastatin transgene slows muscle wasting and obviates changes in myosin isoform expression during murine muscle disuse. J. Physiol. **545:** 819–828.
13. SINGH, R.B. et al. 2004. The sarcoplasmic reticulum proteins are targets for calpain action in the ischemic-reperfused heart. J. Mol. Cell. Cardiol. **37:** 101–110.
14. IWAMOTO, H. et al. 1999. Calpain inhibitor-1 reduces infarct size and DNA fragmentation of myocardium in ischemic/reperfused rat heart. J. Cardiovasc. Pharmacol. **33:** 580–586.

15. LOWELL, B.B., N.B. RUDERMAN & M.N. GOODMAN. 1986. Evidence that lysosomes are not involved in the degradation of myofibrillar proteins in rat skeletal muscle. Biochem. J. **234:** 237–240.
16. TAILLANDIER, D. et al. 1996. Coordinate activation of lysosomal, Ca 2+-activated and ATP-ubiquitin-dependent proteinases in the unweighted rat soleus muscle. Biochem. J. **316:** 65–72.
17. RANNELS, D.E., R. KAO & H.E. MORGAN. 1975. Effect of insulin on protein turnover in heart muscle. J. Biol. Chem. **250:** 1694–1701.
18. WILDENTHAL, K. & E.A. MUELLER. 1974. Increased myocardial cathepsin D activity during regression of thyrotoxic cardiac hypertrophy. Nature **249:** 478–479.
19. WILDENTHAL, K. & J.S. CRIE. 1980. Lysosomes and cardiac protein catabolism. In Degradative Processes in Heart and Skeletal Muscle. K. Wildenthal, Ed.: 113–129. Elsevier/North Holland. New York.
20. GOLDBERG, A.L. 2005. Nobel committee tags ubiquitin for distinction. Neuron **45:** 339–344.
21. CIEHANOVER, A., Y. HOD & A. HERSHKO. 1978. A heat-stable polypeptide component of an ATP-dependent proteolytic system from reticulocytes. Biochem. Biophys. Res. Commun. **81:** 1100–1105.
22. HERSHKO, A., A. CIECHANOVER & I.A. ROSE. 1979. Resolution of the ATP-dependent proteolytic system from reticulocytes: a component that interacts with ATP. Proc. Natl. Acad. Sci. USA **76:** 3107–3110.
23. RAZEGHI, P. et al. 2003. Atrophic remodeling of the heart in vivo simultaneously activates pathways of protein synthesis and degradation. Circulation **108:** 2536–2541.
24. RAZEGHI, P. et al. 2006. Atrophy, hypertrophy, and hypoxemia induce transcriptional regulators of the ubiquitin proteasome system in the rat heart. Biochem. Biophys. Res. Commun. **342:** 361–364.
25. HJALMARSON, A.C. et al. 1975. Effects of hypophysectomy, growth hormone, and thyroxine on protein turnover in heart. J. Biol. Chem. **250:** 4556–4561.
26. LIU, Z. & A.M. GERDES. 1990. Influence of hypothyroidism and the reversal of hypothyroidism on hemodynamics and cell size in the adult rat heart. J. Mol. Cell. Cardiol. **22:** 1339–1348.
27. KATZEFF, H.L., K.M. OJAMAA & I. KLEIN. 1994. Effects of exercise on protein synthesis and myosin heavy chain gene expression in hypothyroid rats. Am. J. Physiol. **267:** E63–E67.
28. KUYKENDALL, R. et al. 1987. Biochemical consequences of protein depletion in the rabbit heart. J. Surg. Res. **43:** 62–67.
29. SAMAREL, A.M. et al. 1987. Protein synthesis and degradation during starvation-induced cardiac atrophy in rabbits. Circ. Res. **60:** 933–941.
30. GOLDSPINK, D.F., S.E. LEWIS & B.J. MERRY. 1986. Effects of aging and long term dietary intervention on protein turnover and growth of ventricular muscle in the rat heart. Cardiovasc. Res. **20:** 672–678.
31. THOMPSON, E.W. et al. 1984. Atrophy reversal and cardiocyte redifferentiation in reloaded cat myocardium. Circ. Res. **54:** 367–377.
32. TOMANEK, R.J. & G.T. COOPER. 1981. Morphological changes in the mechanically unloaded myocardial cell. Anat. Rec. **200:** 271–280.
33. DEPRE, C. et al. 1998. Unloaded heart in vivo replicates fetal gene expression of cardiac hypertrophy. Nat. Med. **4:** 1269–1275.

34. TEVAEARAI, H.T. et al. 2002. Myocardial gene transfer and overexpression of beta2-adrenergic receptors potentiates the functional recovery of unloaded failing hearts. Circulation **106:** 124–129.
35. TSUNEYOSHI, H. et al. 2005. Heterotopic transplantation of the failing rat heart as a model of left ventricular mechanical unloading toward recovery. Asaio J. **51:** 116–120.
36. MCGOWAN, B.S. et al. 2003. Unloading-induced remodeling in the normal and hypertrophic left ventricle. Am. J. Physiol. Heart Circ. Physiol. **284:** H2061–H2068.
37. SCHENA, S. et al. 2004. Effects of ventricular unloading on apoptosis and atrophy of cardiac myocytes. J. Surg. Res. **120:** 119–126.
38. KLEIN, I., C. HONG & S.S. SCHREIBER. 1991. Isovolumic loading prevents atrophy of the heterotopically transplanted rat heart. Circ. Res. **69:** 1421–1425.
39. KLEIN, I. et al. 1991. Heterotopic cardiac transplantation decreases the capacity of rat myocardial protein synthesis. Circ. Res. **68:** 1100–1107.
40. LEWIS, W. et al. 1991. Altered cytoskeletal protein synthesis in rat cardiac isografts. J. Heart Lung Transplant. **10:** 92–99.
41. SHARMA, S. et al. 2006. Atrophic remodeling of the transplanted rat heart. Cardiology **105:** 128–136.
42. SONG, Y.H. et al. 2005. Insulin-like growth factor I-mediated skeletal muscle hypertrophy is characterized by increased mTOR-p70S6K signaling without increased Akt phosphorylation. J. Investig. Med. **53:** 135–142.
43. RAZEGHI, P., N. PALANICHAMY, S. STEPKOWSKI, et al. 2006. Transcriptional regulators of ribosomal biogenesisare increased in the unloaded heart. FASEB J. **20:** 1090–1096.
44. RAZEGHI, P. & H. TAEGTMEYER. 2005. Cardiac remodeling: UPS lost in transit. Circ. Res. **97:** 964–966.
45. BODINE, S.C. et al. 2001. Identification of ubiquitin ligases required for skeletal muscle atrophy. Science **294:** 1704–1708.
46. GOMES, M. et al. 2001. Atrogin-1, a muscle-specific F-box protein highly expressed during muscle atrophy. Proc. Natl. Acad. Sci. USA **98:** 14440–14445.
47. STITT, T.N. et al. 2004. The IGF-1/PI3K/Akt pathway prevents expression of muscle atrophy-induced ubiquitin ligases by inhibiting FOXO transcription factors. Mol. Cell. **14:** 395–403.
48. SKURK, C. et al. 2005. The FOXO3a transcription factor regulates cardiac myocyte size downstream of AKT signaling. J. Biol. Chem. **280:** 20814–20823.
49. LI, H.H. et al. 2004. Atrogin-1/muscle atrophy F-box inhibits calcineurin-dependent cardiac hypertrophy by participating in an SCF ubiquitin ligase complex. J. Clin. Invest. **114:** 1058–1071.
50. ARYA, R. et al. 2004. Muscle ring finger protein-1 inhibits PKC{epsilon} activation and prevents cardiomyocyte hypertrophy. J. Cell. Biol. **167:** 1147–1159.
51. VOISIN, L. et al. 1996. Muscle wasting in a rat model of long-lasting sepsis results from the activation of lysosomal, Ca2+-activated, and ubiquitin-proteasome proteolytic pathways. J. Clin. Invest. **97:** 1610–1617.
52. HUNTER, R.B. & S.C. KANDARIAN. 2004. Disruption of either the Nfkb1 or the Bcl3 gene inhibits skeletal muscle atrophy. J. Clin. Invest. **114:** 1504–1511.
53. SCHOENHEIMER, R. 1942. The Dynamic State of Body Constituents. Harvard University Press. Cambridge, MA.

Role of Cellular Compartmentation in the Metabolic Response to Stress

Mechanistic Insights from Computational Models

LUFANG ZHOU,[a,d] XIN YU,[a,d] MARCO E. CABRERA,[a,b,c,d] AND WILLIAM C. STANLEY[c,d]

[a]*Department of Biomedical Engineering,* [b]*Department of Pediatrics,* [c]*Departments of Physiology and Biophysics, and* [d]*Center for Modeling Integrated Metabolic Systems, Case Western Reserve University, Cleveland, Ohio, 44106-4970 USA*

ABSTRACT: The mechanisms controlling ATP generation in the transition from normal resting conditions to either high work states or ischemia are poorly understood. ATP generation depends upon compartmentation between the mitochondria and cytosol of metabolic pathways and key energy transfer species that cannot be easily assessed experimentally. We developed a multicompartment mathematical model of cardiac metabolism to simulate the metabolic responses to ischemia and increased workload. The model is based on mass balances, transport, and metabolic processes in cardiac tissue, and has three distinct compartments (blood, cytosol, and mitochondria). In addition to distinguishing between cytosol and mitochondria, the model includes a cytosolic subcompartment for glycolytic metabolic channeling. The model simulations predict the rapid activation of glycogenolysis and lactate production at the onset of ischemia, and support the concept of localization of glycolysis to a cytosolic subcompartment. In addition, simulations show that mitochondrial $NADH/NAD^+$ is primarily determined by oxygen consumption during ischemia, while cytosolic $NADH/NAD^+$ and lactate production are largely a function of glycolytic flux during the initial phase, and is controlled by mitochondrial $NADH/NAD^+$ and the malate–aspartate shuttle during the steady state. Finally, the model predicts that metabolic activation with an abrupt increase in workload requires parallel activation of ATP hydrolysis, glycolysis, mitochondrial dehydrogenases, the electron transport chain, and ADP phosphorylation. Taken together, these studies demonstrate the importance of metabolic compartmentation in the regulation of cardiac energetics in response to acute stress, and they highlight the usefulness of computational models in this line of investigation.

Address for correspondence: W.C. Stanley, Department of Physiology and Biophysics, Case Western Reserve University, 10900 Euclid Avenue, Cleveland, OH 44106-4970.
 e-mail: wcs4@case.edu

KEYWORDS: exercise; diabetes; ischemia; glycolysis; mitochondria; NADH; simulations

INTRODUCTION

The regulation of cardiac energy metabolism involves not only metabolites, reactions, and transport processes, but also regional blood flow, work demand, contractility, and hormone levels.[1] Normal contractile function is exquisitely linked to mitochondrial ATP formation by oxidative metabolism, and maintenance of cytosolic ATP for sarcomere shortening and Ca^{2+} uptake into the sarcoplasmic reticulum (FIG. 1). Many *in vivo* and *in vitro* experiments have been done to elucidate the regulatory roles of various components under normal and diseased conditions. These studies have produced an immense amount of biological information, such as enzyme characterization and gene identification; however, accumulation of such knowledge has not led to a quantitative understanding of the factors that regulate fluxes in different pathways in the heart. As a complementary tool, physiologically based mathematical models that incorporate cellular metabolic reactions and transport processes can provide more quantitative insights into the system. In this short article, the progress of metabolic modeling is presented, and then a multicompartment model of cardiac cellular metabolism is developed. Finally, the future work and applications are suggested.

Advantages of Models of Cardiac Metabolism

Although every model is an approximation of the system it represents, a well-developed model can provide significant insight into the processes of the system. One of the potential benefits of a model is prediction of changes that are difficult or impossible to measure in the experimental system. For example, a physiologically based multicompartmental model of cardiac metabolism can predict changes in the key regulatory species that are difficult to measure experimentally, for example, cytosolic and mitochondrial ATP, ADP, NADH, and NAD^+.[2] Another benefit of a mathematical metabolic model is that it can provide dynamic responses for key metabolites and pathway fluxes during the transition from normal to stressed conditions.[3,4] This information can supplement experimental data that can be obtained for only a few discrete time points. Metabolic models can show how different metabolites, reactions, and transport processes interact *in vivo* as an effective network, and provides quantitative and systematic insights into the basic mechanisms of complex metabolic system. Furthermore, such modeling could aid in determining the effects of potential therapeutic approaches for optimizing cardiac metabolism, as well as in the development and evaluation of drugs.

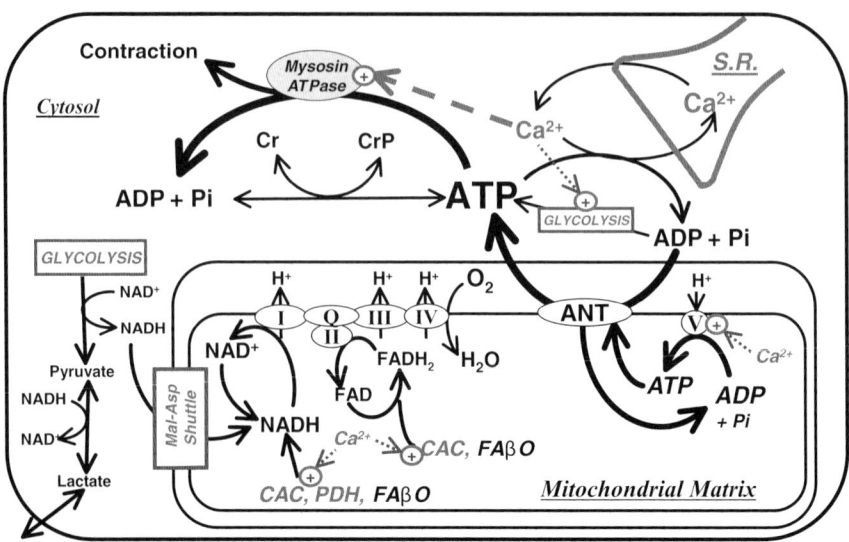

FIGURE 1. Schematic depiction of myocardial energy metabolism. In the cytosol ATP hydrolyzed to fuel contraction and Ca^{2+} uptake into the sarcoplasmic reticulum (SR) to allow for relaxation. Glycolysis forms NADH, which is either reduced to NAD^+ with lactate formation, or shuttled into the mitochondrial matrix. Mitochondrial substrate oxidation generates NADH and $FADH_2$, which drives electron transport chain (ETC) flux and the proton gradient and oxygen consumption at complex IV (also known as the F_0/F_1-ATPase), which provides the energy for ATP formation by complex V. Abbreviations: CAC, citric acid cycle; PDH, pyruvate dehydrogenase; ANT, adenine nucleotide translocase.

EARLIER MODELS OF CARDIAC METABOLISM

The process of developing quantitative models of the heart at various levels of complexity has evolved over last four decades, using the approach of either top-town or bottle-up.[5] Existing models at the cellular level have focused on excitation–contraction coupling,[6–9] substrate delivery, and transmembrane transport.[10,11] At the tissue and whole organ level, Hunter et al. have developed a three-dimensional model of a functional contracting heart with various components.[12] However, those elements necessary to sustain the contractile activity of the heart (e.g., blood flow, substrate and oxygen delivery, and substrate and energy metabolism) have not been incorporated into these models. Current metabolic models lack Ca^{2+} transients, excitation–contraction coupling, cellular biomechanics, and incorporate limited aspects of glycolysis, the citric acid cycle (CAC), and oxidative phosphorylation.[13–16] In the following sections, some examples of mathematical models of metabolic system are reviewed, especially related to cardiac substrate metabolism.

Early mathematical models of cardiac metabolism considered glucose as the sole energy source and focused on the control mechanism of glycolysis. Chance et al.[15] developed a kinetic model that includes each reaction in glycolysis, oxidative phosphorylation, and ATP utilization in ascites tumor cells, and simulated the metabolic responses of these cells to endogenous substrate, the addition of glucose, and inhibition of both sources. Achs et al.[13] further developed this model and applied it to beef heart supernatant. In contrast to the model of Chance et al.,[15] mitochondrial reactions and the conversion of glucose to glucose-6-phosphate (G 6-p) were deleted, but myosin kinase and ATPase were added. Although simulated results agreed well with the experimental data, the values of enzyme properties (K_m and V_{max}) in the model differed from those measured experimentally.

Several groups have modeled glycolysis based on metabolic control analysis (MCA), which uses sensitivity analysis to examine the effects of specific reaction on the fluxes and metabolite concentrations of metabolic system.[17] Using MCA, Kashiwaya et al. studied the control mechanism of glucose utilization in perfused rat hearts.[18] In particular, they investigated the effect of additions of ketone bodies and/or insulin on glucose utilization. Their model included glucose transport, glucose phosphorylation, and all the reactions in glycolytic process, as well as glycogen synthesis and breakdown. Model analysis indicated that the control of the rate of glucose utilization in the rat heart is not exerted by a single enzyme of glycolytic pathway, but is distributed among enzymes depending upon substrate availability, hormonal stimulation, or other changes in metabolic conditions.

Vogt et al.[19] developed a model using MCA to examine the regulation of glycolytic flux in hibernating myocardium. In modeling glycolysis, they included glucose transport and the pathway from glucose phosphorylation through G 6-P to lactate (anaerobic glycolysis). They found that three enzymes (glucose-phosphate isomerase, phosphoglycerate mutase, enolase) produce the greatest effect in flux control. They concluded that the control of anaerobic glycolytic flux in hibernating human myocardium is achieved from flux modulation at several sites in glycolysis. They further addressed the issue of regulation of glycolysis by using enzymatic and metabolite data obtained from pigs subjected to ischemic preconditioning. In this model representation, they did not include glucose uptake because experimentally the hearts were subjected to total ischemia in which glycogen is the sole fuel for glycolysis. Again, their analysis suggested that the control of glycolysis during complete ischemia could not be attributed to substrate availability or to the control of single enzyme, regardless whether the hearts were initially preconditioned or not. With these two different myocardial disease states, their studies employing MCA indicated that regulation of glycolysis occurs at multiple sites, and that the simple concept of a "rate limiting step" in glycolysis does not apply to the heart.

Mathematical Modeling of Cardiac Metabolism During Ischemia

Computational models of physiological systems have been developed as a way to gain a quantitative understanding of the underlying physiological or biochemical mechanisms responsible for the system responses to known inputs. Cabrera et al. developed a mathematical model for muscle metabolism using a top-down approach and studied the regulation of muscle lactate production under hypoxic and ischemic conditions.[20,21] Their model was based on dynamic mass balances and mechanistic kinetics for substrates and control metabolites and contained many key reactions involved in energy metabolism (e.g., glycolysis, glycogeneolysis, glycogenesis, pyruvate oxidation, and oxidative phosphorylation). Ch'en et al. applied a model of glycolysis to study myocardial ischemia and reperfusion using NMR spectroscopy data obtained from isolated perfused rat hearts undergoing global ischemia.[14] This model incorporated changes in pH and several metabolites in order to simulate both Ca^{2+} overload arrhythmias and reperfusion-induced arrhythmias. Their simulations corresponded to a limited set of the experimental data during myocardial ischemia.

Using a more comprehensive model of cardiac cellular metabolism, Salem et al.[22] simulated the dynamics responses of metabolite concentrations and metabolic processes to ischemia (60% reduction in the myocardial blood flow). This model was based on mass balance and chemical reactions and included most key metabolites (glucose, lactate, fatty acids, NADH, NAD, etc.) and pathways (glycolysis, fatty acid oxidation, pyruvate oxidation, oxidative phosphorylation, etc.) involved in cardiac energy metabolism. With this model, potential regulatory mechanisms underlying metabolic changes could be examined. The model parameters were estimated based on experimental data in pigs and dogs. This model was able to simulate the steady-state responses to ischemia that were in agreement with experimental observations from large animal studies, such as the changes in oxygen consumption, glucose and lactate uptake, as well as glycogen, lactate and ATP concentrations. In their following study,[4] they simulated the responses of cardiac metabolism to different levels of ischemia (from 10% to 80% reductions in coronary blood flow) and investigated the regulatory mechanisms responsible for glycolysis and lactate formation under ischemic conditions. They found that changes in phosphorylation state ([ATP]/[ADP]) and glucose uptake affect the initial phase of the glycolytic response to ischemia, while glycogen breakdown exerts control over glycolysis during the entire duration of ischemia. Similarly, changes in the redox state ([NADH]/[NAD^+]) affect the rates of lactate formation and release primarily during the initial transient phase of the response ischemia, while the rate of glycolysis controls the rate of lactate formation throughout the entire period of ischemia.

The models by Salem et al. were limited by the simplified structure of the cell, consisting of a single compartment, with no separation of cytosol from the mitochondria. Therefore, processes that are known to occur only in the cytosol (e.g., glycolysis) could not be distinguished from those that are unique to the mitochondrial matrix (e.g., CAC, electron transport chain [ETC]). As a result, this model could not accurately predict the dynamics at the onset of ischemia, specifically the rapid activation of glycogen breakdown, glycolysis, and the switch from myocardial lactate uptake to production observed in validation studies performed in swine.[3,22]

Modeling Cardiac Metabolism with Increased Power Generation

The basic function of the heart is to pump blood into the circulatory system through the contraction of cardiac myocytes using the energy from ATP hydrolysis. In the transition from normal cardiac workload to the high workloads required during physical exercise, there is up to a fivefold increase in the rates of left ventricular external power, myocardial oxygen consumption (MVO_2), and ATP turnover in the healthy heart.[23] Even with this increased workload, the concentrations of energy transfer species (e.g., ATP and ADP) remain at a relatively constant level,[24,25] reflecting the rapid and simultaneous activation of metabolism of carbon fuels, NADH generation, ETC flux, and oxidative phosphorylation in the mitochondria. The failure of this metabolic homeostasis in the transition from rest to an increase in demand for cardiac power results in myocardial ischemia, as evidenced by activation of anaerobic glycolysis and contractile dysfunction.[26,27] While this complex activation of multiple metabolic processes is necessary for maintaining cell function and the survival of the organism, modeling this phenomenon is a challenge.

The initial hypotheses for the control of the ATP formation by oxidative phosphorylation in response to increased energy demand was the respiratory control mechanism proposed by Chance,[28] where mitochondrial ATP production is limited by the ADP availability in the mitochondrial matrix.[28,29] With increased workload, ATP hydrolysis is activated, ADP concentration increases in the matrix, and the influx of protons through the F_0/F_1-ATPase and ATP synthesis are increased. Consequently, the flux of electrons and extrusion of protons intensifies, causing increased NADH production by the CAC, with greater pyruvate and fatty acids oxidation. Thus feedback from ATP hydrolysis stimulates oxidative phosphorylation. While this hypothesis holds true in isolated mitochondria under some experimental conditions, it is not supported by experimental observations *in vivo*, which show constant concentrations of ATP and ADP during the transition from low to high work states.[29]

An alternative regulatory mechanism, the parallel activation hypothesis, proposes simultaneous direct activation of ATP utilization and production by an increase in Ca^{2+}.[30] The increase in the cytosolic Ca^{2+} transient with the increase in cardiac workload results in an increase in $[Ca^{2+}]$ in the mitochondrial matrix, which activates PDH and the CAC cycle flux.[31,32] Consequently, this produces more reducing equivalents (NADH and $FADH_2$),[32] which increases flux through the ETC and the proton-motive force, and enhances ATP production. Simulations from an integrated computational model of cardiac mitochondrial energy metabolism demonstrate that an increase in Ca^{2+} concentration in the mitochondrial matrix activates NADH generation and oxidative phosphorylation.[33] This model is limited by the lack of inclusion of pyruvate and fatty acids oxidation, nor the exchange of $NADH/NAD^+$ between cytosol and mitochondria, which are important factors of maintaining reducing equivalent balance. Korzeniewski et al. found support for the parallel-activation mechanism in skeletal muscle and the heart using a dynamic computer model of oxidative phosphorylation,[30,34] but this model involved only oxidative phosphorylation, ATP transport and utilization, and did not incorporate metabolic pathways for substrate metabolism and NADH generation. A more comprehensive mathematical model incorporating simultaneous activation of ATP hydrolysis, dehydrogenases, and ATP production with separate cytosolic and mitochondrial compartments is needed in order to test the parallel activation mechanism in the intact cardiac cell.

MULTICOMPARTMENT MODELS OF CARDIAC METABOLISM

At a given energy demand, MVO_2 determines the rates of ETC and ATP formation, which affect the mitochondrial redox state ($NADH/NAD^+$) and phosphorylation state (ATP/ADP). For example, ischemia reduces MVO_2,[35] resulting in a decrease in proton-motive force and the mitochondrial phosphorylation state and an increase in redox state. Ischemia also affects indirectly the cytosolic redox state and phosphorylation state via reduced flux through the malate–aspartate shuttle and ATP–ADP translocase. Decreased cytosolic ATP/ADP activates glycogen breakdown and stimulates glycolysis, while increased cytosolic $NADH/NAD^+$ leads to higher lactate production, and causes cellular acidosis. An increase in mitochondrial $NADH/NAD^+$ can also occur when the rate of fatty acid oxidation is high,[27] which inhibits PDH activity and pyruvate oxidation. When fatty acid oxidation is inhibited (e.g., by pharmacological agent oxfenicine), pyruvate oxidation increases[36] due to the decreased inhibition of PDH. Therefore, a quantitative understanding of the regulation of cardiac energy metabolism during ischemia requires dynamic information on changes in mitochondrial and cytosolic $NADH/NAD^+$. However, current experimental methods of measuring myocardial NADH and NAD^+ concentrations *in vivo* could not provide sufficiently rapid data to track changes in these important regulators during the onset of myocardial ischemia.[37] Furthermore, *in vivo* measurements are based on the whole tissue, without distinguishing the cytosolic and mitochondrial subcellular compartments. Computer simulations from a comprehensive physiologically based mathematical model can provide key information on cytosolic and mitochondrial chemical species, and complement biochemical experiments investigating the regulation of cardiac energy metabolism.

We have developed a multicompartment model of myocardial energy metabolism based on mass balance, transport, and key metabolic reactions.[2,38–40] This model includes most key metabolic pathways (e.g., glycolysis, pyruvate oxidation, fatty acids oxidation, CAC, electric transport chain, ADP phosphorylation) and metabolites (e.g., glucose, glycogen, lactate, ATP, ADP, Pi, NADH, and NAD^+) in the cardiomyocytes, and is based on values from human-like large animal models (e.g., pigs and dogs). Furthermore, this model distinguishes blood, cytosol, and mitochondria compartments, and includes a glycolytic subcompartment to account the metabolic channeling observed in experimental studies.[41–43] Finally, the model incorporates species transport across the cellular membrane and mitochondrial membrane, for example, glucose transport and malate–aspartate shuttle. The model parameters were estimated based on experimental data obtained from *in vivo* experiments (primarily in humans, pigs, and dogs). Model simulations corresponded closely to experimental data (e.g., glycogen and lactate uptake) from open-chest pig studies with reduced blood flow (60% decrease in myocardial blood flow)[3] or increased (fourfold) energy expenditure.[39]

In Silico *Study of Regulation of Cardiac Energy Metabolism during Ischemia*

The primary effect of myocardial ischemia is impaired oxidative phosphorylation due to decreased oxygen delivery to the mitochondria.[27] Reduced aerobic ATP production stimulates glycogen breakdown and increases ATP formation from glycolysis in the cytosol. However, during ischemia, pyruvate and NADH produced by glycolysis do not readily enter the mitochondria to be oxidized like under normal conditions, and there is a high rate of conversion of pyruvate and NADH to lactate and NAD^+ in the cytosol (FIG. 1). This results in accumulation of cellular lactate and H^+ and a switch from net lactate uptake to net lactate release.[44] While moderate ischemia does not cause irreversible tissue damage, severe ischemia may result in tissue necrosis and infarction. The residual MVO_2 during ischemia is primarily supported by fatty acid oxidation,[45,46] nevertheless, lactate production from glycolysis is accelerated dramatically.[45,47–49]

We developed a multicompartment model of cardiac metabolism to simulate the dynamics of cytosolic and mitochondrial redox states, and investigate their roles in the differential regulation of cardiac energy metabolism under ischemic conditions.[2,38] Over a wide range of myocardial blood flow reductions (from 20% to 80%) the model simulated changes of metabolite concentrations and metabolic fluxes during the transition between steady states. Simulations show that under ischemic conditions, especially severe ischemia, the redox states dynamics in the cytosol and mitochondria were very different (FIG. 2). The mitochondrial redox states were reset to higher values immediately in response to ischemia that was proportional to the reduction of MVO_2. In contrast, cytosolic redox states increased initially due to the activation of glycogen breakdown, and then decreased slowly to a steady state corresponding closely to the rate of myocardial lactate production.[2,39] These results indicate that during ischemia, the mitochondrial redox state is determined by MVO_2, while during the initial transition the cytosolic redox state is mainly determined by glycogen breakdown, and in the steady state by mitochondrial redox.

We further applied the model to test the hypothesis that lactate production during ischemia is affected by both glycogen storage and NADH transfer rate into the mitochondria. The effects of the initial glycogen concentration and malate–aspartate shuttle activity on lactate production during ischemia were simulated. Changing glycogen initial concentration only affected cytosolic redox and lactate production during the initial period of ischemia (FIG. 3), and had no effect on mitochondrial redox. On the other hand, alterations in the malate–aspartate shuttle activity controlled the rate of lactate production over the entire ischemic duration (FIG. 4).[2]

Modeling Parallel Activation of Metabolic Processes with Increased Workload

In the transition from rest to exercise the ventricles must generate sufficient power to maintain blood pressure and organ perfusion, which requires the tight coupling of the transfer of chemical energy to mechanical power. This controlled energy transfer during the transition from resting conditions to intense exercise stress can require up to a fivefold increase in cardiac power generation and MVO_2, yet appears to occur without ATP depletion or anaerobic metabolism.[36] Therefore, cardiac metabolism is perfectly controlled so that the transduction of chemical energy matches the need for mechanical energy. However, the mechanisms of this control in the intact heart *in vivo* remain to be quantitatively analyzed.

ATP utilization mainly occurs in the cytosol, which is dependent upon the cytosolic ATP concentration; while most ATP formation in the heart comes from oxidative phosphorylation, which is driven by the availability of ADP and Pi, activity of complex V, the proton-motive force across the mitochondrial inner membrane, and the delivery of NADH and $FADH_2$ to the ETC (FIG. 1). However, concentrations of cytosolic and mitochondrial ATP, ADP, NADH, and NAD^+ change little during the transition from resting to increased workload conditions,[50–52] as demonstrated by a recent *in vivo* experimental study.[36] It has been suggested that independent signaling molecules activate ATP production and utilization as well as NADH generation simultaneously. One possible signaling source between aerobic metabolism and myocardial work is

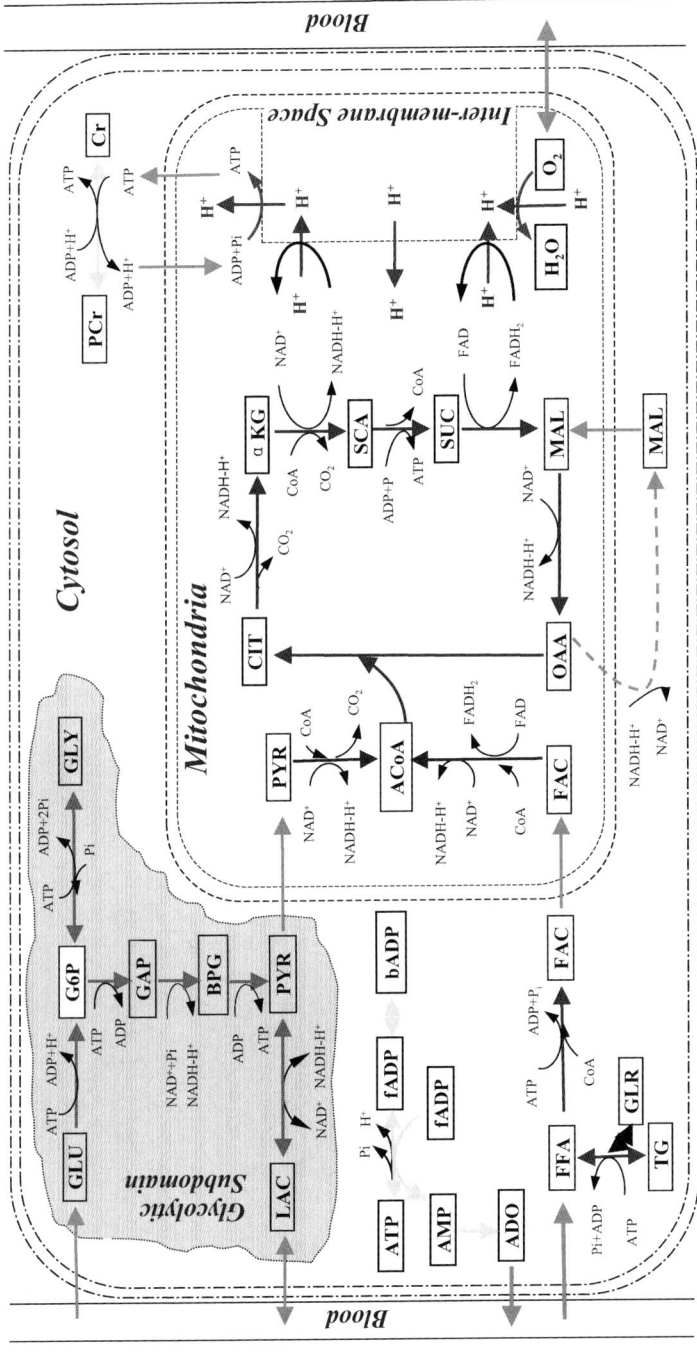

FIGURE 2. Redox state ([NADH]/[NAD$^+$] ratio) in the mitochondria (*top*) and cytosol (*middle*), and the rate of shuttling of NADH between the two compartments. Myocardial blood flow was reduced from a normal value of 1.0 mL g^{-1} min^{-1} to either 0.7, 0.4, or 0.1 mL g^{-1} min^{-1} (decreases of 30%, 60%, or 90%). Simulated from the model presented in Zhou *et al*, J. Physiol. (London) 2005.[39]

Ca^{2+}.[24] Ca^{2+} not only regulates myosin ATPase and sarcoplasmic reticulum (SR) Ca^{2+}-ATPase, but also directly regulates cytosolic ATP hydrolysis[53] and mitochondrial F_0/F_1-ATPase ATP synthesis[54] (FIG. 1). Furthermore, it can also activate PDH phosphatase (and therefore PDH) and the CAC enzymes (isocitrate dehydrogenase and α-ketoglutarate dehydrogenase) that stimulate NADH generation.[32] Moreover, an increase in mitochondrial Ca^{2+} occurs with an increase in extramitochondrial Ca^{2+}, for example, with adrenergic stimulation.[32] These combined effects of Ca^{2+} are expected to have a minimal impact on mitochondrial metabolic intermediates when Ca^{2+} is introduced with an increase in energy demand.[55] Consequently, the heart can change its metabolic rate significantly while maintaining relatively constant cytosolic and mitochondrial intermediate concentrations.[34,56]

To simulate dynamic responses of cardiac metabolism to increased energy expenditure, we modified our model by incorporating parallel activation of various metabolic processes in both cytosol (ATP hydrolysis, glycogen breakdown, and glycolysis) and mitochondria (NADH oxidation, ADP phosphorylation, and dehydrogenase activity).[40] The activations were implemented by increasing the rate coefficients through the Michaelis–Menton equation and myocardial blood flow in proportion to the increase in energy expenditure. Model simulations showed that the rates of MVO_2, ATP production and hydrolysis, fatty oxidation, and pyruvate oxidation were all increased in response to increased blood flow, while the concentrations of ADP and ATP in both cytosol and mitochondria remained constant. These responses are consistent with experimental data. Although cytosolic and mitochondrial NADH and NAD^+ returned to resting values 15 min after increased energy expenditure, moderate changes occurred during the transition. Furthermore, in order to investigate quantitatively the extent of control exerted by various components of "parallel activation" in maintaining the metabolic homeostasis observed in the computational study and other experimental studies, the cardiac responses to increased energy expenditure without activation of specific pathways were simulated. Simulations showed mitochondrial ATP/ADP and cytosolic $NADH/NAD^+$ are mostly affected by the transferring of ATP–ADP and NADH-NAD^+, mitochondrial $NADH/NAD^+$ is mainly regulated by complex I, and cytosolic ATP/ADP is mostly regulated by both mitochondrial dehydrogenases and complex I. These results provided further support for the need for parallel activation of multiple processes in order to maintain the constant levels of regulatory intermediates. Finally, model simulations showed that an elevation in arterial

FIGURE 3. Effect of preischemic glycogen concentration on the dynamics of cytosolic $NADH/NAD^+$ (top), mitochondrial $NADH/NAD^+$ (middle), and lactate production (bottom) in response to moderate severity ischemia (decrease in myocardial blood flow from 1.0 mL g^{-1} min^{-1} to 0.4 mL g^{-1} min^{-1}). Simulated from the model presented in Zhou et al., J. Physiol. (London) 2005.[39]

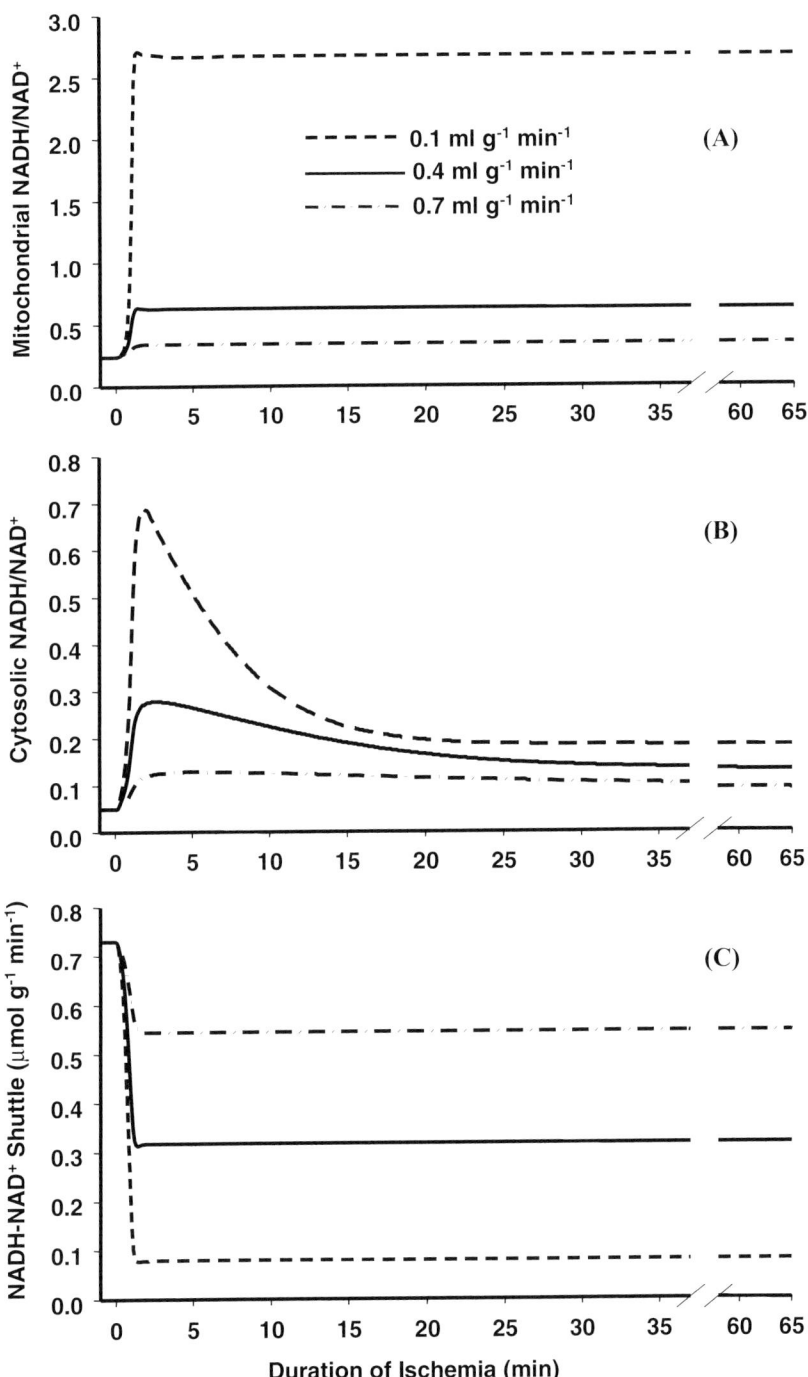

lactate concentration greatly increased the cytosolic NADH/NAD$^+$ ratio, but had a lesser effect on the mitochondria NADH/NAD$^+$ ratio. On the other hand, simulation of diabetic conditions reduced pyruvate oxidation, and the cytosolic NADH/NAD$^+$ ratio, but did not affect mitochondrial NADH/NAD$^+$ ratio, illustrating that alterations in mitochondrial substrate selection can occur independent of large changes in the mitochondrial NADH/NAD$^+$ ratio.

POTENTIAL APPLICATION AND FUTURE DIRECTIONS

To predict changes in mechanical work of the heart in response to metabolic perturbations, such as ischemia and exercise, future models should link substrate metabolism and ATP hydrolysis to mechanical power generation and cardiomyocyte excitation–contraction coupling. Under normal conditions, about two-thirds of energy produced from ATP hydrolysis supports cardiac mechanical work and the reminder supports other functions including Ca^{2+} pumping and protein synthesis.[1,57,58] Under ischemic conditions, power generation is downregulated to match the decreased oxygen consumption, while the energy consumption for ion homeostasis remains at least at the same rate, thus cardiac mechanical efficiency (defined as external power/total energy consumption) is expected to decrease in the ischemic heart. During exercise, however, more energy is required as external power to meet the energy demand, so that cardiac mechanical efficiency should increase. Incorporation of mechanical power generation would allow for the evaluation of mechanical efficiency of cardiac muscle during ischemia or increased energy expenditure.

Incorporating Ca^{2+} into metabolic models is not only important for controlling cardiomyocyte contraction, but also ion homeostasis in both cytosol and mitochondria.[31-33] During cardiac response to increased energy expenditure, Ca^{2+} concentration is expected to increase in both cytosol and mitochondria,[32] where it can activate various enzymes. Following the dynamics of cytosolic hydrogen ions (H$^+$) is important for simulating cellular proton dynamics in response to metabolic stress. Ischemia-induced cellular acidosis reduces the ability of cardiac cardiomyocytes to maintain ion homeostasis (e.g., Ca^{2+}) and use energy from ATP hydrolysis to perform contractile work. When pH is decreased, more ATP is required by the sarcoplasmic Ca^{2+} and higher cytosolic Ca^{2+} concentration is needed during systole to produce a given amount of mechanical power. The efflux of H$^+$ from cardiomyocytes that occur in

FIGURE 4. Effect of the activity of the NADH-NAD+ between the cytosol and mitochondria on the dynamics of cytosolic NADH/NAD$^+$ (top), mitochondrial NADH/NAD$^+$ (middle), and lactate production (bottom) in response to moderate severity ischemia (decrease in myocardial blood flow from 1.0 mL g^{-1} min^{-1} to 0.4 mL g^{-1} min^{-1}). Simulated from the model presented in Zhou et al., J. Physiol. (London) 2005.

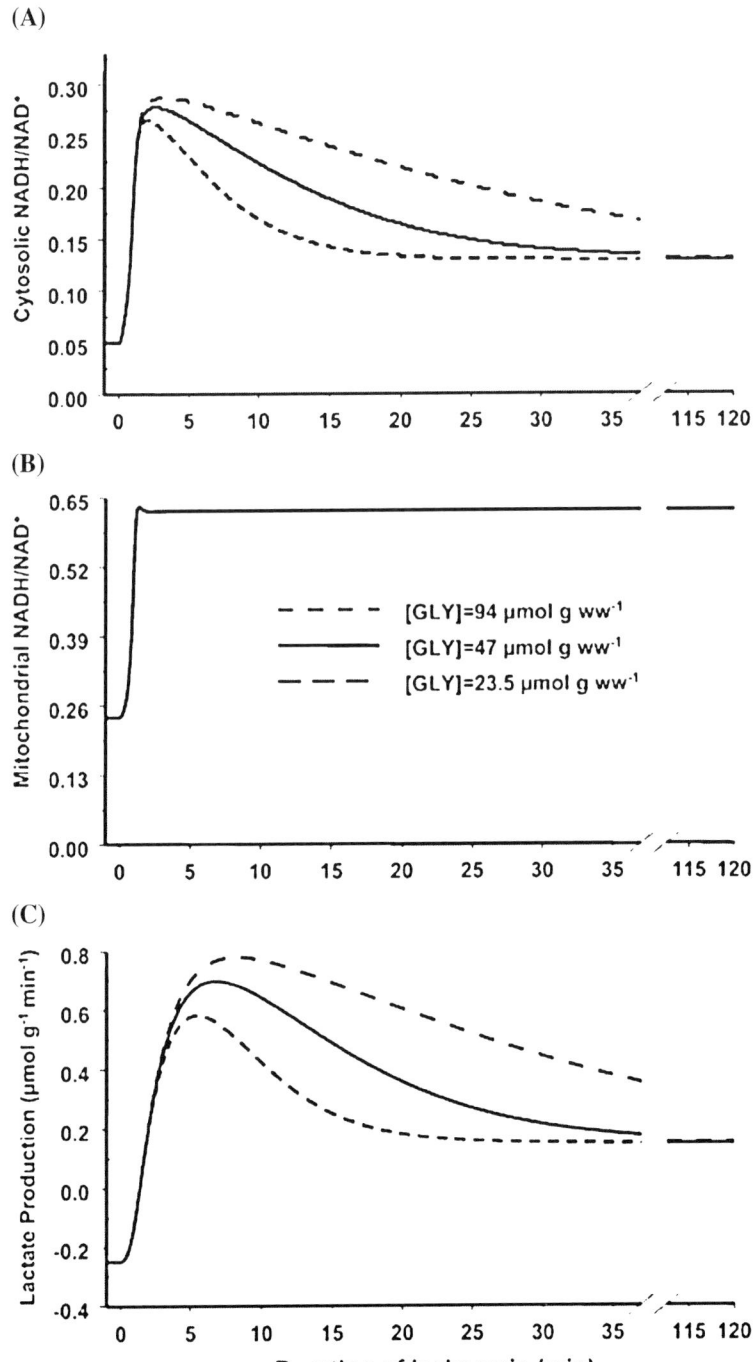

exchange for Na^+ leads to a greater Na^+-Ca^{2+} exchange across the cell membrane, which reduces the availability of ATP to maintain Ca^{2+} homeostasis. Cytosolic H^+ affects the mitochondrial membrane potential associated with the cotransport of ATP and ADP between cytosol and mitochondria and the glycolytic flux. Cytosolic H^+ is involved in numerous reactions (e.g., glycolysis and ATP breakdown) and is maintained in the normal range by cellular (bicarbonate, phosphate, and protein) buffer systems. Model simulation of H^+ in regulating enzymes and reactions, for example, glycolysis, would be important to predict effects when the buffer systems are not sufficient in response to metabolic perturbations.

The compartmentation of metabolites and enzymes between and within cytosol and mitochondria plays an important role in the regulation of energy metabolism.[2,38] Metabolic communication between these compartments is important for achieving optimal substrate utilization, as well as maintaining a balance between ATP production and utilization. The malate–aspartate shuttle is a direct link between the cytosolic and mitochondrial metabolites and serves the function of transferring reducing equivalents (NADH) from the cytosol to the electron transport chain of the inner mitochondrial membrane (FIG. 1). In the process, CAC intermediates exchange with cytosolic metabolites through carrier-mediated transport involving the α-ketoglutarate/malate transporter[59] and the electrogenic glutamate/aspartate transporter.[60] As shown in FIGURE 4, our highly simplified model NADH-NAD^+ exchange between the cytosol and the mitochondria predicts that alterations in the activity of this system has dramatic effects on cytosolic NADH/NAD^+ and lactate production at a given level of myocardial ischemia, and impacts steady-state lactate production during reduced flow conditions.

Previous investigations have suggested altered malate–aspartate shuttle activity under various pathophysiological conditions.[61,62] Studies on isolated mitochondria show that hyperthyroid-induced left ventricular (LV) hypertrophy can lead to an increase in shuttle capacity. Dynamic ^{13}C NMR spectroscopy has revealed depressed metabolite transport in postischemic hearts. However, at present, we have limited experimental means to explore the malate–aspartate shuttle activity due to the difficulties in measuring fluxes and concentrations in these compartments. While pharmacological and physiological studies can describe phenomenological aspects of the role of this shuttle, they provide limited mechanistic insight into the regulatory mechanisms at the subcellular level. Therefore, the impact of altered malate–aspartate shuttle activity on cellular metabolism remains to be elucidated.

As an alternative approach to conducting experimental measurements, mathematical modeling can provide a quantitative analysis of the cellular mechanisms that regulate myocardial metabolism, and can be used to predict non-observable fluxes and metabolite concentrations.[2,38,39] With an appropriate physiologically based mathematical model that incorporates mechanistic details of the malate–asparte shuttle, computer simulations can be made of metabolic dynamics during normal and altered pathophysiological conditions. Such simulation will allow us to gain insight into the impact of altered malate–aspartate shuttle activity on the distribution of metabolites across the mitochondrial membrane, and the regulation of cytosolic versus mitochondrial redox states. By combining model simulation with experimental measurements, hypotheses regarding mechanistic changes and important regulators of cardiac energy metabolism in diseased hearts can be tested.

To this point, the present model was used as an *in silico* tool to investigate the regulatory mechanisms responsible for the changes of substrates and fluxes in response to metabolic stresses. This model with some modifications can be used to analyze cellular metabolism in other cardiac disease states, for example, heart failure and diabetes. Changes in model inputs, (e.g., blood flow, arterial and tissue substrate concentrations, and model parameters) allow investigation of their effects on the whole system responses. For example, the model can be used to study demand-induced ischemia that occurs in coronary artery disease by increasing stress and oxygen demand and restricting coronary flow.

SUMMARY

We have provided an example of metabolic model of cardiac metabolism that illustrates the value of using computational models as a tool for interpreting the metabolic consequence of altered metabolic stress, particularly the importance of cellular compartmentation in the regulation of cardiac energy metabolism. The future direction of cardiac model development would be to incorporate all the components, such as substrate metabolism, ATP hydrolysis, mechanical power generation, cardiac electrophysiology, and myocytes extraction–contraction coupling, and ion channels across mitochondrial membrane. As computational models of the cardiac metabolism become more integrative, comprehensive and mechanistic, their values in the prediction of cardiac response to various diseases will increase significantly.

ACKNOWLEDGMENTS

This work was supported by grant GM-66309 from the National Institute of General Medical Sciences for the establishment of the Center for Modeling Integrated Metabolic Systems (MIMS) at Case Western Reserve University, and NIH grant HL-74237. The authors thank Professor Gerald Saidel for suggestions and discussion.

REFERENCES

1. STANLEY, W.C., F.A. RECCHIA & G.D. LOPASCHUK. 2005. Myocardial substrate metabolism in the normal and failing heart. Physiol. Rev. **85:** 1093–1129.

2. ZHOU, L., W.C. STANLEY, G.M. SAIDEL, X. YU & M.E. CABRERA. 2005. Regulation of lactate production at the onset of ischaemia is independent of mitochondrial NADH/NAD+: insights from in silico studies. J. Physiol. **569:** 925–937.
3. SALEM, J.E., M.E. CABRERA, M.P. CHANDLER, *et al*. 2004. Step and ramp induction of myocardial ischemia: comparison of in vivo and in silico results. J. Physiol. Pharmacol. **55:** 519–536.
4. SALEM, J.E., W.C. STANLEY & M.E. CABRERA. 2004. Computational studies of the effects of myocardial blood flow reductions on cardiac metabolism. Biomed. Eng. Online **3:** 15.
5. CABRERA, M.E., G.M. SAIDEL & S.C. KALHAN. 1998. Modeling metabolic dynamics. From cellular processes to organ and whole body responses. Prog. Biophys. Mol. Biol. **69:** 539–557.
6. GREENSTEIN, J., A.J. TANSKANEN & R. WINSLOW. 2004. Modeling the actions of [beta]-adrenergic signaling on excitation–contraction coupling processes. Ann. N. Y. Acad. Sci. **1015:** 16–27.
7. MATSUOKA, S., N. SARAI, H. JO & A. NOMA. 2004. Simulation of ATP metabolism in cardiac excitation-contraction coupling. Progress Biophys. Mol. Biol. **85:** 279–299.
8. MATSUOKA, S., H. JO, N. SARAI & A. NOMA. 2004. An in silico study of energy metabolism in cardiac excitation-contraction coupling. Jpn. J. Physiol. **54:** 517–522.
9. SOELLER, C. & M.B. CANNELL. 2004. Analysing cardiac excitation-contraction coupling with mathematical models of local control. Prog. Biophys. Mol. Biol. **85:** 141–162.
10. VAN DER VUSSE,G.J., M. VAN BILSEN, J.F. GLATZ, *et al*. 2002. Critical steps in cellular fatty acid uptake and utilization. Mol. Cell. Biochem. **239:** 9–15.
11. CHIU, H.C., A. KOVACS, D.A. FORD, *et al*. 2001. A novel mouse model of lipotoxic cardiomyopathy. J. Clin. Invest. **107:** 813–822.
12. HUNTER, P. & T. ARTS. 1997. Tissue remodeling with micro-structurally based material laws. Adv. Exp. Med. Biol. **430:** 215–225.
13. ACHS, M.J. & D. GARFINKEL. 1977. Computer simulation of energy metabolism in anoxic perfused rat heart. Am. J. Physiol. **232:** R164-R174.
14. CH'EN, F.F., R.D. VAUGHAN-JONES, K. CLARKE & D. NOBLE. 1998. Modelling myocardial ischaemia and reperfusion. Prog. Biophys. Mol. Biol. **69:** 515–538.
15. CHANCE, B., D. GARFINKEL, J. HIGGINS & B. HESS. 1960. Metabolic control mechanisms. 5. A solution for the equations representing interaction between glycolysis and respiration in ascites tumor cells. J. Biol. Chem. **235:** 2426–2439.
16. MCGARRY, J.D., K.F. WOELTJE, J.G. SCHROEDER, *et al*. 1990. Carnitine palmitoyltransferase–structure/function/regulatory relationships. Prog. Clin. Biol. Res. **321:** 193–208.
17. HEINRICH, R. & S. SCHUSTER. 1998. The modelling of metabolic systems. Structure, control and optimality. Biosystems **47:** 61–77.
18. KASHIWAYA, Y., K. SATO, *et al*. 1994. Control of glucose utilization in working perfused rat heart. J. Biol. Chem. **269:** 25502–25514.
19. VOGT, A.M., H. NEF, J. SCHAPER, *et al*. 2002. Metabolic control analysis of anaerobic glycolysis in human hibernating myocardium replaces traditional concepts of flux control. FEBS Lett. **517:** 245–250.
20. CABRERA, M., G. SAIDEL & S. KALHAN. 1998. Role of O2 in regulation of lactate dynamics during hypoxia: mathematical model and analysis. Ann. Biomed. Eng. **26:** 1–27.

21. CABRERA, M., G. SAIDEL & S. KALHAN. 1999. Lactate metabolism during exercise: analysis by an integrative systems model. Am. J. Physiol. **277:** R1522–R1536.
22. SALEM, J.E., G.M. SAIDEL, W.C. STANLEY & M.E. CABRERA. 2002. Mechanistic model of myocardial energy metabolism under normal and ischemic conditions. Ann. Biomed. Eng. **30:** 202–216.
23. GUTH, B.D., R. SCHULZ & G. HEUSCH. 1993. Time course and mechanisms of contractile dysfunction during acute myocardial ischemia. Circulation **87:** IV35–IV42.
24. BALABAN, R.S., S. BOSE, S.A. FRENCH & P.R. TERRITO. 2003. Role of calcium in metabolic signaling between cardiac sarcoplasmic reticulum and mitochondria in vitro. Am. J. Physiol. Cell. Physiol. **284:** C285–C293.
25. HEINEMAN, F.W. & R.S. BALABAN. 1990. Control of mitochondrial respiration in the heart in vivo. Annu. Rev. Physiol. **52:** 523–542.
26. CHANDLER, M.P., H. HUANG, T.A. MCELFRESH & W.C. STANLEY. 2002. Increased nonoxidative glycolysis despite continued fatty acid uptake during demand-induced myocardial ischemia. Am. J. Physiol. Heart Circ. Physiol. **282:** H1871–H1878.
27. STANLEY, W.C., G.D. LOPASCHUK, et al. 1997. Regulation of myocardial carbohydrate metabolism under normal and ischemic conditions. Cardiovasc. Res. **33:** 243–257.
28. CHANCE, B. & G.R. WILLIAMS. 1956. The respiratory chain and oxidative phosphorylation. Adv. Enzymol. Relat. Subj. Biochem. **17:** 65–134.
29. HARRIS, D.A. & A.M. DAS. 1991. Control of mitochondrial ATP synthesis in the heart. Biochem. J. **280**(Pt 3): 561–573.
30. KORZENIEWSKI, B., A. NOMA & S. MATSUOKA. 2005. Regulation of oxidative phosphorylation in intact mammalian heart in vivo. Biophys. Chem. **116:** 145–157.
31. BALABAN, R.S. 2002. Cardiac energy metabolism homeostasis: role of cytosolic calcium. J. Mol. Cell. Cardiol. **34:** 1259–1271.
32. MCCORMACK, J.G., A.P. HALESTRAP & R.M. DENTON. 1990. Role of calcium ions in regulation of mammalian intramitochondrial metabolism. Physiol. Rev. **70:** 391–425.
33. CORTASSA, S., M.A. AON, E. MARBAN, et al. 2003. An integrated model of cardiac mitochondrial energy metabolism and calcium dynamics. Biophys. J. **84:** 2734–2755.
34. KORZENIEWSKI, B. 2000. Regulation of ATP supply in mammalian skeletal muscle during resting state–>intensive work transition. Biophys. Chem. **83:** 19–34.
35. STANLEY, W.C., K.M. KIVILO, et al. 2003. Post-ischemic treatment with dipyruvyl-acetyl-glycerol decreases myocardial infarct size in the pig. Cardiovasc. Drugs Ther. **17:** 209–216.
36. SHARMA, N., I.C. OKERE, D.Z. BRUNENGRABER, et al. 2005. Regulation of pyruvate dehydrogenase activity and citric acid cycle intermediates during high cardiac power generation. J. Physiol. **562:** 593–603.
37. VOGT, A.M., M. POOLMAN, C. ACKERMANN, et al. 2002. Regulation of glycolytic flux in ischemic preconditioning: a study employing metabolic control analysis. J. Biol. Chem. **277:** 24411–24419.
38. CABRERA, M.E., L. ZHOU, W.C. STANLEY & G.M. SAIDEL. 2005. Regulation of cardiac energetics: role of redox state and cellular compartmentation during ischemia. Ann N. Y. Acad. Sci. **1047:** 259–270.

39. ZHOU, L., J.E. SALEM, G.M. SAIDEL, *et al.* 2005. Mechanistic model of cardiac energy metabolism predicts localization of glycolysis to cytosolic subdomain during ischemia. Am. J. Physiol. Heart Circ. Physiol. **288:** H2400–H2411.
40. ZHOU, L., M.E. CABRERA, I.C. OKERE, *et al.* 2006. Regulation of myocardial substrate metabolism during increased energy expenditure: insights from computational studies. Am. J. Physiol. Heart Circ. Physiol. Submitted.
41. ARNOLD, H. & D. PETTE. 1968. Binding of glycolytic enzymes to structure proteins of the muscle. Eur. J. Biochem. **6:** 163–171.
42. JOSHI, A. & B.O. PALSSON. 1989. Metabolic dynamics in the human red cell. Part II–Interactions with the environment. J. Theor. Biol. **141:** 529–545.
43. MASTER, CJ. 1984. Interactions between glycolytic enzymes and the cytomatrix. J. Cell. Biol. **99:** 222s–225s.
44. PANTLEY, G.A., S.A. MALONE, *et al.* 1990. Regeneration of myocardial phosphocreatine in pigs despite continued moderate ischemia. Circ. Res. **67:** 1491–1493.
45. LIEDTKE, A.J. 1981. Alterations of carbohydrate and lipid metabolism in the acutely ischemic heart. Prog. Cardiovasc. Dis. **23:** 321–336.
46. LLOYD, S.G., P. WANG, H. ZENG & J.C. CHATHAM. 2004. Impact of low-flow ischemia on substrate oxidation and glycolysis in the isolated perfused rat heart. Am. J. Physiol. Heart Circ. Physiol. **287:** H351–H362.
47. GUTH, B.D., J.A. WISNESKI, R.A. NEESE, *et al.* 1990. Myocardial lactate release during ischemia in swine. Relat. Reg. Blood Flow Circ. **81:** 1948–1958.
48. MYEARS, D.W., B.E. SOBEL & S.R. BERGMANN. 1987. Substrate use in ischemic and reperfused canine myocardium: quantitative considerations. Am. J. Physiol. **253:** H107–H114.
49. RENSTROM, B., S.H. NELLIS & A.J. LIEDTKE. 1990. Metabolic oxidation of pyruvate and lactate during early myocardial reperfusion. Circ. Res. **66:** 282–288.
50. BALABAN, R.S., H.L. KANTOR, L.A. KATZ & R.W. BRIGGS. 1986. Relation between work and phosphate metabolite in the in vivo paced mammalian heart. Science **232:** 1121–1123.
51. BALABAN, R.S. 1990. Regulation of oxidative phosphorylation in the mammalian cell. Am. J. Physiol. **258:** C377–C389.
52. SCHOLZ, T.D., M.R. LAUGHLIN, R.S. BALABAN, *et al.* 1995. Effect of substrate on mitochondrial NADH, cytosolic redox state, and phosphorylated compounds in isolated hearts. Am. J. Physiol. **268:** H82–H91.
53. SCHOLZ, T.D. & R.S. BALABAN. 1994. Mitochondrial F1-ATPase activity of canine myocardium: effects of hypoxia and stimulation. Am. J. Physiol. **266:** H2396–H2403.
54. TERRITO, P.R., V.K. MOOTHA, S.A. FRENCH & R.S. BALABAN. 2000. Ca(2+) activation of heart mitochondrial oxidative phosphorylation: role of the F(0)/F(1)-ATPase. Am. J. Physiol. Cell. Physiol. **278:** C423–C435.
55. TERRITO, P.R., S.A. FRENCH & R.S. BALABAN. 2001. Simulation of cardiac work transitions, in vitro: effects of simultaneous Ca2+ and ATPase additions on isolated porcine heart mitochondria. Cell. Calcium **30:** 19–27.
56. KORZENIEWSKI, B. 1998. Regulation of ATP supply during muscle contraction: theoretical studies. Biochem. J. **330**(Pt 3): 1189–1195.
57. GIBBS, C.L. 1978. Cardiac energetics. Physiol. Rev. **58:** 174–254.
58. SUGA, H. 1990. Ventricular energetics. Physiol. Rev. **70:** 247–277.
59. ARNOLD, M.K.. 1992. Physiology of the Heart. Raven Press. New York.
60. LANOUE, K.F. & M.E. TISCHLER. 1974. Electrogenic characteristics of the mitochondrial glutamate-aspartate antiporter. J. Biol. Chem. **249:** 7522–7528.

61. LEWANDOWSKI, E.D., X. YU, K.F. LANOUE, *et al*. 1997. Altered metabolite exchange between subcellular compartments in intact postischemic rabbit hearts. Circ. Res. **81:** 165–175.
62. SCHOLZ, T.D., C.J. TENEYCK & B.C. SCHUTTE. 2000. Thyroid hormone regulation of the NADH shuttles in liver and cardiac mitochondria. J. Mol. Cell. Cardiol. **32:** 1–10.

Maintenance of the Metabolic Homeostasis of the Heart

Developing a Systems Analysis Approach

ROBERT S. BALABAN

Laboratory of Cardiac Energetics, National Heart Lung and Blood Institute, Bethesda, Maryland, USA

ABSTRACT: The heart is almost unique in the body with a constant requirement to conduct work well beyond the normal maintenance of cellular integrity. With this constant workload, it is not surprising that cardiac energy conversion is highly specialized to maintain a constant supply of energy. This maintenance of cellular metabolites during alterations in workload has been termed metabolic homeostasis. Here we discuss our efforts to understand the cellular and mitochondrial control network that orchestrates the metabolic homeostasis of the heart. This begins with a better definition of the metabolic pathways, acute posttranslational control sites, and proper kinetic evaluation of the reaction steps in the intact mitochondrial environment. First, a quantitative model of mitochondrial energy conversion is presented and demonstrates several serious gaps in our knowledge of this process. Toward filling these gaps, screens of the entire mitochondrial proteome have been conducted to establish the metabolic pathways that need to be considered. In addition, the dynamic phosphoproteome of intact mitochondria, using 2D gel electrophoresis coupled to ^{32}P labeling, has revealed a remarkably extensive protein phosphorylation network throughout the mitochondrial metabolic network that has essentially been overlooked. Initial studies on evaluating the functional significance of these protein phosphorylations and the kinase–phosphatase system involved will be reviewed. One of the major deficits in the consensus quantitative model of oxidative phosphorylation to explain intact mitochondria activities is in complex I, where even the initiation of Nicotinamide Adenine Dinucleotide (reduced) (NADH) oxidation is problematical using *in vitro* kinetic data. Studies will be described where the NADH binding and oxidation kinetics at complex I in the intact mitochondria were determined using fluorescence lifetime and enzyme dependent-fluorescence recovery after photo-oxidation (ED-FRAP) techniques. These later studies suggest that matrix NADH binding characteristics are much different ($>10^3$ binding constant errors) than isolated proteins. In addition, complex I is far

Address for correspondence: Robert S. Balaban, Ph.D., Laboratory of Cardiac Energetics, National Heart Lung and Blood Institute, National Institute of Health, Bldg 10 Rm B1D-161, 9000 Rockville Pike, Bethesda MD 20892. Voice: 301-496-3658; fax: 301-402-2389.
 e-mail: rsb@nih.gov

from equilibrium and may play an important role in regulating the rate of reducing equivalent delivery to the cytochromes.

KEYWORDS: proteome; phosphoproteome; complex I; NADH; ED-FRAP; oxidative phosphorylation; modeling; protein phosphorylation

INTRODUCTION

The heart continuously pumps blood requiring an output that far exceeds the normal cellular maintenance of homeostasis. One of the hallmarks of this metabolic homeostasis process is the ability to maintain constant the levels of energy conversion metabolites (i.e., ADP, ATP, CrP, and Pi) despite large changes in flux through these pools associated with changes in workload, *in vivo*. Over the last several decades it has become apparent that the heart has developed an energy supply system that can essentially be tuned to maintain the cytosolic potential energy available for contractile activity necessarily constant despite large changes in workload and associated metabolic flux. The principal cytosolic potential energy source is adenosine triphosphate (ATP). Very tightly coupled to ATP levels is the dead-end product, creative phosphate (CrP), which together with its metabolite creatine (Cr) is an important potential energy pool and diffusive flux support.

Many studies over the last several decades have demonstrated that during increases in work demand the levels of ATP, CrP, and other energy metabolites do not change even though the flux through these pools changes manyfold. This phenomenon has been termed as *metabolic homeostasis* where the metabolites of oxidative phosphorylation are held constant, or homeostatic, to support mechanical work. By holding the metabolites constant, changes in workload will not interfere with other cellular processes dependent on these molecules. This phenomenon has been demonstrated using both extraction [1-3] and ^{31}P NMR techniques [4-10] to monitor the phosphate metabolites, *in vivo*, during workload transitions. An example of one of these experiments is shown in FIGURE 1 from Heineman and Balaban.[6] In this example, the heart was paced to increase workload while monitoring the phosphate metabolites with ^{31}P NMR. The steady-state 31-Phosphorus Nuclear Magnetic Resonance, ^{31}P NMR spectrum shows no change in any of the metabolites, as witnessed by the difference spectrum, despite the fact that the flux through these pools has roughly doubled. This is also true in the time course data where not even a transient change is detected (FIG. 1 B).

Does this homeostasis in the cytosol extend to the mitochondria? When one performs an extraction or ^{31}P spectrum, up to 20% of the volume is mitochondria. Since no significant change in these whole tissue extracts is measured, it is unlikely that large changes (twofold or so) occurred in this significant mitochondrial pool. However, it is unclear what contribution the matrix metabolites

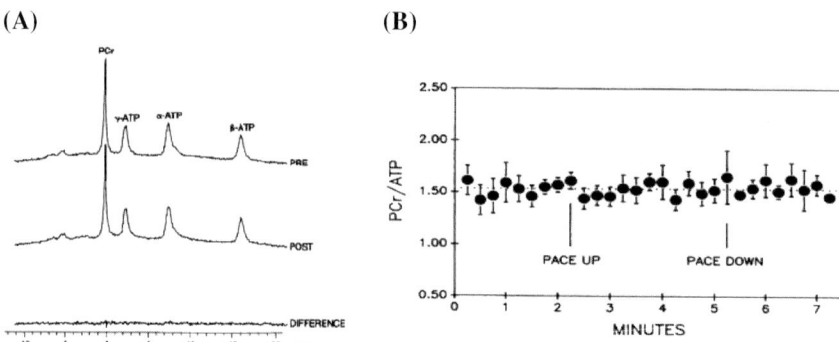

FIGURE 1. Effect of increasing heart rate on ^{31}P NMR detected metabolites, *in vivo*. (**A**) ^{31}P NMR spectra collected from the canine heart *in vivo*. Pre: represents the control period spectrum. Post: represents after increasing the heart rate to increase MVO$_2$ by more than 60%. The difference spectrum is a simple subtraction of Pre and Post spectra. (**B**) The CrP/ATP ratio is plotted as a function of time during the pacing protocol. The pacing initiation and termination are indicated by the arrows. Data from Heineman and Balaban.[6]

make to the total extraction or ^{31}P NMR data. No direct method for determining the ATP, ADP, and Pi in the mitochondrial matrix is currently available in the intact tissue with the potential exception of matrix Pi under specialized conditions.[11] However, other less direct methods are available, such as NADH fluorescence to follow the mitochondrial NADH/NAD ratio, membrane potential, and cytochrome redox state.

An extensive study by Chance *et al.*[12,13] showed that the NADH redox state is highly dependent on the ADP and Pi levels, generally oxidizing with increases in ATP production rate driven by increases in ADP and Pi.[14] However, three studies working around physiological workloads have shown no significant change in NADH/NAD ratio in the whole heart.[3,15–17] Based on the earlier experiments by Chance *et al.* on isolated mitochondria, these data revealed relatively constant mitochondrial NADH levels in the intact heart are not consistent with a change in ADP or Pi levels within the mitochondrial matrix consistent with the metabolic homeostasis extending into the matrix space.

There are at least two experimental results that show large variations in the mitochondrial redox state, but these studies were conducted well away from the normal physiological workloads, likely emphasizing that control systems do not dominate under true *in vivo* conditions. The first study compared vented nonworking and fully working rat hearts[18] far from the physiological range.[19] The second involved a retrograde perfused nonworking mouse heart devoid of myoglobin [20]that at maximum workload only consumed approximately 5.5 μmoles O$_2$/min/g (assuming a 150 mg heart) maximum oxygen consumption that barely approaches the resting oxygen consumption of a resting dog[21] that is doing the same pressure volume work at one-tenth the rate of the mouse.

This analysis also points out one of the problems of working with the mouse for energetic studies. Since the mouse is performing the same pressure volume work (i.e., essentially the same systolic pressure and ejection fraction) as a human or large mammal but at nearly 10 times the rate (550 beats/min), the mitochondrial oxygen consumption can be shown to be much closer to the maximum capacity even at rest. Thus, the mouse is operating in a much different, stressful, metabolic control domain than human and must be interpreted with care on several levels. These studies also point out the importance when using *in vitro* preparations to assure that physiological workloads and metabolic stress are being applied to the tissue to assure that the proper control domain is being evaluated.

The mitochondrial membrane potential is the primary source of energy for ATP generation by the F1-F0-ATPase. As the F1-F0-ATPase depolarizes the membrane potential when activated by ADP and Pi, the polarization of the membrane potential is generally inversely related to ADP and Pi levels. Wan et al.[16] showed that the membrane potential in the intact heart was stable with increases in workload. In our own lab, we used the approach developed by Backus et al.[22] using TC-MIMBI in perfused hearts of the *in vivo* dog heart. In their studies, we did not detect the release of TC-MIMBI using a PET readout with a tripling myocardial workload with dobutamine (Territo et al. unpublished). Since the released technetium-94m Sestamibi (TC-MIMBI) is [sensitive both membrane potential[22]] these data are also consistent with a stable mitochondrial membrane potential with workload, *in vivo*.

The last indirect evidence for the maintenance of the matrix metabolic homeostasis is the cytochrome c (cyto c) redox state determined *in vivo* along with myoglobin/hemoglobin oxygenation by Arai et al.[23] In this study, the epicardial absorbance of cyto c and hemoglobin/myoglobin was monitored during work transitions. Despite a threefold increase in oxygen consumption no change in tissue oxygenation or cyto c redox state was detected. This result is illustrated in FIGURE 2 where two optical difference spectra are presented from this study. The ischemia difference spectrum is a representation of the dynamic range of the measurement. The spectrum labeled **Phe** is the difference between control and the high workload state, phenylephrine infusion, showing no associated absorbance changes despite doubling of flux through **cyto** C and Overall Oxygen Consumption. [Given the plasticity of the cytochrome chain with oxygen and other factors,[24] the data are also consistent with a near homoeostatic metabolic state within the matrix with alterations in workload.]

Most of the available data suggest that the metabolic homeostasis detected in the cytosol projects to the mitochondrial matrix. There are two general models that have been used to explain the apparent metabolic homeostasis within the heart. The first is the proposal that a parallel or feed-forward system in the cytosol is simultaneously activating the metabolic capacity of the tissue and the contractile apparatus. This would result in a balanced increase in ATP production and hydrolysis results in little or no change in ATP or its hydrolysis

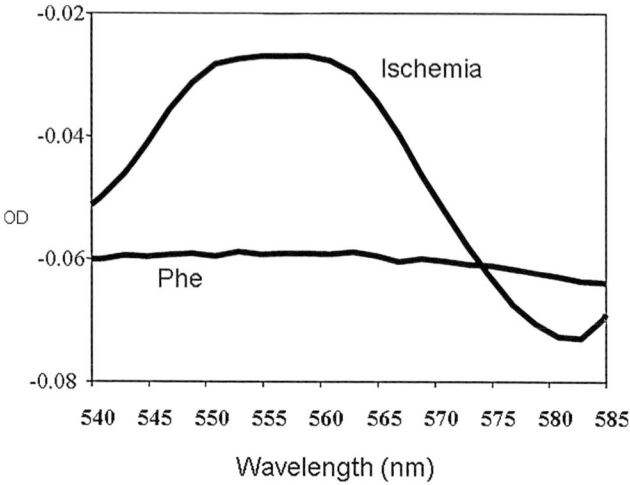

FIGURE 2. Effect of myocardial work on cytochromes c redox state and tissue oxygenation. Optical difference spectra a plotted of control versus ischemia (Ischemia) and control versus phenylephrine infusion (PE). Data from Arai et al.[23]

products. The most popular signaling molecule to accomplish this task is cytosolic Ca^{2+}, that is the major trigger for muscle contractile activity as well as a substrate for one of the major ATPases in the heart, the sarcoplasmic reticulum Ca^{2+} ATPase. Ca^{2+} has also been shown to be an effective modulator of ATP production via activation of dehydrogenase activity[25] as well as the F1-F0-ATPase synthetic activity.[26] A review on the potential role of Ca in the metabolic homeostasis was recently provided.[19]

With the ATP and its reactants, ADP and Pi, held near constant in the cytosol, how can the rate of ATP production be modified? The mechanism seems to rely on modifying the Vmax of the overall ATP synthetic process. That is, at a given ADP and Pi concentration the rate of ATP production can be modified by simply modifying the apparent Vmax of the overall oxidative phosphorylation reaction. To accomplish this, modifications at several levels of the oxidative phosphorylation reaction network must be accomplished as will be described below.

The lack of change in bulk ADP or Pi concentrations during increases in the rate of ATP turnover also implies that the rate of diffusion of these molecules in the cytosol is not rate limiting. Taking a fivefold increase in workload and ATP synthetic rate, the rate of ADP and Pi delivery from the cytosol to the mitochondria has to also increase by a factor of 5. If this process was diffusion limited then the gradients driving diffusion must increase resulting in a net integrated change in concentration, which is not observed, *in vivo*. Thus, a more likely hypothesis is that ADP and Pi delivery is not diffusion limited and the concentrations of these metabolites are essentially equilibrated across the cytosol. Good evidence for this condition, *in vivo,* was found using ketone infusions by Kim *et al.* [27] where the direct infusion of ketones decreased the ADP and Pi concentrations at a constant rate of ATP production. The ketones effectively increased the Vmax of the mitochondria by increasing NADH via hydroxybutyrate dehydrogenase. Thus, the only way to keep the rate of ATP production in line with ATP utilization is to drop the ADP and Pi concentrations in the cytosol, as was observed. The maintenance of the overall ATP synthetic rate while decreasing the ADP and Pi levels in the cytosol implies that the delivery of ADP and Pi are not rate limiting for oxidative phosphorylation. Similar observations have been made in several perfused heart preparations.[7,17,28,29] This study also makes another important point: the ADP and Pi levels are still used in the control network to maintain the balance between ATP production and breakdown. That is, feedback of ADP and Pi is still being used but not dominating under normal physiological conditions. This is especially the case at very high workloads where all the thermodynamic and kinetic forces to increase ATP production are required for what is usually a burst of work that jeopardizes the metabolic homeostasis for a short time.[5,30] That is, as the maximum ATP production capacity is being approached, the cytosolic concentrations of ADP and Pi, with very modest decreases in ATP, provide the added kinetic and thermodynamic driving forces to attain the maximum ATP production rates.

The diffusion coefficient of ATP and CrP has been determined in several muscle systems to be close to the values in free solution[31,32] and is likely not rate limiting given the mM concentration and high affinity of the ATPase reactions for ATP. However, ADP is only $\sim$100 μM and the entire pool turns over at rest every 100 msec[33] making it more susceptible to diffusion limitations. However, ADP diffusion and distribution are facilitated by the Cr kinase reaction and the high mM concentration of Cr.[34,35] Others have been troubled by this question and have suggested that the NMR visible or bulk extracted pools of metabolites are not reflecting the true diffusional driving forces in the cytosol and that microcompartmentation is supporting a diffusion-limited metabolic control on the mitochondria.[34,36–38]

The compartmentation models are rather extensive with compartments being suggested between the inner and outer membrane of the mitochondria[39] and between the SR and the mitochondria[40,41] as well as channeling of metabolites in the cytosol. Many of these compartments have been identified by structural observations, compartmentation of enzymes, or some experimental evidence of the lack of equilibration of some reaction pools with the bulk. These compartments can be used to explain the observed metabolic homeostasis in the bulk measurements of metabolites with NMR or extraction techniques by placing the gradients of the metabolites over very small regions such as the mitochondria inner space. Though these models can mathematically explain the observed bulk metabolic homeostasis, they do not explain the homeostasis extending into the mitochondria matrix. If ADP and Pi were rate limiting and these microcompartments were responsible for the delivery via short steep concentration gradients, then the mitochondria and oxidative phosphorylation elements should be responding to this delivery of metabolites by classical alterations in NADH and membrane polarization, which by most measurements up to now are not consistent with a microcompartmentation.[19] However, much of the experimental data for some metabolite compartments are compelling[41] and a role for metabolite compartmentation will likely be established in this process. Most useful would be direct imaging methods[42] that have been so important in establishing the role of steep cellular gradients in Ca^{2+} signaling in muscle cells.

Mathematical Simulation

Oxidative Phosphorylation Control Network

Taking for fact that the cytosolic levels of ADP and Pi are held near constant with large changes in workload, the question becomes how is mitochondrial ATP synthetic capacity, or apparent Vmax, controlled to match the rate of ATP breakdown in the cytosol? As mentioned earlier, one of the most likely candidates for a cytosolic signaling molecule to accomplish this task is Ca^{2+} that is used by the muscle to trigger muscle contraction while Ca^{2+} SR and plasma membrane transport represents a significant workload. The actions of Ca^{2+} on mitochondria have been recently reviewed and will not be repeated here.[33] What is apparent from this review is that a simple action of Ca^{2+}, or any other cytosolic signaling process that is likely involved in this complex control network, at one or even two sites is not adequate to explain the homeostasis that exists in the mitochondria matrix during work transitions. To model this process, we attempted to formulate a mathematical simulation of oxidative phosphorylation taking the best consensus elements from the literature. This was a forward modeling attempt using consensus data on enzymatic steps. No fitting of parameters was attempted. In this model it was found critical to have an experimentally determined ratio of cytochromes and metabolites to avoid oscillation. Once stable the model would generate an adequate flux with appropriate stoichiometries. However, when actual metabolite values from the matrix were applied the model failed. Naturally, this is not the first time that taking *in vitro*-determined reaction kinetics to model biological metabolic pathways have failed.[43,44] The primary problem at this time was the reaction kinetics for NADH in dehydrogenases. The inhibitory constants for NADH, *in vitro*, is μM while the NADH concentration in the matrix is never much below 1 mM. In addition, the reaction kinetics of complex I has been shown to have an apparent Km of 20 μM, suggesting it was saturated under normal operating conditions. However, numerous intact mitochondria and tissue studies have shown that the oxidation of NADH is linearly dependent on concentration in the mM range and not saturated by any means.[21,45,46] Thus, before progressing further we needed to understand how electrons get into the cytochrome chain from NADH.

To establish what are the appropriate kinetic constants for complex I, we undertook a series of studies to determine the relationship between binding NADH, using fluorescent lifetime studies, and NADH oxidation kinetics in intact mitochondria and isolated mitochondrial membranes as well as direct measures of NADH resynthesis reactions using the enzyme dependent-fluorescence recovery after photo-oxidation (ED-FRAP) technique.[46] Using these approaches, we found that the binding of NADH correlated with NADH oxidation in the intact mitochondria and membranes, however, the binding affinity was increased by three orders of magnitude in the membrane preparations when compared to the >3 mM apparent Km found in intact mitochondria.[47] These data explained why the *in vitro* data were misleading the forward model. These data suggest that the kinetics of NADH binding and oxidation are related, and that the infinity for NADH is several orders of magnitude higher in isolated membranes. These data explained why the **in vitro** data were misleading the mathematical model. The reason for this remarkable shift in affinity is still currently under investigation. The initial study suggested it was not dependent on the membrane potential,[47] but on more complicated interactions in the intact system. Similar corrections will be required for all of the sources of NADH in the citric acid cycle and fatty acid oxidation.

Mitochondria Phosphoproteome and Metabolic Control

Using the corrected values for NADH oxidation kinetics, it became apparent that the mathematical "consensus" model could not generate a metabolic homeostasis with NADH and the membrane potential without the simultaneous modification of several steps of oxidative phosphorylation that affects both the generation of the membrane potential as well as the dissipation by the F1-F0-ATPase and other electrogenic processes. Thus, some type of signaling process is required that can orchestrate changes in the activity of several enzymes simultaneously with a very rapid response time. Protein phosphorylation is the most obvious process to evaluate. Protein phosphorylation in the matrix has been previously established as a powerful tool in regulation dehydrogenases[48] as well as some aspects of apoptosis.[49] However, a large-scale screen for phosphorylation had not been extensively conducted. Using two different methods, Pro-Q Diamond, as originally reported by Schulenberg *et al*.[50] to detect steady-state phosphorylations and ^{32}P labeling to detect the dynamics of phosphorylation, we performed a large-scale screen for protein phosphorylation sites in the mitochondria matrix.[51] The P labeling was done by adding only ^{32}P inorganic phosphate to mitochondria that is transported Kinetics of NADH binding and oxidation in into the mitochondria converted to ^{32}Pγ-ATP with a remarkably high specific

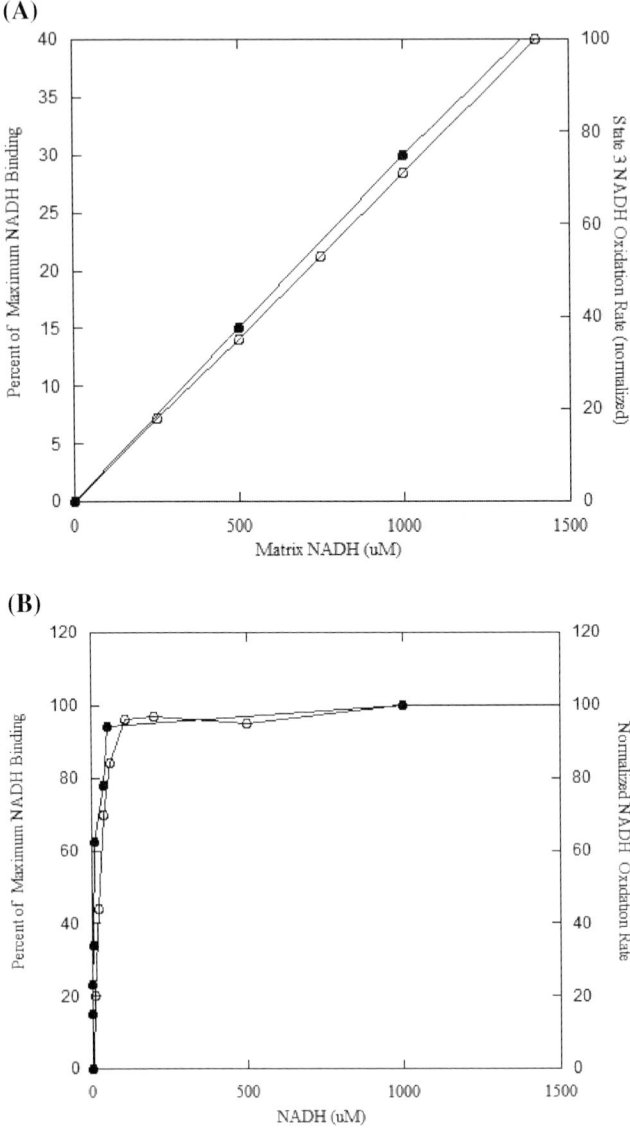

FIGURE 3. Kinetics of NADH binding and oxidation in intact mitochondria and mitochondrial membranes. **(A)** Dependence of NADH oxidation (open symbols) and binding (closed symbols) on matrix NADH concentration in intact mitochondria. The NADH oxidation rate was measured at STATE 3 (maximum ATP synthetic rate) using different carbon substrates as sources of NADH. The maximum concentration of NADH under these conditions was only ~40% of the total NADH/NAD pool. **(B)** Dependence of isolated mitochondria membranes NADH oxidation (open symbols) and binding (closed symbols) on NADH concentration.

(A) 20 minute ³²P incubation   (B)   20 minute incubation: 5 min DNP

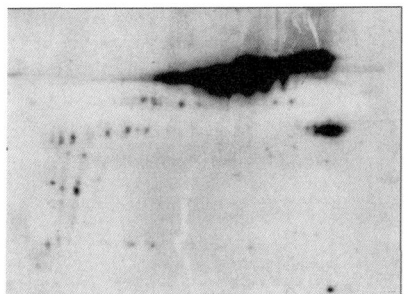
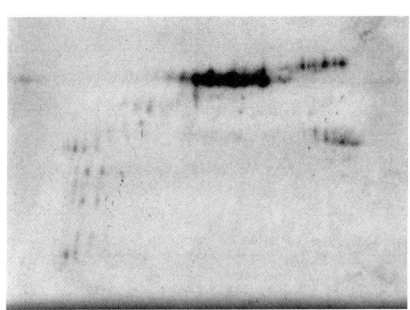

FIGURE 4. Mitochondria matrix phosphoproteone. **(A)** Autoradiogram of a 2D gel electrophoresis of energized porcine heart mitochondria after a 20-minute incubation with ^{32}P inorganic phosphate. **(B)** Autoradiogram of the same conditions with the uncoupler DNP incubated for an additional 5 minutes after the 20-minute ^{32}P phosphate incubation. Data from Hopper et al.[51] where protein assignments are also documented.

activity and a concentration locked to that already present in the matrix. Some examples of these studies are presented in FIGURE 4. Protein phosphorylation in the matrix was found to be extensive and dynamic. De-energizing the mitochondria with uncoupler rapidly decreased the phosphorylation (FIG. 4B) demonstrating the presence of highly active kinases and phosphatases in the matrix. The fact that the phosphorylations were so responsive to the energization state implies that these phosphorylations could be playing numerous roles in the regulation of metabolism during alterations in the high energy phosphates associated with high work states, hypoxia ischemia, or even intermittent ischemia protection schemes. Phosphorylation sites within each one of the complexes of the cytochrome chain along with many of the elements of fatty acid and citric acid cycle metabolic pathways were detected. These data suggest that protein phosphorylation is a very viable mechanism for signaling molecules to orchestrate the production and utilization of the membrane potential for ATP production at several levels resulting in a minimum impact on the NADH redox state or other metabolic intermediates.

SUMMARY

The evidence for the metabolic homeostasis in the cytosol and mitochondrial matrix in the face of changes in workload was reviewed. The most likely cytosolic signaling molecule for orchestrating this process is Ca^{2+} while other candidates are still under investigation. Computer simulation revealed problems with using *in vitro* enzyme kinetic data for modeling *in vivo* processes and indicated that the control of oxidative phosphorylation has to occur at both the level of the generation of the membrane potential and the dissipation processes in a coordinated fashion. Protein phosphorylation studies reveal an extensive and dynamic protein phosphorylation network in the mitochondrial matrix that would provide the mechanism for the coordinated control of oxidative phosphorylation predicted from the computer simulations. Detailed understanding of the effects and control of protein phosphorylation at the individual steps of oxidative phosphorylation will now need to be conducted to establish the role of these phosphorylation events in the control of ATP production.

REFERENCES

1. WOLLENBERGER, A. 1957. Relation between work and labile phosphate content in the isolated dog heart. Circ. Res. **5(2):** 175–178.
2. BOERTH, R.C., J.W. COVELL, S.C. SEAGREN, et al. 1969. High-energy phosphate concentrations in dog myocardium during stress. Am. J. Physiol. **216:** 1103–1106.
3. NEELY, J.R., R.M. DENTON, P.J. ENGLAND & P.J. RANDLE. 1972. The effects of increased heart work on the tricarboxylate cycle and its interactions with glycolysis in the perfused rat heart. Biochem. J. **128:** 147–159.
4. BALABAN, R.S., H.L. KANTOR, L.A. KATZ, et al. 1986. Relation between work and phosphate metabolite in the in vivo paced mammalian heart. Science **232:** 1121–1123.
5. KATZ, L.A., J.A. SWAIN, M.A. PORTMAN, et al. 1989. Relation between phosphate metabolites and oxygen consumption of heart in vivo. Am. J. Physiol. **256:** H265–H274.
6. HEINEMAN, F.W., & R.S. BALABAN. 1990. Phosphorus-31 nuclear magnetic resonance analysis of transient changes of canine myocardial metabolism in vivo. J. Clin. Invest. **85:** 843–852.
7. FROM, A.H.L., M.A. PETEIN, S.P. MICHURSKI, et al. 1986. 31P-NMR studies of respiratory regulation in the intact myocardium. FEBS Lett. **206:** 257–261.
8. ROBITAILLE, P.M., H. MERKLE, B. LEW, et al. 1990. Transmural high energy phosphate distribution and response to alterations in workload in the normal canine myocardium as studied with spatially localized 31P NMR spectroscopy. Mag. Res. Med. **16:** 91–116.
9. DETRE, J.A., A.P. KORETSKY, D.S. WILLIAMS, et al. 1990. Absence of pH changes during altered work in the in vivo sheep heart: a 31P NMR investigation. J. Mol. Cell. Cardiol. **22:** 543–553.
10. SCHAEFER, S., G.G. SCHWARTZ, et al. 1992. Metabolic response of the human heart to inotropic stimulation: in vivo phosphorus-31 studies of normal and cardiomyopathic myocardium. Mag. Res. Med. **25:** 260–272.
11. GARLICK, P.B., S. SOBOLL & G.R. BULLOCK. 1992. Evidence that mitochondrial phosphate is visible in 31P NMR spectra of isolated, perfused rat hearts. NMR Biomed. **5:** 29–36.
12. CHANCE, B. & B. THORELL. 1959. Fluorescence measurements of mitochondrial pyridine nucleotide in aerobiosis and anaerobiosis. Nature **184:** 931–934.
13. CHANCE, B., J.R. WILLIAMSON, D. FAMIESON, et al. 1965. Properties and kinetics of reduced pyridine nucleotide fluorescence of the isolated and in vivo rat heart. Biochemische Zeitschrift **341:** 357–377.
14. CHANCE, B. & C.M. WILLIAMS. 1956. The respiratory chain and oxidative phosphorylation. Adv. Enzymol. **17:** 65–134.

15. HEINEMAN, F.W. & R.S. BALABAN. Effects of afterload and heart rate on NAD(P)H redox state in the isolated rabbit heart. Am. J. Physiol. **264:** H433–H440.
16. WAN, B., C. DOUMEN, J. DUSZYNSKI, *et al.* 1993. Effect of cardiac work on electrical potential gradient across mitochondrial membrane in perfused rat hearts. Am. J. Physiol. **265:** 453–460.
17. VUORINEN, K.H., A. LA-RAMI, Y. YAN, *et al.* 1995. Respiratory control in heart muscle during fatty acid oxidation. Energy state or substrate-level regulation by Ca2+? J. Mol. Cell. Cardiol. **27:** 1581–1591.
18. ASHRUF, J.F., J.M. COREMANS, H.A. BRUINING, *et al.* 1995. Increase of cardiac work is associated with decrease of mitochondrial NADH. Am. J. Physiol. **269:** H856–H862.
19. BALABAN, R.S. 2002. Cardiac energy metabolism homeostasis: role of cytosolic calcium. J. Mol. Cell. Cardiol. **34(10):** 1259–1271.
20. LIIMATTA, E.V., A. GODECKE, J. SCHRADER & I.E. HASSINEN. 2004. Regulation of cellular respiration in myoglobin-deficient mouse heart. Mol. Cell. Biochem. **256–257:** 201–208.
21. MOOTHA, V.K., A.E. ARAI & R.S. BALABAN. 1997. Maximum oxidative phosphorylation capacity of the mammalian heart. Am. J. Physiol. **272:** H769–H775.
22. BACKUS, M., D. PIWNICA-WORMS, D. HOCKETT, *et al.* 1993. Microprobe analysis of TC-MIMBI in heart cells: calculation of mitochondrial membrane potential. Am. J. Physiol. **265:** C178–C187.
23. ARAI, A.E., C.E. KASSERRA, P.R. TERRITO, *et al.* 1999. Myocardial oxygenation in vivo: optical spectroscopy of cytoplasmic myoglobin and mitochondrial cytochromes. Am. J. Physiol. **277:** H683–H697.
24. WILSON, D.F., C.S. OWEN & A. HOLIAN. 1977. Control of mitochondrial respiration: a quantitative evaluation of the roles of cytochrome c and oxygen. Arch. Biochem. Biophys. **182:** 749–762.
25. MCCORMACK, J.G., A.P. HALESTRAP & R.M. DENTON. 1990. Role of calcium ions in regulation of mammalian intramitochondrial metabolism. Physiol. Rev. **70:** 391–425.
26. TERRITO, P.R., V.K. MOOTHA, S.A. FRENCH & R.S. BALABAN. 2000. Ca(2+) activation of heart mitochondrial oxidative phosphorylation: role of F0/F1ATPase. Am. J. Physiol. **278:** C423–C435.
27. KIM, D.K., F.W. HEINEMAN & R.S. BALABAN. 1991. Effects of B-hydroxybutyrate on oxidative metabolism and phosphorylation potential in canine heart in vivo. Am. J. Physiol. **260:** H1767–H1773.
28. LAUGHLIN, M.R. & F.W. HEINEMAN. 1994. The relationship between phosphorylation potential and redox state in the isolated working rabbit heart. J. Mol. Cell. Cardiol. **26:** 1525–1536.
29. SCHOLZ, T.D., M.R. LAUGHLIN, R.S. BALABAN, *et al.* 1995. Effect of substrate on mitochondrial NADH, cytosolic redox state, and phosphorylated compounds in isolated hearts. Am. J. Physiol. **268:** H82–H91.
30. ZHANG, J., D.J. DUNCKER, Y. XU, *et al.* 1995. Transmural bioenergetic responses of normal myocardium to high workstates. Am. J. Physiol. **268:** H1891–H1911.
31. DE GRAAF, R.A., K.A. VAN & K. NICOLAY. 2000. In vivo (31)P-NMR diffusion spectroscopy of ATP and phosphocreatine in rat skeletal muscle. Biophys. J. **78:** 1657–1664.
32. KUSHMERICK, M.J. & R.J. PODOLSKY. 1969. Ionic mobility in muscle cells. Science **166:** 1297–1298.

33. BALABAN, R.S. 2002. Cardiac energy metabolism homeostasis: role of cytosolic calcium. J. Mol. Cell. Cardiol. **34:** 1259–1271.
34. BESSMAN, S.P. & P.J. GEIGER. 1981. Transport of energy in muscle: the phosphorylcreatine shuttle. Science **211:** 448–452.
35. MEYER, R.A., H.L. SWEENEY & M.J. KUSHMERICK. 1984. A simple analysis of the "phosphocreatine shuttle." Am. J. Physiol. **242:** 1–11.
36. BESSMAN, S.P. & A. FONYO. 1966. The possible role of the mitochondrial bound creatine kinase in regulation of mitochondrial respiration Biochem. Biophys. Res. Commun. **22:** 597–602.
37. WALLIMANN, T., M. DOLDER, U. SCHLATTNER, et al. 1998. Some new aspects of creatine kinase (CK): compartmentation, structure, function and regulation for cellular and mitochondrial bioenergetics and physiology. Biofactors **8:** 229–234.
38. SAKS, V.A., O. KONGAS, M. VENDELIN & L. KAY. 2000. Role of the creatine/phosphocreatine system in the regulation of mitochondrial respiration. Acta Physiol. Scand. **168:** 635–641.
39. ALIEV, M.K. & V.A. SAKS. 1993. Quantitative analysis of the 'phosphocreatine shuttle': I. A probability approach to the description of phosphocreatine production in the coupled creatine kinase-ATP/ADP translocase-oxidative phosphorylation reactions in heart mitochondria. Biochim. Biophys. Acta **1143:** 291–300.
40. SEPPET, E.K., T. KAAMBRE, P. SIKK, et al. 2001. Functional complexes of mitochondria with Ca,MgATPases of myofibrils and sarcoplasmic reticulum in muscle cells. Biochim. Biophys. Acta **1504:** 379–395.
41. KAASIK, A., V. VEKSLER, E. BOEHM, et al. 2001. Energetic crosstalk between organelles: architectural integration of energy production and utilization. Circ. Res. **89:** 153–159.
42. ROTHSTEIN, E.C., S. CARROLL, C.A. COMBS, et al. 2005. Skeletal muscle NAD(P)H two-photon fluorescence microscopy in vivo: topology and optical inner filters. Biophys. J. **88:** 2165–2176.
43. WRIGHT, B.E., M.H. BUTLER & K.R. ALBE. 1992. Systems analysis of the tricarboxylic acid cycle in Dictyostelium discoideum. I. The basis for model construction. J. Biol. Chem. **267:** 3101–3105.
44. TEUSINK, B., J. PASSARGE, C.A. REIJENGA, et al. 2000. Can yeast glycolysis be understood in terms of in vitro kinetics of the constituent enzymes? Testing biochemistry. Eur. J. Biochem. **267:** 5313–5329.
45. KORETSKY, A.P. & R.S. BALABAN. 1987. Changes in pyridine nucleotide levels alter oxygen consumption and extramitochondrial phosphates in isolated mitochondria: A 31P NMR and fluorescence study. Biochim. Biophys. **893:** 398–408.
46. JOUBERT, F., H.M. FALES, H. WEN, et al. 2004. NADH enzyme-dependent fluorescence recovery after photobleaching (ED-FRAP): applications to enzyme and mitochondrial reaction kinetics, in vitro. Biophys. J. **86:** 629–645.
47. BLINOVA, K., S. CARROLL, S. BOSE, et al. 2005. Distribution of mitochondrial NADH fluorescence lifetimes: steady-state kinetics of matrix NADH interactions. Biochemistry **44:** 2585–2594.
48. HARRIS, R.A., K.M. POPOV, Y. ZHAO, et al. 1995. A new family of protein kinases— the mitochondrial protein kinases. Adv. Enzyme Regul. **35:** 147–162.
49. NEWMEYER, D.D. & S. FERGUSON-MILLER. 2003. Mitochondria: releasing power for life and unleashing the machineries of death. Cell. **112:** 481–490.

50. SCHULENBERG, B., R. AGGELER, *et al.* 2003. Analysis of steady-state protein phosphorylation in mitochondria using a novel fluorescent phosphosensor dye. J. Biol. Chem. **278:** 27251–27255.
51. HOPPER, R.K., S. CARROLL, A.M. APONTE, *et al.* 2006. Mitochondrial matrix phosphoproteome: effect of extra mitochondrial calcium. Biochemistry **45:** 2524–2536.

Diversity of Ca^{2+} Signaling in Developing Cardiac Cells

EINSLEY JANOWSKI,[a] LARS CLEEMANN,[a] PHILIPP SASSE,[b] AND MARTIN MORAD[a]

[a] *Department of Pharmacology, Georgetown University, 3900 Reservoir Road, NW., Washington, DC 20057, USA*

[b] *Institute of Physiology I, University of Bonn, Sigmund-Freud-Strasse 25, 53105 Bonn, Germany*

ABSTRACT: During embryonic and postnatal development, the mammalian heart undergoes rapid morphological changes with cellular differentiation that at the ultrastructural level encompasses altered expression and organization of the proteins and organelles associated with Ca^{2+} signaling. Here the development and roles of the releasable Ca^{2+} stores located within the sarco/endoplasmic reticulum and possibly within the nuclear envelopes are addressed. Confocal Ca^{2+} imaging experiments were carried out on (i) neonatal rat cardiomyocytes, (ii) pluripotent P19 stem cells, differentiated to a cardiac phenotype by culturing with 1% dimethylsulfoxide (DMSO) in hanging droplets, and (iii) mouse embryonic cardiomyocytes isolated for short-time culture at embryonic day 9–18. The Ca^{2+} release channels in neonatal and "cardiac" P19 cell were activated versus inhibited by targeting ryanodine (Ry) receptors with caffeine versus Ry and IP_3 receptors with adenosine 5'-triphosphate (ATP) or histamine versus U-73122, a phospholipase c (PLC) inhibitor. The neonatal cells displayed four recognizable phenotypes, of which two had specialized Ca^{2+} stores releasable via either Ry or IP_3 receptors, and two had both types of receptors, either controlling functionally separate stores or with some degree of overlap, so that caffeine could deplete the stores releasable by ATP. The P19 cells showed variable presence of IP_3-mediated Ca^{2+} stores, and caffeine releasable stores that gained prominence in the "cardiac" phenotype, but were absent in a "neuronal" phenotype. The different roles of Ca^{2+} stores were seen clearly in the mouse embryonic cells. Some cells from early stages of development (E 9–10) had Ca^{2+} waves that increased in intensity during the diastolic interval and could trigger synchronous electrical excitation (via Na-Ca exchanger [NCX] and excitatory Ca^{2+} and Na^+ channels). At later stages of development (E 18) we observed diastolic Ca^{2+} sparks that appeared to originate from the nuclear envelope, while the Ca^{2+} signals during excitation were faster and stronger in the nuclear region than in the

Address for correspondence: Prof. Martin Morad, Ph.D., Department of Pharmacology, Georgetown University, 3900 Reservoir Road, NW. Washington, DC 20057, USA. Voice: 202-413-8772; fax: 202-687-8458.

e-mail: moradm@georgetown.edu

surrounding cytoplasmic regions. However, we also found cells where the nuclear Ca^{2+} signals were weaker and showed afterglow compared to the cytosolic Ca^{2+} transients. We conclude that the Ca^{2+} stores in cardiac cells during embryogenesis and postnatal development, that is, before the maturation of the t-tubular system and in stem cells with cardiac phenotype, show considerable diversity with respect to the pharmacology of the release channels and that regional differences in Ca^{2+} signaling are observed centered in, at, and around the nucleus. We suggest that the causal relationship excitation and subcellular Ca^{2+} signals in developing cardiac cells is different from that of adult cells and that the developing cardiomyocytes show a diversity that in later stages of development may be reflected in the different properties of atrial, ventricular, and pacemaker cells.

KEYWORDS: embryonic and neonatal cardiac myocytes; P19 cells; pacemaker cells calcium signaling

INTRODUCTION

Ca^{2+} signaling in the adult mammalian heart shows characteristic patterns in different cell types depending on the development of functional intracellular Ca^{2+} stores and their coupling to electrical excitation. The synchronous contractions of mature atria and ventricles are contingent on the rapid spread of excitation between cells, which, through a cascade of events, leads to release of Ca^{2+} from internal stores located in the sarcoplasmic reticulum (SR). In ventricular cells this cascade primarily plays out at dyadic junctions where L-type Ca^{2+} channels in the t-tubular membranes allows Ca^{2+} to enter the cleft space and trigger a much larger release of Ca^{2+} via ryanodine (Ry) receptors in the SR membrane. In atrial cells that lack t-tubules, this basic mechanism is limited to peripheral junctions on the cell surface, but additional pathways may be operative including: (i) fast, (ii) delayed Ca^{2+} release from centrally located corbular SR, (iii) SR release mediated by the IP_3 receptors, and (iv) possibly from mitochondria. In turn, it is also recognized that the elevation of cytosolic Ca^{2+} generates elements of feedback to the electrical excitation. For instance, in dyadic junctions the Ca^{2+} released via Ry receptors plays a dominant role in promoting Ca^{2+}-induced inactivation of the L-type Ca^{2+} channel and the Na^+–Ca^{2+} exchanger may respond to elevated cytosolic Ca^{2+} by generating a potentially arrhythmogenic inward current. In fact, it appears that the primary direction of Ca^{2+} signaling may be reversed in some cases so that Ca^{2+} signals drive the electrical excitation rather than being initiated by them. This situation may arise, for instance, in pacing sinoatrial cells where rhythmic Ca^{2+} oscilliations are seen to persist after membrane depolarizations have been suppressed.[1] To this diversity may be added Ca^{2+} signals originating from other organelles such as nuclei[2] and mitochondria.

In the present report, we survey Ca^{2+} signaling in developing cardiomyocytes where the expression of key Ca^{2+} signaling proteins changes rapidly with development and intracellular Ca^{2+} stores may develop distinct gating and functionality prior to their coupling to membrane depolarization. Experiments were carried out using neonatal rat and embryonic mouse cardiomyocytes as well as human mesenchymal stem cells (hMSC) that were cultured to display a cardiac phenotype and may have potential uses in cell replacement therapies.[3]

Multiplicity of Calcium Pools in Neonatal Rat Cardiomyocytes

During embryonic and postnatal development cardiac cells display marked changes in the expression of multiple proteins and a general transition from cell proliferation to cell growth. The changes affect many cellular processes including energy metabolism, cell-to-cell communication via gap junctions, and Ca^{2+} signaling, which in turn involves the expression of Ca^{2+} channels and transporters and ultrastructural modifications such as maturation of the t-tubular system, reorganization of releasable intracellular Ca^{2+} stores, and formation of macromolecular junctional Ca^{2+} signaling complexes. The understanding of these modifications may also be relevant to the study of cardiac hyperplasia and hypertrophy, partly because they may be evoked by similar factors (hormones, workload, hypoxia, etc.). In addition developing cells appear to display some features, for example, resistance to apoptosis[4] and alternative pathways for regulation of protein expression[5] lacking in diseased myocardium.

In neonatal cardiomyocytes from 1–2-day-old rats we found multiple calcium pools. Cells were dissociated with trypsin and collagenase, plated onto glass cover slips, generally cultured for 24–72 h, and imaged confocally after loading with the Ca^{2+} indicator dye Fluo-4AM (Molecular Probes, Eugene, OR).

To test for the presence of intracellular Ca^{2+} stores we targeted different potential Ca^{2+} release channels with pharmacological agents using, respectively, 10 mM caffeine to activate Ry receptors and 100 μM ATP to trigger IP_3 receptors. We found that the cells with spontaneous activity generated large long-lasting Ca^{2+} transients when exposed to rapid superfusion with solution containing caffeine (FIG. 1, panels EH, cells 1 and 3). When the same group of cells was exposed to ATP, the normally quiescent cells generated similar long-lasting Ca^{2+} transients (panels FI, cells 2 and 4) or produced one or more briefer Ca^{2+} spikes suggesting a tendency for pacemaker activity. This general division is emphasized in FIGURE 1, and it suggests that Ca^{2+} stores in some neonatal cardiomyocytes are primarily gated by Ry receptors while in others they are gated by IP_3 receptors. However, as indicated in TABLE 1 and described below, a more careful analysis indicates that some cells have both types of Ca^{2+} release channels.

The involvement of two types of Ca^{2+} release channels was observed in 151 cultured cells and confirmed in 18 freshly dissociated cells (TABLE 1).

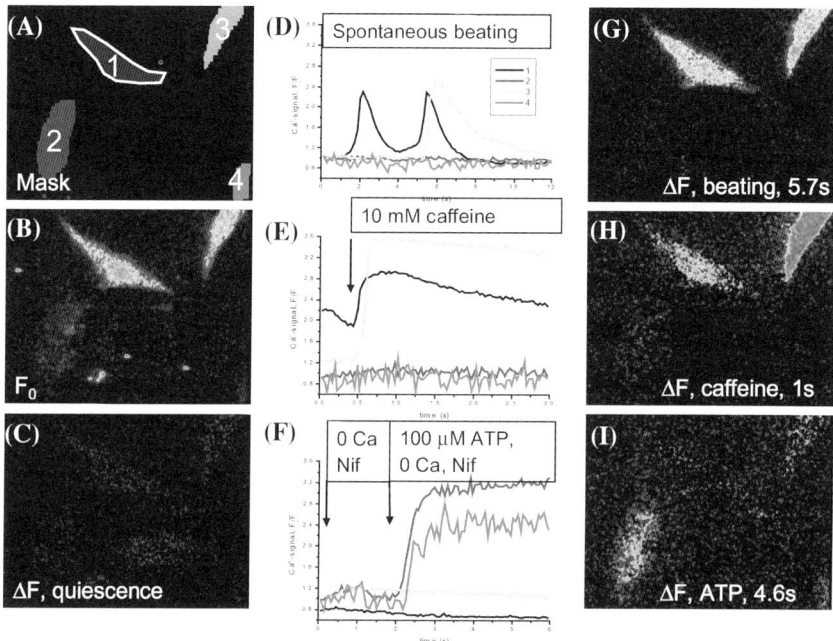

FIGURE 1. Caffeine responsive and beating cells versus adenosine 5′-triphosphate (ATP)-responsive and quiescent neonatal cardiomyocytes. Panel A: Identification of cells and regions of measurement based on colors and numbers as used for traces in panels D–F. Panel B: Background fluorescence, F_0. Panels C, G–I show fluorescence intensity after subtraction of background fluorescence ($\Delta F = F - F_0$) measured as indication of the noise level. Panels D–F show changes in fluorescence intensity for the four identified cells during: (**D**) spontaneous beating of some cells, (**E**) rapid addition of 10 mM caffeine, and (**F**) exposure to 100 μM ATP while the cell was superfused with a Tyrode's solution without Ca^{2+}, but with 10 μM nifedipine. (1–2 day old rat cardiomyocytes cultured 2 days; fluo-4 staining; confocal imaging at 30 frames/sec). As shown in panels D and G, some cells generated spontaneous rhythmic Ca^{2+} transients with an initial rapid rise indicative of electrical depolarization.

The observed Ca^{2+} transients did not require influx of Ca^{2+} across the cell membrane via the L-type Ca^{2+} channel as they persisted when Ca^{2+} was removed and/or 10 μM nifedipine was added well in advance of the exposure to the Ca^{2+}-releasing agent (FIG. 1F). The ATP-triggered Ca^{2+} releases were abolished by 5-min exposure to a PLC inhibitor (10 μM U-73122) while caffeine-induced Ca^{2+} releases, on average, were suppressed in 65% of the cells by 40 μM Ry. Collectively these results provide strong evidence that neonatal cardiomyocytes have substantial intracellular Ca^{2+} stores that can be released via Ry or IP_3 receptors.

We further found that a subset of the spontaneously beating cells released Ca^{2+} in response to both caffeine and ATP and that this fraction was somewhat

TABLE 1. Ca²⁺ stores in neonatal rat cardiomyocytes and P19 pluripotent stem cells

	Beating (spont.)	Ca²⁺ release via Ry receptor (Caffeine 10 mM)		Ca²⁺ release via IP₃ receptor (ATP 100 μM)				RyR_IP₃R interaction	n
		F/F_0	Block by 40 μM Ry	F/F_0	Block by 10 μM U-73122	Histamine	Glutamate	ATP response blocked by 10 mM caff.	
Cardiomyocytes, from 1–2 old rat	+	2.1	65%	—					37c + 10a
	—	—	—	1.6	95%			—	74c + 6a
				2.1	100%			+	40c + 2a
P19 stem cells Undiff.	→	→	++	++	→	+	—		
"cardiac"	++	++	(+)	(+)		(+)	—		
"neuronal"	++	—	(+)	(+)		(+)	++		

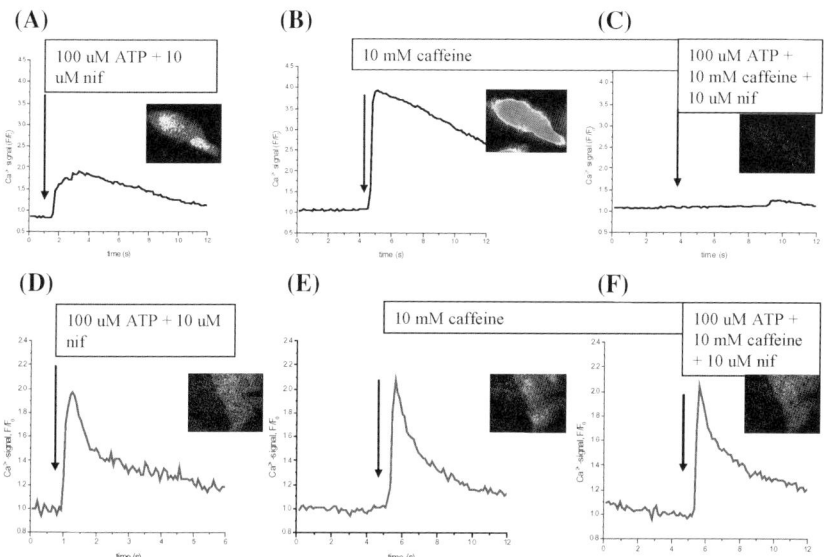

FIGURE 2. Two ATP-sensitive phenotypes among neonatal cardiomyocytes with responsiveness to both caffeine and ATP. Panels A–C: Recordings from a cell where the initial ATP response (**A**) was abolished (**C**) following a caffeine-induced Ca^{2+} release. Panels D–F: Recordings from cell where the ATP response was similar before (**D**) and after (**F**) the addition of caffeine (**E**). Arrows indicate the timing of solution changes. Insets show rise in Ca^{2+} (ΔF). (1–2 day old rat cardiomyocytes cultured 2 days; Fluo-4AM staining; confocal imaging at 30 frames/sec).

larger in cultured (65% = 74 cells/(74 cells + 107 cells)) than in freshly dissociated cells (38% = 6 cells /(6 cells + 10 cells)). This finding might indicate the presence in the same cell of two independent types of Ca^{2+} store, where one was controlled by Ry receptors and the other one by IP_3 receptors, but it might also suggest that Ca^{2+} pools in the same SR compartments could be released by either Ry or IP_3 receptors. These possibilities were tested as shown in FIGURE 2, which compares the responses of two cultured cardiomyocytes to ATP in the absence and presence of 10 mM caffeine. The cell illustrated in the upper row of panels in FIGURE 2 (panels A, B, C) had a small but distinct response to ATP (panel A) that was completely abolished (panel C) after the caffeine releasable pool had been emptied (panel B). In contrast the cell in the lower row of panels produced similar ATP-triggered Ca^{2+} releases before (panel D) and after (panel F) caffeine was added and had produced a Ca^{2+} transient of similar magnitude (panel E). Similar recordings were obtained with freshly dissociated cardiomyocytes.

In summary, we identified four types of neonatal cardiomyocytes based on measurements of triggered release of Ca^{2+} from intracellular pools that are: (i) gated exclusively by Ry receptors, (ii) gated exclusively by IP_3 receptors,

(iii) organized as functionally distinct Ca^{2+} pools that are either gated by either Ry receptors or IP_3 receptors, but not both, or (iv) integrated in such a way that the Ry receptors and IP_3 receptors appear to provide alternate routes of releasing Ca^{2+} from the same functional compartment.

Calcium Signaling Characterization of P19 Pluripotent Stem Cells that are Differentiated into Neuronal and Cardiac Cell Types

Pluripotent P19 embryonal carcinoma cells are known to differentiate into neuronal and cardiac cells, but the role of development or loss of different Ca^{2+} signaling pathways in these phenotypes has not been fully explored. Here we report on Ca^{2+} signaling cascades in cardiac, neuronal, and undifferentiated cell types. Undifferentiated cells were grown either with retinoic acid (3 days) in aggregates or with dimethylsulfoxide (DMSO) (8 days) in hanging drops to promote differentiation of neuronal or cardiac cells, respectively. As in neonatal cardiomyocytes, confocal Ca^{2+} imaging was used to assess the presence of different Ca^{2+} signaling pathways. We used: (i) caffeine and Ry to target Ry receptors, (ii) histamine, ATP, and U-73122 to control activation of IP_3 receptors via the phospholipase C pathway, (iii) KCl, nifedipine, and Ca^{2+} withdrawal to assess the roles of membrane depolarization and plasmalemmal L-type Ca^{2+} channels, and (iv) thapsigargin, Ca^{2+} withdrawal, and La^{+3} to assess Ca^{2+} influx linked to depletion of intracellular Ca^{2+} stores.

FIGURE 3 shows typical responses of undifferentiated, "neuronal," and "cardiac" type P19 cells to histamine, ATP, and caffeine. In undifferentiated cells, Ca^{2+} release occurred consistently only on exposure to 100 μM histamine (FIG. 3A), but less frequently to 100 μM ATP (FIG. 3D) and hardly at all to 10 mM caffeine (FIG. 3G). Small rises in cytosolic Ca^{2+} were also observed on depolarization or depletion of Ca^{2-} stores, but not with 100 μM glutamate exposure. The histamine and ATP responses were inhibited by the PLC inhibitor U-73122, the caffeine response by Ry, and a prominent store-operated Ca^{2+} signal by La^{3+}.

Ca^{2+} signals were generally smaller in neuronal phenotypes where responses were infrequently evoked by histamine (FIG. 3B), more often by ATP (FIG. 3E), but never with caffeine (FIG. 3H). Glutamate and store depletion produced larger Ca^{2+} rises than KCl depolarizations.

The P19 cells differentiated to "cardiac" phenotype responded almost in every cell robustly to caffeine (FIG. 3I), and less frequently to histamine (FIG. 3C) and ATP (FIG. 3F). It may be noted that those "cardiac" cells that responded to ATP rarely responded to caffeine, and that this feature is shared both with undifferentiated P19 cells and neonatal cardiomyocytes. Small rises in Ca^{2+} were also observed on depolarization with KCl, but not on exposure to glutamate.

We conclude that differentiation of P19 cells parallels changes in their unique Ca^{2+} signaling pathways. Whether this differentiation is related to development or deletion of a specific Ca^{2+} signaling cascades remains to be explored.

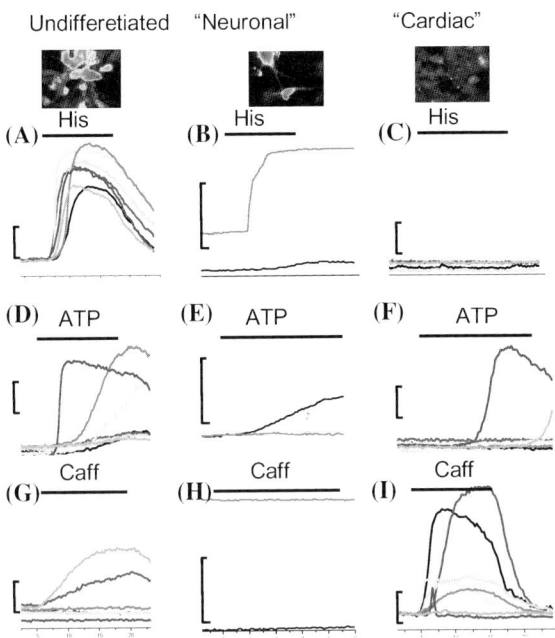

FIGURE 3. Responses of differentially cultured P19 cells to histamine, ATP, and caffeine (vertical scale bar: $\Delta F/F_0 = 1$; 25 sec recordings; staining with Fluo-4AM: confocal imaging at 4 frames per sec.)

Ca^{2+} Signaling in Mouse Embryonic Cardiomyocytes

As shown above, intracellular Ca^{2+} stores are quite varied from cell to cell at the same stage of development and significantly change their characteristics during a few days of culturing. In case of P19 cells, these changes were guided intentionally by culture conditions, but even the neonatal cells appeared to change during the 1–3 days of culture normally allowed for the cells to stabilize following enzymatic dissociation. With such diverse properties of Ca^{2+} stores, it is pertinent to ask what the functional implications may be. We explored this question using high-speed (240 frames per sec) confocal Ca^{2+} imaging of mouse embryonic cardiomyocytes that were harvested at day 9–19 of gestation, dispersed enzymatically, and cultured 1–5 days prior to experimentation.

The embryonic cells produced strong synchronized Ca^{2+} transients similar to those triggered by action potentials in adult atrial and ventricular cells, but in addition they produced Ca^{2+} sparks and waves that were independent of membrane depolarization or Ca^{2+} influx and were often centered around the nucleus, which in turn might either participate in or be excluded from the general cellular response during depolarization. FIGURE 4 shows Ca^{2+} signals from a cell where a spontaneous action potential gave rise to a nuclear Ca^{2+}

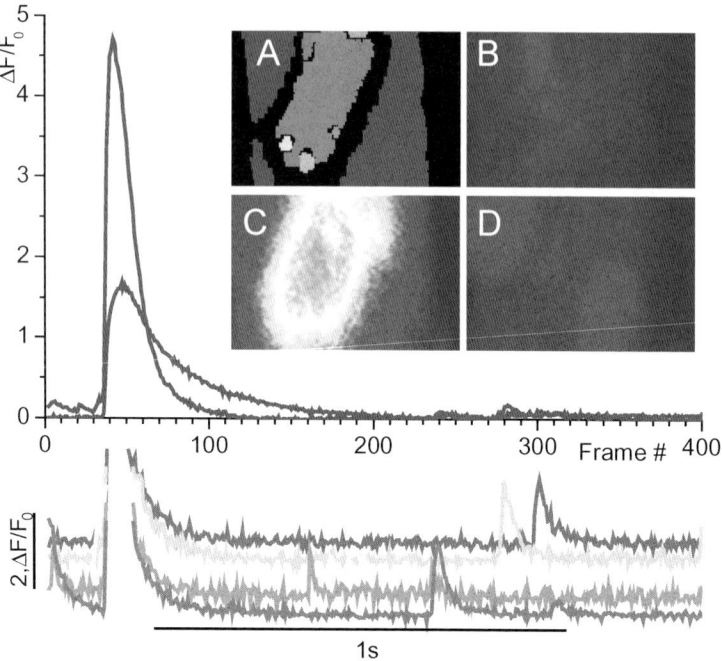

FIGURE 4. Ca^{2+} sparks around the nucleus of a mouse embryonic cell. Upper traces show Ca^{2+} signals ($\Delta F/F_0$) in the nuclear region (purple) and in the remaining cytosol (blue) (shown in color online). The lower traces show local Ca^{2+} signals from color-coded spots around the nucleus at locations where Ca^{2+} sparks were observed during diastolic intervals. Inset panels show a map of selected, color-coded regions (**A**), background fluorescence (**B**), the Ca^{2+} signal during the action potential (**C**, frame no. 50), and the more slowly decaying fluorescence around the nucleus (**D**, frame no. 100). (Confocal Ca^{2+} imaging at 240 frames per sec, mouse cell harvested at embryonic day 18).

signal that was stronger and more rapidly decaying than in the cytosol in general. Furthermore, the prominent role of the nucleus was underscored by numerous Ca^{2+} sparks that, in the subsequent diastolic interval, appear to cluster around its perimeter. These Ca^{2+} sparks were typical of cardiac cells with regard to amplitude and time course, but their distribution was markedly different from those of atrial and ventricular cells where Ca^{2+} sparks generally are found, respectively, near the sarcolemma [6,7] and along z-lines.[8]

In some other cells that rarely produced ordinary Ca^{2+} sparks, we observed Ca^{2+} waves that were of low intensity, prominent around the nucleus, and increased in intensity toward the end of the diastolic interval, and therefore could trigger electrical excitation. Such pacemaker activity centered around the nucleus would clearly be different from the more conventional scheme where the heart rate is thought to be controlled by time- and voltage-dependent ionic channels in the cell membrane. In addition, it raises the question of whether the nuclear envelope during embryonic development may serve as a significant intracellular store for releasable Ca^{2+}.

SUMMARY

We have emphasized here the diversity of intracellular Ca^{2+} stores in developing cells and have raised questions regarding their role. The reported findings demonstrate a high degree of plasticity that may also come into play during normal physiological responses as well as in disease states. In fact, it seems likely that the impetus to provide clear understanding of normal atrial and ventricular function has lead to an underestimation of the multiple E–C coupling pathways that may exist in these tissues. For instance, we and others have found that activator Ca^{2+} in adult atrial cardiomyocytes does not derive solely from Ca^{2+} influx and Ca^{2+}-induced release of Ca^{2+} from subsarcolemmal Ca^{2+} stores, but also involves IP_3-gated stores, more centrally located Ca^{2+} stores triggered by fast–slow mechanisms, and even mechanically triggered Ca^{2+} stores.

It should also be emphasized that the Ca^{2+} stores do not operate in isolation, but in coordination with many other cellular processes of which some of the more pertinent clearly are the other Ca^{2+}-transporting, -buffering, and -sensing proteins, and ultrastructural modification involved in the organization of macromolecular signaling complexes. From developmental perspective and with increased appreciation of the diversity of cardiac cells, it is both challenging and rewarding to explore the details of cellular and subcellular cardiac Ca^{2+} signaling during embryogenesis and postnatal maturation.

ACKNOWLEDGMENT

This study was supported by NIH Grant R0116152.

REFERENCES

1. VINOGRADOVA, T.M., V.A. MALTSEV, K.Y. BOGDANOV, et al. 2005. Rhythmic Ca^{2+} oscillations drive sinoatrial nodal cell pacemaker function to make the heart tick. Ann. N. Y. Acad. Sci. **1047:** 138–156.
2. BKAILY, G., N. EL-BIZRI, M. NADER, et al. 2005. Angiotensin II induced increase in frequency of cytosolic and nuclear calcium waves of heart cells via activation of AT1 and AT2 receptors. Peptides **26:** 1418–1426.
3. HEUBACH, J.F., E.M. GRAF, J. LEUTHEUSER, et al. 2004. Electrophysiological properties of human mesenchymal stem cells. J. Physiol. **554:** 659–672.
4. DE WINDT, L.J., H.W. LIM, T. TAIGEN, et al. 2000. Calcineurin-mediated hypertrophy protects cardiomyocytes from apoptosis in vitro and in vivo: an apoptosis-independent model of dilated heart failure. Circ. Res. **86:** 255–263.

5. JU, H., T. SCAMMEL-LA FLEUR & I.M. DIXON. 1996. Altered mRNA abundance of calcium transport genes in cardiac myocytes induced by angiotensin II. J. Mol. Cell Cardiol. **28:** 1119–1128.
6. WOO, S.H., L. CLEEMANN & M. MORAD. 2005. Diversity of atrial local Ca2+ signalling: evidence from 2-D confocal imaging in Ca2+-buffered rat atrial myocytes. J. Physiol. **567:** 905–921.
7. WOO, S.H., L. CLEEMANN & M. MORAD. 2003. Spatiotemporal characteristics of junctional and nonjunctional focal Ca2+ release in rat atrial myocytes. Circ. Res. **92:** e1–e11.
8. CLEEMANN, L., W. WANG & M. MORAD. 1998. Two-dimensional confocal images of organization, density, and gating of focal Ca2+ release sites in rat cardiac myocytes. Proc. Natl. Acad. Sci. USA **95:** 10984–10989.

Regulation of Ca^{2+} and Na^+ in Normal and Failing Cardiac Myocytes

DONALD M. BERS, SANDA DESPA, AND JULIE BOSSUYT

Department of Physiology, Loyola University Chicago, Maywood, Illinois 60153, USA

ABSTRACT: Ca^{2+} in cardiac myocytes regulates contractility and relaxation, and Ca^{2+} and Na^+ regulation are linked via Na^+/Ca^{2+} exchange (NCX). Heart failure (HF) is accompanied by contractile dysfunction and arrhythmias, both of which may be due to altered cellular Ca^{2+} handling. Smaller Ca^{2+} transient and sarcoplasmic reticulum (SR) Ca^{2+} content cause systolic dysfunction in HF. The reduced SR Ca^{2+} content is due to: (*a*) reduced SR Ca^{2+}-ATPase function (which also contributes to diastolic dysfunction), (*b*) increased expression and function of NCX (which competes with SR Ca^{2+}-ATPase during relaxation, but preserves diastolic function), and (*c*) enhanced diastolic SR Ca^{2+} leak. Relative contributions of these may vary with HF etiology and stage. Triggered arrhythmias (e.g., delayed afterdepolarizations [DADs]) are prominent in HF. DADs are due to spontaneous SR Ca^{2+} release and consequent activation of transient inward NCX current, which in HF allows DADs to more readily trigger arrhythmogenic action potentials. Thus NCX and Na^+ are critical in systolic and diastolic function and arrhythmias. $[Na^+]_i$ is elevated in HF, which may limit SR unloading and provide some Ca^{2+} influx during the HF action potential, thus limiting the depression of systolic function. High $[Na^+]_i$ in HF is due to enhanced Na^+ influx. Cellular Na^+/K^+-ATPase (NKA) function appears unaltered, despite reduced NKA expression. This dichotomy led us to test NKA regulation by phospholemman (PLM). We find that PLM regulates NKA in a manner analogous to phospholamban regulation of SR Ca^{2+}-ATPase (i.e., inhibition that is relieved by PLM phosphorylation). We measured intermolecular FRET between PLM and NKA, which is reduced upon PLM phosphorylation. The lower expression level of more phosphorylated PLM in HF may explain the above dichotomy. Thus, altered Ca^{2+} and Na^+ handling contributes to altered contractile function and arrhythmogenesis in HF.

KEYWORDS: calcium; heart failure; Na^+–Ca^{2+} exchange; SR Ca^{2+}-ATPase; Na^+/K^+-ATPase; phospholemman

Address for correspondence: Dr. Donald M. Bers, Ph.D., Department of Physiology, Stritch School of Medicine, Loyola University Chicago, 2160 South First Avenue, Maywood, IL 60153–5500. Voice: 708-216-1018; fax: 708-216-6308.
  e-mail: dbers@lumc.edu

INTRODUCTION: $[Ca^{2+}]_i$ REGULATION AND CONTRACTILE DYSFUNCTION IN HEART FAILURE

Ca^{2+} ions play an essential role in cardiac myocyte contraction and relaxation.[1] During the cardiac action potential, Ca^{2+} enters the myocyte via voltage-dependent L-type Ca^{2+} channels, located primarily at sarcolemmal–sarcoplasmic reticulum (SR) junctions where the SR Ca^{2+} release channels (or ryanodine receptors [RyRs]) exist. Ca^{2+} entry triggers Ca^{2+} release from the SR. This raises the free intracellular $[Ca^{2+}]$ ($[Ca^{2+}]_i$), allowing Ca^{2+} to bind to the myofilaments and trigger contraction. For relaxation to occur, $[Ca^{2+}]_i$ must decline, allowing Ca^{2+} dissociation from the myofilaments. This requires Ca^{2+} transport out of the cytosol, mainly via the SR Ca^{2+}-ATPase (SERCA), which takes Ca^{2+} back into the SR, and by the sarcolemmal Na^+/Ca^{2+} exchange (NCX), which exchanges one Ca^{2+} ion for three Na^+ ions.[1] The direction (i.e., Ca^{2+} efflux or influx) and activity of NCX depends on the internal and external concentration of both Na^+ and Ca^{2+}, as well as on the membrane potential.[2] High $[Ca^{2+}]_i$ favors Ca^{2+} efflux whereas positive membrane potential and high $[Na^+]_i$ favor Ca^{2+} influx. Thus, Ca^{2+} and Na^+ regulation are linked via NCX.

Heart failure (HF) is accompanied by contractile dysfunction and arrhythmia, both of which may be due to altered cellular Ca^{2+} handling. Myocyte Ca^{2+} transients are depressed in HF and this causes systolic dysfunction. The reduced Ca^{2+} transients are due to lower SR Ca^{2+} content,[3–8] while Ca^{2+} entry via Ca^{2+} channels and the SR fractional release are generally not altered.[7–12] There are three factors that result in a reduced SR Ca^{2+} content in HF (FIG. 1): (a) reduced SR Ca^{2+}-ATPase function, (b) increased expression and function of NCX, and (c) enhanced diastolic SR Ca^{2+} leak. Relative contributions of these may vary with HF etiology and stage. SERCA expression is decreased by ~24% and NCX expression and function are increased by 100% in a nonischemic, arrhythmogenic rabbit heart failure model.[7] Nevertheless, the mild reduction in SERCA coupled with the increased NCX allows NCX to compete better with the SR Ca^{2+}-ATPase in extruding Ca^{2+} from the cytosol during relaxation, thus resulting in a lower SR Ca^{2+} content.[7] At the other extreme, Piacentino et al.[8] found a 40% reduction of SERCA function, but unaltered NCX extrusion in human end-stage HF, resulting again in lower SR Ca^{2+} content. Intermediate results, with increased NCX and decreased SERCA function, were observed in a rapid pacing-induced HF in dogs.[11] Hasenfuss et al.[13] found a spectrum of increase in NCX and decrease in SERCA2 expression in individual HF patients, suggesting that there is individual variation as to how much of the decrease in SR Ca^{2+} load in HF is due to increased NCX and decreased SERCA function. Hearts with decreased SERCA and unchanged NCX had diastolic dysfunction, whereas increased NCX expression and relatively unaltered SERCA was associated with preserved diastolic function. Thus, while downregulation of SERCA and upregulation of NCX both result in a lower SR Ca^{2+} content and

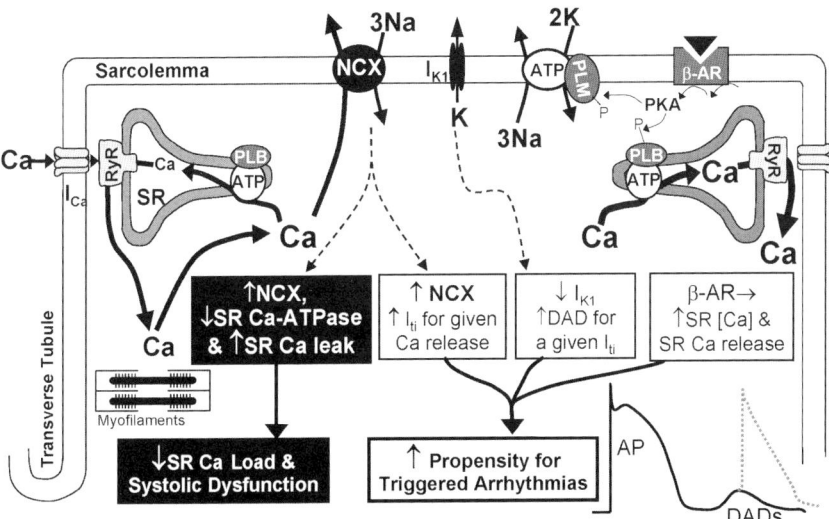

FIGURE 1. Ca^{2+} and Na^+ transport in cardiac myocytes. Ca^{2+} entry via Ca^{2+} current (I_{Ca}) activates SR Ca^{2+} release via RyR, which activates the myofilaments and Ca^{2+} is cleared from the cytoplasm by the SR Ca^{2+}-ATPase (ATP) and NCX. Three factors contribute to reduced SR Ca^{2+} load in HF (left), while enhanced NCX function, reduced I_{K1}, and residual β-adrenergic receptor (β-AR) responsiveness contribute to arrhythmogenesis via induction of delayed afterdepolarizations (DADs).

impaired contractility, reduced SERCA function also contributes to diastolic dysfunction. Increased expression and function of NCX preserves diastolic function but, as will be discussed below, also leads to a higher propensity for triggered arrhythmias in HF.

Enhanced diastolic SR Ca^{2+} leak was first demonstrated in ventricular myocytes from an arrhythmogenic rabbit HF model by Shannon et al.,[6] who showed how this might contribute to lower SR Ca^{2+} content in HF. This is probably the cellular correlate of the enhanced single-channel RyR gating previously seen in HF by Marx et al.[14] That group has published a long series of articles[14–18] that have all been consistent with the following working hypothesis. In HF the hyperadrenergic state causes RyR2 hyperphosphorylation (via RyR associated protein kinase A [PKA], abetted by less RyR-associated phosphatase and phosphodiesterase 4D), which causes dissociation of the FK-506 binding protein (FKBP12.6; which normally stabilizes RyR in the closed state), resulting in enhanced RyR open probability and diastolic SR Ca^{2+} leak. While they make a compelling case for most of these steps, there are numerous groups which have been unable to confirm certain key aspects (e.g., that PKA does not hyper-phosphorylate RyR2 in HF or cause FKBP12.6–RyR2 dissociation, that PKA activation does not increase steady state RyR2 activation and that there are additional PKA sites on RyR2).[19–22]

RyR2 can also be phosphorylated by CaMKII (which is also bound to the RyR2) and this activates RyR opening and diastolic SR Ca^{2+} release.[23–25] Ai et al.[26] found that CaMKII expression, association with RyR2 and activation state were higher in HF rabbits and that the enhanced SR Ca^{2+} leak could be prevented by CaMKII blockade, but not PKA inhibition. Interestingly, CaMKII blockade restored SR Ca^{2+} content, but had little effect on systolic function.[26] This may be because the increased RyR Ca^{2+}-sensitivity that caused the leak also enhanced the fractional SR Ca^{2+} release during E–C coupling.[27] Thus, while enhanced SR Ca^{2+} leak contributes to reduced SR Ca^{2+} content in HF, details of the proximal cause are controversial, and it may not contribute much to the systolic dysfunction in HF. However, this sensitization of RyR to Ca^{2+} in HF may play a very important role in diastolic dysfunction and triggered arrhythmias (see below). Thus, we think that the systolic dysfunction in HF is due mainly to lowered SR Ca^{2+} content as a consequence of reduced SERCA2 function and enhanced NCX function. As we will see, the enhanced SR Ca^{2+} leak and NCX function may both contribute to an increased propensity for arrhythmias.

Ca^{2+} AND INCREASED PROPENSITY FOR ARRHYTMIAS IN HF

In nonischemic HF, arrhythmias initiate mainly by nonreentrant mechanisms, or triggered activity (which may include early and delayed afterdepolarizations; EADs and DADs). EADs are more common at very low heart rates, but at higher heart rates (and SR Ca^{2+} content) DADs are more common. Our nonischemic rabbit HF model[7,12,28] demonstrates mainly tachyarrhythmias and we will focus here on how DADs are likely to occur in HF. DADs are initiated by spontaneous SR Ca^{2+} release at diastolic membrane potentials causing a Ca^{2+}-activated transient inward current (I_{ti}), which depolarizes the membrane toward the threshold for a triggered action potential. We have shown that this I_{ti} is virtually entirely attributable to NCX current in both rabbit and human HF and have developed the following working hypothesis (FIG. 1).[7,29]

When a spontaneous SR Ca^{2+} release occurs, the upregulated NCX in HF causes more inward I_{ti} (NCX current) for a given SR Ca^{2+} release. There is also a large reduction in the inward rectifier K^+ current that is responsible for stabilizing the resting membrane potential (I_{K1}), which means that any given I_{ti} will cause more membrane depolarization. These changes in NCX and I_{K1} combine to increase the likelihood that an SR Ca^{2+} release event will induce a DAD that is sufficiently large to trigger a full action potential.

These classical "spontaneous" Ca^{2+} waves that underlie DADs (at least in normal ventricular myocytes) are due to increased SR Ca^{2+} content (e.g., Ca^{2+} overload) and there is a steep relationship between SR Ca^{2+} content and SR Ca^{2+} leak and wave generation.[6] Thus, in HF where SR Ca^{2+} content is reduced, it would seem that these events would be less common. However, in HF at least before the real end stage, there is residual β-adrenergic responsiveness and high sympathetic tone, such that local (and probably heterogeneous) β-adrenergic stimulation may cause regions where local SR Ca^{2+} content is elevated to the point of activating spontaneous SR Ca^{2+} release events. We have also seen that the amount of SR Ca^{2+} leak at any level of SR Ca^{2+} content is higher in HF myocytes,[6] such that DADs could occur at a lower-than-normal SR Ca^{2+} content. This is consistent with a recent finding concerning human RyR2 mutations that are linked with catecholaminergic polymorphic ventricular tachycardia (CPVT), and where the mutant RyR has been shown to have increased the Ca^{2+}-dependence of activation.[30]

$[Na^+]_i$ IN MYOCYTES FROM CONTROL AND FAILING HEARTS

In cardiac myocytes, $[Ca^{2+}]_i$ and $[Na^+]_i$ are linked through NCX. In normal myocytes, under physiological conditions NCX works almost exclusively in the Ca^{2+} extrusion mode, driven mostly by the high subsarcolemmal Ca^{2+} transient.[1] However, when $[Na^+]_i$ is elevated, the amount of Ca^{2+} influx through NCX can increase greatly. This will raise the cellular and SR Ca^{2+} content, resulting in larger Ca^{2+} transients and therefore enhanced contractility. Indeed, the inotropic effect of increasing $[Na^+]_i$ is well known. In cardiac Purkinje fibers, the developed tension doubles with a 1 mM increase in Na^+ activity.[31] The effect is smaller but still prominent in ventricular myocytes.[32] $[Na^+]_i$ may have an even bigger impact on contractility in HF because NCX has a more prominent role in Ca^{2+} extrusion from the cytosol during relaxation (due to NCX upregulation/SERCA downregulation, see above).

$[Na^+]_i$ is elevated in myocytes from rabbits with pressure and volume overload-induced HF[33,34] as well as in human heart failure.[32] As higher $[Na^+]_i$ shifts the balance of fluxes through NCX to favor more Ca^{2+} influx in HF, this may better maintain SR Ca^{2+} load and thus contractility in HF. That is, if $[Na^+]_i$ did not increase, then systolic function and SR Ca^{2+} content could be even worse. The prolongation of action potential duration and smaller Ca^{2+} transients in HF will also more strongly favor Ca^{2+} influx via NCX, again limiting the extent of systolic dysfunction.

Higher $[Na^+]_i$ in HF may be due to either decreased Na^+ extrusion via the Na^+/K^+ pump (NKA) or increased Na^+ influx. Decreased NKA expression and/or isoform shifts have been found in several, but not all HF models. Part of the disagreement may reflect differences in species, HF models and differences in human HF population. Protein levels of α_1- and α_3-subunit isoforms as well as β_1-subunit are decreased in failing human myocardium,[35] whereas no changes were found at the mRNA level.[36] Protein and mRNA expression of the dominant α_1-isoform are unchanged in most HF models in rat, whereas α_2-isoform is generally reduced and α_3-isoform is increased.[37] In myocytes from our volume and pressure overload-induced HF model in rabbits, the protein expression of all three α-subunit isoforms was reduced.[38] When assessed with an antibody that recognizes all α-isoforms equally, NKA protein expression was reduced by 36%.[38] Most prior studies were performed in tissue homogenates and could reflect changes in non-myocytes.[38] Moreover, such expression measurements cannot differentiate between internalized versus sarcolemmal NKA, nor between functional and inactive pumps. Thus, it is difficult to correlate such biochemical findings to cellular function.

Despite the considerable expression data, there are few functional NKA studies in HF myocytes, and results are equivocal. Myocytes from rats with HF following myocardial infarction showed a reduction in the maximal Na^+ extrusion rate but unchanged $[Na^+]_i$-affinity.[39] On the contrary, myocytes from dogs with chronic atrioventricular block and hypertrophy have unaltered maximal NKA pump current and reduced $[Na^+]_i$ affinity.[40] We found that neither the maximal Na^+ transport rate nor the affinity of NKA for internal Na^+ was affected in myocytes from HF rabbits.[33] Moreover, since $[Na^+]_i$ was approximately 3 mM higher in HF, our data suggest that under normal conditions, NKA activity was actually higher in HF. Thus, Na^+ influx must also be higher in our HF model. Indeed, we found that the initial slope of $[Na^+]_i$ rise upon NKA inhibition was twice as large as in myocytes from normal hearts.[33] Most of this elevated Na^+ entry was TTX-sensitive, suggesting a role for Na^+ channels. Indeed, an increased slowly inactivating Na^+ current was found in ventricular myocytes from a canine ischemic model of HF[41] and more recently in dogs with pacing-induced HF.[42] The latter study also reports an increased slowly inactivating Na^+ current in human HF. Using essentially the same animal model we used, Baartscheer *et al.*[34] also found that higher $[Na^+]_i$ is caused by elevated Na^+ influx. However, in their case the enhanced Na^+ influx was inhibited by cariporide, suggesting an important role for the Na^+/H^+ exchanger (NHE), which was upregulated. Furthermore, chronic cariporide treatment prevented the onset of HF in rabbits with pressure and volume overload.[43] Although cariporide at the concentrations used in these studies might also inhibit slowly inactivating Na^+ channels,[44] this raises another potential explanation for elevated $[Na^+]_i$ in HF. The close interplay between Na^+ and Ca^{2+} in heart (via NCX) makes it especially important to understand this point better.

Na^+/K^+ ATPase AND PHOSPHOLEMMAN IN THE HEART

Na^+/K^+ ATPase is the main pathway for Na^+ extrusion from the cells and thus is essential in controlling $[Na^+]_i$. NKA expression and function is modulated by several factors, including variations in substrate, interaction with membrane-associated compounds, glycoside binding, and hormonal stimulation.[45] There is evidence that sympathetic transmitters can adjust the NKA activity to the functional demands of the heart (reviewed in Refs. 45,46) This may limit the rise in $[Na^+]_i$ in the face of greater Na^+ influx due to more frequent and larger Na^+ current and enhanced Na^+ entry via NCX (which has to extrude more Ca^{2+} to balance the larger Ca^{2+} entry via L-type Ca^{2+} channels). However, there is controversy at present because studies in single myocytes using Na^+/K^+ pump current found either stimulation,[47–49] inhibition[50,51] or no change[52] upon β-AR stimulation. Controversy extends also to the molecular target on the NKA. The NKA α-subunit can be phosphorylated by PKA, but *only* in the presence of detergents, while *in situ* the phosphorylation site may be inaccessible to the kinase.[53] There is a larger consensus that α-AR stimulation and protein kinase C (PKC) activate cardiac NKA,[54–56] but the mechanism involved is unclear.

Recently, the FXYD protein family has emerged as tissue-specific modulators of NKA. FXYD are single-membrane spanning proteins containing a conserved Pro-Phe-X-Tyr-Asp motif in the extracellular N terminus domain.[57] There are seven FXYD proteins (FXYD-1 to -7), including phospholemman (FXYD-1), the NKA γ-subunit (FXYD-2), and the regulator of renal Na^+/K^+-ATPase (FXYD-4, or CHIF). All family members, but FXYD-6, have been shown to co-immunoprecipitate with NKA α-subunits and to modulate NKA function.[58–63] Of the FXYD proteins, FXYD-1, known also as phospholemman (PLM), is highly expressed in the heart. PLM, a 72 amino acid sarcolemmal protein, is unique in the FXYD family in having multiple phosphorylation sites at its cytosolic carboxyl terminus. Indeed, PLM is a major cardiac target for α- and β-adrenergic agonist-mediated phosphorylation in myocytes.[64,65] PKA and PKC share a common phosphorylation site (at position Ser 68), and PKC has an additional site (at Ser 63).

Using myocytes from mice in which the PLM gene was targeted (PLM-KO) versus wild-type littermates we found that PLM inhibits NKA, mainly by reducing its affinity for internal Na^+ (but we could not rule out a smaller effect on the maximum Na^+ extrusion rate).[66] Furthermore, we found that β-adrenergic stimulation activated NKA function in myocytes from wild-type mice (by reducing the K_m for internal Na^+) and had no effect in PLM-KO mice.[66] β-adrenergic stimulation of wild-type myocytes made the $[Na^+]_i$-dependence of NKA similar to that found in the PLM-KO mice. These data suggest that PLM affects NKA function in a manner similar to the way PLB affects SERCA, i.e., inhibition, relieved by phosphorylation. It is as yet unclear what role NKA activation plays in the sympathetic *fight or flight* response. We found that β-adrenergic stimulation reduces resting $[Na^+]_i$ in myocytes from wild-type but not PLM-KO mice.[66] We can speculate that in beating myocytes, NKA activation will limit the rise in $[Na^+]_i$ expected to occur during sympathetic stimulation, which would otherwise greatly reduce the energy in the $[Na^+]_i$ gradient and thus limit the ability of NCX to extrude Ca^{2+}.

Interestingly, the association between PLM and α-subunit of NKA, as determined by co-immunoprecipitation experiments, appears to be unaffected by PKA phosphorylation.[38,67] Thus we looked for more subtle changes in the NKA–PLM association by using fluorescence resonance energy transfer

(FRET) in HEK cells expressing fusion proteins of α1-NKA fused to a cyan fluorescent protein (NKA-CFP) and PLM fused to a yellow fluorescent protein (PLM-YFP).[68] We saw clear membrane colocalization and robust FRET at base line that was dramatically decreased upon PLM phosphorylation by either PKA or PKC. Thus, PLM phosphorylation by PKA and PKC changes the PLM–NKA interaction but does not necessarily result in a complete dissociation. In the analogous PLB-SERCA system it was long thought that PLB phosphorylation caused PLB to dissociate from SERCA, but more recent results show that PLB remains bound to SERCA even after phosphorylation and abolition of SERCA inhibition.[69]

PHOSPHOLEMMAN-REGULATION OF THE Na^+/K^+ ATPase IN HF

NKA protein expression was reduced by 36% in ventricular myocytes from HF rabbits.[38] However, the characteristics of NKA-mediated Na^+ extrusion were unchanged.[33] To explain this dichotomy, we investigated whether PLM expression and phosphorylation level are altered in HF. We found that PLM expression was reduced by 42%.[38] This is a more extensive decrease than that for NKA expression, thus the PLM:NKA ratio is reduced in HF. Furthermore, a higher percentage of PLM was phosphorylated in HF and both findings were also found in human HF.[38] The combination of reduced amount and more phosphorylated PLM results in less overall NKA inhibition by PLM in HF. Thus, downregulation of NKA expression in this rabbit HF model may be functionally offset by less PLM-dependent inhibition. Different models of hypertrophy and HF may vary in PLM alterations. For example, short-term postmyocardial infarction rat hearts show increased PLM expression.[70]

CONCLUSION

The numerous ion transport pathways involved in the regulation of $[Ca^{2+}]_i$ and $[Na^+]_i$ are critical individually in mediating both contractile and electrical activity of cardiac myocytes. However, the integrated cellular handling of each ion must be borne in mind in order to understand and predict the consequences of drugs or pathophysiological changes. $[Ca^{2+}]_i$ and $[Na^+]_i$ regulation are also highly interdependent, due to NCX and also complex dependences on membrane potential. The dynamic interplay of $[Ca^{2+}]_i$ and $[Na^+]_i$ regulation can also be perturbed in pathophysiological situations such as heart failure and are involved in contractile dysfunction and arrhythmogenesis.

ACKNOWLEDGMENTS

Supported by grants from the National Institutes of Health HL-81526 and HL-64724 (DMB).

REFERENCES

1. BERS, D.M. 2001. Excitation-Contraction Coupling and Cardiac Contractile Force, 2nd ed. Kluwer Academic Press. Dordrecht, The Netherlands.
2. BERS, D.M., W.H. BARRY & S. DESPA. 2003. Intracellular Na^+ regulation in cardiac myocytes. Cardiovasc. Res. **57:** 897–912.
3. LINDNER, M., E. ERDMANN & D.J. BEUCKELMANN. 1998. Calcium content of the sarcoplasmic reticulum in isolated ventricular myocytes from patients with terminal heart failure. J. Mol. Cell Cardiol. **30:** 743–749.
4. PIESKE, B., L.S. MAIER, D.M. BERS, et al. 1999. Ca^{2+} handling and sarcoplasmic reticulum Ca^{2+} content in isolated failing and nonfailing human myocardium. Circ. Res. **85:** 38–46.
5. HOBAI, I.A. & B. O'ROURKE. 2001. Decreased sarcoplasmic reticulum calcium content is responsible for defective excitation-contraction coupling in canine heart failure. Circulation **103:** 1577–1584.
6. SHANNON, T.R., S.M. POGWIZD & D.M. BERS. 2003. Elevated sarcoplasmic reticulum Ca^{2+} leak in intact ventricular myocytes from rabbits in heart failure. Circ. Res. **93:** 592–594.
7. POGWIZD, S.M., K. SCHLOTTHAUER, L. LI, et al. 2001. Arrhythmogenesis and contractile dysfunction in heart failure: roles of sodium-calcium exchange, inward rectifier potassium current, and residual beta-adrenergic responsiveness. Circ. Res. **88:** 1159–1167.
8. PIACENTINO, V., III, C.R. WEBER, X. CHEN, et al. 2003. Cellular basis of abnormal calcium transients of failing human ventricular myocytes. Circ. Res. **92:** 651–658. 9.
9. BEUCKELMANN, D.J. & E. ERDMANN. 1992. Ca^{2+} currents and intracellular Ca^{2+} transients in single ventricular myocytes isolated from terminally failing human myocardium. Basic Res. Cardiol. **87:** 235–243.
10. GOMEZ, A.M., H.H. VALDIVIA, H. CHENG, et al. 1997. Defective excitation-contraction coupling in experimental cardiac hypertrophy and heart failure. Science **276:** 800–806.
11. O'ROURKE, B., D.A. KASS, G.F. TOMASELLI, et al. 1999. Mechanisms of altered excitation-contraction coupling in canine tachycardia-induced heart failure. Circ. Res. **84:** 562–570.
12. POGWIZD, S.M., M. QI, W. YUAN, et al. 1999. Upregulation of Na^+/Ca^{2+} exchanger expression and function in an arrhythmogenic rabbit model of hear failure. Circ. Res. **85:** 1009–1019.
13. HASENFUSS, G., W. SCHILLINGER, S.E. LEHNART, et al. 1999. Relationship between Na^+-Ca^{2+}-exchanger protein levels and diastolic function of failing human myocardium. Circulation **99:** 641–648.
14. MARX, S.O., S. REIKEN, Y. HISAMATSU, et al. 2000. PKA phosphorylation dissociates FKBP12.6 from the calcium release channel (ryanodine receptor): defective regulation in failing hearts. Cell **101:** 365–376.
15. LEHNART, S.E., X.H. WEHRENS, S. REIKEN, et al. 2005. Phosphodiesterase 4D deficiency in the ryanodine-receptor complex promotes heart failure and arrhythmias. Cell **123:** 25–35.
16. WEHRENS, X.H., S.E. LEHNART & A.R. MARKS. 2005. Intracellular calcium release and cardiac disease. Annu. Rev. Physiol. **67:** 69–98.
17. WEHRENS, X.H., S.E. LEHNART, S. REIKEN, et al. 2006. Ryanodine receptor/ calcium release channel PKA phosphorylation: a critical mediator of heart failure progression. Proc. Natl. Acad. Sci. USA. **103:** 511–518.

18. WEHRENS, X.H., S.E. LEHNART, S.R. REIKEN, et al. 2004. Protection from cardiac arrhythmia through ryanodine receptor-stabilizing protein calstabin2. Science **304:** 292–296.
19. JIANG, M.T., A.J. LOKUTA, E.F. FARRELL, et al. 2002. Abnormal Ca^{2+} release, but normal ryanodine receptors, in canine and human heart failure. Circ. Res. **91:** 1015–1022.
20. STANGE, M., L. XU, D. BALSHAW, et al. 2003. Characterization of recombinant skeletal muscle (Ser-2843) and cardiac muscle (Ser-2809) ryanodine receptor phosphorylation mutants. J. Biol. Chem. **278:** 51693–51702.
21. LI, Y., E.G. KRANIAS, G.A. MIGNERY, et al. 2002. Protein kinase A phosphorylation of the ryanodine receptor does not affect calcium sparks in mouse ventricular myocytes. Circ. Res. **90:** 309–316.
22. XIAO, B., M.T. JIANG, M. ZHAO, et al. 2005. Characterization of a novel PKA phosphorylation site, serine-2030, reveals no PKA hyperphosphorylation of the cardiac ryanodine receptor in canine heart failure. Circ. Res. **96:** 847–855.
23. ZHANG, T., L.S. MAIER, N.D. DALTON, et al. 2003. The deltaC isoform of CaMKII is activated in cardiac hypertrophy and induces dilated cardiomyopathy and heart failure. Circ. Res. **92:** 912–919.
24. MAIER, L.S., T. ZHANG, L. CHEN, et al. 2003. Transgenic CaMKIIdeltaC overexpression uniquely alters cardiac myocyte Ca^{2+} handling: reduced SR Ca^{2+} load and activated SR Ca^{2+} release. Circ. Res. **92:** 904–911.
25. WEHRENS, X.H., S.E. LEHNART, S.R. REIKEN, et al. 2004. Ca^{2+}/calmodulin-dependent protein kinase II phosphorylation regulates the cardiac ryanodine receptor. Circ. Res. **94:** e61–70.
26. AI, X., J.W. CURRAN, T.R. SHANNON, et al. 2005. Ca^{2+}/calmodulin-dependent protein kinase modulates cardiac ryanodine receptor phosphorylation and sarcoplasmic reticulum Ca^{2+} leak in heart failure. Circ. Res. **97:** 1314–1322.
27. LI, L., G. CHU, E.G. KRANIAS, et al. 1998. Cardiac myocyte calcium transport in phospholamban knockout mouse: relaxation and endogeneous CaMKII effects. Am. J. Physiol. **274:** H1335–H1347.
28. POGWIZD, S.M. 1995. Nonreentrant mechanism underlying spontaneous ventricular arrhythmias in a model of nonischemic heart failure in rabbits. Circulation **92:** 1034–1048.
29. BERS, D.M., S.M. POGWIZD & K. SCHLOTTHAUER. 2002. Upregulated Na^+/Ca^{2+} exchange is involved in both contractile dysfunction and arrhythmogenesis in heart failure. Basic Res. Cardiol. **97**(Suppl 1): 36–42.
30. PRIORI, S.G. & C. NAPOLITANO. 2005. Cardiac and skeletal muscle disorders caused by mutations in the intracellular Ca^{2+} release channels. J. Clin. Invest. **115:** 2033–2038.
31. LEE, C.O. & M. DAGOSTINO. 1982. Effect of strophanthidin on intracellular Na^+ ion activity and twitch tension on constantly driven canine cardiac Purkinje fibers. Biophys. J. **40:** 185–198.
32. PIESKE, B., L.S. MAIER, V. PIACENTINO, 3RD. et al. 2002. Rate dependence of $[Na^+]i$ and contractility in nonfailing and failing human myocardium. Circulation **106:** 447–453.
33. DESPA, S., M.A. ISLAM, C.R. WEBER, et al. 2002. Intracellular Na^+ concentration is elevated in heart failure, but Na^+/K-pump function is unchanged. Circulation **105:** 2543–2548.
34. BAARTSCHEER, A., C.A. SCHUMACHER, M.M. VAN BORREN, et al. 2003. Increased Na^+/H^+-exchange activity is the cause of increased $[Na^+]i$ and underlies

disturbed calcium handling in the rabbit pressure and volume overload heart failure model. Cardiovasc. Res. **57:** 1015–1024.
35. SCHWINGER, R.H., J. WANG, K. FRANK, et al. 1999. Reduced sodium pump α1, α3 and β1-isoform protein levels and Na^+,K^+-ATPase activity but unchanged Na^+-Ca^{2+} exchanger protein levels in human heart failure. Circulation **99:** 2105–2112.
36. ALLEN, D., T.A. SCHIMDT, J.D. MARSH, et al. 1992. Na^+,K^+-ATPase expression in normal and failing human left ventricle. Basic Res. Cardiol **87**(Suppl1): 87–94.
37. VERDONCK, F., P.G. A. VOLDERS, M.A. VOS, et al. 2003. Intracellular Na^+ and altered Na^+ transport mechanisms in cardiac hyperhtrophy and failure. J. Mol. Cell Cardiol. **35:** 5–25.
38. BOSSUYT, J., X. AI, R.J. MOORMAN, et al. 2005. Expression and phosphorylation the Na^+-pump regulatory subunit phospholemman in heart failure. Circ. Res. **97:** 558–565.
39. SEMB, S.O., P.K. LUNDE, et al. 1998. Reduced myocardial Na^+, K^+ pump capacity in congestive heart failure following myocardial infarction in rats. J. Mol. Cell Cardiol. **30:** 1311–1328.
40. VERDONCK, F., P.G. VOLDERS, M.A. VOS, et al. 2003. Increased Na^+ concentration and altered Na^+/K^+ pump activity in hypertrophied canine ventricular cells. Cardiovasc. Res. **57:** 1035–1043.
41. UNDROVINAS, A.I., V.A. MALTSEV & H.N. SABBAH. 1999. Repolarization abnormalities in cardiomyocytes of dogs with chronic heart failure: role of sustained inward current. Cell. Mol. Life Sci. **55:** 494–505.
42. VALDIVIA, C.R., W.W. CHU, J. PU, et al. 2005. Increased late sodium current in myocytes from a canine heart failure model and from failing human heart. J. Mol. Cell Cardiol. **38:** 475–483.
43. BAARTSCHEER, A., C.A. SCHUMACHER, M.M. VAN BORREN, et al. 2005. Chronic inhibition of Na^+/H^+–exchanger attenuates cardiac hypertrophy and prevents cellular remodeling in heart failure. Cardiovasc. Res. **65:** 83–92.
44. CHATTOU, S., A. COULOMBE, J. DIACONO, et al. 2000. Slowly inactivating component of sodium current in ventricular myocytes is decreased by diabetes and partially inhibited by known Na^+-H^+ Exchange blockers. J. Mol. Cell Cardiol. **32:** 1181–1192.
45. THERIEN, A.G. & R. BLOSTEIN. 2000. Mechanisms of sodium pump regulation. Am. J. Physiol. Cell Physiol. **279:** C541–566.
46. GLITSCH, H.G. 2001. Electrophysiology of the sodium-potassium-ATPase in cardiac cells. Physiol. Rev. **81:** 1791–1826.
47. DOBRETSOV, M., S.L. HASTINGS & J.R. STIMERS. 1998. Na^+-K^+ pump cycle during beta-adrenergic stimulation of adult rat cardiac myocytes. J. Physiol. **507:** 527–539.
48. KOCKSKÄMPER, J., S. ERLENKAMP & H.G. GLITSCH. 2000. Activation of the cAMP-protein kinase A pathway facilitates Na^+ translocation by the Na^+-K^+ pump in guinea-pig ventricular myocytes. J. Physiol. **523:** 561–574.
49. SILVERMAN, B.D., W. FULLER, P. EATON, et al. 2005. Serine 68 phosphorylation of phospholemman: acute isoform-specific activation of cardiac Na^+/K^+ ATPase. Cardiovasc. Res. **65:** 93–103.
50. GAO, J., I.S. COHEN, R.T. MATHIAS, et al. 1998. The inhibitory effect of beta-stimulation on the Na/K pump current in guinea pig ventricular myocytes is mediated by a cAMP-dependent PKA pathway. Pflugers Arch. **435:** 479–484.

51. GAO, J., R.T. MATHIAS, I.S. COHEN, et al. 1992. Isoprenaline, Ca^{2+} and the Na^+-K^+ pump in guinea-pig ventricular myocytes. J. Physiol. **449:** 689–704.
52. ISHIZUKA, N. & J.R. BERLIN. 1993. Beta-adrenergic stimulation does not regulate Na^+ pump function in voltage-clamped ventricular myocytes of the rat heart. Pflugers Arch. **424:** 361–363.
53. SWEADNER, K.J. & M.S. FESCHENKO. 2001. Predicted location and limited accessibility of protein kinase A phosphorylation site on Na^+-K-ATPase. Am. J. Physiol. **280:** C1017–C1026.
54. WILLIAMSON, A.P., R. H. KENNEDY, E. SEIFEN, et al. 1993. Alpha 1b-adrenoceptor-mediated stimulation of Na-K pump current in adult rat ventricular myocytes. Am. J. Physiol. **264:** H1315–1318.
55. WANG, Y., J. GAO, R.T. MATHIAS, et al. 1998. Alpha-adrenergic effects on Na^+-K^+ pump current in guinea-pig ventricular myocytes. J. Physiol. **509:** 117–128.
56. ERLENKAMP, S., H.G. GLITSCH & J. KOCKSKAMPER. 2002. Dual regulation of cardiac Na^+-K^+ pumps and CFTR Cl- channels by protein kinases A and C. Pflugers Arch. **444:** 251–262.
57. SWEADNER, K.J. & E. RAEL. 2000. The FXYD gene family of small ion transport regulators or channels: cDNA sequence, protein signature sequence, and expression. Genomics **68:** 41–56.
58. CRAMBERT, G., M. FUZESI, H. GARTY, et al. 2002. Phospholemman (FXYD1) associates with Na,K-ATPase and regulates its transport properties. Proc. Natl. Acad. Sci. USA. **99:** 11476–11481.
59. ARYSTARKHOVA, E., C. DONNET, N.K. ASINOVSKI, et al. 2002. Differential regulation of renal Na,K-ATPase by splice variants of the gamma subunit. J. Biol. Chem. **277:** 10162–10172.
60. CRAMBERT, G., C. LI, D. CLAEYS, et al. 2005. FXYD3 (Mat-8), a new regulator of Na,K-ATPase. Mol. Biol. Cell. **16:** 2363–2371.
61. GARTY, H., M. LINDZEN, R. SCANZANO, et al. 2002. A functional interaction between CHIF and Na-K-ATPase: implication for regulation by FXYD proteins. Am. J. Physiol. Renal. Physiol. **283:** F607–F615.
62. LUBARSKI, I., K. PIHAKASKI-MAUNSBACH, S.J. KARLISH, et al. 2005. Interaction with the Na,K-ATPase and tissue distribution of FXYD5 (related to ion channel). J. Biol. Chem. **280:** 37717–37724.
63. CRAMBERT, G., C. LI, L.K. SWEE, et al. 2004. FXYD7, mapping of functional sites involved in endoplasmic reticulum export, association with and regulation of Na,K-ATPase. J. Biol. Chem. **279:** 30888–30895.
64. PRESTI, C.F., L.R. JONES & J.P. LINDEMANN. 1985. Isoproterenol-induced phosphorylation of a 15-kilodalton sarcolemmal protein in intact myocardium. J. Biol. Chem. **260:** 3860–3867.
65. LINDEMANN, J.P. 1986. Alpha-adrenergic stimulation of sarcolemmal protein phosphorylation and slow responses in intact myocardium. J. Biol. Chem. **261:** 4860–4867.
66. DESPA, S., J. BOSSUYT, F. HAN, et al. 2005. Phospholemman-phosphorylation mediates the beta-adrenergic effects on Na^+/K^+ pump function in cardiac myocytes. Circ. Res. **97:** 252–259.
67. FULLER, W., P. EATON, J.R. BELL, et al. 2004. Ischemia-induced phosphorylation of phospholemman directly activates rat cardiac Na^+/K^+-ATPase. FASEB J. **18:** 197–199.

68. BOSSUYT, J., S. DESPA, J.L. MARTIN, et al. 2006. Phospholemman (PLM) phosphorylation modulates its association with the Na/K pump (NKA) assessed by FRET. Biophys. J. **90:** 19a.
69. ASAHI, M., E. MCKENNA, K. KURZYDLOWSKI, et al. 2000. Physical interactions between phospholamban and sarco(endo)plasmic reticulum Ca^{2+}-ATPases are dissociated by elevated Ca^{2+}, but not by phospholamban phosphorylation, vanadate, or thapsigargin, and are enhanced by ATP. J. Biol. Chem. **275:** 15034–15038.
70. ZHANG, X.Q., J.R. MOORMAN, B.A. AHLERS, et al. 2006. Phospholemman overexpression inhibits Na^+-K^+-ATPase in adult rat cardiac myocytes: relevance to decreased Na^+ pump activity in post-infarction myocytes. J. Appl. Physiol. **100:** 212–220.

The Integration of Spontaneous Intracellular Ca^{2+} Cycling and Surface Membrane Ion Channel Activation Entrains Normal Automaticity in Cells of the Heart's Pacemaker

EDWARD G. LAKATTA, TATIANA VINOGRADOVA, ALEXEY LYASHKOV, SYEVDA SIRENKO, WEIZONG ZHU, ABDUL RUKNUDIN, AND VICTOR A. MALTSEV

Laboratory of Cardiovascular Science, Gerontology Research Center, National Institute on Aging Intramural Research Program, National Institutes of Health, Baltimore, Maryland 21224, USA

ABSTRACT: Although the ensemble of voltage- and time-dependent rhythms of surface membrane ion channels, the membrane "Clock", is the immediate cause of a sinoatrial nodal cell (SANC) action potential (AP), it does not necessarily follow that this ion channel ensemble is the formal cause of spontaneous, rhythmic APs. SANC also generates intracellular oscillatory spontaneous Ca^{2+} releases that ignite excitation (SCaRIE) of the surface membrane via Na^+/Ca^{2+} exchanger activation. The idea that a rhythmic intracellular Ca^{2+} Clock might keep time for normal automaticity of SANC, however, has not been assimilated into mainstream pacemaker dogma. Recent experimental evidence, derived from simultaneous, confocal imaging of submembrane Ca^{2+} and membrane potential of SANC, and supported by numerical modeling, indicates that normal automaticity of SANC is entrained and stabilized by the tight integration of the SR Ca^{2+} Clock that generates rhythmic SCaRIE, and the surface membrane Clock that responds to SCaRIE to immediately produce APs of an adequate shape. Thus, tightly controlled, rhythmic SCaRIE does not merely fine tune SANC AP firing, but is the formal cause of the basal and reserve rhythms, insuring pacemaker stability by rhythmically integrating multiple Ca^{2+}-dependent functions, and effects normal automaticity by rhythmic ignition of the surface membrane Clock.

KEYWORDS: spontaneous local Ca^{2+} release; sarcoplasmic reticulum; Na^+/Ca^{2+} exchanger; ryanodine receptor; cardiac pacemaker; normal automaticity

Address for correspondence: Edward G. Lakatta, M.D., National Institute on Aging, Gerontology Research Center, Intramural Research Program, 5600 Nathan Shock Drive, Baltimore, MD 21224. Voice: 410-558-8202; fax: 410-558-8150.
e-mail: LakattaE@grc.nia.nih.gov

Ann. N.Y. Acad. Sci. 1080: 178–206 (2006). © 2006 New York Academy of Sciences.
doi: 10.1196/annals.1380.016

INTRODUCTION

Evidence that an intracellular "clock" is implicated in the initiation of the cardiac impulse stems from the turn of the last century. Multiple additional clues subsequently indicated that this intracellular clock was a Ca^{2+} oscillator, and that it produced an (oscillatory) inward current[1] that could result in spontaneous Ca^{2+} release ignited excitation (SCaRIE) of the cell membrane, initiating an action potential (AP).[2] But the "brut force" experimental Ca^{2+} overload that was employed in these studies relegated the relevance of SCaRIE to "abnormal automaticity."[3] Indeed, under such Ca^{2+} overload conditions, SCaRIE is "scary."

Recent experimental evidence, derived from simultaneous, confocal imaging of submembrane Ca^{2+} and membrane potential of sinoatrial nodal cells (SANC), and supported by numerical modeling, indicates that sarcoplasmic reticulum (SR)-generated SCaRIE occurs within SANC in the absence of Ca^{2+} overload and underlies their normal automaticity. Rhythmic, SR-generated local Ca^{2+} releases (LCRs) begin to occur beneath the surface membrane during the later part of diastolic depolarization, and ignite an inward Na^+/Ca^{2+} exchange current, which imparts an exponential increase to the late diastolic depolarization, leading to activation of L-type Ca^{2+} channel current that generates the AP upstroke. Thus, tightly controlled, rhythmic SCaRIE does not merely fine tune SANC AP firing, but is the formal cause of the basal and reserve rhythms, integrating multiple Ca^{2+}-dependent functions. High levels of intrinsic, basal cAMP, and protein kinase A (PKA)-dependent protein phosphorylation, and the attendant modulation of intracellular Ca^{2+} regulate (*a*) the timing of LCR occurrence following a prior AP-triggered SR Ca^{2+} release, which is set by the functional state of the SR Ca^{2+} cycling or "SR Ca^{2+} clock," and (*b*) the voltage- and time-dependent kinetics of the components of the surface membrane ion channel ensemble or "membrane clock." This latter effect results in APs with characteristics (e.g., repolarization kinetics) commensurate with a given membrane excitation rate set by the rhythmic Ca^{2+} "clock." Thus, normal automaticity of SANC is entrained and stabilized by the tight integration of an SR Ca^{2+} clock that generates rhythmic SCaRIE, and the surface membrane clock that responds to SCaRIE to immediately produce APs of an adequate shape.

THE SURFACE MEMBRANE ION CHANNEL "CLOCK" IN CARDIAC PACEMAKER CELLS

An external membrane depolarizing event is not required to initiate the sinoatrial nodal pacemaker cell duty cycle, as these cells normally "auto excite." The ensemble of surface membrane ion channel and exchanger currents ("membrane clock") that determine the instantaneous membrane potential change of

SANC is clearly the immediate cause of their AP. But the idea that the surface membrane clock is also a formal, that is, a primary, cause of normal pacemaker automaticity became dogma that has gripped the pacemaker research field in an "intellectual and experimental phase lock" for nearly five decades. The entire, normal duty cycle of pacemaker cells has been portrayed simply as repetitive APs that are both initiated and generated by a simple reciprocal activation of surface membrane ion currents. This reductionist approach to unravel the pacemaker riddle has been largely "reduced" to electrophysiology studies of ion channel currents in the absence of normal pacemaker function, in part, to discover new ion channel currents, and in part, to dissect identified ion currents into their specific ion current subcomponents.[3–8] Numerous numerical models, based upon gating schema of ensembles of SANC currents, have been devised, and these models can indeed generate spontaneous APs.[9–12] Was there a need to search for additional, intracellular mechanisms?

Early Clues That Intracellular Ca^{2+} Is Involved in Normal Automaticity of Cardiac Pacemaker Cells

But perhaps not all of the crucial mechanisms that are implicated in spontaneous excitation of pacemaker cells are embodied in this ensemble of cell surface ion channels. Could it be that the formal cause of spontaneous rhythmic APs in SANC, i.e., of their normal automaticity, is an intracellular process? Evidence that an "intracellular clock" is implicated in the initiation of the cardiac impulse stems from the turn of the last century (c.f. review[13]). Multiple, additional clues subsequently indicated that this intracellular clock was a Ca^{2+} oscillator,[3,13–16] but that it related solely to "abnormal" pacemaker function.

Observations of pacemaker tissue during spontaneous firing (as distinct from voltage clamp studies) under various experimental conditions provided clues to the potential importance of Ca^{2+} in regulation of normal spontaneous firing rate of pacemaker cells. For example, graded suppression or blockade of L-type Ca^{2+} channel function by Ca^{2+} channel blockers that also suppresses or blocks the AP-triggered Ca^{2+} transient, has long been known to reduce and abolish SANC spontaneous beating. But until recently, this has been interpreted to be due to the fact that AP cannot occur, because L-type Ca^{2+} channel activation drives the AP upstroke. This interpretation is certainly correct, and this function of L-type Ca^{2+} channels is crucial to normal automaticity. But other actions of L-type Ca^{2+} current, that is, to trigger SR Ca^{2+} release and sustain the SR Ca^{2+} load[17,18] are not considered in this narrow interpretation of L-type Ca^{2+} channel blockade.

Other important, earlier observations were that an increase in bathing $[Ca^{2+}]$ (Ca_0) or stimulation of β-adrenergic receptors (β-ARs) markedly increases rhythmic pacemaker firing rates.[19,20] But these effects were attributed to mechanisms limited to the surface membrane clock, rather than to the enhanced intracellular Ca^{2+} cycling in SANC, as widely documented in other cardiac cell types.[21] Thus, a relationship between changes in intracellular Ca^{2+} and normal automaticity in pacemaker cells, elicited by L-type Ca^{2+} channel blockers, or a change in Ca_0 or β-AR stimulation, went largely unappreciated. The idea that an internal Ca^{2+} clock within pacemaker cells could drive the membrane clock to ignite a normal AP seemed not to have been seriously entertained, and thus did not become assimilated into mainstream pacemaker dogma.

Subsequent studies have made a compelling argument that SR Ca^{2+} cycling in AV nodal cells,[22] latent pacemaker cells,[23] Purkinje cells,[24] and SANC[25–29] is involved in their normal firing. Ca^{2+} cycling proteins previously identified in atrial or ventricular cells, that is, SERCA, ryanodine receptors (RyRs), Na^+/Ca^{2+} exchanger (NCX), were also identified in nodal pacemaker cells, including SANC.[30,31] When it became possible to measure routinely intracellular Ca^{2+} in single nodal pacemaker cells, it was observed that a cytosolic Ca^{2+} transient is evoked by the AP[22,25,31,32] and that Ca^{2+} influx via L-type Ca^{2+} channels affects Ca^{2+} loading of the SR.[22,27,29,31] That chelation of intracellular Ca^{2+}, by BAPTA but not EGTA applied intracellularly, markedly slowed or abolished spontaneous SANC beating,[33] underscoring the crucial requirement of intracellular Ca^{2+} in pacemaker function (see for example FIG. 8 B). EGTA, a slow Ca^{2+} buffer, is relatively ineffectual at buffering rapid Ca^{2+} fluxes in confined spaces; BAPTA, a fast Ca^{2+} buffer is more effective at buffering Ca^{2+} in this context.[34] Changes in the AP-induced cytosolic Ca^{2+} transient in response to β-AR stimulation were correlated with corresponding changes in the beating rate.[31,32]

CARDIAC SR IS A CA^{2+} OSCILLATOR

The cardiac SR is "wired" to physiologically oscillate Ca^{2+}. The normal duty cycle of a cardiac ventricular myocyte features a synchronized, intracellular Ca^{2+} oscillation, generated by the SR that is triggered or initiated by an AP in response to excitation of the cell membrane from an external source. *In vivo*, the source of the rhythmic excitations is the SANC. In the experimental realm of isolated, cardiac ventricular muscle or single cells, the external source is an electrical stimulation that produces inward current to trigger an AP. The potential for spontaneous SR Ca^{2+} release, however, is inherent in the design of this organelle. When disconnected from the surface membrane, cardiac ventricular SR is not entrained by rhythmic APs but becomes "free running," that is, generating spontaneous, roughly periodic Ca^{2+} releases, even in the context of physiologic intracellular $[Ca^{2+}]$.[2,35] Isolated cardiac SR vesicles,[36] cardiac cell fragments in which the sarcolemma had been mechanically removed,[37,38] but SR function preserved, and electrochemically shunted cardiac myocytes[39] exhibit such spontaneous SR Ca^{2+} release. In cardiac ventricular preparations with intact surface membranes, spontaneous SR Ca^{2+} release can be detected noninvasively in the absence of experimental Ca^{2+} loading by disconnecting the internal Ca^{2+} cycling apparatus from externally driven APs, that is, by simply discontinuing electrical stimulation, or by acutely switching from higher to lower stimulation rates.[2,35,40–50] Cardiac ventricular SR spontaneously cycles Ca^{2+}, i.e. generates spontaneous, roughly periodic Ca^{2+} releases even in the context of physiologic intracellular $[Ca^{2+}]$.[35,37–39]

The period or time required for spontaneous SR Ca^{2+} release to occur following a prior SR Ca^{2+} release reflects the speed at which the SR Ca^{2+} cycling clock "ticks" in a given condition.[51,52] Since spontaneous SR-generated Ca^{2+} releases in ventricular cells are thought to occur when luminal SR Ca^{2+} achieves a threshold level,[51,53,54] their frequency is determined, in part, at least, by how fast the SR can reload with Ca^{2+}. This depends upon how much Ca^{2+} is available for pumping, and the speed of the SR Ca^{2+} pump. Interventions effecting an increase in cell and SR Ca^{2+} loading, that is, β-AR stimulation, an increase in bathing $[Ca^{2+}]$, or cardiac glycosides, reduce the restitution time, and increase the frequency of successive SR Ca^{2+} releases. The frequency range of spontaneous SR Ca^{2+} releases, <0.1 Hz to about 10 Hz, brackets the physiologic frequencies at which the heart can beat.[2]

In contrast to the synchronized, or "systolic," SR Ca^{2+} release triggered by an AP, spontaneous SR Ca^{2+} release occurs locally within cells. Variable types of spontaneous, SR-generated, LCR exhibiting varying degrees of synchronization have been observed, ranging from Ca^{2+} sparks,[55,56] to Ca^{2+} wavelets[18,57–59] or Ca^{2+} waves, which are more synchronized, and are roughly periodic. It is important to note that while a Ca^{2+} wave may travel the length of the cell, depleting the entire SR cell throughout, at any given time the wave-related Ca^{2+} release occurs within a relatively small part of the cell, that is, in the form of LCRs.[41,45]

Confocal imaging has documented the occurrence of submembrane LCRs in spontaneously firing SANC (FIG. 1 A).[57] These LCRs are locally propagating wavelets,[57] larger than the spontaneous Ca^{2+} sparks in ventricular cells, but markedly less well organized than Ca^{2+} waves that can propagate the length of ventricular cells.[2] While LCRs occur during the spontaneous diastolic depolarization in spontaneously firing rabbit SANC, they are not triggered by the depolarization: rhythmic LCRs in SANC occur in the absence of membrane potential changes, i.e., during voltage clamp, or following "chemical skinning" of the surface membrane with the detergent saponin.[58] Of note, in cat, latent atrial pacemaker cells, T-type Ca^{2+} current, activated during diastolic depolarization, are thought to trigger LCRs, as these are blocked by 50 μM Ni^{2+} in concentrations that inhibit T-type Ca^{2+} channels[17]; in contrast, in primary rabbit SANC, Ni^{2+} at these concentrations does not inhibit LCRs.[59] When intact rabbit SANC membrane potential is clamped at the maximum diastolic potential (–60 mV), Ca^{2+} extrusion from the cell occurs via NCX. Rhythmic LCRs continue to occur, increase to a maximum (FIG. 2 A, iv), but

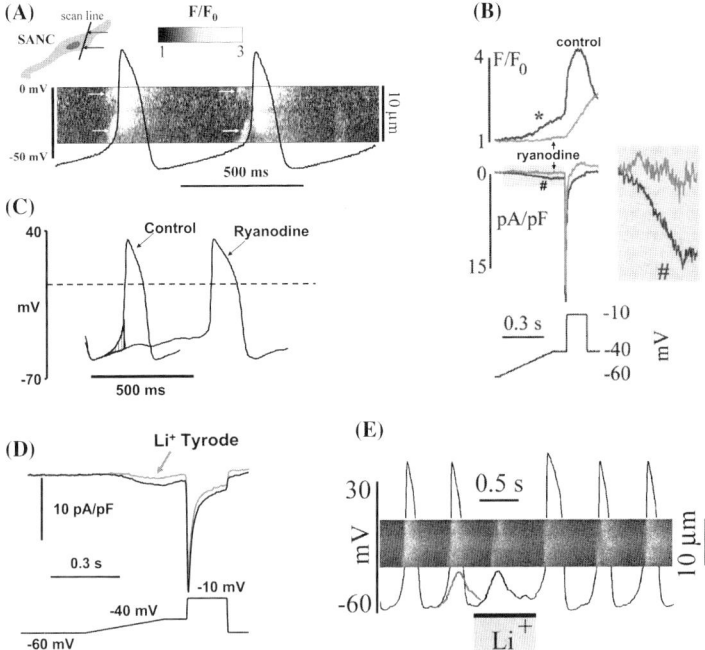

FIGURE 1. (**A**) Superimposed, confocal linescan image and membrane potential in a representative rabbit SANC. Scanning the crossed the longitudinal axis of the cell depth. Arrows on the confocal image show LCRs in the submembrane space during diastolic depolarization. (**B**) Ryanodine inhibits submembrane Ca^{2+} increase and inward current during a simulated diastolic depolarization without affecting peak $I_{Ca,L}$. Normalized fluorescence (top) and membrane current (middle) under voltage clamp before (black) and 4 min after (gray) addition of 3 μmol/L ryanodine; voltage clamp protocol is shown in the bottom panel. Inset shows the indicated part of the current record at greater magnification to more optimally show the inhibitory effect of ryanodine on inward current during the voltage ramp. (∗) Local $[Ca^{2+}]_i$ increase in the absence of ryanodine and corresponding inward current (#). Both are inhibited by ryanodine. (**C**) The ryanodine abolition of the LCR-ignited, inward current eliminates the late, exponential part of diastolic depolarization. (**D**) Membrane current during voltage clamp before (black) and 10 sec after (gray) superfusion with Na^+-free, Li^+-containing solution during voltage protocol (bottom). The gray arrow shows an inhibitory effect of Na^+-free Li^+ spritz on inward current during the voltage ramp. (**E**) Linescan image of Ca^{2+} release with superimposed AP records during rapid and brief superfusion with a solution in which Na^+ was replaced by Li^+. Note that the maneuver blocked the subsequent AP firing. The line superimposed on the last AP preceding spritz of Na^+-free solution is a copy of the residual membrane potential oscillation observed during the Li^+ solution spritz.[57]

then become damped, and cease after a few seconds, as the cytosol and SR become Ca^{2+} depleted in the absence of Ca^{2+} influx via L-type Ca^{2+} channels (FIG. 2 B, i–iv). The characteristics of LCR in SANC that occur when clamped near the maximum diastolic potential, mirrors the rest potentiation and decay of

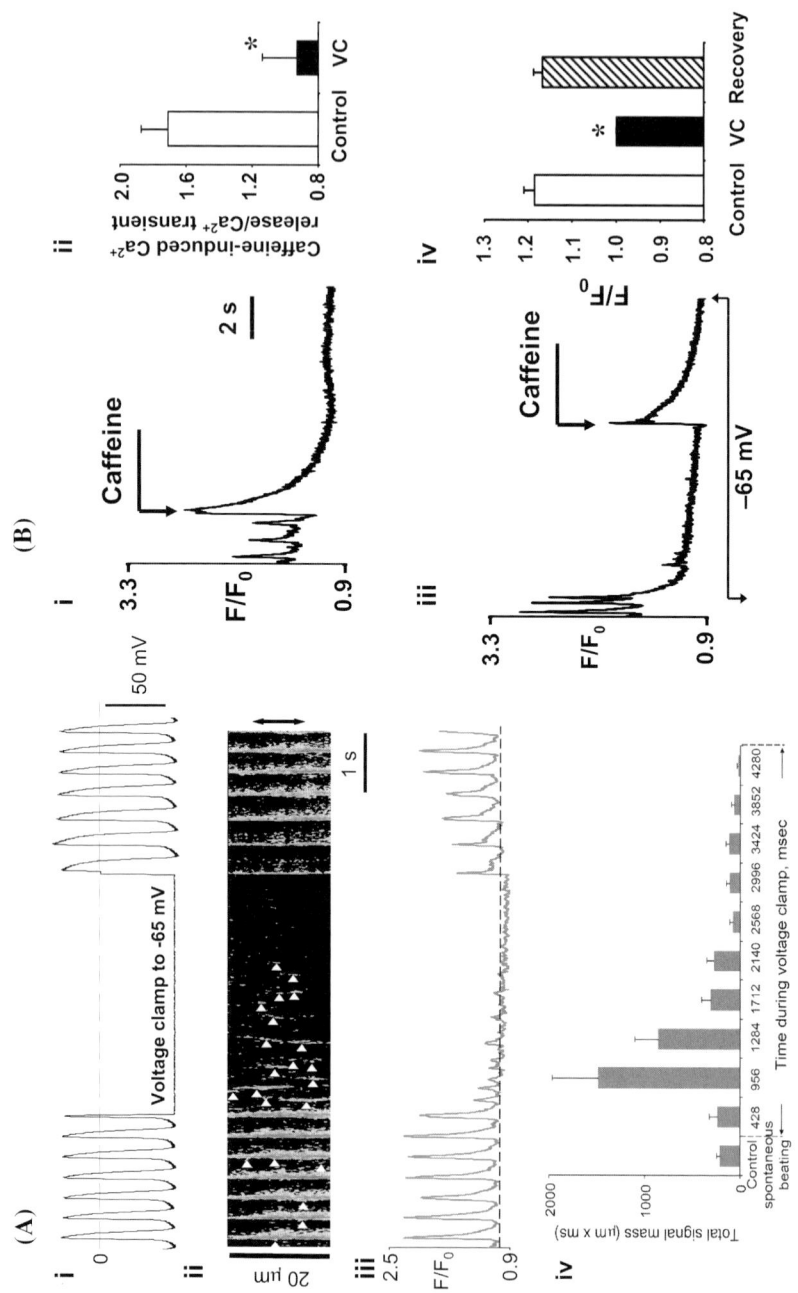

spontaneous Ca^{2+} sparks in rabbit ventricular cells when regular stimulation is stopped.[60]

In contrast to voltage clamping SANC at their maximum diastolic potential, a voltage clamp to a potential closer to the NCX reversal potential prevents cell Ca^{2+} extrusion by NCX and, therefore, SR Ca^{2+} depletion; rhythmic LCRs persist throughout the voltage clamp (FIG. 3). This mimics the behavior of Ca^{2+} sparks or waves in rabbit ventricular cells when stimulation is stopped and NCX is inhibited.[2,44,48,60]

SPONTANEOUS LOCAL CA^{2+} RELEASE INTERACTS WITH SURFACE MEMBRANE ELECTROGENIC PROCESSES

During normal heart beating, repeated SR Ca^{2+} depletion of ventricular cells by rhythmically occurring APs, emanating from the SANC, resets the SRs rhythmic clock. Under most conditions, this prevents the occurrence of spontaneous SR Ca^{2+} release between heartbeats (in diastole), by depleting the SR Ca^{2+} load at the onset of systole, and by the RyR inactivation that SR Ca^{2+} release effects. When the SR Ca^{2+} clock ticks faster than the regularly occurring APs, diastolic spontaneous Ca^{2+} release occurs between beats. Spontaneous Ca^{2+} release occurrence in the absence of electrical stimulation, or during diastole between successive beats, usually produces a small depolarization of the cell membrane via activation of an inward current.[35] This does not usually initiate a spontaneous AP in ventricular cells, due, in part, to the presence of an outwardly directed current (I_{K1}), which stabilizes the diastolic membrane potential. Under a variety of inotropic interventions, as the period of spontaneous Ca^{2+} releases decreases, spontaneous LCRs occur more often during a given epoch, that is, the ensemble of LCRs become synchronized within cells (multifocal spontaneous Ca^{2+} release), and this exposes a greater

←

FIGURE 2. (**A**) LCR occurrence in the absence of changes in membrane potential in SANC with intact sarcolemma (iii). Recordings of APs (i), linescan image (ii), and normalized subsarcolemmal fluorescence averaged spatially over the band indicated by double headed arrow in a representative cell measured before, during, and after voltage clamp (VC) at the maximum diastolic potential. (iv) Average total signal mass of LCRs during spontaneous beating and during voltage clamp ($n = 14$). (**B**) Voltage clamp (CV) at the maximum diastolic potential decreases SR Ca^{2+} content and intracellular [Ca^{2+}] in SANC. Spontaneous Ca^{2+} transients and caffeine-induced Ca^{2+} releases, indexed by F/F$_0$, in a representative cell during spontaneous beating (i) and in a representative cell after several seconds of voltage clamp (iii). (ii) Average response to caffeine in cells during spontaneous beating and cells subjected to several seconds of voltage clamp. Initial rapid component of the caffeine-induced Ca^{2+} transient in each cell is normalized to the amplitude of Ca^{2+} transient during spontaneous beating. (iv) Averages of submembrane diastolic [Ca^{2+}] during spontaneous beating before, during, and after voltage clamp in nine cells.[58] *$P < 0.05$. Error bars indicate standard error of mean.

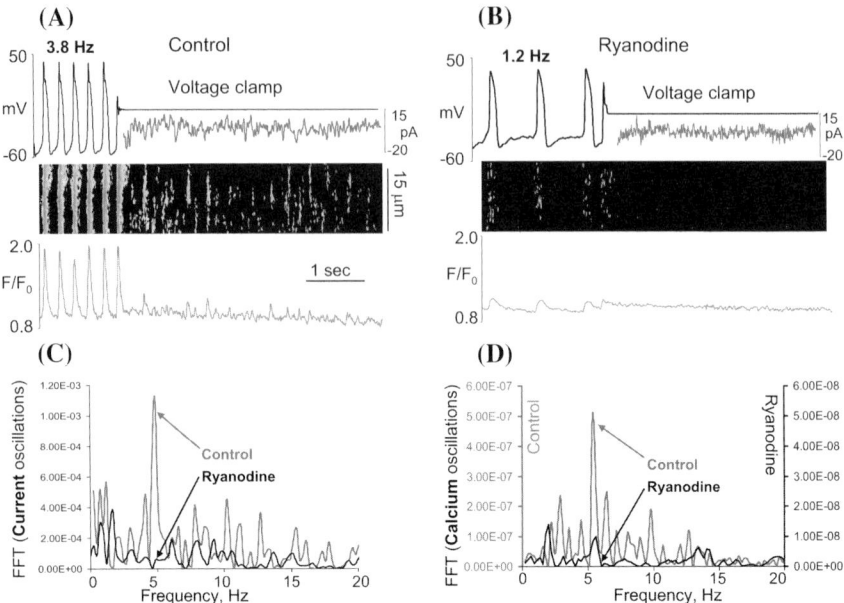

FIGURE 3. (**A, B**) Simultaneous recordings of membrane potential or current (top), confocal linescan image (middle), and normalized fluo-3 fluorescence (bottom) averaged over the linescan image, in a representative spontaneously beating SANC with intact sarcolemma prior to and during voltage clamp to -10 mV in control (**A**) and following inhibition of RyR with 3 µmol/L ryanodine (**B**). The local increase in submembrane [Ca^{2+}], resulting from LCRs during voltage clamp, generates an inward current via NCX. The gray lines in panels **A** and **B** under voltage clamp depict membrane current fluctuations generated by LCR occurrence. (**C, D**) Fast Fourier Transform (FFT) of Ca^{2+} (**D**) and membrane current (**C**) fluctuations during voltage clamp in control and after ryanodine. Note that the periodicity of these current fluctuations is the same as that of LCRs and is similarly suppressed by ryanodine.

area of the sarcolemma to high Ca^{2+}. The NCX inward current that is ignited by multifocal spontaneous Ca^{2+} release, even in the absence of Ca^{2+} overload,[35] is often sufficient to depolarize the ventricular cell surface membrane to the level required to activate Na^+ channels, and to generate a spontaneous AP, a process that could be described as a SCaRIE.

A SCARIE TALE ABOUT AN INTRACELLULAR CA^{2+} CLOCK WITHIN CARDIAC PACEMAKER CELLS

SCaRIE had been, in fact, also observed in pacemaker cells nearly 30 years ago.[1,3] But, with the relatively insensitive techniques available at that time, the "brut force" experimental Ca^{2+} overload that was employed in these studies to enable detection of spontaneous Ca^{2+} release relegated the relevance of

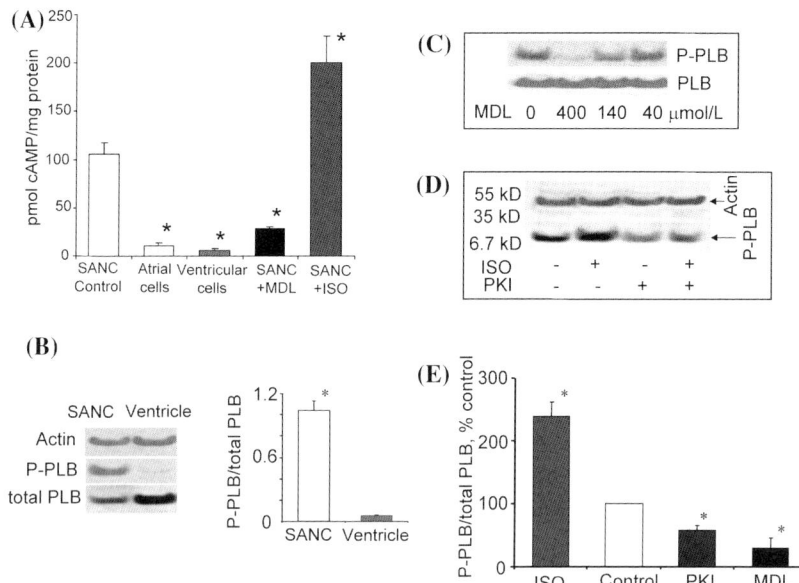

FIGURE 4. High basal level of cAMP and PKA-dependent phospholamban (PLB) phosphorylation in SANC. (**A**) Average content of cAMP in suspensions of SANC, atrial or ventricular myocytes, and changes in cAMP level in SANC following suppression of adenylyl cyclase activity with 400 μmol/L MDL (an adenylyl cyclase inhibitor) or β-AR stimulation (1 μmol/L isoproterenol [ISO]). (**B**) Left, Western blots of the basal level of phosphorylated at serine16 (P-PLB) and total PLB in SANC and ventricular myocytes; right, average values of phosphorylated PLB normalized to total PLB. (**C**) Phosphorylated PLB and total PLB at base line and in response to graded increases in AC inhibition by MDL (note that the concentration of MDL increases from right to left). (**D**) Typical Western blots of the basal level of PLB phosphorylation and that following PKA inhibition (15 μmol/L PKI, a specific peptide inhibitor of PKA catalytic subunit), β-AR stimulation (1 μmol/L ISO). (**E**) Average changes in phosphorylated PLB induced by maneuvers in (**C** and **D**) (MDL concentration was 400 μmol/L).[18] *$P < 0.05$. Error bars indicate standard error of means.

SCaRIE to "abnormal automaticity."[3] Under such Ca^{2+} overload conditions, SCaRIE is indeed "scary," because, in the intact organism, it may initiate life-threatening arrhythmias. The "scare" in such studies, however, emanates not from the intrinsic spontaneous SR Ca^{2+} release process, *per se*, but rather from the experimenter, who controls the superfusate concentrations of ions or drugs.

Other studies in the 1980s provided evidence for the involvement of SCaRIE in normal pacemaker automaticity. Evidence for the occurrence of spontaneous Ca^{2+} release in the absence of Ca^{2+} overload conditions was demonstrated, not only in intact ventricular and atrial cells, but also in Purkinje fibers.[62,63] Additional data in latent Ca^{2+} pacemaker cells[64] provided evidence that an intracellular Ca^{2+} oscillator could be a formal cause of normal rhythmic APs in

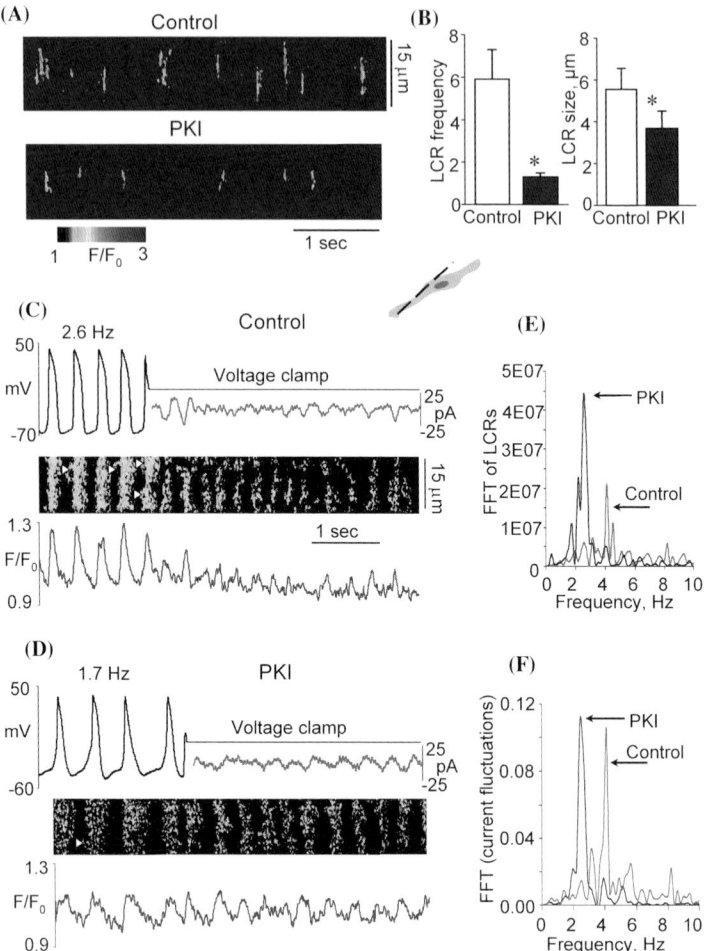

FIGURE 5. Suppression of cAMP-mediated, PKA-dependent signaling in SANC decreases frequency and size of LCRs in permeabilized and intact SANC. (**A**) Confocal linescan images of a representative saponin-permeabilized SANC bathed in 100 nmol/L free [Ca^{2+}] before (top) and after (bottom) superfusion with 15 μmol/L PKI, a specific peptide inhibitor of PKA catalytic submit. (**B**) The average frequency (normalized per 1 s and 100 μm) and size of LCR in skinned SANC in control conditions (72 LCR, $n = 4$) and 15 μmol/L PKI (20 LCR) $^*P < 0.05$. Error bars indicate standard error of mean. (**C** and **D**) Simultaneous recordings of membrane potential or current (top), confocal linescan image (middle), and normalized fluo-3 fluorescence (bottom) averaged over the linescan image, in a representative spontaneously beating SANC with intact sarcolemma before and during voltage clamp to −10 mV in control (**A**) and following PKA inhibition (8 μmol/L PKI) (**D**). Fast Fourier transform (FFT) of Ca^{2+} (**E**) and membrane current (**F**) fluctuations during voltage clamp in control and after PKI. Because current fluctuations during voltage clamp were imposed on the total membrane current, each data set was fit with a nonlinear regression line that was subtracted to give a difference signal to minimize frequency interference.[18]

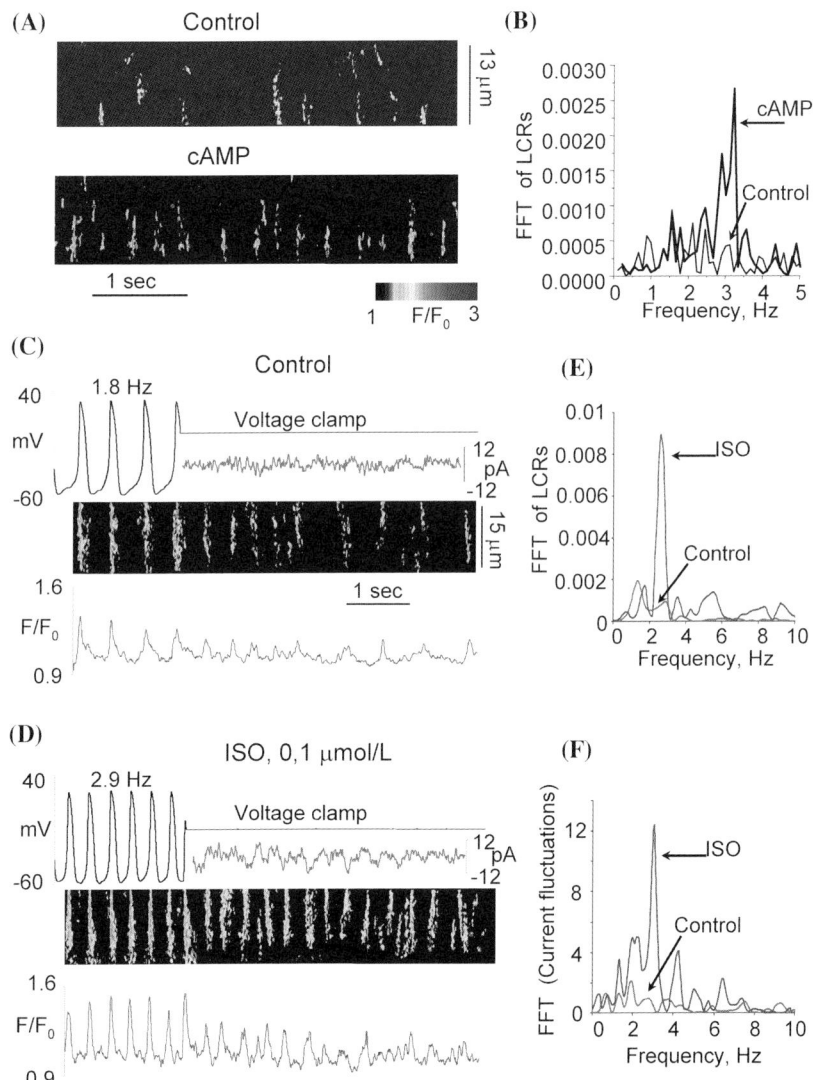

FIGURE 6. Stimulation of cAMP-mediated, PKA-dependent signaling in SANC increases internal Ca^{2+} oscillation frequency. (**A**) Confocal linescan images of a representative saponin-skinned SANC bathed in 100 nmol/L free $[Ca^{2+}]$ before (top) and after (bottom) superfusion with 10 μmol/L cAMP. (**B**) Fast Fourier transform (FFT) of Ca^{2+} fluctuations of the cell in (**A**) in control conditions and during superfusion with cAMP. (**C** and **D**) Simultaneous recordings of membrane potential or current (top), linescan image (middle), and normalized fluo-3 fluorescence (bottom) averaged over the linescan image, in a representative spontaneously beating cell with intact sarcolemma before and during voltage clamp to −10 mV in control (**C**) and following β-AR agonist (0.1 μmol/L isoproterenol [ISO]) (**D**). FFT of Ca^{2+} (**E**) and membrane current (**F**) fluctuations during voltage clamp in control and after ISO.[18]

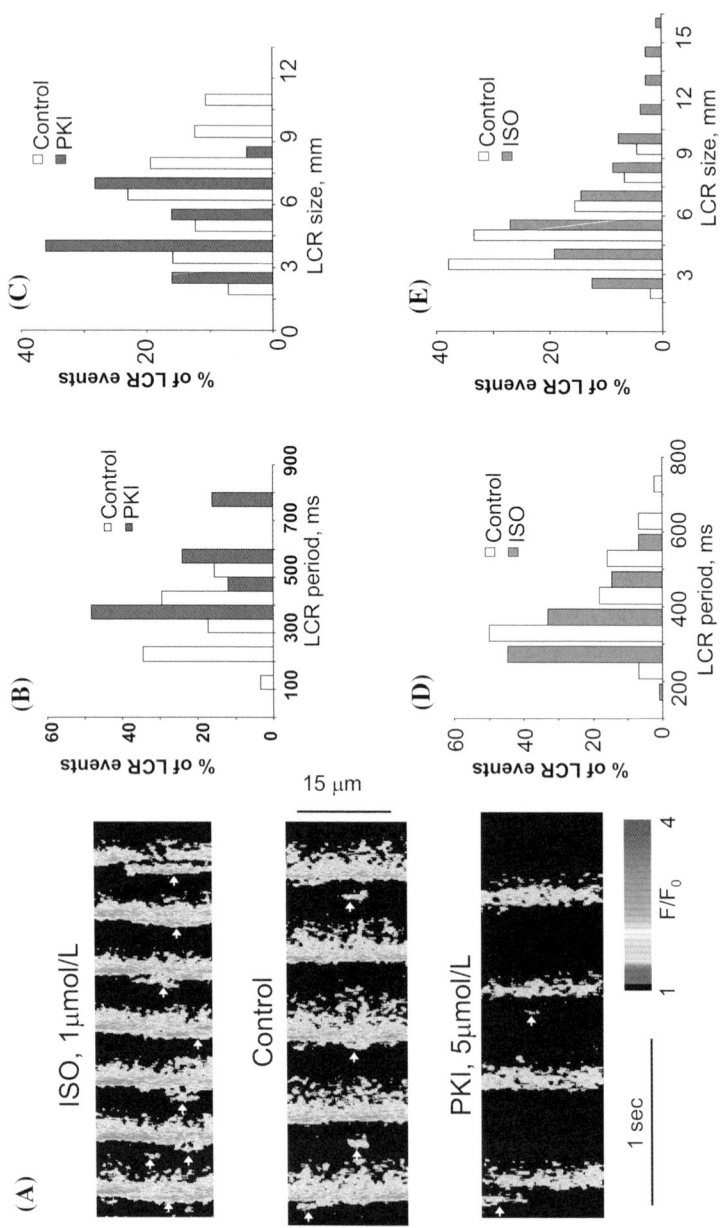

these cells: activation of an inward NCX current was abolished by ryanodine,[64] which disables RyRs, depletes the SR Ca^{2+} load, and prevents spontaneous SR Ca^{2+} release.

SCaRIE in Primary SANC

Recent, robust experimental evidence derived from simultaneous confocal linescan Ca^{2+} imaging and measurement of membrane potential in spontaneously firing, rabbit SANC[18,57–59,65,66] shows that, LCRs, which begin to occur during the later part of diastolic depolarization, ignite an NCX inward current (FIG. 1). This imparts an exponential increase to the later part of diastolic depolarization, (FIG. 1 C)[57] prompting activation of surface membrane, voltage-gated, L-type Ca^{2+} channels to initiate an AP. Blocking LCRs with ryanodine (FIG. 1 B) or blocking NCX by brief, rapid Na^+-free superfusion (FIG. 1 D, E) reduces the LCR-initiated inward current (and markedly slows or abolishes spontaneous SANC AP firing). In voltage clamped SANC, persistent, rhythmic LCRs generate rhythmic membrane current fluctuations with the same periodicity (FIG. 3). Both periodic LCRs and current fluctuations are abolished by ryanodine (FIG. 3).

SCaRIE Is Normally Tightly Regulated in SANC and Is not "Scary"

The Ca^{2+} cycling proteins of the SR, the NCX, L-type Ca^{2+} channels, and other sarcolemmal ion channels mutually entrain each other during spontaneous SANC firing. L-type Ca^{2+} current is a crucial factor in the SR Ca^{2+} clock, as well as a member of the ensemble, surface membrane, ion channel clock. In contrast to ventricular myocytes, the electrical excitation in primary SANC is mediated via activation of L-type Ca^{2+} channels rather than Na^+ channels. Moreover, the relatively synchronous SR Ca^{2+} release triggered by L-type Ca^{2+} channels causes a global SR Ca^{2+} depletion that quenches the spontaneous LCRs and resets the SR Ca^{2+} clock, as in ventricular cells. While L-type Ca^{2+} current does not trigger LCRs (FIG. 2 A), it is essential for LCR persistence, because Ca^{2+} influx via these channels offsets Ca^{2+} loss from the cell via NCX during each cycle, thus maintaining the SR Ca^{2+} load during spontaneous beating. In this sense, Ca^{2+} influx via L-type Ca^{2+} channels, by

---

FIGURE 7. Suppression (PKI, a specific inhibitor of PKA, 14–22 amide) or stimulation (isoproterenol [ISO]) of PKA-dependent phosphorylation have opposite effects on frequency and spatiotemporal properties of LCRs in intact, spontaneously firing SANC. (**A**) Confocal linescan images in a representative nodal cells depicting AP-induced Ca^{2+} transients and LCRs during spontaneous beating in control and when PKA phosphorylation was inhibited by PKI or stimulated by ISO. (**B** and **C**) Histograms of LCR period and size (FWHM) in control ($n = 4$ cells, 58 LCRs) and after superfusion with 5 μmol/L PKI ($n = 4$ cells, 25 LCRs). (**D** and **E**) Histograms of LCR period and size in control (8 cells, 42 LCRs) and after superfusion with 0.1 μmol/L ISO (8 cells, 89 LCRs).[18]

supplying Ca^{2+} to be pumped into the SR,[51] "rewinds" the SR Ca^{2+} clock. The magnitude of L-type Ca^{2+} channel-mediated, Ca^{2+} influx is finely tuned by the channel inactivation by the cytosolic Ca^{2+} transient that it triggers, and, during the AP, the electrogenic NCX ion flux is finely tuned by the membrane depolarization induced by L-type Ca^{2+} channels and by membrane repolarization due to K^+ channels. Thus, rhythmic LCR occurrence, by entrainment of rhythmic NCX current, leads to entrainment of voltage-gated, L-type Ca^{2+}, K^+, I_f, and other ion channels of the membrane clock, and this entrainment produces rhythmic APs. In the process of this entrainment of sarcolemmal protein activation, the SR Ca^{2+} clock entrains itself: the AP that it initiates resets the LCR period by triggering global SR Ca^{2+} release via RyRs, synchronizing both RyR activation status and the SR load at a low level following release, and also provides Ca^{2+} for the SR to pump to replenish its load, a crucial determinant of spontaneous LCR occurrence. This tight, mutual entrainment of the SR Ca^{2+} clock and the surface membrane clock integrates their functions to form a robust, stable pacemaker, preventing normal SCaRIE from becoming "scary!"

High Levels of Basal cAMP and PKA-dependent Phosphorylation in SANC Regulate the Time the Ca^{2+} Clock Keeps

The LCR period is the delay between the prior AP-induced, L-type Ca^{2+} channel-triggered, relatively synchronized cytosolic Ca^{2+} transient and LCR emergence later in diastole (FIGS. 1 A and 9 A). The speed at which the rhythmic SR Ca^{2+} clock "ticks" determines the LCR period, and thus determines the rate at which rhythmic SCaRIE occurs. A key point to note is that the LCR period is not fixed, but rather depends upon the speed at which SR Ca^{2+} cycling mechanisms have restituted following the Ca^{2+} release and SR Ca^{2+} depletion, and RyR inactivation effected by the prior AP, similar to what has been observed in ventricular cells.[52] Neither the SR Ca^{2+} load, nor Ca^{2+} cycling restitution status is fixed, but each change in response to variations in (*a*) rate or pattern of APs, which determine net cell Ca^{2+} balance, (*b*) the velocity and extent of SR Ca^{2+} pumping into the SR, and (*c*) activation status of SR release mechanisms. Stimulation of β-AR via cAMP-mediated, PKA-dependent phosphorylation of the L-type Ca^{2+} channel and of SR Ca^{2+} cycling proteins increases both Ca^{2+} flux into the cell and SR Ca^{2+} loading, and enhances the restitution kinetics of SR Ca^{2+} cycling, and the amplitude of SR Ca^{2+} release.[21,52,67-69]

While, basal, diastolic Ca^{2+} levels in rabbit SANC and ventricular cells do not differ,[58,60,66] the basal SR Ca^{2+} cycling clock within spontaneously firing SANC restitutes and generates LCRs following a delay period (FIGS. 5–10) that is substantially less than in ventricular myocytes.[2] A recent discovery provides the clue as to why the SANC SR Ca^{2+} clock runs so fast in the basal state: high basal levels of cAMP and cAMP-dependent phosphorylation are

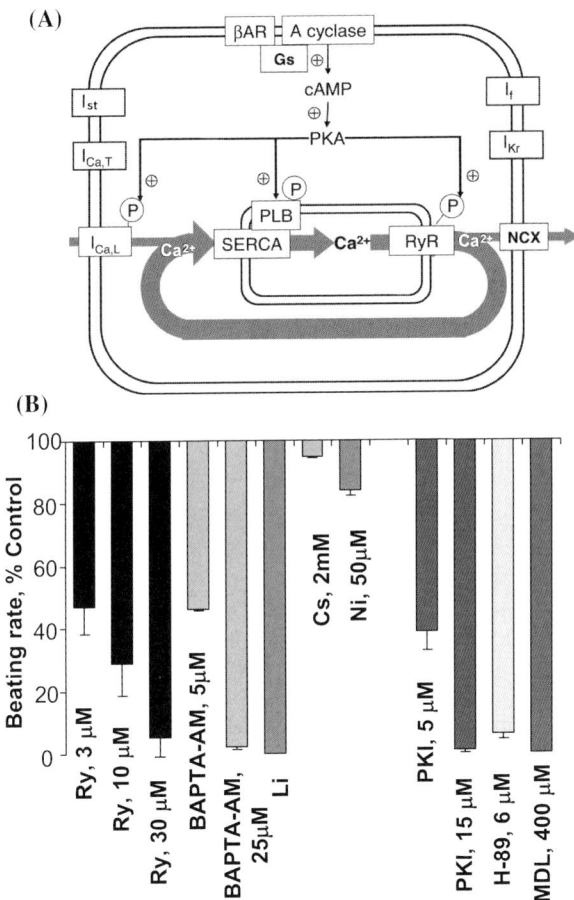

FIGURE 8. (**A**) cAMP-mediated, PKA-dependent phosphorylation controls Ca^{2+} influx via L-type Ca^{2+} channels, $I_{Ca,L}$, internal Ca^{2+} pumping into SR via SERCA2, and local submembrane SR Ca^{2+} release via RyRs during the latter part of the diastolic depolarization. The thick red line indicates spontaneous SR Ca^{2+} cycling. The spontaneous LCR, which requires SR Ca^{2+} loading by $I_{Ca,L}$, is linked to diastolic depolarization via an inward current induced by Ca^{2+} activation of the NCX (see text for details).[18,57] (**B**) Spontaneous beating of SANC is critically dependent upon Ca^{2+}-related mechanisms and protein phosphorylation. Bars show a decrease in the beating rate (% control) induced by different drugs that affect Ca^{2+} cycling; [ryanodine (Ry), BAPTA-AM, Li^+], protein phosphorylation (PKI, H-89, MDL), or ion currents: I_f (Cs^+) or T-type Ca^{2+} current (Ni^+).

present within SANC, that is, even in the absence of β-AR stimulation (FIG. 4). The high levels of basal cAMP are due to high constitutive adenylyl cyclase activity that is not driven by constitutive β-AR activation.[18] Preliminary evidence indicates that two adenylyl cyclase isoforms, type 2 and type 8, a Ca^{2+}-activated

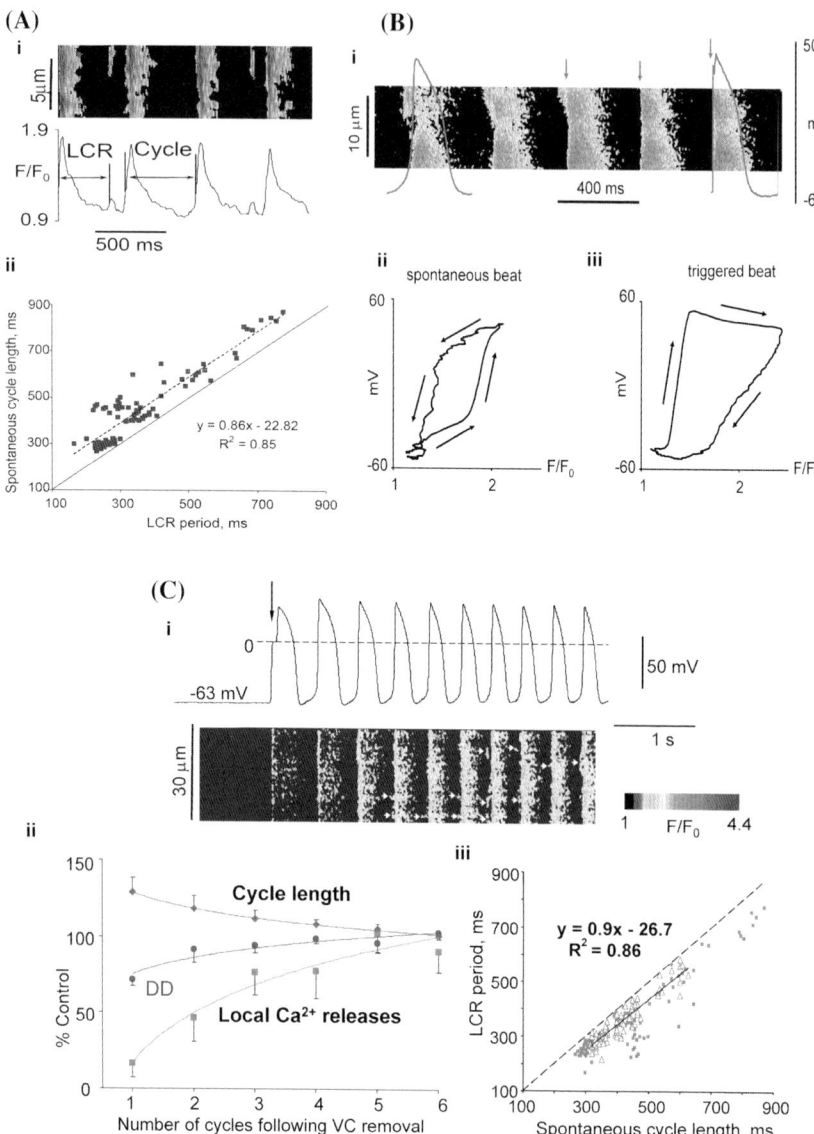

FIGURE 9. (**A**) (i) Confocal linescan image and normalized subsarcolemmal fluorescence averaged over the image width in a representative SANC. Double-headed arrows delineate the LCR period and cycle length during spontaneous beating. (ii) Squares, relationship between cycle length and the LCR period during spontaneous beating (10 cells, 86 LCRs).[58] (**B**) External pacemaker captures the beating rate of an isolated, spontaneously beating SANC. (i) Linescan image of fluo-3 fluorescence with superimposed APs of the first and last beats in a representative SANC. External electrical stimulation through a patch pipette was initiated at beat 3, at a rate just higher than the spontaneous beating rate (see black arrows). The two spontaneous beats before initiation of external stimulation reveal

isoform highly expressed in the brain, are expressed in SANC, but not in other cardiomyocytes.[70] Interestingly, basal phosphodiesterase activity also appears to be elevated in SANC,[71] likely as a mechanism to keep basal cAMP levels in check. Among proteins highly phosphorylated in the basal state are phospholamban (FIG. 4) and RyRs,[18] and L-type Ca^{2+} channels are likely to be as well.[72] Basal PKA-dependent phosphorylation of numerous other proteins, yet to be identified, also likely participate in functions that insure the occurrence of basal LCRs, i.e., insures that the SR Ca^{2+} clock runs, and runs at a physiologic, basal rate.[18]

The speed at which the SR Ca^{2+} clock "ticks," is under tight regulation by the degree of PKA-dependent phosphorylation.[18] In skinned (FIG. 5 A, B) or voltage clamped SANC (FIG. 5 C–F), inhibition of PKA-dependent phosphorylation by PKI, a specific peptide PKA inhibitor, reduces or abolishes LCRs, indicating a crucial role of PKA-dependent phosphorylation of SR Ca^{2+} cycling proteins in the generation of basal LCRs in SANC. In contrast, the LCR period is reduced and signal mass of LCRs is increased when cAMP is added directly to skinned cells (FIG. 6 A, B) or when β-ARs are stimulated during voltage clamping (FIG. 6 C–F).

In spontaneously firing SANC, PKA-dependent phosphorylation of the L-type Ca^{2+} channels determines the Ca^{2+} influx via these channels during spontaneous firing, and thus the amount of Ca^{2+} available for SR pumping, underscoring the notion that L-type Ca^{2+} channels are a *bona fide* component of the Ca^{2+} clock. Inhibition of PKA slows down the SR Ca^{2+} clock (FIG. 7 A–C), presumably via a reduction in L-type Ca^{2+} channel phosphorylation,[72] as well as a reduction in the phosphorylation of SR Ca^{2+} cycling proteins. Stimulation of β-AR extends the range of PKA-dependent control of the SR Ca^{2+} clock speed (FIG. 7 A, D, E).

←

the occurrence of the subsarcolemmal Ca^{2+} increase during the diastolic depolarization (i) which drives the trajectory of membrane potential versus calcium concentration (F/F_0) in a counterclockwise loop (ii). Note that by beat 5, the pre-AP increase in Ca^{2+} is precluded by the early occurrence of the externally driven AP, shifting the trajectory of membrane potential versus Ca^{2+} to a clockwise loop, similar to that seen during the duty cycle of normal ventricular myocytes (iii).[65] (C) Simultaneous recovery of LCR period and cycle length after removal of voltage clamp. (i) Simultaneous recordings of APs (top) and linescan image (bottom, SANC) in a representative during recovery from voltage clamp. Arrow indicates the moment of voltage clamp removal. (ii) Average relative recovery of total signal mass of LCRs, cycle length, and diastolic depolarization rate after removal of voltage clamp ($n = 5$). Recovery of total signal mass and diastolic depolarization rate of LCRs was highly correlated ($R^2 = 0.78$), as was the recovery of total signal mass and spontaneous cycle length of LCRs ($R^2 = 0.92$). (iii) Relationship of the recovery of the LCR period and that of the cycle length after removal of voltage clamp (triangles) was highly correlated ($R^2 = 0.86$). Dashed line is the line of identity.[58]

Rhythmic SCaRIE Drive Normal Automaticity in SANC

Robust experimental evidence,[18,57–59,65] supported by computational modeling,[18,59,65,66] demonstrates that factors that influence the speed of the SR Ca^{2+} clock, and thus the LCR period and the magnitude of the LCR signal mass regulate the rate at which SCaRIE drives SANC APs: when the SR Ca^{2+} clock restitutes more slowly, prolonging the LCR period, or when LCRs are blocked, the spontaneous cycle length becomes prolonged and spontaneous beating usually ceases.

The scheme in the (FIG. 8 A) integrates findings of multiple studies and illustrates the control points, at which five distinct maneuvers, each of which directly or indirectly markedly inhibits SR Ca^{2+} cycling to produce LCRs and global Ca^{2+} transients, blocks rabbit SANC pacemaker function.

(1) Graded suppression or complete blockade of Ca^{2+} cycling by buffering intracellular Ca^{2+} (FIG. 8 B) slows and blocks beating. In addition to abolishing Ca^{2+} release following excitation and abolishing LCRs, chelation of Ca^{2+} by BAPTA may inhibit Ca^{2+} calmodulin-dependent facilitation of L-type Ca^{2+} current.[33]

(2) Ryanodine, a specific inhibitor of normal RyR function, produces graded suppression or blockade of LCRs, and, in a concentration-dependent manner ($IC_{50} = 3$ μM), reduces the spontaneous SANC beating rate; at higher concentrations, ryanodine can abolish beating[57] (FIG. 8 B). This occurs in the presence of normal, as well as β-AR stimulation-augmented, L-type Ca^{2+} channel function.[59] In contrast to ryanodine, which specifically blocks the Ca^{2+} clock, a nifedipine blockade of L-type Ca^{2+} channel directly blocks the membrane ion channel ensemble clock and Ca^{2+}-induced Ca^{2+} release (CICR), and indirectly inhibits the SR Ca^{2+} clock too, because L-type Ca^{2+} channel inhibition begets SR Ca^{2+} depletion and LCR and SCaRIE abolition. Acutely blocking NCX current blocks spontaneous APs (FIGS. 1 E and 8 B) while leaving LCRs intact (FIG. 1 E).

(3) Variations in the basal LCR period among different cells are tightly linked to variations in their spontaneous cycle length (FIG. 9 A). The LCRs drive the spontaneous APs, because the LCR period is slightly shorter than the cycle length (FIG. 9 A). Application of external, rhythmic depolarizations, with a period length just less than the LCR period, suppresses ("overdrives") LCRs, and within a few cycles rhythmic APs become entrained at the external depolarization rate (FIG. 9 B).

(4) Cessation of spontaneous APs, by voltage clamp at the maximum diastolic potential (i.e., as in FIG. 2), leads to SR Ca^{2+} depletion and LCR abolition. Removal of the voltage clamp is followed by the gradual recovery of the control spontaneous cycling rate, and this gradual recovery is highly correlated with the return of LCRs and the recovery of the control LCR period (FIG. 9 C).

(5) There is tight coupling among the degree of PKA-dependent protein phosphorylation, the speed at which the SR clock generates LCRs, and the

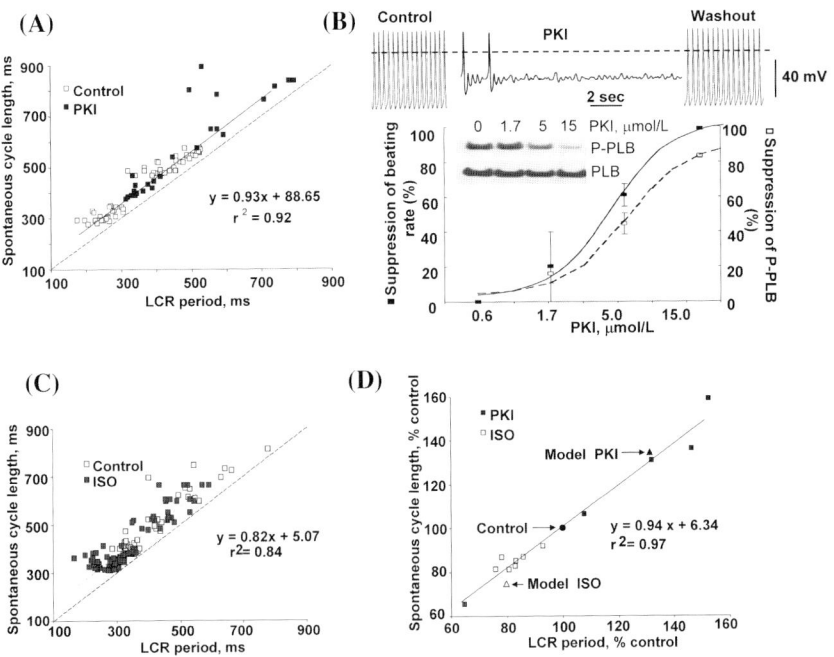

FIGURE 10. (**A**) The PKI effect to increase the spontaneous cycle length is linked to its effect on the LCR period. Note that this relationship lies above the line of identity (dashed line), indicating that the period of LCRs is shorter than the spontaneous cycle length. (**B**) (top) Typical example of APs recorded in a single, isolated SANC before (Control), during superfusion with 15 μmol/L PKI, and during washout of the drug. (bottom) The relationship of PKI-induced suppression of SANC beating rate (solid line) and PLB phosphorylation of SANC suspensions (dashed line). Inset shows Western blots of phosphorylated PLB and total PLB in response to increasing PKI concentrations. Error bars indicate standard error of mean. (**C**) Relationship between LCR period and spontaneous cycle length is shifted to shorter periods by β-AR stimulation with 0.1 μmol/L ISO. Dashed line is the line of identity. (**D**) The relative PKI and ISO effects to alter spontaneous cycle length over a wide range are linked to their effects on the LCR period within the same cells. Note that this relationship conforms to the line of identity. Square filled symbols and solid line depict the experimentally obtained data; unfilled symbols depict the average data simulated by numerical model using experimentally measured changes in LCR characteristics and phase (see text for details).[18]

rate at which spontaneous APs are generated (FIG. 10). Graded reduction of PKA-dependent phosphorylation via graded effects on L-type Ca^{2+} channel to reduce Ca^{2+} influx and cytosolic Ca^{2+}, and on SR Ca^{2+} cycling proteins (FIG. 8 A), prolong the LCR period or abolish LCRs and produces parallel effects on the spontaneous AP cycle length of SANC (FIG. 8 B). The dose response of the suppression of the spontaneous beating rate, due to the inhibition of PKA phosphorylation, closely parallels that of the suppression of phospholamban phosphorylation at serine 16 (FIG. 10 B). Submaximal basal PKA inhibition, in slowing the basal SR Ca^{2+} clock and prolonging the LCR

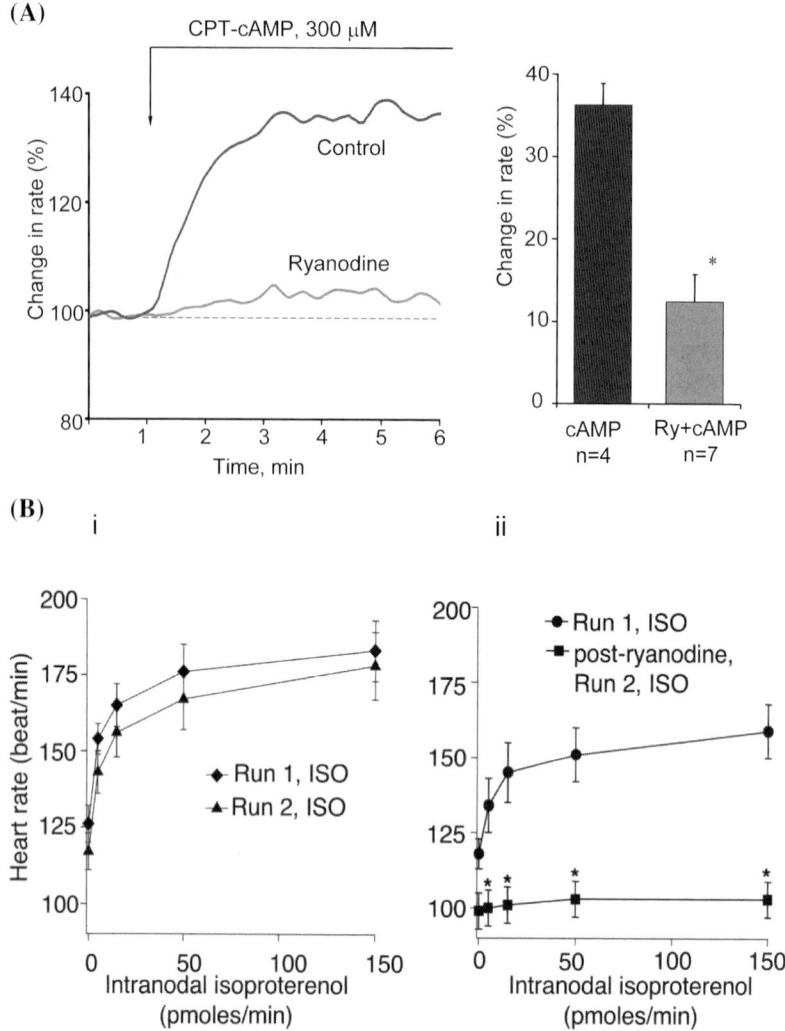

FIGURE 11. (**A**) A typical example of the change in the spontaneous beating rate of an isolated SANC in response to CTP-cAMP before and after exposure to ryanodine; The average effects of 300 μmol/L CTP-cAMP on beating rate of isolated SANC in the absence and presence of ryanodine are illustrated in the right panel. Note, that the CPT-cAMP-induced acceleration of the SANC beating rate is reduced in the presence of ryanodine. In control conditions, CPT-cAMP accelerated SANC rate beating rate by 36.3 ± 2.65 % (from 2.62 to 3.56 Hz), when CPT-cAMP was applied after exposure to ryanodine, the acceleration of SANC beating rate was only $12.5 \pm 3.3\%$, $^*P < 0.05$.[18] (**B**) Disabling RyRs dramatically reduces the effects of cAMP signaling to increase the heart rate *in vivo*. (i) Increased heart rate responses to sequential ISO dose responses delivered by microdialysis into the SA node of anesthetized open-chest dogs. Dogs underwent two sequential dose–response effects of ISO ($n = 5$). ISO produced a brisk, reproducible tachycardia, and sequential dose responses

period (FIG. 7), concomitantly slows the spontaneous AP firing rate (FIG. 10). The extent to which the LCR period in individual, isolated SANC becomes increased by PKA inhibition is highly correlated with the concomitant prolongation of the spontaneous AP cycle length (FIG. 10). The time-dependent effects on beating rate, of submaximal, basal PKA inhibition and its reversal in individual SANC, are also highly correlated with the concomitant time-dependent changes in LCR period.[18,73] After a prolonged time of submaximal PKA inhibition or following higher levels of PKA inhibition, LCRs are no longer detectable, and the rate of spontaneous APs markedly slows, becomes highly irregular, and often ceases.[18]

Increasing PKA-dependent phosphorylation by adding cell permeable cAMP analogs to the bathing fluid, or by stimulating β-ARs (FIGS. 6 and 8 A), speeds up the Ca^{2+} clock, reducing the LCR period. The extent to which this occurs is highly correlated with the concomitant increase in the spontaneous beating rate (FIG. 10 C). The relative change in AP firing rate among cells and the relative LCR period prolongation by PKI, or relative LCR period reduction by β-AR stimulation are extremely highly correlated ($r^2 = 0.97$), and this relationship lies on the line of identity (FIG. 10 D).

The crucial role of normal RyR function in mediating the chronotropic response to cAMP-dependent signaling by β-AR stimulation can be demonstrated by employing these perturbations in the presence and absence of ryanodine. *In vitro*, in single SANC, the effects of the cell-permeant cAMP (FIG. 11 A), or β-AR stimulation,[59] and in the intact organism, *in vivo* (FIG. 11 B), to increase the spontaneous AP firing rate or heart rate are markedly blunted in the presence of ryanodine. Moreover, although augmentation of the L-type Ca^{2+} current is necessary for the β-AR-cAMP PKA-dependent effect to increase beating rate, it is not sufficient to produce the effect, because blocking RyR function markedly reduces the cAMP-dependent increase of the SANC AP firing rate, while leaving β-AR stimulation-dependent L-type Ca^{2+} current augmentation intact.[59]

NUMERICAL PACEMAKER MODELS

An Internal Ca^{2+} Clock Ignites the Membrane Ion Channels Clock to Initiate an AP and to Sustain Rhythmic Spontaneous APs (Normal Automaticity)

Initial tests of the ability of LCRs during the diastolic depolarization to command the AP firing rate used a recently developed SANC model.[12] Experimen-

---

← in controls were superimposable. (ii) Following initial dose response to ISO, ryanodine (5 nmol/min) was introduced ($n = 5$). Local dialysis with ryanodine reduced resting heart rate before ISO by 12% (from 108 ± 5 to 96 ± 6 bpm; $P < 0.05$) and suppressed the response to subsequently added ISO by 75%. *$P < 0.05$. Error bars indicate SEM.[18]

tally measured, submembrane, oscillatory Ca^{2+} waveform introduced into the model easily entrained the spontaneous AP firing rate.[65] Subsequently, a pacemaker model,[61] modified to include a local oscillatory Ca^{2+} release function,[66] reproduced, for the first time, the negative chronotropic effect of ryanodine, and predicted a new powerful mechanism of rate regulation by varying Ca^{2+} release rate and phase: the larger release resulted in the larger NCX current that, in turn, allowed wider rate regulation range by the phase of the release covering basically the entire physiologic range. In terms of the fine diastolic depolarization structure, the model showed that the LCR-activated NCX current imparts exponentially rising part to the late diastolic depolarization that culminates in an AP upstroke.[66]

The most recent upgrade of this local Ca release model[18] reproduced individual stochastic LCRs (a multicompartment SR model). Varying frequency, size, and phase of the LCRs according to experimental data, this model predicted the wide range of chronotropic effects observed with graded PKA activity, that is, basal and reserve rate regulation (FIG. 12 D).[18] This most recent model, which includes interactions of SR and surface membrane oscillator, reproduces the entire range of basal and reserve (β-AR) rate regulation (FIG. 10 D).[18]

This model identified numerous benefits of interactions of the rhythmic LCRs and the membrane ion channel clock. Under conditions, in which ion channels operating alone in numerical models fail to generate rhythmic APs, stable and rhythmic AP firing resumes when the timely and powerful prompt to the membrane sent by SR via LCRs and NCX is introduced into the model.[73] In turn, the stability of the SR Ca^{2+} clock, itself, is insured by the interactive L-type Ca^{2+} current activation that supplies Ca^{2+} to the SR, and very importantly, by the L-type Ca^{2+} channel global CICR that resets the phases of multiple individual oscillatory LCRs. SERCA, RyR, NCX, and L-type Ca^{2+} channels work together to insure that LCRs reappear about the same time during next late diastolic depolarization and thus produce a powerful cumulative NCX current depolarization signal for next L-type Ca^{2+} current activation, and so on. The LCR and L-type Ca^{2+} current interaction is critical, as the SR Ca^{2+} clock slows markedly or stops shortly after either of its interacting components are reduced or become blocked, that is, under ryanodine (FIG. 8 B) or under voltage clamp at maximum diastolic potential (FIG. 2 A), respectively. Thus, two oscillatory processes of a different nature, the ensemble membrane ion channel clock and the SR Ca^{2+} clock, when left to operate alone become relatively unstable and fail. During spontaneous AP firing, these two unstable clocks become integrated and entrain each other, and the regulated, combined system results in stable, robust, normal automaticity.

SUMMARY

While the SANC sarcolemmal membrane clock is necessary to effect an AP, it is not sufficient in our opinion to ignite an AP, or to generate rhythmic

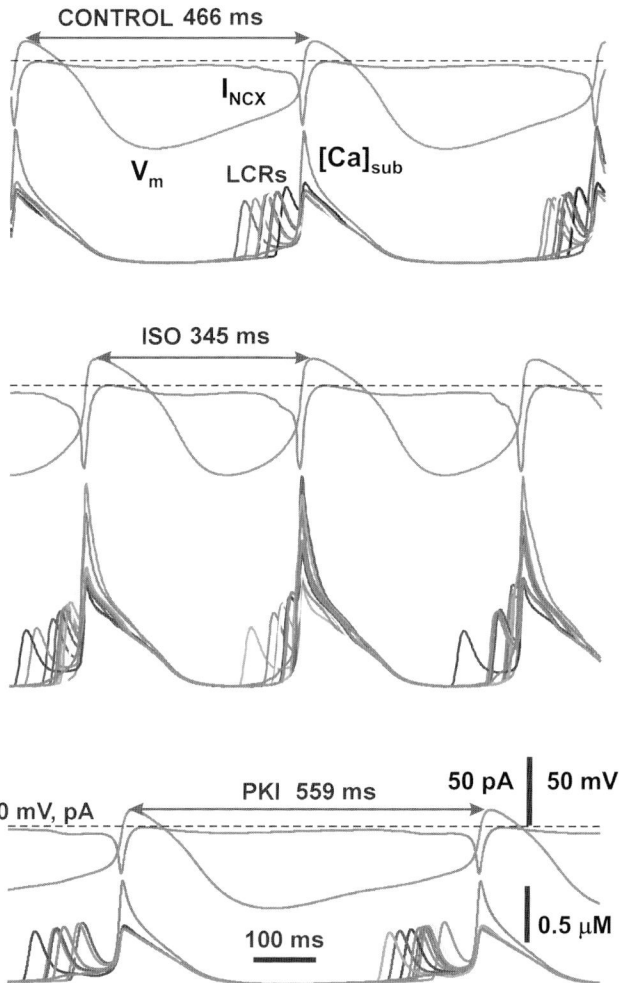

FIGURE 12. Numerical model simulations in primary rabbit SANC of chronotropic interventions with ISO or PKI compared to "CONTROL." Shown are AP (Vm), NCX current (I_{NCX}), overlapped, arbitrary eight LCRs, and average submembrane $[Ca^{2+}]_{sub}$. The arrows show respective cycle lengths together with their numerical values for comparison. Cycle length was linked to appearance of LCR associated with an increase of NCX current shortly followed by the AP upstroke. The respective model parameters are given in Table 2 of Online supplement in Reference 18.

APs at normal rates. Rather, the data in FIGURES 8, 10, 11, and 12 demonstrate that intracellular Ca^{2+} and rhythmic SCaRIE do not merely "fine tune" the normal automaticity of SANC, but represent the formal cause of APs, and thus they control rhythmic, spontaneous AP firing across the broad range of physiologic firing rates. Interfering with SR internal Ca^{2+} cycling interferes with normal pacemaking functions, just as does interfering with membrane ion channels that generate the AP upstroke and repolarization. In short, variations of internal Ca^{2+} cycling within SANC result in corresponding variations of SCaRIE that are tightly linked to gradations in their normal automaticity. The spontaneous, but tightly controlled, rhythmic, SR Ca^{2+} clock insures the stability of the basal rhythm by integrating multiple Ca^{2+}-dependent functions and rhythmically interacting with one, igniting the surface membrane clock to effect APs. Variable degrees of intrinsic PKA-dependent protein phosphorylation, and its attendant variations in intracellular Ca^{2+} regulate the time that the SR Ca^{2+} clock keeps, thus regulating the rate at which SCaRIE occurs, and modulate the voltage- and time-dependent kinetics of the components of the surface membrane clock, thus insuring that it produces APs with characteristics commensurate with given rhythmic ignition rates commanded by SCaRIE.

In the intact organism, integrated autonomic nervous system signals confer another layer of regulation of the intrinsic cAMP/PKA/Ca^{2+} signaling and of the SANC, SR Ca^{2+} clock and membrane clocks of SANC: vagal stimulation of cholinergic receptors predominates in the basal state, keeping the SR clock in check; in response to a demand for higher heart rates, stimulation of cholinergic receptors wanes, and sympathetic stimulation of β-adrenergic waxes; at the maximum chronotropic rate, β-AR activation of PKA-dependent phosphorylation is maximal, and the SR clock runs at full speed, producing SCaRIE at a maximum rate in order to achieve the maximum heart rate.

ACKNOWLEDGMENT

This research was supported by the Intramural Research Program of the NIH, National Institute on Aging.

REFERENCES

1. KASS, R.S. & R.W. TSIEN. 1982. Fluctuations in membrane current driven by intracellular calcium in cardiac Purkinje fibers. Biophys. J. **38:** 259–269.
2. LAKATTA, E.G. 1992. Functional implications of spontaneous sarcoplasmic reticulum Ca^{2+} release in the heart. Cardiovasc. Res. **26:** 193–214.
3. NOBLE, D. 1984. The surprising heart: a review of recent progress in cardiac electrophysiology. J. Physiol. **353:** 1–50.
4. HAGIWARA, N., H. IRISAWA & M. KAMEYAMA. 1998. Contribution of two types of calcium currents to the pacemaker potentials of rabbit sino-atrial node cells. J. Physiol. **395:** 233–253.
5. VERHEIJCK, E.E., *et al.* 1999. Contribution of L-type Ca^{2+} current to electrical activity in sinoatrial nodal myocytes of rabbits. Am. J. Physiol. **276:** H1064–H1077.

6. DiFrancesco, D. & M. Mangoni. 1994. Modulation of single hyperpolarization-activated channels (I_f) by cAMP in the rabbit sino-atrial node. J. Physiol. **474:** 473–482.
7. Guo, J., K. Ono & A. Noma. 1995. A sustained inward current activated at the diastolic potential range in rabbit sino-atrial node cells. J. Physiol. **483:** 1–13.
8. Hagiwara, N., et al. 1992. Background current in sino-atrial node cells of the rabbit heart. J. Physiol. **448:** 53–72.
9. Demir, S.S., et al. 1994. A mathematical model of a rabbit sinoatrial node cell. Am. J. Physiol. **266:** C832–C852.
10. Brown, H.F., et al. 1984. The ionic currents underlying pacemaker activity in rabbit sino-atrial node: experimental results and computer simulation. Proc. R. Soc. B. **222:** 329–347.
11. Dokos, S., B. Celler & N. Novell. 1996. Ion currents underlying sinoatrial node pacemaker activity: a new single cell mathematical model. J. Theor. Biol. **181:** 245–272.
12. Zhang, H., et al. 2000. Mathematical models of action potentials in the periphery and center of the rabbit sinoatrial node. Am. J. Physiol. **279:** H397–H421.
13. Cranfield, P.F. 1977. Action potentials, afterpotentials, and arrhythmias. Circ. Res. **41:** 415–423.
14. Noble, D. 2002. Modeling the heart—from genes to cells to the whole organ. Science **295:** 1678–1682.
15. Kass, R.S., R.W. Tsien & R. Weingart. 1978. Ionic basis of transient inward current induced by strophanthidin in cardiac Purkinje fibres. J. Physiol. (Lond.) **281:** 209–226.
16. Lederer, W.J. & R.W. Tsien. 1976. Transient inward current underlying arrhythmogenic effects of cardiotonic steroids in Purkinje fibres. J. Physiol.(Lond.) **262:** 73–100.
17. Huser, J., L.A. Blatter & S.L. Lipsius. 2000. Intracellular Ca^{2+} release contributes to automaticity in cat atrial pacemaker cells. J. Physiol. **524:** 415–422.
18. Vinogradova, T.M., et al. 2006. High basal protein kinase A-dependent phosphorylation drives rhythmic internal Ca^{2+} store oscillations and spontaneous beating of cardiac pacemaker cells. Circ. Res. **98:** 505–514.
19. Seifen, E., H. Schaer & J.M. Marshall. 1964. Effects of calcium on the membrane potentials of single pacemaker fibers and atrial fibers in isolated rabbit atria. Nature **202:** 1223–1224.
20. Cranffield, P.F. 1975. The Conduction of the Cardiac Impulse. Futura Publishing Company. Mount Kisco, NY.
21. Bers, D.M. 2001. Excitation-Contraction Coupling and Cardiac Contractile Force, 2nd ed. Kluwer Academic Publishers. Norwell, Mass.
22. Hancox, J.C., A.J. Levi & P. Brooksby. 1994. Intracellular calcium transients recorded with Fura-2 in spontaneously active myocytes isolated from the atrioventricular node of the rabbit heart. Proc. Biol. Sci. **255:** 99–105.
23. Rubenstein, D.S. & S.L. Lipsius. 1989. Mechanisms of automaticity in subsidiary pacemakers from cat right atrium. Circ. Res. **64:** 648–657.
24. Stuyvers, B.D., et al. 2005. Ca^{2+} sparks and waves in canine Purkinje cells: a triple layered system of Ca^{2+} activation. Circ. Res. **97:** 35–43.
25. Li, J., J. Qu & R.D. Nathan. 1997. Ionic basis of ryanodine's negative chronotropic effect on pacemaker cells isolated from the sinoatrial node. Am. J. Physiol. **273:** H2481–H2489.

26. RIGG, L. & D.A. TERRAR. 1996. Possible role of calcium release from the sarcoplasmic reticulum in pacemaking in guinea-pig sino-atrial node. Exp. Physiol. **81:** 877–880.
27. HATA, T., et al. 1996. The role of Ca^{2+} release from sarcoplasmic reticulum in the regulation of sinoatrial node automaticity. Heart Vessels **11:** 234–241.
28. SATOH, H. 1997. Electrophysiological actions of ryanodine on single rabbit sinoatrial nodal cells. Gen. Pharmacol. **28:** 31–38.
29. JU, Y.K. & D.G. ALLEN. 1998. Intracellular calcium and Na^+- Ca^{2+} exchange current in isolated toad pacemaker cells. J. Physiol. **508:** 153–166.
30. MUSA, H., et al. 2002. Heterogeneous expression of Ca^{2+} handling proteins in rabbit sinoatrial node. J. Histochem. Cytochem. **50:** 311–324.
31. RIGG, L., et al. 2000. Localisation and functional significance of ryanodine receptors during beta-adrenoceptor stimulation in the guinea-pig sino-atrial node. Cardiovasc. Res. **48:** 254–264.
32. JU, Y.K. & D.G. ALLEN. 1999. How does beta-adrenergic stimulation increase the heart rate? The role of intracellular Ca^{2+} release in amphibian pacemaker cells. J. Physiol. **516:** 793–804.
33. VINOGRADOVA, T.M., et al. 2000. Sinoatrial node pacemaker activity requires Ca^{2+}/calmodulin-dependent protein kinase II activation. Circ. Res. **87:** 760–767.
34. STERN, M.D. 1992. Buffering of calcium in the vicinity of a channel pore. Cell. Calcium **13:** 183–192.
35. CAPOGROSSI, M.C., et al. 1987. Synchronous occurrence of spontaneous localized calcium release from the sarcoplasmic reticulum generates action potentials in rat cardiac ventricular myocytes at normal resting membrane potential. Circ. Res. **61:** 498–503.
36. SCHWARTZ, A., et al. 1973. Abnormal biochemistry in myocardial function. Am. J. Cardiol. **32:** 407–422.
37. FABIATO, A. & F. FABIATO. 1978. Calcium-induced release of calcium from the sarcoplasmic reticulum of skinned cells from adult human, dog, cat, rabbit, rat, and frog hearts and from fetal and new-born rat ventricles. Ann. N. Y. Acad. Sci. **307:** 491–522.
38. FABIATO, A. & F. FABIATO. 1972. Excitation contraction coupling of isolated cardiac fibers with distributed or closed sarcolemma: calcium dependent cyclic and tonic contractions. Circ. Res. **32:** 293–307.
39. CHIESI, M., et al. 1981. Primary role of sarcoplasmic reticulum in phasic contractile activation of cardiac myocytes with shuttled myolemma. J. Cell. Biol. **91:** 728–742.
40. LAKATTA, E.G. & D.L. LAPPE. 1981. Diastolic scattered light fluctuation, resting force and twitch force in mammalian cardiac muscle. J. Physiol. (Lond.) **315:** 369–394.
41. STERN, M.D., et al. 1983. Scattered light intensity fluctuations in diastolic rat cardiac muscle caused by spontaneous Ca^{++}-dependent cellular mechanical oscillations. J. Gen. Physiol. **82:** 149–153.
42. LAKATTA, E.G., et al. 1985. Spontaneous myocardial Ca oscillations: an overview with emphasis on ryanodine and caffeine. Fed. Proc. **44:** 2977–2983.
43. LAPPE, D.L. & E.G. LAKATTA. 1980. Intensity fluctuation spectroscopy monitors contractile activation in "resting" cardiac muscle. Science **207:** 1369–1371.
44. CAPOGROSSI, M.C., et al. 1986. Single adult rabbit and rat cardiac myocytes retain the Ca^{2+}- and species-dependent systolic and diastolic properties of intact muscle. J. Gen. Physiol. **88:** 589–613.

45. KORT, A.A., M.C. CAPOGROSSI & E.G. LAKATTA. 1985. Frequency, amplitude, and propagation velocity of spontaneous Ca^{2+}-dependent contractile waves in intact adult rat cardiac muscle and isolated myocytes. Circ. Res. **57:** 844–855.
46. STERN, M.D., et al. 1989. Laser backscatter studies of intracellular Ca^{2+} oscillations in isolated hearts. Am. J. Physiol. **257:** H665–H673.
47. CAPOGROSSI, M.C. & E.G. LAKATTA. 1985. Frequency modulation and synchronization of spontaneous oscillations in cardiac cells. Am. J. Physiol. **248:** H412–H418.
48. CAPOGROSSI, M.C., B.A. SUAREZ-ISLA & E.G. LAKATTA. 1986. The interaction of electrically stimulated twitches and spontaneous contractile waves in single cardiac myocytes. J. Gen. Physiol. **88:** 615–633.
49. KORT, A.A. & E.G. LAKATTA. 1988. Biomodal effect of stimulation on light fluctuation transients monitoring spontaneous sarcoplasmic reticulum calcium release in rat cardiac muscle. Circ. Res. **63:** 960–968.
50. KORT, A.A. & E.G. LAKATTA. 1988. The relationship of spontaneous sarcoplasmic reticulum calcium release in twitch tension in rat and rabbit cardiac muscle. Circ. Res. **63:** 969–979.
51. FABIATO, A. 1985. Simulated calcium current can both cause calcium loading in and trigger calcium release from the sarcoplasmic reticulum of a skinned canine cardiac Purkinje cell. J. Gen. Physiol. **85:** 291–320.
52. FABIATO, A. 1985. Time and calcium dependence of activation and inactivation of calcium-induced release of calcium from the sarcoplasmic reticulum of a skinned canine cardiac Purkinje cell. J. Gen. Physiol. **85:** 247–289.
53. GYORKE, S., et al. 2002. Regulation of sarcoplasmic reticulum calcium release by luminal calcium in cardiac muscle. Front. Biosci. **7:** d1354–d1363.
54. JIANG, D., et al. 2004. RyR2 mutations linked to ventricular tachycardia and sudden death reduce the threshold for store-overload-induced Ca^{2+} release (SOICR). Proc. Natl. Acad. Sci. USA **101:** 13062–13067.
55. CHENG, H., W.J. LEDERER & M.B. CANNELL. 1993. Calcium sparks: elementary events underlying excitation-contraction coupling in heart muscle. Science **262:** 740–744.
56. LUKYANENKO, V. & S. GYORKE. 1999. Ca^{2+} sparks and Ca^{2+} waves in saponin-permeabilized rat ventricular myocytes. J. Physiol. **521:** 575–585.
57. BOGDANOV, K.Y., T.M. VINOGRADOVA & E.G. LAKATTA. 2001. Sinoatrial nodal cell ryanodine receptor and Na^+-Ca^{2+} exchanger: molecular partners in pacemaker regulation. Circ. Res. **88:** 1254–1258.
58. VINOGRADOVA, T.M., et al. 2004. Rhythmic ryanodine receptor Ca^{2+} releases during diastolic depolarization of sinoatrial pacemaker cells do not require membrane depolarization. Circ. Res. **94:** 802–809.
59. VINOGRADOVA, T.M., K.Y. BOGDANOV & E.G. LAKATTA. 2002. Beta-adrenergic stimulation modulates ryanodine receptor Ca^{2+} release during diastolic depolarization to accelerate pacemaker activity in rabbit sinoatrial nodal cells. Circ. Res. **90:** 73–79.
60. SATOH, H., L.A. BLATTER & D.M. BERS. 1997. Effects of $[Ca^{2+}]i$, SR Ca^{2+} load, and rest on Ca^{2+} spark frequency in ventricular myocytes. Am. J. Physiol. **272:** H657–H668.
61. KURATA, Y., et al. 2002. Dynamical description of sinoatrial node pacemaking: improved mathematical model for primary pacemaker cell. Am. J. Physiol. Heart. Circ. Physiol. **283:** H2074–H2101.

62. KORT, A.A. & E.G. LAKATTA. 1984. Calcium-dependent mechanical oscillations occur spontaneously in unstimulated mammalian cardiac tissues. Circ. Res. **54:** 396–404.
63. LIPSIUS, S. & W.R. GIBBONS. 1982. Membrane currents, contractions, and aftercontractions in cardiac Purkinje fibers. Am. J. Physiol. **243:** H77–H86.
64. ZHOU, Z. & S.L. LIPSIUS. 1993. Na^+- Ca^{2+} exchange current in latent pacemaker cells isolated from cat right atrium. J. Physiol. **466:** 263–285.
65. LAKATTA, E.G., et al. 2003. Cyclic variations of intracellular calcium: a critical factor for cardiac pacemaker cell dominance. Circ. Res. **92:** e45–e50.
66. MALTSEV, V.A., et al. 2004. Diastolic calcium release controls the beating rate of rabbit sinoatrial node cells: numerical modeling of the coupling process. Biophys. J. **86:** 2596–2605.
67. FABIATO, A. & F. FABIATO. 1975. Relaxing and iontropic effects of cyclic AMP on skinned cardiac cells. Nature (Lond.) **253:** 556–558.
68. TAKASAGO, T., T. IMAGAWA & M. SHIGEKAWA. 1989. Phosphorylation of the cardiac ryanodine receptor by cAMP-dependent protein kinase. J. Biochem. **106:** 872–877.
69. HAIN, J., et al. 1995. Phosphorylation modulates the function of the calcium release channel of sarcoplasmic reticulum from cardiac muscle. J. Biol. Chem. **270:** 2074–2081.
70. VINOGRADOVA, T.M., et al. 2006. High basal cAMP content markedly elevates pka-dependent protein phosphorylation and sustains spontaneous beating in rabbit sinoatrial nodal pacemaker cells (SANC), [abstract] Biophysic. J. (Suppl.) 155a.
71. VINOGRADOVA, T.M., et al. 2005. Constitutive phosphodiesterase activity confers negative feedback on intrinsic cAMP-PKA regulation of local rhythmic subsarcolemmal calcium releases and spontaneous beating in rabbit sinoatrial nodal, [abstract] Biophysic. J. **88**(Suppl.): 303a.
72. PETIT-JACQUES, J., et al. 1993. Mechanism of muscarinic control of the high-threshold calcium current in rabbit sino-atrial node cells. Pflugers Arch. **423:** 21–27.
73. MALTSEV, V.A., et al. 2005. Local subsarcolemmal Ca^{2+} releases within rabbit sinoatrial nodal cells not only regulate beating rate but also ensure normal rhythm during protein kinase A inhibition. Biophys. J. **88:** 89a–90a.

Calcium Handling in Embryonic Stem Cell–Derived Cardiac Myocytes

Of Mice and Men

ILANIT ITZHAKI,[a] JACKIE SCHILLER,[a] RAFAEL BEYAR,[a,b] JONATHAN SATIN,[c] AND LIOR GEPSTEIN[a,b]

[a]*Department of Physiology, the Bruce Rappaport Faculty of Medicine, Technion, Israel Institute of Technology Haifa, Israel*

[b]*Rambam Health Care Campus, Haifa, Israel*

[c]*Department of Physiology, University of Kentucky College of Medicine, Lexington, Kentucky, USA*

ABSTRACT: Excitation–contraction (EC) coupling is fundamental to the function of cardiac myocytes (CMs). In mature myocytes plasma membrane (PM) L-type Ca^{2+} channels function in close juxtaposition to ryanodine receptors (RyR) on the sarcoplasmic reticulum (SR) membrane. Action potentials (APs) cause the opening of PM L-type Ca^{2+} channels, which in turn provide trigger Ca^{2+} for a larger RyR-mediated SR Ca^{2+} release. In contrast, developing myocytes have a less well-developed SR. This incomplete development is observed in early stage and mid-maturation stages of murine embryonic stem cell–derived cardiac myocytes (ESC-CMs). Despite the absence of a well-developed t-tubule system, murine ESC-CMs use internal Ca^{2+} stores for EC coupling. Direct measures of Ca^{2+} handling, including pharmacological studies and investigation of genetically modified mouse ESC-CMs, established an important contribution of RyR-mediated internal Ca^{2+} store to cell function. Similarly, early-stage human ESC-CMs use internal Ca^{2+} store and partially share Ca^{2+} handling characteristics with murine ESC-CMs. For example, elementary Ca^{2+} release events are present in both murine and human ESC-CMs, and it is likely that Ca^{2+} handling contributes to automatic rhythm generation in these cells. However, in human ESC-CMs, a unique voltage-gated Na^{+} channel window current is critical for spontaneous, rhythmic depolarization. The advent of the murine and human ES cardiomyocyte differentiating systems has provided initial insights into the early steps of development of excitability and electromechanical coupling in the mammalian heart, including patterns of gene expression, myofibrillogenesis, ion channel development and function, and Ca^{2+} handling. Here we discuss the information gained from these models to describe the nexus of voltage-gated channel currents and Ca^{2+} handling on rhythmic activity.

KEYWORDS: ion channel; calcium channel; heart development; voltage-gated ion channel; cardiac electrophysiology; excitation–contraction

INTRODUCTION

Excitability and excitation–contraction (EC) coupling are essential functions of cardiac myocytes and have distinctive signatures in mature myocardium. The cellular processes responsible for the regulation of these functions undergo important changes during the maturation of the heart. Embryonic stem cell–derived cardiac myocytes (ESC-CMs) may provide an opportunity to study the development of these processes in early-stage cardiac tissue. Comparing the development of excitability and EC coupling between murine and human ES-derived cardiomyocytes is of importance due to the central role that the mouse species plays in the design of human disease models. Whereas the mouse ESC-CMs, denoted mESC-CM, model has been extensively used to study cardiac developmental paradigms, very little is known regarding the development of excitability and EC coupling in early-stage human cardiac tissue due to obvious ethical and practical reasons. The establishment of a cardiomyocyte differentiating system from human embryonic stem cells (hESC) may provide a unique model to study these processes. The acquired knowledge will also be essential for the successful future implementation and engineering of human ESC-CMs, denoted hESC-CMs, in cell replacement therapy strategies.

The aim of this review is to discuss recent work that has increased our understanding of the development of excitability and EC coupling in developing cardiac myocytes, with an emphasis on those derived from mouse and human embryonic stem cells.

EC COUPLING

Mature EC Coupling

Mature EC coupling follows a well-defined sequence. During the cardiac action potential (AP), Ca^{2+} enters the cell through depolarization-activated L-type Ca^{2+} channels. This inward Ca^{2+} current contributes to phase 2 of the AP plateau. This Ca^{2+} influx is the key event, leading to the transition from the resting diastolic state to contraction. The relatively small amount of Ca^{2+} that enters the cell in this fashion is not sufficient to cause a large contraction of the myofibrils. In most species, this initial Ca^{2+} signal is amplified several-fold by provoking additional Ca^{2+} release from an intracellular Ca^{2+} store, the sarcoplasmic reticulum (SR). This positive feedback mechanism is known as the Ca^{2+}–induced Ca^{2+} release (CICR) mechanism.[1-3]

The L-type Ca^{2+} current activates the Ca^{2+} release channels in the SR via ryanodine receptors (RyR), specifically RyR2.[4] The Ca^{2+}–sensitive RyRs are located in the immediate vicinity of the transverse tubule L-type Ca^{2+} channels and are activated by the local increase in Ca^{2+} from the transsarcolemmal Ca^{2+} influx. Once activated, the channels open and release Ca^{2+} from the SR into the cytosol. The membranous Ca^{2+} influx and the SR Ca^{2+} release raise the $[Ca^{2+}]_i$[5,6] and facilitate Ca^{2+} binding to the myofilament regulatory protein, troponin C, which then switches on the contractile filaments. Overall, the Ca^{2+} transient exhibits a transient increase of $[Ca^{2+}]_i$ from a resting concentration of approximately 0.15 µM to a peak level of approximately 1 µM.[3] The whole cell $[Ca^{2+}]_i$ transient is thought to represent the recruitment and summation of many Ca^{2+} sparks, localized discrete SR Ca^{2+} release events.[3,5,6]

Ca^{2+} must be removed from the cytosol to allow relaxation, which is essential for diastolic refilling of the heart. SR Ca^{2+} ATPase (SERCA) and Na^+/Ca^{2+} exchanger (NCX) serve as the main Ca^{2+} uptake pathways.[7] The relative role of these two transport systems is species-dependent[3,7] and is mainly determined by the abundance and activity of SERCA and NCX, by the intracellular Na^+ concentration ($[Na^+]_i$), and by the membrane potential.[8]

Distinct chamber-specific spatial and temporal Ca^{2+} handling characteristics exist within the heart. For example, ventricular myocytes have an extensive transverse tubule system, possessing L-type Ca^{2+} channels extending into the interior of the cells, thereby enabling a temporally and spatially uniform CICR pattern. In contrast to cardiac ventricular cells, cardiac atrial cells lack a regular system of transverse tubules. Many atrial cells display an irregular internal transverse-axial tubular system. As a consequence of this arrangement atrial myocytes, in response to depolarization, tend to display a spatial–temporal CICR pattern indicated by a spread of a Ca^{2+} wave from the periphery to the center of the cell.[9]

Fetal EC Coupling

In contrast to the adult mammalian heart, the contribution of SR Ca^{2+} release to EC coupling during fetal cardiac development is present, but is rather reduced compared to that of the adult ventricular myocytes. Indeed, several studies have reported that the SR in the fetal heart is structurally and functionally underdeveloped.[10] In addition, the SR vesicles have a lower volume resulting in a limited capacity to load Ca^{2+}.[11] The utilization of ryanodine, a RyR2 inhibitor, appears to have no effect on Ca^{2+} transients in fetal cells.[11-13] It was, therefore, suggested that fetal cardiomyocytes are mostly dependent on transsarcolemmal Ca^{2+} influx for tension generation rather than on Ca^{2+} release from the SR. However, recent reports challenge these findings. For example, ryanodine and thapsigargin, a SERCA2a inhibitor, decrease Ca^{2+} transient amplitude in fetal cardiomyocytes.[14] Moreover, studies show that the SR SERCA2a and RyR2 mRNAs/proteins are already abundantly expressed during the earliest stages of myocyte beating.[15,16]

MOUSE AND HUMAN ESC-CMs EC COUPLING

It is obviously interesting to compare human and mouse ESC-CMs excitability and EC coupling. Here we consider three salient features:(1) Ca handling proteins, (2) the presence of a functional SR, and (3) the nexus of excitability and Ca handling. Although mouse and human gestation periods are different[17] (21 vs. 270 days), approximations of comparable stages are possible based on cardiac morphology. Mouse ESC-CMs are well characterized and are often classified into very early (<20 days human equivalent), early (20–50 day human equivalent), and mature, which develop properties within 20 days of *in vitro* differentiation and maturation (270 day human equivalent). In parallel, hESC-CMs, at 20 days of *in vitro* differentiation, show immature-like ion channel expression.[18] At this early stage, hESC-CMs display molecular,[18] structural,[19] and functional[20] properties of early-stage cardiomyocytes. The cellular morphology of isolated hESC-CMs, differentiated about 1 month *in vitro*, is dramatically different from that of mature heart cells. The majority of the dispersed spontaneously beating cells studied have a roughly spherical area centered on a flatter apron (FIG.1, left panel).[18] The hESC-CMs are small (20–30 μm in diameter) and relatively featureless, displaying no discernable transverse tubules with myofilaments existing in a disorganized arrangement typical of immature cardiomyocytes (FIG. 1, right panel).[19]

Ca^{2+} Handling Proteins

Studies of the developmental changes of Ca^{2+} handling in mouse ventricular cells, from early embryo to adulthood, showed that from early embryonic to late fetal stage, mRNA for RyR2, SERCA2a, and phospholamban (PLB) increased by 3- to 15-folds. After birth there was a further increase in the mRNA of these proteins by 18- to 33-folds.[13] In mouse ESC-CMs, it has been reported that several SR mRNAs/proteins, such as RyR2, SERCA2a, and PLB are expressed before the initiation of the earliest contraction.[21,22] Similarly, early-stage human ESC-CMs express RyR2 mRNA[23] as well as SERCA2a, which are expressed in contracting embryoid bodies, differentiated about 2 months *in vitro*, in levels comparable to those detected in the left ventricle of a porcine heart, but lack PLB expression.[24]

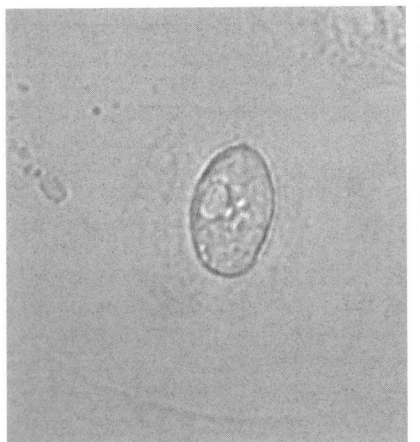 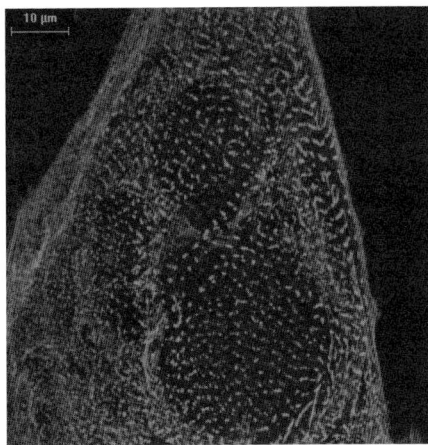

FIGURE 1. An isolated hESC-CM (left panel). Immunocytochemistry probing sarcomeric α-actinin (right panel) in a monolayer hESC-CMs cluster displaying disorganized sarcomeric arrangement.

The Presence of a Functional SR

Although EC coupling proteins' expression has been detected in mouse and human ESC-CMs, it remains to be determined whether these proteins are functional in comparable stages of maturation.

Evidence for SR activity in mESC-CMs is expressed in the form of spontaneous Ca^{2+} sparks representing Ca^{2+} release through RyRs channels.[25] The amplitude and frequency of these Ca^{2+} sparks, the expression of RyRs, and the volume of RyR-positive SR are reported to increase with time of differentiation. Furthermore, a time-dependent developmental elevation of caffeine-releasable Ca^{2+} was also observed.[25]

There is only scant information on internal Ca^{2+} handling in hESC-CMs. In contrast to the mature myocardium, hESC-CMs display a negative force frequency relationship.[24] Healthy mature myocardium tends to display a positive force frequency relationship induced by a net uptake of Ca^{2+} into the cells as the frequency of stimulation is increased.[26,27] In contradiction, the increase in stimulation rate in hESC-CMs is reported to cause a reduction in the amplitude of both the intracellular Ca^{2+} transient and the contraction, thus presenting a negative force–frequency relationship. Postrest potentiation of contraction, another index for a mature SR, is also absent in hESC-CMs.[24]

We are presently assessing the basic mechanisms underlying EC coupling in early-stage hESC-CMs differentiated up to 1 month *in vitro*, and the possible impact of the structure–function interactions on this process. Our studies show that relatively immature hESC-CMs exhibit prominent local Ca^{2+} transients. We have also observed that internal Ca^{2+} traverses the cell interior via propagated waves. Such mature-like Ca^{2+} waves suggest that hESC-CMs express mature Ca^{2+} handling molecules. Future studies will delineate the interaction of these elements and will determine the spatiotemporal relationships between sarcolemmal, SR Ca^{2+} channels, exchangers, and ion pump activity.

The Nexus of Excitability and Ca^{2+} Handling

A balanced interplay of ion channel activity is responsible for the activity of cardiac pacemaker cells. The means by which initiation of rhythmic beating takes place during early stages of cardiomyogenesis is unknown. The most apparent functional difference between a mature versus immature ventricular myocyte is the spontaneous excitability of the latter. Embryonic stem cells often differentiate into spontaneously contracting myocytes.[18,22] In the adult heart, RyR-mediated Ca^{2+} release governs the strength of contraction and contributes to the beating rate of the cells. In adult rabbit pacemaker cells, during diastolic depolarization and before an AP, SR Ca^{2+} release via RyR is reported[28] to trigger the NCX, inducing an inward current that causes the acceleration of spontaneous membrane depolarization rate, resulting in an increased rate of contraction. The mechanism for automaticity, however, may be different in immature ventricular myocytes compared to mature pacemaker cells.

In mESC-CMs, RyR2 is critical to the control of spontaneous activity. mESC-CMs with a functional knockout of RyR2 display a slowing of spontaneous diastolic depolarization rate and an absence of Ca^{2+} sparks. This occurrence can be mimicked in wild-type mESC-CMs by ryanodine-induced slowing of spontaneous beat rate,[22] underscoring the dual role of the SR as a source of Ca^{2+} for contraction as well as for the internal Ca^{2+} contribution to spontaneous excitability. Consistent with this view, Viatchenko-Karpinski et al.[29] observed intracellular Ca^{2+} concentration oscillations from RyR-sensitive Ca^{2+} stores in mESC-CMs. These intracellular Ca^{2+} oscillations are reported to have the ability to evoke small membrane depolarizations that have the potential of triggering L-type Ca^{2+} channel-driven APs.[29]

Immature hESC-CMs, differentiated about 1 month *in vitro*, express a prominent Na+ current with a current density that approaches mature levels.[18] These cells also express a hyperpolarization-activated current (HCN) yet lack an inward rectifier K^+ current (Kir). The absence of an inward rectifying K^+ current conductance is a phenomenon that provides the substrate for a relatively large voltage-gated Na^+ current to drive activity and, therefore, is the basis for the spontaneous depolarization in hESC-CMs. This has been displayed by the sensitivity of spontaneous activity to tetrodotoxin (TTX) in the same range as the partial block of $Na_V 1.5$.[18] Future investigations will explore whether additional mechanisms, including rhythmic store Ca^{2+} release,[30] also contribute to hESC-CMs automaticity.

SUMMARY

Results from our preliminary experiments with hESC-CMs were compared to literature data of mature murine cardiac cells. The adult mouse and the adult human cardiac myocytes differ in their EC-coupling properties when compared to developing human embryonic-derived cardiomyocytes. These data will be important in understanding the basic physiological processes of excitability and EC coupling in developing human embryonic cells.

The knowledge gained here may serve the long-term goal of using hESC-CMs as a cell source for tissue replacement therapies.[31] Nonetheless, mouse and human show different molecular mechanisms of spontaneous excitability at comparable embryonic stages.[18] We do not as yet know the degree of divergence between mouse and human mechanisms of embryonic EC coupling. Given the observed difference in mature mouse versus human EC coupling, we note that there must be important molecular changes at some point in maturation that determine species-specific function.

ACKNOWLEDGMENTS

We gratefully acknowledge the support of the Lady Davis Fellowship Trust (J.S.). This work is also supported in part by NIH grants (J.S.), the Israel Science Foundation, and the Nahum Guzik Research Fund (L.G.).

REFERENCES

1. FABIATO, A. 1983. Calcium-induced release of calcium from the cardiac sarcoplasmic reticulum. Am. J. Physiol. **245:** C1–C14.
2. BERS, D.M. & E. PEREZ-REYES. 1999. Ca^{2+} channels in cardiac myocytes: structure and function in Ca^{2+} influx and intracellular Ca^{2+} release. Cardiovasc. Res. **42:** 339–360.
3. BERS, D.M. 2002. Cardiac excitation-contraction coupling. Nature **415:** 198–205.
4. MARKS, A.R.. 1997. Intracellular calcium-release channels: regulators of cell life and death. Am. J. Physiol. **272:** 597–605.
5. CHENG, H., W.J. LEDERER & M.V. CANNELL. 1993. Calcium sparks: elementary events underlying excitation-contraction coupling in heart muscle. Science **262:** 740–744.
6. NIGGLI, E. 1999. Localized intracellular calcium signaling in muscle: calcium sparks and calcium quarks. Annu. Rev. Physiol. **61:** 311–335.
7. BASSANI, J.W.M., R.A. BASSANI & M.D. BERS. 1994. Relaxation in rabbit and rat cardiac cells: species-dependent differences in cellular mechanisms. J. Physiol. **476:** 279–293.
8. BLAUSTEIN, M.P. & W.J. LEDERER. 1999. Sodium/calcium exchange: its physiological implications. Physiol. Rev. **79:** 763–854.

9. KIRK, M.M., L.T. IZU, Y. CHEN-IZU, et al. 2003. Role of transverse-axial tubule system in generating calcium sparks and calcium transients in rat atrial myocytes. J. Physiol. **547:** 441–451.
10. PEGG, W. & M. MICHALAK. 1987. Differentiation of sarcoplasmic reticulum during cardiac myogenesis. Am. J. Physiol. **252:** H22–H31.
11. NAKANISHI, T., M. SEGUCHI & A. TAKAO. 1988. Development of the myocardial contractile system. Experientia **44:** 936–944.
12. TAKESHIMA, H., S. KOMAZAKI, K. HIROSE, et al. 1998. Embryonic lethality and abnormal cardiac myocytes in mice lacking ryanodine receptor type 2. EMBO J. **17:** 3309–3316.
13. LIU, W., K. YASUI, T. OPTHOF, et al. 2002. Developmental changes of Ca^{2+} handling in mouse ventricular cells from early embryo to adulthood. Life Sci. **71:** 1279–1292.
14. SEKI, S., M. NAGASHIMA, Y. YAMADA, et al. 2003. Fetal and postnatal development of Ca^{2+} transients and Ca^{2+} sparks in rat cardiomyocytes. Cardiovasc. Res. **58:** 535–548.
15. MOORMAN, A.F., J.L. VERMEULEN, M.U. KOBAN, et al. 1995. Patterns of expression of sarcoplasmic reticulum Ca^{2+}-ATPase and phospholamban mRNAs during rat heart development. Circ. Res. **76:** 616–625.
16. MOORMAN, A.F., C.A. SCHUMACHER, P.A. DE BOER, et al. 2000. Presence of functional sarcoplasmic reticulum in the developing heart and its confinement to chamber myocardium. Dev. Biol. **223:** 279–290.
17. REPPEL, M., C. BOETTINGER & J. HESCHELER. 2004. Beta-adrenergic and muscarinic modulation of human embryonic stem cell-derived cardio-myocytes. Cell. Physiol. Biochem. **14:** 187–196.
18. SATIN, J., I. KEHAT, O. CASPI, et al. 2004. Mechanism of spontaneous excitability in human embryonic stem cell derived cardiomyocytes. J. Physiol. **559:** 479–496.
19. SNIR, M., I. KEHAT, A. GEPSTEIN, et al. 2003. Assessment of the ultrastructural and proliferative properties of human embryonic stem cell-derived cardiomyocytes. Am. J. Physiol. Heart Circ. Physiol. **285:** 2355–2363.
20. KEHAT, I., L. KHIMOVICH, O. CASPI, et al. 2004. Electromechanical integration of cardiomyocytes derived from human embryonic stem cells. Nat. Biotechnol. **22:** 1282–1289.
21. BOHELER, K.R., J. CZYZ, D. TWEEDIE, et al. 2002. Differentiation of pluripotent embryonic stem cells into cardiomyocytes. Circ. Res. **91:** 189–201.
22. YANG, H.T., D. TWEEDIE, S. WANG, et al. 2002. The ryanodine receptor modulates the spontaneous beating rate of cardiomyocytes during development. Proc Natl Acad. Sci. USA **99:** 9225–9230.
23. MUMMERY, C., D. WARD-VAN OOSTWAARD, P. DOEVENDANS, et al. 2003. Differentiation of human embryonic stem cells to cardiomyocytes - role of coculture with visceral endoderm-like cells. Circulation **107:** 2733–2740.
24. DOLNIKOV, K., M. SHILKRUT, N. ZEEVI-LEVIN, et al. 2006. Functional properties of human embryonic stem cell-derived cardiomyocytes: intracellular ca handling and the role of sarcoplasmic reticulum in the contraction. Stem Cells **24:** 236–245.
25. SAUER, H., T. THEBEN, J. HESCHELER, et al. 2001. Characteristics of calcium sparks in cardiomyocytes derived from embryonic stem cells. Am. J. Physiol. Heart Circ. Physiol. **281:** H411–H421.
26. LEWARTOWSKI, B. & B. PYTKOWSKI. 1987. Cellular mechanisms of the relationship between myocardial force and frequency of contractions. Pro. Biophys. Mol. Biol. **50:** 97–120.

27. LAYLAND, J. & J.C. KENTISH. 1999. Positive force- and $[Ca^{2+}]_i$-frequency relationships in rat ventricular trabeculae at physiological frequencies. Am. J. Physiol. Heart Circ. Physiol. **276:** H9–H18.
28. BOGDANOV, K.Y., T.M. VINOGRADOVA & E.G. LAKATTA. 2001. Sinoatrial nodal cell ryanodine receptor and Na-Ca exchanger. Circ. Res. **88:** 1254–1258.
29. VIATCHENKO-KARPINSKI, S., B.K. FLEISCHMANN, Q. LIU, et al. 1999. Intracellular Ca^{2+} oscillations drive spontaneous contractions in cardiomyocytes during early development. Proc. Natl. Acad. Sci. USA **96:** 8259–8264.
30. VINOGRADOVA, T.M., A.E. LYASHKOV, W. ZHU, et al. 2006. High basal protein kinase A-dependent phosphorylation drives rhythmic internal Ca^{2+} store oscillations and spontaneous beating of cardiac pacemaker cells. Circ. Res. **98:** 505–514.
31. GEPSTEIN, L. 2002. Derivation and potential applications of human embryonic stem cells. Circ. Res. **91:** 866–876.

Cellular Alternans

A Mechanism Linking Calcium Cycling Proteins to Cardiac Arrhythmogenesis

LANCE D. WILSON, XIAOPING WAN, AND DAVID S. ROSENBAUM

Heart and Vascular Research Center, MetroHealth Campus of Case Western Reserve University, Cleveland, Ohio 44109-1998, USA

ABSTRACT: Essentially all previous research on alternans has been restricted to normal myocardium, whereas sudden cardiac death (SCD) occurs most commonly in patients with ventricular dysfunction (i.e., heart failure), which is associated with marked disruption of proteins responsible for normal calcium cycling in myocytes. Several lines of evidence from studies in normal hearts suggest a link between impaired calcium cycling which characterizes ventricular mechanical dysfunction and impaired calcium cycling that is responsible for alternans. In normal myocardium, cells which exhibit the slowest calcium cycling, and not the slowest repolarization, are most susceptible to alternans. Decreased expression of key calcium cycling proteins is observed in alternans-prone cells. Sarcoplasmic reticulum ATPase (SERCA2a) expression is decreased, suggesting a mechanism for the slower sarcoplasmic reticulum (SR) calcium reuptake observed in alternans-prone cells. In addition, diminished ryanodine receptor (RyR) function leading to abnormal calcium release from the SR is also linked to cellular alternans. Although impaired contractile function clearly predisposes to SCD, the mechanisms linking mechanical to electrophysiological dysfunction in the heart are unclear. We propose that cellular calcium alternans may be an important mechanism linking mechanical dysfunction to cardiac arrhythmogenesis.

KEYWORDS: arrhythmias; alternans; calcium cycling; heart failure; repolarization

INTRODUCTION

The complex sequence of events which incite electrical instability in the heart leading to sudden cardiac death (SCD) are poorly understood. Consequently, most patients at risk go unrecognized and SCD remains a major unresolved

Address for correspondence: David S. Rosenbaum, MetroHealth Campus, Case Western Reserve University, 2500 MetroHealth Drive, Hamann 330, Cleveland, OH 44109-1998. Voice: 216-778-2005; fax: 216-778 4924.
e-mail: drosenbaum@metrohealth.org

public health problem. Subtle beat-to-beat alternation of cardiac repolarization (manifest clinically as T-wave alternans [T-ALT]) is a highly sensitive marker of susceptibility to SCD in patients. Moreover, cellular alternans is linked to a mechanism of reentrant arrhythmogenesis by forming spatial gradients of repolarization causing conduction block. There is compelling evidence that alternans of repolarization arises from beat-to-beat alternations in intracellular calcium cycling, and that calcium alternans is transduced to repolarization alternans by electrogenic feedback mechanisms.

SUDDEN CARDIAC DEATH

SCD is the most devastating manifestation of heart disease and accounts for at least 50% of deaths in patients with heart failure.[1] The structural and electrophysiological changes that predispose to SCD in chronically diseased hearts have been studied extensively.[2,3] Yet, surprisingly little is known of the complex sequence of events that incite malignant arrhythmias in some patients but not in others. This presents a major obstacle to ongoing efforts aimed at developing clinical strategies for identifying those patients at greatest risk.[4-8] Also, the only effective therapy available is the implantable defibrillator, which shocks ongoing fibrillation but does nothing to alter the natural history of SCD. Consequently, SCD remains a major unresolved public health problem.

It is well recognized that the vast majority of SCDs occur in patients with ventricular contractile dysfunction, that is, heart failure.[9,10] However, the mechanisms linking mechanical to electrophysiological dysfunction in the heart are unclear. *Impaired calcium cycling is the most striking abnormality of failing myocytes, and is most directly responsible for contractile dysfunction; yet it remains unclear how this influences susceptibility to arrhythmias.*[11] Improved understanding of the fundamental relationships between mechanical and electrophysiological cardiac dysfunction is critical for developing better approaches for identifying and treating patients at risk for SCD.

CARDIAC ALTERNANS AS A MARKER FOR SCD

T-ALT is defined as a beat-to-beat fluctuation in the amplitude of the ECG T-wave that repeats every other beat. T-ALT was first recognized nearly 100 years ago, shortly after the ECG was introduced into clinical medicine.[12] Visible T-ALT has been associated with ventricular arrhythmias in diverse experimental and clinical settings[13-15] raising speculation that T-ALT is a universal precursor to cardiac arrhythmias.[16,17] In 1994 the first evidence was provided that subtle (microvolt level) and visually inapparent T-ALT is actually quite common (80% incidence) in high-risk patients and importantly, the absence of T-ALT was associated with very low risk (2–5%) of events.[18] Numerous subsequent clinical trials in more than 2500 patients have reaffirmed these

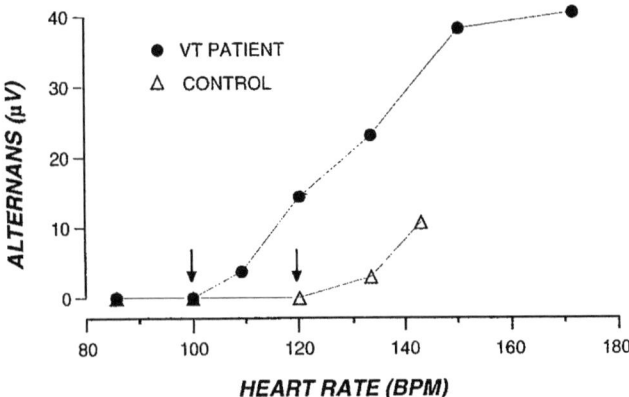

FIGURE 1. T-ALT—heart rate relation in a patient with history of VT (•) is shifted to lower heart rate threshold (arrows) compared to controls (△) (from Ref. 29).

findings,[4,19–24] and have demonstrated that when compared directly to other indices, such as ejection fraction, signal averaged ECG, and heart rate variability, T-ALT is currently the most sensitive noninvasive marker for SCD risk.[22,25–27] Importantly, multiple studies have demonstrated that in patients at risk for sudden death, particularly those with left ventricular dysfunction, increased susceptibility to T-ALT independently predicts SCD.[4] Interestingly, two recent clinical trials demonstrated that a negative T-ALT test obtained in patients who would otherwise be considered candidates for preventative defibrillator therapy (ejection fraction < 0.35 and no previous arrhythmias) have such low event rates that the benefit to therapy is questionable.[4,28] These findings imply that *resistance to T-ALT somehow confers protection against SCD in humans, further suggesting that understanding mechanisms of T-ALT can provide fundamentally new insights to the pathophysiology of SCD.*

T-ALT is a rate-dependent property of the heart, such that there is a patient-specific heart rate threshold above which T-ALT increases monotonically, independent of autonomic state.[29] Moreover, patients at risk for SCD (FIG. 1, ventricular tachycardia [VT] patient) exhibit a fundamental leftward shift in their alternans–heart rate relation compared to controls. *The mechanism responsible for the shift in the alternans–heart rate relation may have significant bearing on susceptibility to SCD, and is a major focus of this review.*

MECHANISM LINKING REPOLARIZATION ALTERNANS TO GENESIS OF ARRHYTHMIAS

The mechanisms linking alternans to arrhythmogenesis was established through detailed measurements of the time course of membrane voltage (V_m) throughout the ventricle at a time when T-ALT was elicited on the surface

ECG. To accomplish this, high-resolution voltage-sensitive dye mapping was applied to a guinea pig model of pacing-induced T-ALT.[24,30,31] This model is particularly suited to investigate the cellular basis for T-ALT because: (*a*) it possesses repolarization properties that are more comparable to humans than mouse, rat, or rabbit, (*b*) heterogeneities of repolarization across the epicardial surface are well characterized, and (*c*) the proportion of cytoplasmic calcium extrusion by the sodium–calcium exchanger (NCX) versus the sarcoplasmic reticulum ATPase (SERCA2a) in guinea pig is comparable to human.[32] T-ALT was induced in a controlled fashion by steady-state pacing over a broad range of heart rates (120–333 bpm), and by reducing perfusion temperature (27–33°C).[30] T-ALT in this model exhibits several important characteristics of T-ALT in humans[18]: (*a*) T-ALT is induced reproducibly above a heart rate threshold, (*b*) the magnitude of alternans is titratable and persists at a constant heart rate (i.e., does not require abrupt rate change), (*c*) T-ALT affects primarily the peak of the T wave rather than the ST segment or QRS complex, and (*d*) T-ALT is a consistent (actually requisite) precursor to ventricular fibrillation (VF).

There is compelling evidence from our laboratory[24,30,31] and others[33,34] that T-ALT results from beat-to-beat alternation in the time course of repolarization at the cellular level (V_m-ALT).[24,30,31,35,36] In addition to being the electrophysiological basis for T-ALT, V_m-ALT is several orders of magnitude larger in amplitude than T-ALT, indicating that relatively small T-ALT on the surface ECG actually corresponds to large V_m-ALT at the cellular level. These findings may explain why detection of very subtle (microvolt level) T-ALT has physiological and clinical significance in patients.

A novel mechanism linking cellular alternans to reentrant arrhythmogenesis was recently described by our laboratory.[37] When V_m-ALT is first initiated, it occurs with identical phase in all cells of a particular region of ventricular myocardium (i.e., concordant alternans). However, as illustrated in FIGURE 2 (panel A) above a critical heart rate threshold V_m-ALT switches phase in some cells but not others, such that some cells undergo a prolongation of action potential duration (APD) while other populations of cells undergo APD shortening on the same beat (i.e., discordant alternans).[30,31] The transformation from concordant alternans to discordant alternans has significant consequences on the spatial organization of repolarization across the ventricle. As shown in FIGURE 2 (panel B), during discordant alternans, marked spatial dispersion of repolarization emerged. Discordant alternans amplified physiological heterogeneities of repolarization present at baseline into pathophysiological heterogeneities of sufficient magnitude to produce conduction block and reentrant excitation.[24,30,31] Consequently, discordant alternans is key to the mechanism linking T-ALT to cardiac arrhythmogenesis, and in fact VF never occurred without discordant alternans. The same paradigm was used to explain the initiation of a variety of arrhythmias including polymorphic and monomorphic VT, as the resultant arrhythmias were determined by structural discontinuities

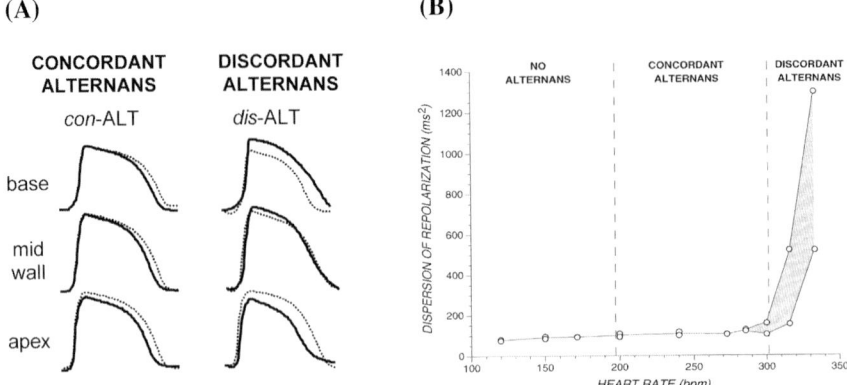

FIGURE 2. (**A**) Optical action potentials from epicardial cells on base, apex, and midwall of guinea pig during two consecutive beats (solid and stippled) of Vm-ALT. Above a critical heart rate, con-ALT is transformed to dis-ALT between apex and base. (**B**) dis-ALT amplifies spatial gradients of repolarization (from Ref. 30).

in the tissue, but in each case discordant alternans was required to initiate reentry.[31]

CELLULAR, SUBCELLULAR, AND MOLECULAR BASIS FOR CARDIAC ALTERNANS

Although a variety of sarcolemmal currents can exhibit alternating-type activity including I_{to},[38] I_{Ca},[39] I_{Kr},[40] few have been definitively shown to be mechanistically responsible for producing V_m-ALT. However, there are convincing data for a primary role of sarcoplasmic reticulum (SR) calcium cycling in the mechanism of V_m-ALT.[35,41–49] For example, inhibiting calcium cycling by blocking the ryanodine receptor (RyR), I_{Ca}, or by depleting SR calcium stores with caffeine, eradicates V_m-ALT.[45,46,50] Given the complex regulatory feedback between cytosolic calcium and sarcolemmal ion channels governing the action potential, deciphering the role of SR versus sarcolemmal currents in the mechanism of V_m-ALT is a challenging "chicken and egg" problem. However, the seminal observations of Chudin et al.,[51] (FIG. 3) that beat-to-beat alternation of calcium transient amplitude (Ca-ALT) is similarly induced under current-clamp (where V_m-ALT occurs) and voltage-clamp (i.e., where V_m-ALT is prevented) conditions proved that Ca-ALT, is not dependent on V_m-ALT, and strongly supported the notion that cellular alternans arises from SR calcium cycling.

Dual V_m-calcium imaging was recently used by our laboratory to generate an independent line of evidence supporting a primary role of calcium cycling

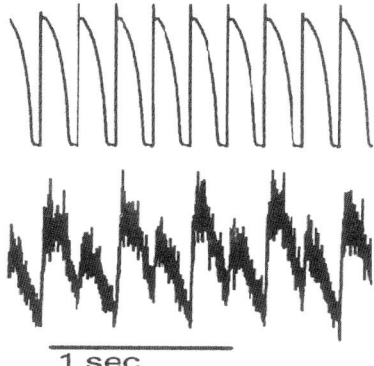

FIGURE 3. Induction of Ca-ALT (bottom trace) by constant action potential clamp (top trace) suggesting that Ca-ALT causes V_m-ALT, but V_m-ALT does not cause Ca-ALT (adapted from Ref. 51).

rather than APD restitution in the mechanism of V_m-ALT.[35] The "restitution hypothesis" states that V_m-ALT occurs when the slope of the APD restitution curve is > 1, which has been taken as evidence that sarcolemmal rather than SR calcium cycling determine V_m-ALT.[17,52–56] The guinea pig model of T-ALT includes an epicardial gradient of APD restitution, thus providing an opportunity to determine if myocytes with steepest restitution slope are most susceptible to V_m-ALT. To the contrary, we found that when compared to V_m-ALT-resistant myocytes, V_m-ALT-susceptible myocytes failed to exhibit steep restitution or prolonged APD,[35] (FIG. 4, panels B and C). Instead, V_m-ALT-susceptible myocytes had the slowest time constant for diastolic calcium reuptake, and greatest propensity for rate-dependent cytosolic calcium accumulation, strongly suggesting that calcium cycling rather than restitution properties dictates cellular alternans. In analogous fashion, applying dual V_m-calcium imaging to the transmural surface of canine wedge preparations, transmural heterogeneities of calcium handling were used to determine mechanisms of alternans in normal canine heart. Analogous to the guinea pig epicardium, susceptibility to V_m-ALT is heterogeneous across the transmural surface of the canine heart, with endocardial cells more susceptible to alternans than epicardial cells. Again, these alternans-susceptible endocardial cells exhibit significantly slower calcium reuptake kinetics[57] (FIG. 4, panel A). We used a similar experimental approach to also demonstrate (FIG. 5) that that V_m-ALT-susceptible myocytes express significantly less SERCA2a[30,57,58] and RyR[58] compared to V_m-ALT-resistant myocytes, suggesting a molecular basis for cellular alternans[58] and specifically implicating calcium cycling proteins in this mechanism. *These findings support the contention that calcium cycling proteins in general, and SERCA2a and RyR specifically, are key to understanding the mechanisms of cellular alternans.*

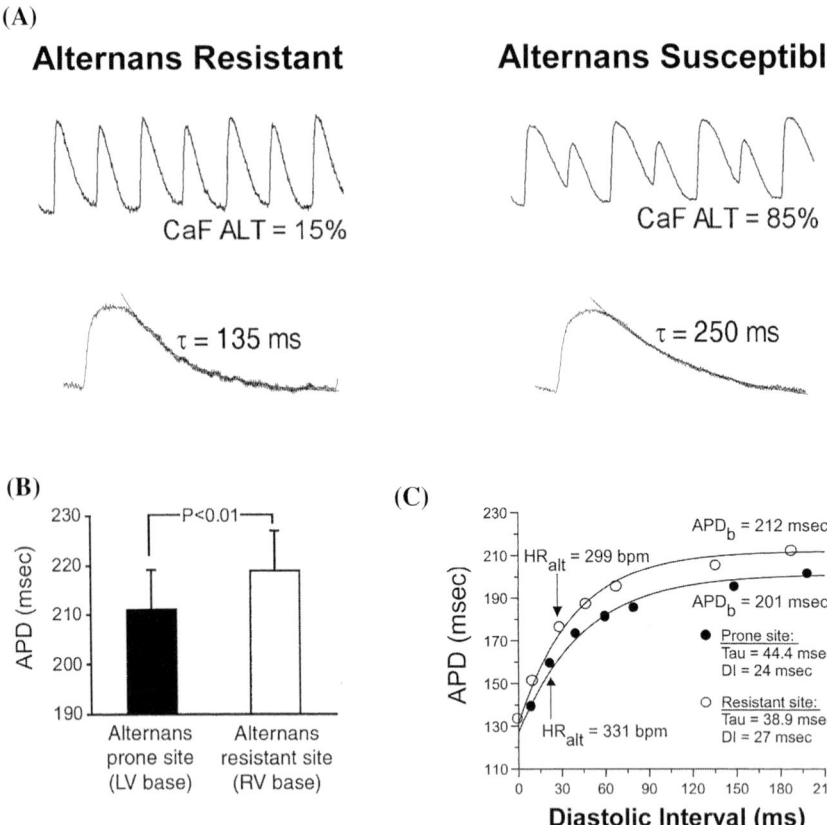

FIGURE 4. Development of calcium alternans is related to calcium handling properties of cells and not repolarization properties. Panel A. In alternans-resistant canine cells (left panel) calcium transient alternans (upper) is small and in these cells the rate of decline of the calcium transient is faster (smaller Tau, lower); however, alternans-susceptible cells (right panel), exhibit greater calcium transient alternans (upper) and have a slower rate of decline of the calcium transient, (larger Tau, lower) (from Ref. 57). Panels B and C. In guinea pig epicardium, alternans-prone cells have shorter baseline APD compared to alternans-susceptible cells and both alternans-susceptible and -resistant cells have similar restitution properties, suggesting susceptibility to alternans is not determined by cellular repolarization properties (from Ref. 35).

The advent of confocal imaging in living tissues has led to numerous exciting observations on subcellular mechanisms of alternans in normal myocytes. This review will not attempt to deal comprehensively with the many complex calcium regulatory mechanisms that are operative in cardiac myocytes. Instead, the most fundamental mechanisms ascribed to the genesis of Ca-ALT are consid-

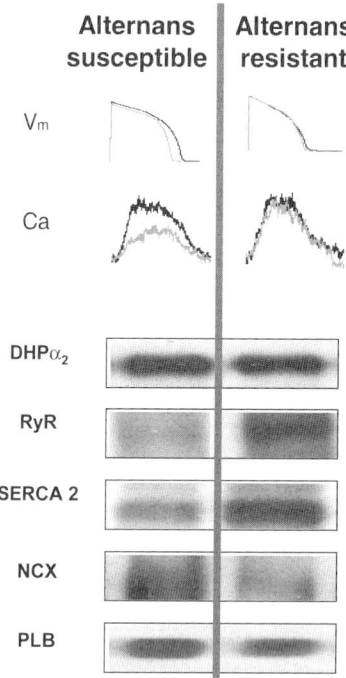

FIGURE 5. Molecular profile of alternans-susceptible versus resistant myocytes. Endocardial myocyte (left) undergoes significant V_m-ALT and Ca-ALT (black and orange traces) while under identical conditions the epicardial myocyte (right) does not. Western immunoblots show decreased RyR and SERCA2a in alternans-susceptible myocytes (from Ref. 58).

ered. With initiation of the action potential, myocyte depolarization is followed promptly by influx of calcium via I_{Ca} located in sarcolemmal protrusions into the cell termed T-tubules. T-tubules are directly adjacent to the RyR on the SR membrane, facilitating calcium binding to the RyR. RyR releases abundant SR calcium into the cytosol via the calcium-induced calcium-release mechanism.[59] Importantly, in normal myocytes calcium release is tightly regulated by SR calcium content.[60–64]

Experiments performed in normal myocytes subjected to pharmacological inhibition of either RyR or SERCA2a have demonstrated, at least conceptually, that dysfunction of either of these key calcium cycling proteins can cause Ca-ALT.[58,60,65] However, it is quite likely that the actual subcellular and molecular mechanisms for T-ALT vary, depending on which of the multitude of disease models it occurs in (long QT syndrome, ischemia, heart failure, etc.). Here we consider potential mechanisms associated with either impairment of SR calcium release or reuptake.

Subcellular Mechanisms of Ca-ALT Associated with Impaired SR Calcium Reuptake

Although there is considerable interspecies variation, approximately 70% of calcium is removed by sequestration into the SR by SERCA2a, 30% by sarcolemmal NCX, and a minor fraction by sarcolemmal calcium ATPase.[61] SERCA2a is concentrated in the longitudinal component of the SR[66] where its activity is tonically inhibited by the protein phospholamban.[67] After uptake by SERCA2a, calcium is bound to calsequestrin located primarily in the junctional SR. It is postulated that the SR is comprised of two compartments whereby calcium uptake occurs in one compartment and is then translocated to a release compartment following a brief time delay.[68] SERCA2a maintains a calcium gradient between the SR matrix and the cytosol which is close to the theoretical limit based on the free energy available from ATP hydrolysis.[69] Therefore, one would predict that elevations in heart rate could easily overcome the capability of SERCA2a, leading to alternation in calcium reuptake as subpopulations of SERCA2a fully respond on alternating beats only. To maintain homeostasis, the amount of calcium released from the SR to initiate contraction must be equaled by the amount of calcium reclaimed from the cytosol by SERCA and NCX. When SERCA2a is impaired or underexpressed, the amount of released calcium can only be fully reclaimed on an alternating beat basis, giving rise to Ca-ALT. Various compensatory mechanisms act to prevent Ca-ALT under normal circumstances. For example, as heart rate increases, cytosolic calcium rises causing activation of calcium calmodulin kinase II (CaMKII), which, in turn, phosphorylates the SERCA2a inhibitory protein phospholamban, increasing SERCA2a function, and allowing more rapid calcium removal into the SR at rapid heart rates. This mechanism is augmented when heart rate is increased by beta-sympathetic stimulation as protein kinase A signaling further releases SERCA2a from phospholamban inhibition, causing greater resistance to Ca-ALT. Interestingly, the CaMKII-mediated pathway is deficient in heart failure,[70] suggesting that in heart failure, there is an inability to compensate for increasing heart rate.

Subcellular Mechanisms of Ca-ALT Associated with Impaired SR Calcium Release

Two important mechanisms have been proposed for Ca-ALT attributable to RyR dysfunction, based on whether Ca-ALT, due to RyR dysfunction, is associated with alternating SR calcium content or is not.[65] Using metabolic inhibition in cat atrial and ventricular myocytes to inhibit RyR phosphorylation, Huser et al.[65] reported Ca-ALT without beat-to-beat fluctuations in SR content, suggesting that refractory-like properties of RyR can produce alternating open probabilities of the channel irrespective of SR calcium load. Of course, the relevance of this experimental model of Ca-ALT to heart failure

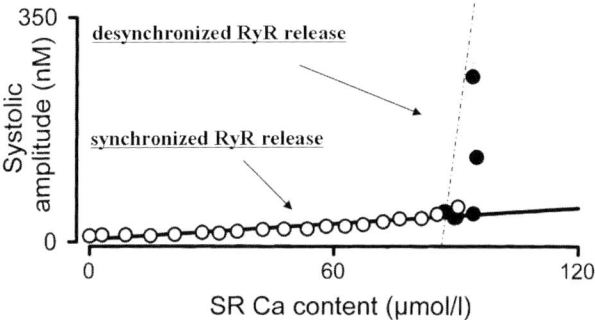

FIGURE 6. Under conditions of desynchronized calcium release, the relationship between SR calcium content and release becomes markedly steepened. Under these conditions, small perturbations in SR calcium load cause large fluctuations in release causing alternans dynamics (adapted from Ref. 60).

is questionable. Recently, Diaz et al.[60] used an innovative, albeit nonphysiological, stimulation protocol to induce Ca-ALT without pharmacological inhibition of RyR (thereby avoiding nonselective drug effects). Ventricular myocytes were repetitively voltage-clamped just at the minimum activation voltage for I_{Ca}. The resulting weak calcium-induced calcium release produced desynchronized RyR release, which dramatically steepened the relationship (feedback gain) between SR calcium content (i.e., luminal calcium) and the subsequent SR calcium release (FIG. 6). These subcellular conditions highly favored the development of Ca-ALT dynamics, as a small transient increase in luminal SR calcium produced relatively large RyR release, leading to depletion of SR calcium, and a small calcium release on the subsequent beat, leading to restoration of SR calcium, and a large RyR release, as the alternating pattern continued. Under these circumstances, Ca-ALT is associated with beat-to-beat alternation of SR calcium content. Importantly, these findings strongly suggested that conditions that produce desynchronized RyR release can lead to Ca-ALT.

The aforementioned mechanisms are obviously not mutually exclusive. As SR calcium release and reuptake processes are tightly coupled and share many regulatory mechanisms, their effects on Ca-ALT may not be independent. In fact, their effects are likely to be synergistic because reduced SERCA2a function will: (*a*) increase cytosolic calcium which will inactivate I_{Ca} and attenuate RyR release, and (*b*) reduce SR calcium, thereby reducing calsequestrin binding to RyR and impairing RyR release.

Electrogenic Mechanisms for Transducing Ca-ALT to V_m-ALT

It is important to understand how Ca-ALT is gives rise to V_m-ALT, because V_m-ALT is the mechanism of arrhythmogenesis. There are two important electrogenic feedback mechanisms by which Ca-ALT may be transduced to V_m-ALT: (*a*) SR calcium release enhances inactivation of sarcolemmal I_{Ca}, shown as negative feedback because it results in lowering membrane voltage (shortening APD), and (*b*) SR calcium release enhances calcium extrusion by NCX, shown as positive feedback because it increases membrane voltage (lengthens APD because electrogenic NCX drives three sodium into the cell for every one calcium extruded). Also, I_{to} and I_{Ks} are calcium-dependent ion channels which can modulate V_m in response to changing calcium. All these mechanisms are not mutually exclusive. We hypothesize that alternating activity of NCX is the most likely electrogenic mechanism for V_m-ALT based on our dual V_m-calcium-imaging experiments, which have consistently revealed similar phase of Ca-ALT and V_m-ALT (i.e., the APD prolonging beat of alternans is associated with a large SR calcium release, while APD shortening is associated with small calcium release). The opposite would be expected if I_{Ca}, I_{Ks}, or I_{to}, were the electrogenic mechanism.

IMPAIRED CALCIUM CYCLING AND ALTERNANS IN HEART FAILURE

Heart failure is associated with multiple pathophysiological changes which can influence electrophysiological properties of the heart. In addition to remodeling numerous ion channels,[11,71–73] heart failure alters the extracellular matrix,[71,74,75] intercellular gap junctions,[71,73,74] and neurohumoral reflexes.[76–78] Heart failure is associated with slow conduction attributable to remodeling of both extracellular matrix and gap junctions.[71,73] Prolongation of cardiac repolarization[11] is another hallmark of heart failure, but the causative ionic mechanisms are controversial. However, the most fundamental abnormality in heart failure is impaired calcium cycling. As the mechanism of cardiac alternans in normal myocytes is related to impaired calcium cycling, it is likely that heart failure myoctes are especially susceptible to alternans. Interestingly, more than a century ago, Traube described pulsus alternans in patients with severe heart failure, recognizing a fundamental relationship between Ca-ALT and heart failure.[12] Recently, we demonstrated experimentally that heart failure increases susceptibility to alternans (FIG. 7).[79] Transmural optical mapping ($n = 7$) was performed in wedges of myocardium from normal dogs and dogs in which heart failure was induced by rapid pacing.[71] Heart failure hearts demonstrated markedly increased susceptibility to V_m-ALT from epicardial, midmyocardial, and endocardial myocytes. FIGURE 7 (panel A) illustrates the leftward shift in V_m-ALT to cycle length relationship of midmyocardial cells, indicating greater susceptibility to V_m-ALT in heart failure.

Particular heart failure-induced changes that are directly responsible for contractile dysfunction are consistently observed in experimental and human heart failure. These include reduced expression and altered regulation of SERCA2a

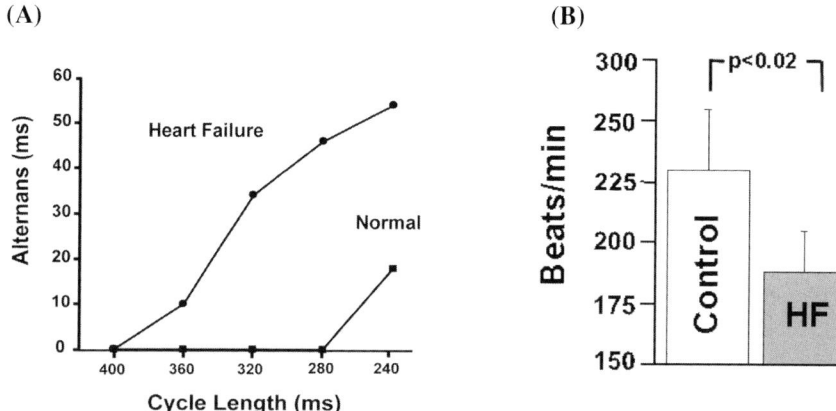

FIGURE 7. Panel A. Cycle length dependence of V_m-ALT recorded from midmyocardial cells using transmural optical mapping in normal and heart failure canine wedge preparation. Heart failure produced a profound leftward shift in V_m-ALT to cycle length relationship, demonstrating that heart failure myocytes have greater susceptibility to alternans. Panel B summarizes heart rate threshold for V_m- ALT ($n = 7$) (from Ref. 79).

and RyR and increased expression of electrogenic NCX. It is reasonable to hypothesize that changes in some of these calcium cycling proteins may critically effect alternans and, therefore, electrophysiological stability of the failing heart. It is abundantly clear that heart failure is associated with significant blunting of SR calcium reuptake, caused by reduced SERCA2 expression.[11,80–82] Expression of the SERCA2a regulatory protein phospholamban is also diminished.[83–85] Heart failure causes decreased SR calcium content due to both decreased SERCA2a function and expression as well as increased NCX expression, both leading to less cytosolic calcium being taken up into the SR.[85,86] In addition, faster stimulation rates result in decreased SR calcium uptake in heart failure versus normal hearts, indicating a decreased ability for calcium cycling to keep up with increasing heart rates.[87] Therefore, it is likely that diminished SERCA2a function increases susceptibility to Ca-ALT in failing myocytes. In heart failure, abnormal excitation-contraction coupling is manifest by impaired calcium release from RyR during calcium-induced calcium release. Heart failure directly and indirectly disrupts normal function of RyR.[88–95] As in normal myocytes, it is also likely that heart failure-induced abnormalities of RyR expression or function can also increase susceptibility to Ca-ALT in heart failure. In addition, upregulation of NCX is almost uniformly reported in human and animal models of heart failure.[11,96] In heart failure, increased NCX may be a compensatory response to decreased SERCA2a expression in order to extrude calcium and improve diastolic function.[97] Because NCX is upregulated in heart failure, it is possible that there is also enhanced electrogenic "gain" (i.e., any given amount of Ca-ALT will produce greater

V_m-ALT), providing an additional mechanism for enhanced susceptibility to V_m-ALT in heart failure.

SUMMARY

Over the past 10 years, there is increasing recognition that subtle beat-to-beat alternation of cardiac repolarization, manifested clinically as T-ALT,[18] is a highly sensitive marker of susceptibility to SCD. Remarkably, in the absence of T-ALT, patients with heart failure exhibit resistance to SCD.[4] Importantly, although ventricular dysfunction is clearly related to the development of SCD, the mechanisms relating mechanical dysfunction to electrical dysfunction and arrhythmogenesis remain to be elucidated. We have recently discovered that alternans of cellular repolarization is linked to a mechanism of arrhythmogenesis in normal hearts, where spatially discordant alternans between myocytes amplify repolarization gradients to produce conduction block and reentrant excitation.[30] Cellular alternans has been determined by us[24,30,31,36] and others[17,55,98] to be a consistent precursor to cardiac fibrillation in the mammalian heart. We propose cellular alternans as a key mechanism linking calcium cycling proteins with susceptibility to arrhythmias. Although it has yet to be demonstrated that repolarization alternans links electrical and mechanical dysfunction, several lines of evidence from studies in normal hearts suggest a link between the abnormal function and expression of calcium cycling proteins which characterize ventricular mechanical dysfunction, and abnormalities in calcium cycling that are responsible for alternans. In normal myocardium, cells which exhibit the slowest calcium cycling are most prone to alternans and a decreased expression of key calcium cycling proteins is observed in these cells. Heart failure causes: (*a*) reduced SERCA2a expression and impaired SR calcium reuptake[11] and (*b*) impaired RyR function and abnormal SR calcium release.[88,97,99] Both of these perturbations have been implicated as mechanisms of alternans in nonfailing myocytes.[58] However, essentially all previous research on alternans has focused on normal hearts, rather than heart failure, and hence the role of cellular alternans in the most common setting for SCD, that is, heart failure, is unknown. Therefore, much has to be done to determine the link between mechanical and electrical dysfunction in the heart and the subceullar mechanisms establishing the relationship.

ACKNOWLEDGMENTS

This work was supported by a grant from the National Institutes of Health No. RO1- HL54807 (DSR) and a grant from the Emergency Medicine Foundation (LW).

REFERENCES

1. COHN, J., D. ARCHIBALD, S. ZIESCHE, et al. 1986. Effect of vasodilator therapy on mortality in chronic congestive heart failure: results of a Veterans Administration cooperative study. N. Engl. J. Med. **314:** 1547–1552.
2. ZIPES, D.P. & H.J.J. WELLENS. 1998. Sudden cardiac death. Circulation. **98:** 2334–2351.
3. MYERBURG, R.J., K.M. KESSLER & A. CASTELLANOS. 1992. Sudden cardiac death: structure, function, and time-dependence of risk. Circulation **85**(1 Suppl): I2–10.
4. BLOOMFIELD, D.M., R.C. STEINMAN, P.B. NAMEROW, et al. 2004. Microvolt T-wave alternans distinguishes between patients likely and patients not likely to benefit from implanted cardiac defibrillator therapy: a solution to the Multicenter Automatic Defibrillator Implantation Trial (MADIT) II conundrum. Circulation **110:** 1885–1889.
5. MOSS, A.J., W.J. HALL, D.S. CANNOM, et al. 1996. For the MADIT Investigators: improved survival with an implanted defibrillator in patients with prior myocardial infarction, low ejection fraction, and asymptomatic non-susatined ventricular tachycardia. The Multicenter Automatic Defibrillator Trial (MADIT). N. Engl. J. Med. **335:** 1933–1940.
6. PRYSTOWSKY, E.N. & S. NISAM. 2000. Prophylactic implantable cardioverter defibrillator trials: MUSTT, MADIT, and beyond. Am. J. Cardiol. **86:** 1214–1215.
7. PRIORI S.G., P.J. SCHWARTZ, G.H. BARDY, et al. 1997. Survivors of out-of-hospital cardiac arrest with apparently normal heart—need for definition and standardized clinical evaluation. Circulation **95:** 265–272.
8. BIGGER, J.T. JR., W. WHANG, J.N. ROTTMAN, et al. 1999. Mechanisms of death in the CABG Patch trial—a randomized trial of implantable cardiac defibrillator prophylaxis in patients at high risk of death after coronary artery bypass graft surgery. Circulation **99:** 1416–1421.
9. SOLOMON, S.D., S. ZELENKOFSKE, J.J. MCMURRAY, et al. 2005. Sudden death in patients with myocardial infarction and left ventricular dysfunction, heart failure, or both. N. Engl. J. Med. **352:** 2581–2588.
10. BARDY, G.H., K.L. LEE, D.B. MARK, et al. 2005. Clapp-Channing N, Davidson-Ray LD, Fraulo ES, Fishbein DP, Luceri RM, Ip JH: amiodarone or an implantable cardioverter-defibrillator for congestive heart failure. N. Engl. J. Med. **352:** 225–237.
11. TOMASELLI, G.F. & E. MARBÁN. 1999. Electrophysiological remodeling in hypertrophy and heart failure. Cardiovasc Res. **42:** 270–283.
12. TRAUBE, L. 1872. Ein Fall von Pulsus Bigeminus nebst Bemerkungen uber die Leberschwellungen bei Klappenfehlern und uber acute Leberatrophie. Berlin Klin Wochenschr **9:** 185–188.
13. MARTÍNEZ, J.M., R.R. PAPPALARDO, E.S. MARCOS, et al. 1998. Dynamics of a highly charged ion in aqueous solutions: MD simulations of dilute $CrCl_3$ aqueous solutions using interaction potentials based on the hydrated ion concept. J. Phys. Chem. B. **102:** 3272–3282.
14. VERRIER, R.L. & B.D. NEARING. 1994. Electrophysiologic basis for T wave alternans as an index of vulnerability to ventricular fibrillation. J. Cardiovasc. Electrophysiol. **5:** 445–461.
15. EULER, D.E. 1999. Cardiac alternans: mechanisms and pathophysiological significance. Cardiovasc. Res. **42:** 583–590.

16. ECHEBARRIA, B. & A. KARMA. 2002. Instability and spatiotemporal dynamics of alternans in paced cardiac tissue. Phys. Rev. Lett. **88:** 208101-1–208101-4.
17. WATANABE, M.A., F.H. FENTON, S. EVANS, et al. 2001. Mechanisms for discordant alternans. J. Cardiovasc. Electrophysiol. **12:** 196–206.
18. ROSENBAUM, D.S., L.E. JACKSON, J.M. SMITH, et al. 1994. Electrical alternans and vulnerability to ventricular arrhythmias. N. Eng. J. Med. **330:** 235–241.
19. VERRIER, R.L., B.D. NEARING, M.T. LA ROVERE, et al. 2003. Ambulatory electrocardiogram-based tracking of T wave alternans in postmyocardial infarction patients to assess risk of cardiac arrest or arrhythmic death. J. Cardiovasc. Electrophysiol. **14:** 705–711.
20. HOHNLOSER, S.H., T. IKEDA, D.M. BLOOMFIELD, et al. 2003. T-wave alternans negative coronary patients with low ejection and benefit from defibrillator implantation. Lancet **362:** 125–126.
21. HOHNLOSER, S.H., T. KLINGENHEBEN, D. BLOOMFIELD, et al. 2003. Usefulness of microvolt T-wave alternans for prediction of ventricular tachyarrhythmic events in patients with dilated cardiomyopathy: results from a prospective observational study. J. Am. Col. Cardiol. **41:** 2220–2224.
22. HOHNLOSER, S.H., T. KLINGENHEBEN, M. ZABEL, et al. 1997. T wave alternans during exercise and atrial pacing in humans. J. Cardiovasc. Electrophysiol **8:** 987–993.
23. IKEDA, T., H. SAITO, K. TANNO, et al. 2002. T-wave alternans as a predictor for sudden cardiac death after myocardial infarction. Am. J. Cardiol. **89:** 79–82.
24. WALKER, M.L. & D.S. ROSENBAUM. 2003. Repolarization alternans: implications for the mechanism and prevention of sudden cardiac death. Cardiovasc. Res. **57:** 599–614.
25. HOHNLOSER, S.H., T. KLINGENHEBEN, Y.G. LI, et al. 1998. T wave alternans as a predictor of recurrent ventricular tachyarrhythmias in ICD recipients: prospective comparison with conventional risk markers. J. Cardiovasc. Electrophysiol. **9:** 1258–1268.
26. HOHNLOSER, S. & R.J. COHEN. 1999. T wave alternans and left ventricular ejection fraction, but not QT variability index, predict appropriate ICD discharge. J. Cardiovasc. Electrophysiol. **10:** 626–626.
27. HOHNLOSER, S.H. Macroscopic T wave alternans as a harbinger of sudden death. J. Cardiovasc. Electrophysiol.**10:** 625–625.
28. KLINGENHEBEN, T., M. ZABEL, R.B. D'AGOSTINO, et al. 2000. Predictive value of T-wave alternans for arrhythmic events in patients with congestive heart failure. Lancet **356:** 651–652.
29. KAUFMAN, E.S., J.A. MACKALL, B. JULKA, et al. 2000. Influence of heart rate and sympathetic stimulation on arrhythmogenic T wave alternans. Am. J. Physiol. Heart Circ. Physiol. **279:** H1248-H1255.
30. PASTORE, J.M., S.D. GIROUARD, K.R. LAURITA, et al. 2000. Mechanism linking T-wave alternans to the genesis of cardiac fibrillation. Circulation **99:** 1385–1394.
31. PASTORE, J.M. & D.S. ROSENBAUM. 2000. Role of structural barriers in the mechanism of alternans-induced reentry. Circ. Res. **87:** 1157–1163.
32. BERS, D. 2001. Excitation-contraction coupling and cardiac contractile force. *In* Cardiac Inotrophy and Ca Mismanagement. D.M., Bers, Ed.: 273–331. Kluwer Academic Publishers. Dordrecht.
33. EL-SHERIF, N., E.B. CAREF, H. YIN, et al. 1996. The electrophysiological mechanism of ventricular arrhythmias in the long QT syndrome—tridimensional mapping of activation and recovery patterns. Circ. Res. **79:** 474–492.

34. CHINUSHI, M., D. KOZHEVNIKOV, et al. 2003. Mechanism of discordant T wave alternans in the in vivo heart. J. Cardiovasc. Electrophysiol. **14:** 632–638.
35. PRUVOT, E.J., R.P. KATRA, D.S. ROSENBAUM, et al. 2004. Role of calcium cycling versus restitution in the mechanism of repolarization alternans. Circ. Res. **94:** 1083–1090.
36. WALKER, M.L., X. WAN, G.E. KIRSCH, et al. 2003. Hysteresis effect implicates calcium cycling as a mechanism of repolarization alternans. Circulation **108:** 2704–2709.
37. ZHAO, Z. & S.A. RIVKEES. 2000. Programmed cell death in the developing heart: regulation by BMP4 and FGF2. Dev. Dyn. **217:** 388–400.
38. LUKAS, A. & C. ANTZELEVITCH. 1993. Differences in the electrophysiological response of canine ventricular epicardium and endocardium to ischemia: role of the transient outward current. Circulation **88:** 2903–2915.
39. KONTA, T., K. IKEDA, M. YAMAKI, et al. 1990. Significance of discordant ST alternans in ventricular fibrillation. Circulation **82:** 2185–2189.
40. LUO, C. & Y. RUDY. 1991. A model of the ventricular cardiac action potential: depolarization, repolarization, and their interaction. Circ. Res. **68:** 1501–1526.
41. DAVEY, P., S. BRYANT & G. HART. 2001. Rate-dependent electrical, contractile and restitution properties of isolated left ventricular myocytes in guinea-pig hypertrophy. Acta Physiol. Scand. **171:** 17–28.
42. HIRAYAMA, Y., H. SAITOH, H. ATARASHI, et al. 1993. Electrical and mechanical alternans in canine myocardium in vivo: dependence on intracellular calcium cycling. Circulation **88:** 2894–2902.
43. LAB, M.J. & J.A. LEE. 1990. Changes in intracellular calcium during mechanical alternans in isolated ferret ventricular muscle. Circ. Res. **66:** 585–595.
44. LEE, H.C., R. MOHABIR, N. SMITH, et al. 1988. Effect of ischemia on calcium-dependent fluorescence transients in rabbit hearts containing Indo-1: correlation with monophasic action potentials and contraction. Circulation **78:** 1047–1059.
45. SAITOH, H., J. BAILEY & B. SURAWICZ. 1988. Alternans of action potential duration after abrupt shortening of cycle length: differences between dog purkinje and ventricular muscle fibers. Circ. Res. **62:** 1027–1040.
46. SAITOH, H., J. BAILEY & B. SURAWICZ. 1989. Action potential duration alternans in dog purkinje and ventricular muscle fibers. Circulation **80:** 1421–1431.
47. SPENCER, C.I., S.E.J.N. MÖRNER, M.I.M. NOBLE, et al. 1993. Effects of nifedipine and low [Ca^{2+}] on mechanical restitution during hypothermia in guinea pig papillary muscles. Basic Res. Cardiol. **88:** 111–119.
48. MILLER, W.L., F.A. SGURA, et al. 2001. Characteristics of presenting electrocardiograms of acute myocardial infarction from a community-based population predict short- and long-term mortality. Am. J. Cardiol. **87:** 1045–1050.
49. LAURITA, K.R., A. SINGAL, J.M. PASTORE, et al. 1988. Spatial heterogeneity of calcium transients may explain action potential dispersion during T-wave alternans [abstract]. Circulation **98**(Suppl I): I-187.
50. HIRATA, Y., I. KODAMA, et al. 1979. Effects of verapamil on canine Purkinje fibers and ventricular muscle fibers with particular reference to the alternation of action potential duration after a sudden increase in driving rate. Cardiovasc. Res. **13:** 1–8.
51. CHUDIN, E., J.I. GOLDHABER, J. WEISS, et al. 1999. Intracellular Ca2 dynamics and the stability of ventricular tachycardia. Biophys. J. **77:** 2930–2941.
52. RASHBA, E.J., A.F. OSMAN, et al. 2002. Influence of QRS duration on the prognostic value of T wave alternans. J. Cardiovasc. Electrophysiol. **13:** 770–775.

53. GARFINKEL, A., Y.H. KIM, et al. 2000. Preventing ventricular fibrillation by flattening cardiac restitution. Proc. Natl. Acad. Sci. USA **97:** 6061–6066.
54. DONAHUE, J.K. 2004. Gene therapy for cardiac arrhythmias. Ann. N. Y. Acad. Sci. **1015:** 332–337.
55. QU, Z., A. GARFINKEL, P. CHEN, et al. 2000. Mechanisms of discordant alternans and induction of reentry in simulated cardiac tissue. Circulation **102:** 1664–1670.
56. RICCIO, M.L., M.L. KOLLER & R.F. GILMOUR. 1999. Electrical restitution and spatiotemporal organization during ventricular fibrillation. Circ. Res. **84:** 955–963.
57. LAURITA, K.R., R. KATRA, B. WIBLE, et al. 2003. Transmural heterogeneity of calcium handling in canine. Circ. Res. **92:** 668–675.
58. WAN, X., K.R. LAURITA, E. PRUVOT, et al. 2005. Molecular correlates of repolarization alternans in cardiac myocytes. J. Mol. Cell. Cardiol. **39:** 419–428.
59. MEISSNER, G. 1994. Ryanodine receptor/Ca^{2+} release channels and their regulation by endogenous effectors. Annu. Rev. Physiol. **56:** 485–508.
60. DIAZ, M.E., S.C. O'NEILL & D.A. EISNER. 2004. Sarcoplasmic reticulum calcium content fluctuation is the key to cardiac alternans. Circ. Res. **94:** 650–656.
61. BASSANI, J.W., W. YUAN & D.M. BERS. 1995. Fractional SR Ca release is regulated by trigger Ca and SR Ca content in cardiac myocytes. Am. J. Physiol. **268:** C1313–C1319.
62. LUKYANENKO, V., I. GYÖRKE & S. GYÖRKE. 1996. Regulation of calcium release by calcium inside the sarcoplasmic reticulum in ventricular myocytes. Pflugers Arch. **432:** 1047–1054.
63. BERS, D.M., L. LI, H. SATOH, E. MCCALL, et al. 1998. Factors that control sarcoplasmic reticulum calcium release in intact ventricular myocytes. Ann. N. Y. Acad. Sci. **853:** 157–177.
64. TERENTYEV, D., S. VIATCHENKO-KARPINSKI, et al. 2002. Luminal Ca^{2+} controls termination and refractory behavior of Ca^{2+}-induced Ca^{2+} release in cardiac myocytes. Circ. Res. **91:** 414–420.
65. HUSER, J., Y.G. WANG, et al. 2000. Functional coupling between glycolysis and excitation-contraction coupling underlies alternans in cat heart cells. J. Physiol. (Lond.) **524:** 795–806.
66. JORGENSEN, A.O., A.C. SHEN, P. DALY, et al. 1982. Localization of Ca^{2+}-Mg^{2+}-ATPase of the sarcoplasmic reticulum in adult rat papillary muscle. J. Cell. Biol. **93:** 883–892.
67. RAVENS, U. & D. DOBREV. 2000. Regulation of sarcoplasmic reticulum Ca^{2+}-ATPase and phospholamban in the failing and nonfailing heart. Cardiovasc. Res. **45:** 245–252.
68. WIER, W.G. & D.T. YUE. 1986. Intracellular calcium transients underlying the short-term force-interval relationship in ferret ventricular myocardium. J. Physiol. (Lond.) **376:** 507–530.
69. CHEN, W., C. STEENBERGEN, L.A. LEVY, et al. 1996. Measurement of free Ca^{2+} in sarcoplasmic reticulum in perfused rabbit heart loaded with 1,2-bis(2-amino-5,6-difluorophenoxy)ethane-N,N,N',N'-tetraacetic acid by 19 F NMR. J. Biol. Chem. **271:** 7398–7403.
70. WEHRENS, X.H., S.E. LEHNART, S.R. REIKEN, et al. 2004. Ca^{2+}/calmodulin-dependent protein kinase II phosphorylation regulates the cardiac ryanodine receptor. Circ. Res. **94:** e61–e70.

71. AKAR, F.G., D.D. SPRAGG, R.S. TUNIN, et al. 2004. Mechanisms underlying conduction slowing and arrhythmogenesis in nonischemic dilated cardiomyopathy. Circ. Res. **95:** 717–725.
72. PAK, P.H., H.B. NUSS, R.S. TUNIN, et al. 1997. Repolarization abnormalities, arrhythmia and sudden death in canine tachycardia-induced cardiomyopathy. J. Am. Coll. Cardiol. **30:** 576–584.
73. AKAR, F.G., R.C. WU, G.J. JUANG, et al. 2005. Molecular mechanisms underlying potassium current down-regulation in canine tachycardia-induced heart failure. Am. J. Physiol. Heart Circ. Physiol. **288:** H2887–H2896.
74. KOSTIN, S., M. RIEGER, S. DAMMER, et al. 2003. Gap junction remodeling and altered connexin43 expression in the failing human heart. Mol. Cell. Biochem. **242:** 135–144.
75. HELING, A., R. ZIMMERMANN, S. KOSTIN, et al. 2000. Increased expression of cytoskeletal, linkage, and extracellular proteins in failing human myocardium. Circ. Res. **86:** 846–853.
76. ATHERTON, J.J., H.L. THOMSON, T.D. MOORE, et al. 1997. Diastolic ventricular interaction—a possible mechanism for abnormal vascular responses during volume unloading in heart failure. Circulation **96:** 4273–4279.
77. THAMES, M.D., T. KINUGAWA & M.E. DIBNER-DUNLAP. 1993. Reflex sympathoexcitation by cardiac sympathetic afferents during myocardial ischemia: role of adenosine. Circulation **87:** 1698–1704.
78. DIBNER-DUNLAP, M.E. & M.D. THAMES. 1992. Control of sympathetic nerve activity by vagal mechanoreflexes is blunted in heart failure. Circulation **86:** 1929–1934.
79. WILSON, L.D., D. JEYARAJ, K.R. LAURITA, et al. 2004. Spatially discordant cellular alternans as a novel mechanism of arrhythmogenesis in heart failure [abstract]. Circulation **110**(Suppl.): III-98.
80. DAVIES, C.H., K. DAVIA, J.G. BENNETT, et al. 1995. Reduced contraction and altered frequency response of isolated ventricular myocytes from patients with heart failure. Circulation **92:** 2540–2549.
81. KIHARA, Y., J.P. MORGAN, et al. 1991. Abnormal Ca_i^{2+} handling is the primary cause of mechanical alternans: study in ferret ventricular muscles. Am. J. Physiol. **261:** H1746–H1755.
82. DE LA BASTIE, D., D. LEVITSKY, L. RAPPAPORT, et al. 1990. Function of the sarcoplasmic reticulum and expression of it's Ca2 (+)-ATPase gene in pressure overload-induced cardiac hypertrophy in the rat. Circ. Res. **66:** 554–564.
83. STUDER, R., H. REINECKE, J. BILGER, et al. 1994. Gene expression of the cardiac Na-Ca exchanger in end-stage human heart failure. Circ. Res. **75:** 443–453.
84. FLESCH, M., R.H.G. SCHWINGER, F. SCHIFFER, et al. 1996. Evidence for functional relevance of an enhanced expression of the Na^+-Ca^{2+} exchanger in failing human myocardium. Circulation **94:** 992–1002.
85. SCHWINGER, R.H.G., M. BÖHM, U. SCHMIDT, et al. 1995. Unchanged protein levels of SERCA II and phospholamban but reduced Ca^{2+} uptake and Ca^{2+}-ATPase activity of cardiac sarcoplasmic reticulum from dilated cardiomyopathy patients compared with patients with nonfailing hearts. Circulation **92:** 3220–3228.
86. SHANNON, T.R., S.M. POGWIZD & D.M. BERS. 2003. Elevated sarcoplasmic reticulum Ca^{2+} leak in intact ventricular myocytes from rabbits in heart failure. Circ. Res. **93:** 592–594.

87. PIESKE, B., B. KRETSCHMANN, M. MEYER, et al. 1995. Alterations in intracellular calcium handling associated with the inverse force-frequency relation in human dilated cardiomyopathy. Circulation **92:** 1169–1178.
88. MARX, S.O., S. REIKEN, Y. HISAMATSU, et al. 2000. PKA phosphorylation dissociates FKBP12.6 from the calcium release channel (ryanodine receptor): defective regulation in failing hearts. Cell **101:** 365–376.
89. YANO, M., K. ONO, T. OHKUSA, et al. 2000. Altered stoichiometry of FKBP12.6 versus ryanodine receptor as a cause of abnormal Ca^{2+} leak through ryanodine receptor in heart failure. Circulation **102:** 2131–2136.
90. ZHAO, L., A. SEBKHI, D.J.R. NUNEZ, et al. 2001. Right ventricular hypertrophy secondary to pulmonary hypertension is linked to rat chromosome 17—evaluation of cardiac ryanodine Ryr2 receptor as a candidate. Circulation **103:** 442–447.
91. MARKS, A.R. 2003. A guide for the perplexed—towards an understanding of the molecular basis of heart failure. Circulation **107:** I456–I459.
92. MARKS, A.R. 2000. Cardiac intracellular calcium release channels—role in heart failure. Circ. Res. **87:** 8–11.
93. WEHRENS, X.H.T., S.E. LEHNART, F. HUANG, et al. 2003. FKBP12.6 deficiency and defective calcium release channel (ryanodine receptor) function linked to exercise-induced sudden cardiac death. Cell **113:** 829–840.
94. O'ROURKE, B., D.A. KASS, G.F. TOMASELLI, et al. 1999. Mechanisms of altered excitation-contraction coupling in canine tachycardia-induced heart failure, I—experimental studies. Circ. Res. **84:** 562–570.
95. HASENFUSS, G., W. SCHILLINGER, S.E. LEHNART, et al. 1999. Relationship between Na^+-Ca^{2+}-exchanger protein levels and diastolic function of failing human myocardium. Circulation **99:** 641–648.
96. HASENFUSS, G. 1998. Alterations of calcium-regulatory proteins in heart failure. Cardiovasc. Res. **37:** 279–289.
97. HOBAI, I.A. & B. O'ROURKE. 2000. Enhanced Ca(2+)-activated Na(+)-Ca(2+) exchange activity in canine pacing-induced heart failure. Circ. Res. **87:** 690–698.
98. WATANABE, M., N.F. OTANI & R.F. GILMOUR. 1995. Biphasic restitution of action potential duration and complex dynamics in ventricular myocardium. Circ. Res. **76:** 915–921.
99. LEHNART, S.E., X.H. WEHRENS, S. REIKEN, et al. 2005. Phosphodiesterase 4D deficiency in the ryanodine-receptor complex promotes heart failure and arrhythmias. Cell **123:** 25–35.

The Mechanoelectric Feedback: A Novel "Calcium Clamp" Method, Using Tetanic Contraction, for Testing the Role of the Intracellular Free Calcium

YAEL YANIV, CARMIT LEVY, AND AMIR LANDESBERG

Department of Biomedical Engineering, Technion, Israel Institute of Technology, Haifa 32000, Israel

ABSTRACT: Mechanical perturbations affect the membrane action potential, a phenomenon denoted as the mechanoelectric feedback (MEF), and may elicit cardiac arrhythmias. Two plausible mechanisms were suggested to explain this phenomenon: (i) stretch-activated channels (SACs) within the cell membrane and (ii) modulation of the action potential by the intracellular Ca^{2+} (the Calcium hypothesis). The intracellular Ca^{2+} varies mainly due to the effects of the mechanical perturbations on the affinity of troponin for calcium. The present study concentrates on the unique experimental methods that allow differentiating between the effects of SAC and Ca^{2+} on the action potential. This is achieved by controlling the sarcomere lengths (SLs) independently of the intracellular Ca^{2+} concentration, in the intact fiber. A dedicated experimental setup allowed simultaneous measurements of the membrane potential and the mechanical performance (Force and SL). The action potential was measured by voltage-sensitive dye (Di-4-ANEPPS). The SL was measured by laser diffraction technique and was controlled by a fast servomotor. The intracellular Ca^{2+} was controlled (calcium clamp) by imposing stable tetanic contractions at various extracellular calcium concentrations ($[Ca^{2+}]_0$s). Tetanus was obtained by 8 Hz stimulation in the presence of cyclopiazonic acid (CPA) (30 μM). Isolated trabeculae from a rat's right ventricle were studied at different SLs and $[Ca^{2+}]_0$s. The experimental data strongly support the calcium hypothesis. Although the action potential duration (APD) decreases at longer SL, the $[Ca^{2+}]_0$ has a significantly larger effect on the APD. The APD decreases as the $[Ca^{2+}]_0$ increases. Understanding the underlying mechanism opens new research avenues for the development of therapeutic modalities for cardiac arrhythmias.

KEYWORDS: excitation-contraction coupling; calcium; membrane potential; arrhythmia; action potential duration; delayed after depolarization; sudden death; cooperativity; sarcomere

Address for correspondence: Prof. Amir Landesberg, M.D., Ph.D., Department of Biomedical Engineering, Technion, IIT, Haifa 32000, Israel. Voice: 972-4-829-4143; fax: 972-4-829-4599.
 e-mail: amir@bm.technion.ac.il

INTRODUCTION

The Mechanoelectric Feedback

Cardiac arrhythmia is one of the leading causes of death in the Western world. Each year about 300,000 people in the United States suffer from sudden death.[1] Sudden death commonly occurs due to the existence of some underlying structural abnormalities.[2] The predominant structural abnormality is attributed to coronary artery disease.[2] Other leading structural and function abnormalities that cause sudden death are myocardial hypertrophy and heart failure. The precise underlying mechanisms that elicit the lethal arrhythmias remain unclear.

There exists significant clinical and experimental evidence that mechanical perturbations and mechanical inhomogeneity play a significant role in the development of cardiac arrhythmia. It is striking that there is a tight correlation between the prevalence of sudden death and the severity of the myocardial mechanical dysfunction.[3] The prevalence of lethal arrhythmias is extremely high in patients with chronic heart failure, and about 50% of these patients die from arrhythmia.[2] Mechanical loading conditions affect the myocyte action potential, leading to changes in repolarization that affect the QT interval and the T wave amplitude.[4] An increase in the afterload is associated with a smaller action potential duration (APD) and a smaller T wave. The effect of the mechanical perturbation on the action potential depends on the time onset of perturbation. A larger effect is observed at mid contraction, and the effect diminishes when the perturbations are imposed earlier or later during the twitch.[4] These phenomena were related to the existence of a "Mechanoelectric Feedback" (MEF) in the cardiac myocytes.[4,5]

Great efforts are directed to explore the membrane function. The prevailing explanation suggests the existence of stretch-activated channels (SAC) within the membrane, whereby stretch increases the open probability of these channels.[6,7] However, there is evidence that strongly suggests that the intracellular control of excitation-contraction coupling, and specifically the free calcium, play key roles in mediating the MEF (Calcium hypothesis). The evidence is based on the effects of changes in the intracellular control of excitation-contraction coupling on the membrane potential. Nonuniformity in the intracellular control of contraction, even without any structural damage, can produce Ca^{2+} waves and delayed after depolarization.[8–10] ter Keurs *et al.*[10] generated reversible inhomogeneity in a restricted segment (300 μm) along the trabeculae by exposing this segment to different solutions using a glass pipette. The jet from the pipette affected the small segment without damaging the trabeculae. Four different solutions were used: (i) standard HEPES solution as in the adjacent "normal" segments; (ii) caffeine that opens the SR ryanodine channels and depletes the SR; (iii) 2,3-butanedione monoxime (BDM) that inhibits crossbridge (XB) cycling; and (iv) low extracellular Ca^{2+} ($[Ca^{2+}]_0 = 0.2$ mM) that reduces the SR Ca^{2+} content. Application of BDM, caffeine, or low $[Ca^{2+}]_o$ through the pipette on the segment produced striking mechanical inhomogeneity. Interestingly, Ca waves appeared in all three cases and the Ca^{2+} waves always originated in the border zone between the normal and the weak segments during the relaxation (lengthening) phase of the normal segments. It is noteworthy that various mutations in the SR[11–13] and the sarcomere contractile proteins[14–16] are associated with an increased risk of developing lethal arrhythmias.

The XB-Ca^{2+} Cooperativity Modulates the Intracellular Calcium

The proposed Calcium hypothesis is supported by extensive data. Rapid shortening produces fast release of calcium from troponin, leading to the conspicuous increase ("extra") in the free calcium transient.[17,18] This extra calcium transient can directly affect the membrane potential by Ca^{2+}-dependent depolarizing currents.[19,20] This "extra" calcium can also elicit calcium release from the SR by the calcium-induced calcium-release (CICR) mechanism, which further amplifies the calcium surge and produces calcium waves and propagating contractions.[8–10,19] The calcium waves always start in the vicinity of the damaged area, immediately following the rapid shortening of these damaged areas during the contraction relaxation phase.[8] These observations strongly suggest that calcium dissociation from troponin initiates the calcium surge.

The kinetics of calcium binding and dissociation from troponin are tightly coupled to the regulation of cardiac force–length relationship (FLR) and the related Frank-Starling Law of the heart. The cardiac FLR is steep: a 10% sarcomere lengthening yields a 30–70% increase in the isometric force.[21–23] Sarcomere lengthening also increases the contractile filaments' sensitivity to calcium.[22,23] These phenomena relate to cooperative interactions between contractile proteins.[18,20,22–24] The opinions vary as to whether the increase in calcium sensitivity at longer sarcomere length (SL) is determined by a XB-Ca^{2+} cooperativity, whereby the number of strong XBs determines the affinity of troponin for calcium,[20,21,24–28] or by other mechanisms that depend on the SL[21,29] or interfilament lattice spacing.[30] An increase in calcium affinity with an increase in the number of strong XBs was shown in skeletal[26,29] and cardiac muscles[20–23,27] by using fluorescently labeled Troponin-C,[26] measurement of isotopic Ca^{2+} binding to Troponin,[27] or by monitoring the effects of length and force changes on the free Ca^{2+} transients.[17,20] This cooperativity mechanism was strongly supported in our recent studies[31–33] where we have studied the plausible hypotheses and have shown that the cooperativity is force dependent.[32] To decipher whether the dominant cooperativity mechanism that regulates XB recruitment is length, interfilament spacing, or force dependent, we have developed a unique procedure that allows us to control the SL independently of the intracellular free Ca^{2+} concentration. This enigma was resolved by showing that the kinetic of XB recruitment is directly force (number of strong XBs) dependent. SL and calcium have only indirect effects through the modulation of the force.[32]

The present report focuses on the development of the tools for exploring and differentiating between the above mentioned two notions: (i) The SAC hypothesis, whereby SACs in the sarcolemma, which are modulated by the SL, directly affect the membrane potential, and (ii) The Calcium hypothesis, whereby the loading conditions modulate the action potential by the loading conditions through the effect of the XB-Ca^{2+} cooperativity mechanism on the intracellular calcium. Thus the aim was to differentiate between the direct effects of the SL (SACs) and Ca^{2+} (cooperativity mechanism) on the action potential.

METHODS

The developed experimental setup allows us to study the cardiac fiber mechanical function simultaneously with the action potential. Force is measured with a silicon strain gauge (SensoNor AE801, Sensor One Technologies Corp., Sausalito, CA). The SL is determined by laser diffraction technique using HeNe laser (632.8 nm, Model 1135P, Uniphase, CA). Striations of the cardiac muscle act as an optical grating to incident light. The diffractions pass through the objective to the side port of an inverted microscope (Nikon, Eclipse TE300, DALSA, DALSA Eindhoven, High Tech Campus 12a M/S 02 5656 AE Eindhoven, The Netherlands). Two cylindrical lenses focus the laser diffraction on a linear CCD array (Dalsa camera, with 2048 pixels and frame rate of 7500 Hz, Nikon Corp. Co. Ltd., Kawasaki, Kanagawa, Japan). The system tracks the centers of the two first-order diffractions from both sides of the zero order and calculates the SL from the distance between them. The spatial resolution of the SL measurements is of 3 nm. Muscle length (ML) is controlled by a fast servomotor (Aurora Scientific Inc. 308B, Aurora Scientific, Richmond Hill, Ontario, Canada) with a rise time of 250 μsec.

The action potential is measured by using the voltage-sensitive dye di-4 ANEPPS.[34] The trabeculae are stained for 15 min at room temperature. The dye is washed out with Krebs-Henseleit (K-H) solution. Excitation light comes from a xenon light source. The light is filtered at 480 ± 60 nm by a filter within the filter box of the inverted microscope, and passes through the objective toward the preparation. A second filter (600 nm Low-Pass) in the filter box allows the laser light (632 nm) and the emitted fluorescence to pass to the microscope side port, where the light is focused on a photomultiplier (Hamamatsu PMT H3906, Japan).

The trabeculae were isolated from the rat right ventricle (Spargue Dawley, 250–300 g). The dissection and the technique of mounting the trabeculae in the experiment setup followed the procedures developed by ter Keurs.[35] Rats were anesthetized and the hearts were quickly removed and transferred to a dissection dish, where the hearts were perfused retrogradely through a cannulated aorta (horizontal Langendorff setup). Thin, long, and unbranched trabeculae that run between the atrioventricular ring and the right ventricle free wall were isolated. The ventricular end of the trabecula was mounted in a basket attached to the force transducer, while the valvular end was nailed to a hook attached to the motor lever-arm. The fibers were perfused with modified K-H solution, containing (in mM): Na^+ 143.7; K^+ 5.0; Cl^- 130.4; Mg^{2+} 1.2; PO_4^- 2.26; SO_4^- 1.2; HCO_3^- 19.0; and glucose 10. The pH was set at 7.40 by adjusting the flow of 95% O_2 and 5% CO_2 (25°C, $[Ca^{2+}]0 = 1.5$ mM). The trabeculae were stimulated at 0.5 Hz. Passive and twitch FLR were measured after 1 h of stabilization and were used as a control for evaluating the viability of the trabeculae. A trabecula was discarded when the twitch force dropped by more than 15% relative to the baseline at the same $[Ca^{2+}]_0$ and SL.

The protocol used to control the intracellular free Ca^{2+} was designed to differentiate between the effects of SL and Ca^{2+}. The action potentials and the force were studied at constant intracellular calcium levels by using tetanic contractions.[31,32] Stable fused tetanii were achieved at different extracellular Ca^{2+} concentrations ($[Ca^{2+}]_0 = 1.5, 3, 4.5,$ and 6 mM) by using 8 Hz stimulation and 30 μM cyclopiazonic acid (CPA) (Sigma Aldrich, St. Louis, MO), which blocks the sarcoplasmic reticulum (SR) calcium ATPase.[31,32] The twitch frequency was 0.2 Hz and tetanii were elicited every 10 twitches (i.e., every 50 sec). The tetanus duration was 3.5 sec.

The tetanic SL was determined by stretching the trabecula during the first second of the tetanic contraction until the desired SL was reached. Length perturbations, as large oscillations, were imposed 1s after a stable tetanus was reached (FIG. 1). These perturbations and oscillations were imposed at various tetanic SLs and Ca^{2+} concentrations to assess the effects of the SL and calcium on the APD (not shown here). FIGURE 1 presents identical length oscillations imposed at the same tetanic SL at different $[Ca^{2+}]_0$ concentrations (4.5 and 6 mM). The $[Ca^{2+}]_0$ concentrations studied were: 1.5, 3, 4.5, and 6 mM and the SL ranged from 1.75 to 2.20 μM. The ML, force, and SL were sampled at 5000 Hz. Each oscillation was repeated five times and the results were averaged to reduce random noise.

Although we have not measured directly the intracellular free Ca^{2+}, the steady tetanic force (FIG. 1) implies that the intracellular free calcium has reached a certain level ("calcium clamp") around which small fluctuations may exist during the action potential.

RESULTS AND DISCUSSION

Validation of the Cooperativity Mechanism

The idea of studying the action potential at apparently constant intracellular Ca^{2+} ("Calcium Clamp") and controlled SL using tetanic contraction stems

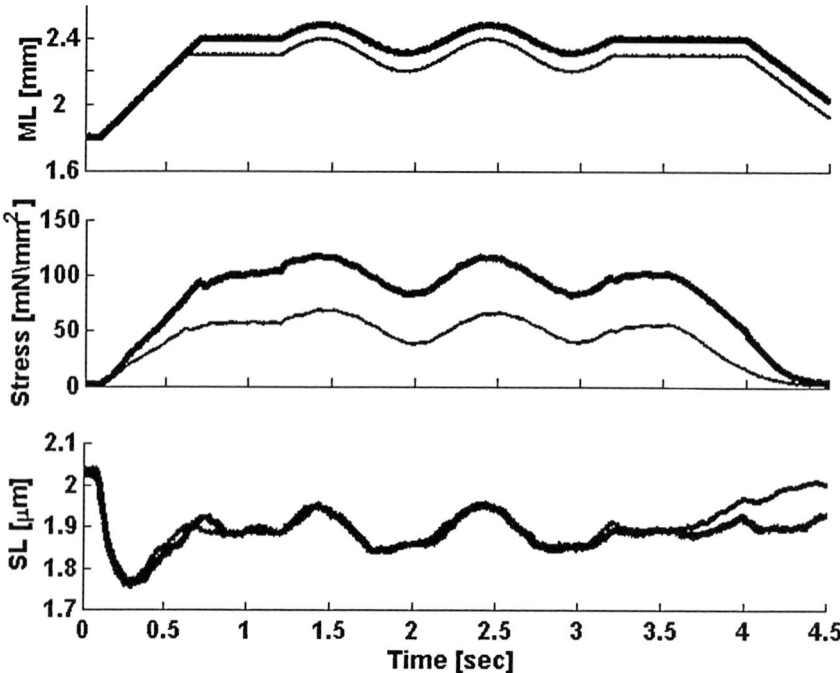

FIGURE 1. The stress responses to oscillations at identical tetanic SL but with different $[Ca^{2+}]_0$, $[Ca^{2+}]_0 = 4.5$ (thin lines) and 6 mM (thick lines). The ML was stretched during the first second of the tetanic contraction to yield identical SL (1.9 μm). Large (56 nm/sarcomere) 1-Hz oscillations were imposed after a steady tetanic stress was reached. The force lagged the length oscillation and the phase delay in the force response was smaller at higher $[Ca^{2+}]_0$.

from our recent investigation of the cooperativity mechanism.[31–33] We have studied the intact fiber force response to length oscillations at different tetanic SLs and intracellular Ca^{2+} levels using the tetanus technique to differentiate between the effects of the length and the free calcium concentration.

The stress response to slow (1 Hz) SL oscillations imposed during tetanus lagged behind the SL oscillations.[31,32] This phase delay yielded counterclockwise (CCW) hystereses in the stress-length plane (FIG. 2), indicating that the stress was higher during shortening than during lengthening. The muscle generates external work during shortening while work is done upon the muscle during lengthening. Thus the muscle generated external work during the observed CCW hystereses. A larger external work was generated by the trabeculae during shortening than the work required for stretching the fiber. The area inside the hysteresis loop is equal to the work done by the trabeculae during each oscillation. This external work originated from recruitment of new XBs (conversion of energy form ATP hydrolysis to external work) during the

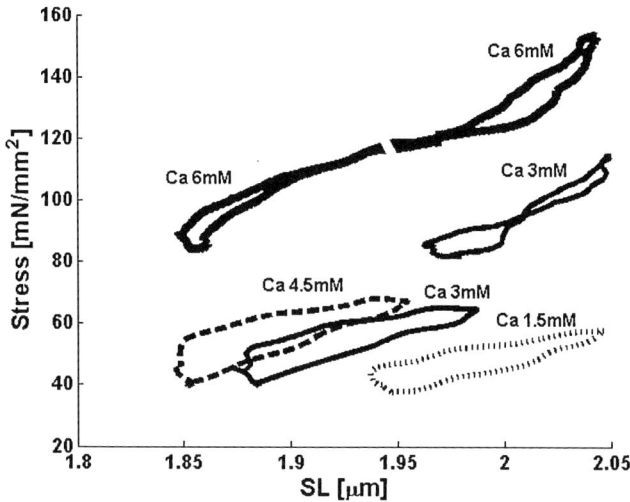

FIGURE 2. The phase of the hysteresis depends differently on SL, calcium concentration, and stress level. The hystereses, at three different SLs (from 1.89 μm to 1.98 μm) and three stress levels (from 50 to 134 mN/mm^2), were recorded from one trabecula. The phase decreased as $[Ca^{2+}]_0$ increased at the same SL. The phase decreased at longer SL at the same $[Ca^{2+}]_0$. However, similar phases were obtained at identical stress levels.

oscillation. Note that the area within the hysteresis is determined by the phase delay between the force and the length.

The dependencies of the phase of the hysteresis on the tetanic SL, the Ca^{2+} concentration, and the tetanic force were quantified. An increase in extracellular calcium ($[Ca^{2+}]_0$) increased the mean tetanic stress and was associated with a decrease in the phase of the stress-SL hysteresis (FIG. 2). A CCW hysteresis was observed at low calcium levels ($[Ca^{2+}]_0 = 1.5, 3.0$, and 4.5 mM) but a clockwise (CW) hysteresis (negative phase) was obtained at high calcium level ($[Ca^{2+}]_0 = 6.0$ mM). The phase decreased by 15° ± 5.7° ($P < 0.01$) for an increase of 1.5 mM in $[Ca^{2+}]_0$, at constant SL, for all the data points.[32] However, at constant $[Ca^{2+}]_0$ the phase decreased with sarcomere lengthening. The phase decreased by 25.7° ± 17.0° for 0.1 μM sarcomere lengthening ($P < 0.01$) at constant $[Ca^{2+}]_0$. Thus the phase is both SL and Ca^{2+} dependent. Lengthening the sarcomere or raising $[Ca^{2+}]_0$ levels independently decreases the phase of the hysteresis.[32] However, both effects are associated with force augmentation.

We have consequently studied the effects of SL and $[Ca^{2+}]_0$ at constant stress. We balanced decreases in $[Ca^{2+}]_0$ by increasing the SL to obtain identical tetanic stress (FIG. 2). For each fiber, a similar phase of hysteresis was obtained at constant stress levels, although different pairs of SL and $[Ca^{2+}]_0$ were used. FIGURE 2 presents hystereses obtained at two different stress levels,

50 and 98 mN/mm^2 with various pairs of SL and $[Ca^{2+}]_0$ (1.5, 3.0, and 4.5 mM at 50 mN/mm^2, 3.0 and 6.0 mM at 98 mN/mm^2). The phase was 27° ± 1° at 50 ± 3 mN/mm^2 and 5.1° ± 2.4° at 98 mN/mm^2. Although a similar phase was observed at constant stress level for different pairs of SL and $[Ca^{2+}]_0$, the phase always decreased as the stress increased.[32] The same phase obtained at identical force level when using different pairs of $[Ca^{2+}]_0$ and SL, and the dependence of the phase on the force level are conceivably explained by the hypothesis that the dominant cooperativity is force (number of strong XBs) dependent.[32,33]

Any regulatory mechanism whereby the kinetic rates of XB cycling or calcium binding to troponin are modulated by SL, calcium, or the number of strong XBs (force) requires the existence of some time delay in the force response to changes in the SL[31,32] or calcium[32,36] due to the involved biochemical kinetics. The phase decreased with sarcomere lengthening (FIG. 2)[31,32] at constant calcium. Similarly, the phase decreased at higher $[Ca^{2+}]_0$ levels (FIG. 2) at constant SL. Changes in the phase of the hystereses at constant calcium or constant SL are incongruent with the hypotheses that the dominant cooperativity is either exclusively Ca^{2+} or SL dependent.

The described hystereses in the force–length plane are consistent with the described hysteresis in the force–calcium relation, at constant SL, in intact and skinned skeletal muscles[36] and in skinned cardiac[37] muscles. The suggested XB-Ca^{2+} cooperativity can also explain the observed[36,37] hysteresis in the force–calcium plane.[33]

The MEF

We have extended the application of the same technique to study the mechanisms underlying the MEF. Furthermore, establishing the XB-Ca^{2+} cooperativity[24,32,33,38,39] allows us to suggest that changes in the loading conditions modulate the intracellular free calcium.

FIGURE 3 presents the action potential fluorescence observed during tetanic contractions. The tetanic contraction started at the same initial SL (2.05 μm) at different calcium concentrations ($[Ca^{2+}]_0 = 1.5$ and 4.5 mM). Although there were motion artifacts during the initial phase of the tetanic contraction, stable action potentials were obtained during the steady tetanic contractions. Conspicuous difference between the action potentials was observed at the different $[Ca^{2+}]_0$s. As seen in FIGURE 3, smaller APD was observed at higher $[Ca^{2+}]_0$. The SL also affects the APD, and a smaller APD was obtained at longer SL at the same $[Ca^{2+}]_0$. However, the effect of the SL was significantly smaller than the effect of $[Ca^{2+}]_0$. Intriguingly, a tight dependence of the APD on the stress was obtained, similar to the observed dependence of the phase of the hysteresis on the stress[32]; the APD decreased with an increase in the stress. These observations strongly support the "calcium hypothesis," whereby

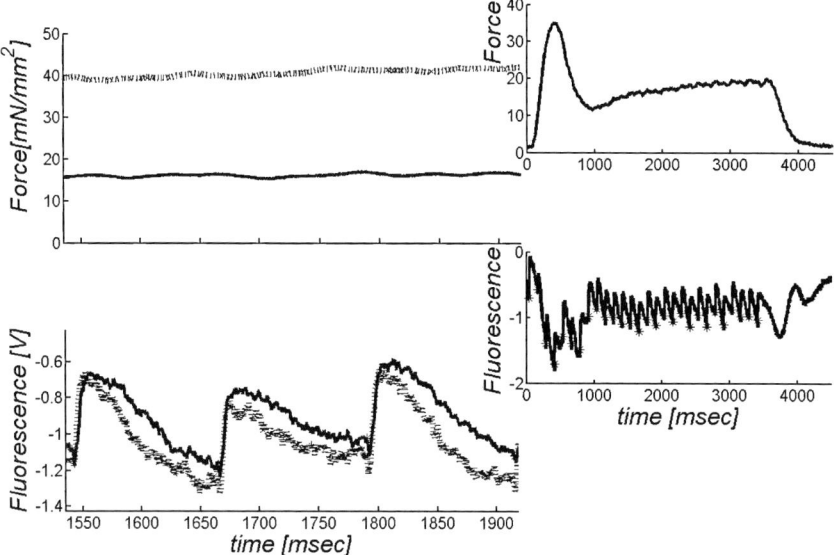

FIGURE 3. The action potential fluorescence during the tetanic contractions starting from the same initial SL (2.05 μm) in the presence of different extracellular calcium concentrations: $[Ca^{2+}]_0 = 1.5$ mM (continuous lines) and 4.5 mM (dashed lines). The tetanic contractions allow studying the effects of calcium and SL on the APD without having motion artifacts during the steady tetanic contractions. Note the motion artifacts during the tetanic initial phase (inset). The APD is significantly smaller at higher extracellular calcium.

the intracellular control of contraction plays a key role in mediating the MEF phenomenon and the effect of the afterload on the membrane potential.

The sodium–calcium exchanger (NCX) can conveniently explain modulation of the APD by calcium. Calcium extrusion out of the cell through the NCX produces inward current as three sodium ions are exchanged for each calcium ion. Although an increase in the $[Ca^{2+}]_0$ increases the intracellular calcium, the ratio of the extracellular to the intracellular Ca^{2+} increases. Therefore, the current through the NCX decreases as $[Ca^{2+}]_0$ increases, leading to a smaller APD.

The role of the inhibition of L-type channel inflow by the intracellular tetanic calcium, and the activation of other currents as the chloride currents by the intracellular calcium, are presently under investigation using different SLs and $[Ca^{2+}]_0$s and by using Indo-1 for quantifying the changes in the intracellular calcium. The observed smaller APD at longer SL at the same $[Ca^{2+}]_0$, where the force increases and the intracellular calcium decreases, are incongruent with suggestions that either the L-type channels or calcium-activated chloride channel play a significant role. The results strongly suggest that NCX, which is the main route of calcium sequestration out of the cell, is the key player that accounts for the effect of calcium on the membrane potential.

Opposing effects of calcium and SAC on the intracellular calcium concentration and APD were predicted. The results support the calcium hypothesis and the cooperativity pathway as $[Ca^{2+}]_0$ has a significantly larger effect on the APD. Smaller APD was observed at higher $[Ca^{2+}]_0$, although the tetanic SL was shorter (incongruent with the SAC hypothesis). Moreover, the effects of the SL can be explained through the FLR and the cooperativity mechanism: sarcomere lengthening increases the force and the affinity of troponin to calcium. Thus lengthening at constant $[Ca^{2+}]_0$ decreases the intracellular calcium [35] and decreases the APD.

Deciphering the role of the intracellular control of excitation-contraction coupling in modulating the membrane action potential and initiating life-threatening arrhythmias addresses the hitherto quite unclear pathogenesis of sudden death. The suggested role of the intracellular control of contraction is based on solid experimental and clinical evidences. The study describes a novel experimental tool and allows testing, validating, or voiding the suggested roles of the intracellular control of excitation contraction and the SACs. The suggested mechanism has significant clinical implication to heart failure, where the prevalence of lethal arrhythmias is high, the myocardium is inhomogeneous, and the NCX sequestrates most of the calcium out of the cytosol. Better understanding of the mechanisms underlying the MEF will open new avenues of research toward the development of new therapeutic modalities.

SUMMARY

The utility of our technique of using tetanic contraction (calcium clamp) was presented here. The advantages are in the separate assessment of the roles of SL, calcium, or the number of strong XBs (stress level), by keeping one variable constant at various values, while observing the effects of the other variables. The ability to differentiate between the effects of the SL, $[Ca^{2+}]_0$, and the stress allows us to test plausible hypotheses and suggests that: (i) the dominant mechanistically appealing explanation for the observed hystereses in the force–length plane is the dependence of the cooperativity on the number of strong XBs[32] and (ii) the MEF is mediated by Ca^{2+} during systole, and the SL has only an indirect effect through the stress and the cooperativity mechanism. The study strongly supports the hypothesis that the MEF phenomenon during muscle contraction is determined by the cooperativity and the NCX.

ACKNOWLEDGMENTS

The study was supported by the Fund for the Promotion of Research at the Technion (AL) and a grant from the United States-Israel Binational Science Foundation (BSF Research Project No. 2003399).

REFERENCES

1. MYERBURG, R.J., K.M. KESSLER & A. CASTELLANOS. 1993. Sudden cardiac death: epidemiology, transient risk, and intervention assessment. Ann. Intern. Med. **119:** 1187.
2. BRAUNWALD, E. 1997. Heart disease—A textbook of cardiovascular medicine. W.B. Saunders. Philadelphia, PA.
3. SHULZE, R.A., J. ROULEAU, et al. 1975. Ventricular arrhythmia in the late hospitalization phase of acute myocardial infarction relates to left ventricular function detected by gated cardiac blood pool scanning. Circulation **52:** 1006–1011.
4. LAB, M.J. 1980. Transient depolarization and action potential alterations following mechanical changes in isolated myocardium. Cardiovasc. Res. **14:** 624–637.
5. LAB, M.J. 1982. Contraction-excitation feedback in myocardium: physiological basis and clinical relevance. Circ. Res. **50:** 757–766.
6. KOHL, P., K. DAY & D. NOBLE. 1998. Cellular mechanisms of cardiac mechanoelectric feedback in a mathematical model. Can. J. Cardiol. **14:** 111–119.
7. KOHL, P., F. SACHS & M.R. FRANZ. 2005. Cardiac Mechanoelectric Feedback and Arrhythmias. W.B. Saunders. Philadelphia, PA.
8. DANIELS, M.C.G., D. FEDIDA, C. LAMONT & H.E.D.J. TER KEURS. 1991. Role of the sarcolemma in triggered propagated contractions in rat cardiac trabeculae. Circ. Res. **68:** 1408–1421.
9. TER KEURS, H.E.D.J., Y.M. ZHANG & M. MIURA. 1988. Damage induced arrhythmias: reversal of excitation-contraction coupling. Cardiovasc. Res. **40:** 444–455.
10. TER KEURS, E.E.J., Y. WAKAYAMA, M. MIURA, et al. 2006. A. arrhythmogenic calcium release from cardiac myofilaments. Prog. Biophysics. Mol. Biol. **90:** 151–171.
11. JIANG, D., B. XIAO, D. YANG, et al. 2004. RyR2 mutations linked to ventricular tachycardia and sudden death reduce the threshold for store-overload-induced Ca^{2+} release (SOICR). Proc. Nat. Acad. Sci. USA **31:** 13062–13067.
12. LAHAT, H., E. PRAS, et al. 2001. Missense mutation in a highly conserved region of CASQ2 is associated with autosomal recessive catecholamine-induced polymorphic ventricular tachycardia in Bedouin families from Israel. Am. J. Hum. Genet. **69:** 1378–1384.
13. WEHRENS, X.H., S.E. LEHNART, et al. 2003. FKBP12.6 deficiency and defective calcium release channel (ryanodine receptor) function linked to exercise-induced sudden cardiac death. Cell 27 **113:** 829–840.
14. KNOLLMANN, B.C., P. KIRCHOF, et al. 2003. Familial hypertrophic cardiomyopathy-linked mutant troponin T causes stress-induced ventricular tachycardia and Ca depended action potential remodeling. Circ. Res. **92:** 428–436.
15. RICHARD, P., P. CHARRON, et al. 2005. Hypertrophic cardiomyopathy: distribution of disease genes, spectrum of mutations, and implications for a molecular diagnosis strategy. Circulation **19:** e39–e44.
16. VENKATRAMAN, G., A.V. GOMES, W.G. KERRICK & J.D. POTTER. 2005. Characterization of troponin T dilated cardiomyopathy mutations in the fetal troponin isoform. J. Biol. Chem. **280:** 17584–17592.
17. ALLEN, D.G. & J.C. KENTISH. 1988. Calcium concentration in the myoplasm of skinned ferret ventricular muscle following changes in muscle length. J. Physiol. **407:** 489–503.
18. KENTISH, J.C. & A. WRZOSEK. 1998. Changes in force and cytosolic calcium concentration after length changes in isolated rat ventricular trabeculae. J. Physiol. **506:** 431–444.

19. CLUSIN, W.T. 2003. Calcium and cardiac arrhythmias: DADs, EADs, and alternans. Crit. Rev. Clin. Lab. Sci. **40:** 337–375.
20. KURIHARA, S. & K. KOMUKAI. 1995. Tension dependent changes of intracellular calcium transient in ferret ventricular muscle. J. Physiol. **489:** 617–625.
21. ALLEN, D.G. & J.C. KENTISH. 1985. The cellular basis of the length-tension relation in cardiac muscle. J. Mol. Cell Cardiol. **17:** 821–840.
22. HIBBERD, M.G. & B.R. JEWELL. 1979. Length-dependence of the sensitivity of the contractile system to calcium in rat ventricular muscle [proceedings]. J. Physiol. Lond. **290:** 30–31.
23. KENTISH, J.C., H.E. TER-KEURS, L. RICCIARDI, et al. 1986. Comparison between the sarcomere length-force relations of intact and skinned trabeculae from rat right ventricle. Influence of calcium concentrations on these relations. Circ. Res. **58:** 755–768.
24. LANDESBERG, A. & S. SIDEMAN. 1994. Coupling calcium binding to troponin-C and cross-bridge cycling in skinned cardiac cells. Am. J. Physiol. **266:** H1260–H1266.
25. GRABAREK, Z., J. GRABAREK, P.C. LEAVIS & J. GERGELY. 1983. Cooperative binding to the Ca^{2+}-specific sites of troponin C in regulated actin and actomyosin. J. Biol. Chem. **258:** 14098–14102.
26. GUTH, K. & J.D. POTTER. 1987. Effect of rigor and cycling cross-bridges on the structure of troponin-C and on the Ca^{2+} affinity of the Ca^{2+}-specific regulatory sites in skinned rabbit psoas fibers. J. Biol. Chem. **262:** 13627–13635.
27. HOFMANN, P.A. & F. FUCHS. 1987. Effect of length and cross-bridge attachment on Ca^{2+} binding to cardiac troponin C. Am. J. Physiol. **253:** C90–C96.
28. SHNIER, J.S. & J. SOLARO. 1982. Activation of thin-filament-regulated muscle by calcium ion: considerations based on nearest-neighbor lattice statistics. Proc. Natl. Acad. Sci. USA **79:** 4637–4641.
29. STEPHENSON, D.G. & I.R. WENDT. 1984. Length dependence of changes in sarcoplasmic calcium concentration and myofibrillar calcium sensitivity in striated muscle fibers. J. Muscle Res. Cell. Motil. **5:** 243–272.
30. FUCHS, F. & Y.P. WANG. 1996. Sarcomere length versus interfilament spacing as determinants of cardiac myofilament Ca^{2+} sensitivity and Ca^{2+} binding. J. Cardiol. Mol. Cell. **28:** 1375–1383.
31. LEVY, C. & A. LANDESBERG. 2004. Hysteresis in the force-length relation and the regulation of cross-bridge recruitment in the tetanized rat trabeculae. Am. J. Physiol. Heart Circ. Physiol. **286:** H434–H441.
32. LEVY, C. & A. LANDESBERG. 2006. Cross-bridge dependent cooperativity determines the cardiac force-length relationship. J. Mol. Cell Cardiol. **40:** 639–647.
33. YANIV, Y., R. SIVAN & A. LANDESBERG. 2005. Analysis of hystereses in force length and force calcium relations. Am. J. Physiol. **288:** H389–H399.
34. ROSENBAUM, D.S. & J. JALIFE. 2001. Optical mapping of cardiac excitation and arrhythmias. Futura Publishing Co., Armonk, NY.
35. BACKX, P. & H.E.D.J. TER KEURS. 1993. Fluorescent properties of rat cardiac trabeculae microinjected with fura-2 salt. Am. J. Physiol. **264:** H1098–H1110.
36. RIDGWAY, E.B., A.M. GORDON & D.A. MARTYN. 1983. Hysteresis in the force-calcium relation in muscle. Science **219:** 1075–1077.
37. HARRISON, S.M., C. LAMONT & D.J. MILLER. 1988. Hysteresis and the length dependence calcium sensitivity in chemically skinned rat cardiac muscle. J. Physiol. **401:** 115–143.

38. GIBBS, C.L. 2003. Cardiac energetics: sense and nonsense. Clin. Exp. Pharmacol. Physiol. **30:** 598–603.
39. LANDESBERG, A. & S. SIDEMAN. 1999. Regulation of energy consumption in the cardiac muscle: analysis of isometric contractions. Am. J. Physiol. **276:** H998–H1011.

Role of Sarcomere Mechanics and Ca^{2+} Overload in Ca^{2+} Waves and Arrhythmias in Rat Cardiac Muscle

HENK E.D.J. TER KEURS,[a] YUJI WAKAYAMA,[b] YOSHINAO SUGAI,[b] GUY PRICE,[a] YUTAKA KAGAYA,[b] PENELOPE A. BOYDEN,[c] MASAHITO MIURA,[b] AND BRUNO D.M. STUYVERS[a]

[a]University of Calgary, Canada
[b]Tohoku University Graduate School of Medicine, Japan
[c]Columbia University, New York, USA

ABSTRACT: Ca^{2+} release from the sarcoplasmic reticulum (SR) depends on the sarcoplasmic reticulum (SR) Ca^{2+} load and the cytosolic Ca^{2+} level. Arrhythmogenic Ca^{2+} waves underlying triggered propagated contractions arise from Ca^{2+} overloaded regions near damaged areas in the cardiac muscle. Ca^{2+} waves can also be induced in undamaged muscle, in regions with nonuniform excitation–contraction (EC) coupling by the cycle of stretch and release in the border zone between the damaged and intact regions. We hypothesize that rapid shortening of sarcomeres in the border zone during relaxation causes Ca^{2+} release from troponin C (TnC) on thin filaments and initiates Ca^{2+} waves. Elimination of this shortening will inhibit the initiation of Ca^{2+} waves, while SR Ca^{2+} overload will enhance the waves. Force, sarcomere length (SL), and $[Ca^{2+}]_i$ were measured and muscle length was controlled. A small jet of Hepes solution with an extracellular $[Ca^{2+}]$ 10 mM (HC), or HC containing BDM, was used to weaken a 300 μm long muscle segment. Trains of electrical stimuli were used to induce Ca^{2+} waves. The effects of small exponential stretches on triggered propagatory contraction (TPC) amplitude and propagation velocity of Ca^{2+} waves (V_{prop}) were studied. Sarcomere shortening was uniform prior to activation. HC induced spontaneous diastolic sarcomere contractions in the jet region and attenuated twitch sarcomere shortening; HC+ butanedione monoxime (BDM) caused stretch only in the jet region. Stimulus trains induced Ca^{2+} waves, which started inside the HC jet region during twitch relaxation. Ca^{2+} waves started in the border zone of the BDM jet. The initial local $[Ca^{2+}]_i$ rise of the waves by HC was twice that by BDM. The waves propagated at a V_{prop} of 2.0 ± 0.2 mm/sec. Arrhythmias occurred frequently in trabeculae following exposure to the HC jet. Stretch early during relaxation, which reduced sarcomere shortening in the weakened regions, substantially decreased

Address for correspondence: Prof. Henk E.D.J. Ter Keurs, M.D., Ph.D., School of Medicine, Department of Physiology, University of Calgary, 3330 Hospital Dr, N.W., Calgary, Alberta T2N 4N1, Canada. Voice: 403-220-4525; fax: 403-270-0313.
e-mail: terkeurs@ucalgary.ca

force of the TPC (F_{TPC}) and delayed Ca^{2+} waves, and reduced V_{prop} commensurate with the reduction F_{TPC}. These results are consistent with the hypothesis that Ca^{2+} release from the myofilaments initiates arrhythmogenic propagating Ca^{2+} release. Prevention of sarcomere shortening, by itself, did not inhibit Ca^{2+} wave generation. SR Ca^{2+} overload potentiated initiation and propagation of Ca^{2+} waves.

KEYWORDS: arrhythmogenic; Ca^{2+} waves; shortening; SR; Ca^{2+} overload.

INTRODUCTION

Currently proposed molecular mechanisms underlying sarcomere length (SL) dependence of Ca^{2+} binding to troponin C (TnC) suggest that cross-bridge force exerted on the actin filament deforms the TnC molecule, thus retarding the dissociation of Ca^{2+} from TnC.[1,2] This effect is bound to be SL-dependent since the number of myosin cross-bridges attaching to actin increases with SL over the range of operation of cardiac muscle. Thus, the mechanical load on a sarcomere will influence the dissociation of Ca^{2+} from TnC. In fact, it has been shown that rapid removal of an external load on a muscle during the twitch causes a robust additional $[Ca^{2+}]_i$ transient.[3] This phenomenon may be important when the ECC properties of the myocardium are nonuniform (such as in disease), since nonuniformity of contraction may be accompanied by such unloading-related $[Ca^{2+}]_i$ transients. It is well known that a large amount of Ca^{2+} is bound to TnC during contraction. Hence, Ca^{2+} release from TnC upon rapid unloading may be large enough to activate Ca^{2+}-dependent mechanisms including SR Ca^{2+} release and Ca^{2+}-dependent membrane currents.

REVERSE EXCITATION–CONTRACTION (EC) COUPLING IN A NONUNIFORM CARDIAC MUSCLE

During our work on cardiac sarcomere dynamics we have discovered that when cardiac muscle is damaged locally, Ca^{2+} waves start near the damaged region and propagate rapidly in a coordinated fashion into adjacent tissue.[4] These aftercontractions in multicellular preparations occur as the combined result of the mechanical effects and elevated cellular $[Ca^{2+}]_i$ levels owing to the regional damage and thus may give rise to premature beats as well as triggered arrhythmias. These aftercontractions appear to be initiated by stretch and release of the damaged region during the regular twitch and they propagate into neighboring myocardium; hence the term triggered propagated contractions (TPCs). Damage-induced TPCs may, therefore, serve as the mechanism that couples regional damage with the initiation of premature beats and arrhythmias in the adjacent myocardium. The displacement of the TPC occurs at a velocity of propagation (V_{prop}), which varies at room temperature from

0.1 to 15 mm/sec[5] and is correlated tightly with the amplitude of the twitch preceding the TPC, suggesting that the Ca^{2+} load of the sarcoplasmic reticulum (SR) dictates V_{prop}. In contrast, sarcomere stretch, which increases the twitch force for any level of loading of the SR, does not increase V_{prop} of the TPC.[6] Studies of the effects of interventions such as varied $[Ca^{2+}]_o$, Ca^{2+} channel agonists and antagonists also support the idea that the SR Ca^{2+} load is an important determinant of V_{prop}.[7] On the other hand, interventions that cause a leak of Ca^{2+} from the SR (caffeine and ryanodine) increase V_{prop}, suggesting that V_{prop} also depends on diastolic cytosolic $[Ca^{2+}]_i$.[8] Finally, the rate of initiation of TPCs is tightly correlated with V_{prop} when the SR Ca^{2+} load is modulated, suggesting that the triggering process and the propagation process share closely related mechanisms.

We have recently investigated Ca^{2+} waves underlying TPCs in rat's cardiac trabeculae under experimental conditions that simulate the functional nonuniformity caused by local mechanical or ischemic damage of the myocardium. A mechanical discontinuity along the trabeculae was created by exposing the preparation to a small jet of solution with a composition that reduces ECC in myocytes within that segment. The jet solution contained either caffeine (CF), 2,3-butanedione monoxime (BDM), or low Ca^{2+} concentration ($[Ca^{2+}]$) (LC). Each of these solutions was chosen to render the exposed segment weaker than the normal muscle parts, by either depleting the SR of Ca^{2+} ions (CF) or inhibiting the cross-bridges (BDM) or by lowering the Ca^{2+} load of the cell (LC). The jet of solution was applied perpendicularly to a small muscle region (200 to 300 μm) at constant flow. When the jet contained caffeine, BDM, or low $[Ca^{2+}]$ during the stimulated twitch, muscle-twitch force decreased and the sarcomeres in the exposed segment were stretched by shortening normal regions outside the jet. Repeated stimulation at 2.5 Hz, room temperature, and physiological $[Ca^{2+}]_o$, reproducibly generated Ca^{2+} waves that arose from the border between shortening and stretched regions. Such Ca^{2+} waves started during force relaxation of the last stimulated twitch of the train and propagated into segments both inside and outside of the jet. Arrhythmias, in the form of non-driven rhythmic activity, were induced when the amplitude of the Ca^{2+}-wave was increased by raising $[Ca^{2+}]_o$. Arrhythmias disappeared rapidly when the uniformity of ECC throughout the muscle was restored by turning the jet off. These results showed, for the first time, that nonuniform ECC can cause Ca^{2+} waves underlying TPCs and suggest that Ca^{2+} dissociated from myofilaments plays an important role in the initiation of Ca^{2+} waves.

SPONTANEOUS SR CA^{2+} RELEASE

Normal Ventricular Muscle

Spontaneous release of Ca^{2+} from the SR is evident in the form of Ca^{2+} "sparks,"[9] which are, as "evoked Ca^{2+} sparks" induced during action potentials,[10] or voltage-clamp pulses,[11] probably by Ca^{2+} entering via single L-type Ca^{2+} channels.[12–14] Ca^{2+} sparks may also trigger each other to produce Ca^{2+} waves, which propagate through the cell.[15] Ca^{2+} sparks evoked by L-type Ca^{2+} currents are believed to summate, spatially and temporally, constituting the electrically evoked whole cell $[Ca^{2+}]_i$ transient[10–13,16] that couples excitation to contraction. The relevance of Ca^{2+} sparks to normal ECC in cardiac muscle was proven by similar observations using confocal microscopy of working ventricular trabeculae under physiological conditions ($[Ca^{2+}]_i$ and temperature). Also, microscopic Ca^{2+} waves were found in these trabeculae, which had been recorded previously only in single isolated cells.[17–19] The peak amplitude Ca^{2+} sparks is ~200 nmol/L, which is below the level at which cross-bridges are activated in the intact trabeculae. Furthermore, Ca^{2+} sparks are spatially restricted, suggesting that the $[Ca^{2+}]$ in the myofilament space during and after the peak of the Ca^{2+} spark must have been substantially lower than 170 nM, which makes it even more unlikely that cross-bridges are activated by individual Ca^{2+} sparks. The observation that Ca^{2+} sparks and micro-Ca^{2+} waves occur in microscopically quiescent muscles is therefore not surprising.

SR Ca^{2+} Overload and Spontaneous Ca^{2+} Release

Spontaneous SR Ca^{2+} release was first observed by Fabiato and Fabiato[20] in the form of spontaneous oscillatory contractions in skinned myocyte fragments. The spontaneous contractions were initiated by loading the SR with Ca^{2+}, while the $[Ca^{2+}]$ used for the loading was by itself insufficient to induce Ca^{2+} release. This observation led to the concept that a heavily Ca^{2+}-loaded SR is characterized by spontaneous Ca^{2+} release.[21] The mechanism for increased probability of opening of the SR-Ca^{2+} channel when the SR is heavily loaded with Ca^{2+} is still uncertain, but suggests that the channel is directly or indirectly sensitive to the luminal $[Ca^{2+}]$ of the SR. Intact cells with a high SR Ca^{2+} load show similar phenomena.[22,23]

Spontaneous SR Ca^{2+} release in intact multicellular preparations can take on forms that range from an increased rate of Ca^{2+} spark generation to Ca^{2+} waves that propagate throughout individual cells accompanied by propagating contractile waves[24] or even waves that traverse borders between cells and ultimately repetitive oscillatory Ca^{2+} release occurring synchronously throughout the preparation. The importance of this phenomenon is that the propensity of cardiac muscle in CHF, as was shown in rat, may generate spontaneous cellular contractile waves at increased stimulation frequency or following catecholamine activation. This phenomenon appeared to result in a decrease in force of the driven contraction. These spontaneous contractile waves render failing cardiac muscle unable to augment force in response to increased heart rate and sympathetic stimulation.[24]

Another important observation has been that spontaneous cytosolic $[Ca^{2+}]_i$ transients[25,26] are accompanied by spontaneous depolarizing transmembrane currents in single myocytes as well as in nondriven multicellular cardiac preparations.[23,27] The resulting depolarization may be large enough to trigger an action potential. Ca^{2+} entry during the ensuing action potential may cause even more Ca^{2+} loading of the SR. Consequently, as soon as the release process has recovered after the electrically induced Ca^{2+} release, the overloaded SR again releases a fraction of its Ca^{2+} leading to another action potential and a so-called triggered arrhythmia. Agents that reduce Ca^{2+} load of the SR (e.g., ryanodine, caffeine, EGTA buffer) abolish spontaneous $[Ca^{2+}]_i$ oscillations as well as the oscillatory depolarizations and contractions.[28,29] Therefore, it is thought that spontaneous $[Ca^{2+}]_i$ oscillations are not secondary to transmembrane potential changes, but may cause depolarization and give rise to nondriven action potentials.[30,31]

The Aim of this Study

It is clear that mechanical nonuniformity of cardiac muscle can be induced by mechanisms (e.g., local differences in catecholamine levels or local ischemia) that differ from nonuniformity due to spontaneous Ca^{2+} release (e.g., local postischemic damage). What we do not know is the contribution and/or interaction of these two mechanisms of nonuniformity to the induction of arrhythmogenic Ca^{2+} waves.

The purpose of the studies reported here was to explore whether local Ca^{2+} overload induces Ca^{2+} waves in nonuniform myocardium and whether the reduction of force generating capacity of Ca^{2+} overloaded cardiac muscle during the electrically driven twitch is involved in the generation of propagated Ca^{2+} waves in normal myocardium.

METHODS

Dissection of the Trabeculae

For the studies of the effect of reduced contractile force in the presence of an overloaded SR, 14 trabeculae were dissected from the right ventricle of Lewis Brown Norway rats (length 2.5 ± 0.13, width 0.25 ± 0.03, thickness 0.10 ± 0.01 mM). For the studies of the effect of muscle length, 17 muscles (length: 2.26 ± 0.11 mM, width: 227 ± 18 μM, thickness: 114 ± 7 μM in slack conditions) were used.[32,33] The muscles were mounted in a bathe on an inverted microscope (Nikon Canada Inc., Missisauga, Ontario, Canada) between a silicon strain gauge and a servo-controlled motor arm. Force and

SL were measured respectively by the strain gauge and laser diffraction techniques.[34] Muscle length was changed using a servo-controlled motor and set at 2.0 μM of resting SL (SL_0). The muscle was stimulated in HEPES buffer solution ((in mM): 137.2 NaCl, 5KCl, 1.2$MgCl_2$ 2.8 Na-Acetate, 1 Taurine, 10 HEPES, 10 Glucose, $[Ca^{2+}]_o = 0.7$, 100% O_2 at pH 7.4. at 25°C) at 0.5 Hz until contractions were stable.

Local Jet Exposure

To suppress regional activation of the muscle, the restricted region was exposed to a small "jet" of solution as reported previously.[33] Briefly, the jet was continuously applied using a syringe pump (≈ 0.06 mL/min) from a glass pipette (≈ 100 μm tip) perpendicularly to the trabecula (FIG. 1 A). Alignment and position of the jet flow with the muscle was adjusted using fluorescein (< 0.01 mg/mL). The jet solution was composed of standard HEPES solution containing: (1) caffeine (5 mmol/L) to deplete Ca^{2+} content in the SR[35,36] and (2) 2,3-butanedione monoxime (BDM; 20 mmol/L) to suppress the activation of cross-bridges.[37–40] Ca^{2+} concentrations in the jet ($[Ca^{2+}]_{jet}$) were set at 2.0 mmol/L, as those in the bath ($[Ca^{2+}]_o$). Using this method, sarcomeres in the jet-exposed region were stretched during the stimulated twitches (FIG. 1 B) as has been shown previously.[33]

The effect of the combination of Ca^{2+} overload of the SR was studied by exposing the muscle to a jet of a standard HEPES solution with added Ca^{2+}: high (10 mM) $[Ca^{2+}]_o$ (HC jet) or the combination of HC and 2,3-butanedione monoxime (BDM;20 mM) to inhibit cross-bridge action (HC+BDM jet).

Fura-2 Loading and $[Ca^{2+}]_i$ Measurement

Measurements of cytosolic Ca^{2+} concentration in trabeculae ($[Ca^{2+}]_i$) have been described in detail.[32,41] Briefly, Fura-2 salt was microinjected iontophoretically into the trabecula. Fluorescence signals evoked by excitation lights of 340, 360, or 380 nm were collected using (1) a photomultiplier tube (PMT), which provides average regional $[Ca^{2+}]_i$ using 340/380 nm ratio and *in vitro* calibration or (2) an image intensified CCD camera (IIC) at 30 frames/sec to assess local $[Ca^{2+}]_i$.

The local $[Ca^{2+}]_i$ was analyzed from fluorescence images (8 bit BMP, 512 × 512 pixels; pixel size:2.94 × 2.17 μM), which consisted of one fluorescence image at 360 nm in the resting condition (Im_{Ref}) and a sequence of images at 380 nm.[42] (Im_{380}) recorded continuously during stimulus protocols. The overall kinetics of $[Ca^{2+}]_i$ were obtained from pixel-to-pixel ratios Im_{Ref}/Im_{380} (ratio images) after subtraction of the autofluorescence. Longitudinal ratio profiles

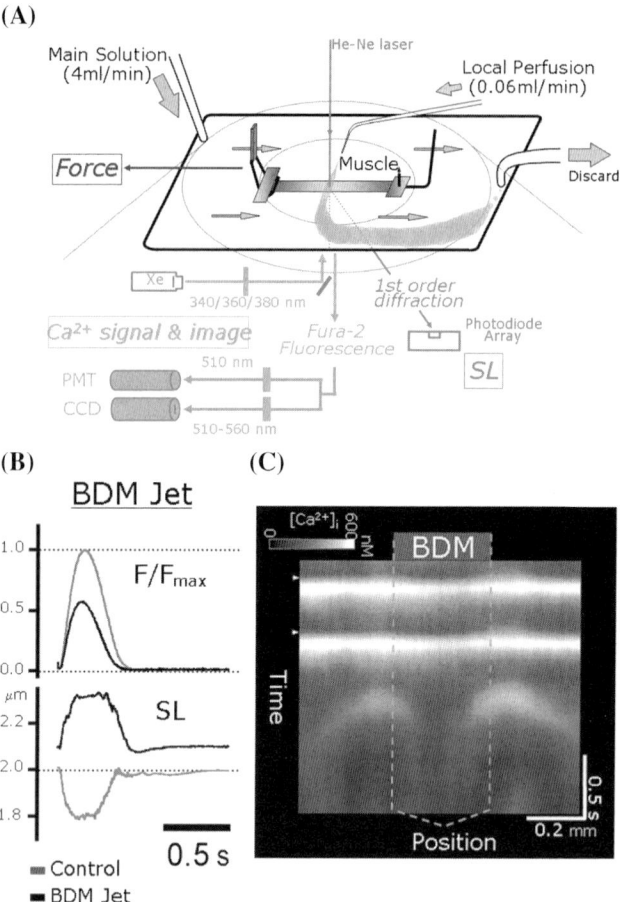

FIGURE 1. Panel **A** shows the experimental paradigm to study nonuniform contraction in rat cardiac trabeculae. The muscle is mounted in an epifluorescent microscope and exposed to a HEPES solution flowing through the bath, together with a jet of modified HEPES solution (see text) that renders the segment in the jet weaker than the remainder of the muscle. SL is measured by laser diffraction, F by strain gauge, and $[Ca^{2+}]_i$ by Fura fluorescence using a PMT and image-intensified camera (CCD). Panel **B** shows the effects of a local jet with BDM: a jet containing BDM inhibits the activation of sarcomeres in the jet resulting in regional stretch of the muscle in the jet. Panel **C**. The spatiotemporal Ca^{2+} distribution shows that Ca^{2+} waves arise from the border between regions with and without the BDM jet following a repeated stimulation (2.5 Hz–7.5 sec). Arrowhead: moment of electrical stimulation.

along the long axis of the trabecula were calculated from the mean ratio across the region of interest (ROI: 250–300 × 25 pixels) and then expressed as $[Ca^{2+}]_i$ using linear regression between PMT and IIC ratio.[43] Finally, variations in local $[Ca^{2+}]_i$ along the trabeculae were studied through spatiotemporal diagrams as represented in FIGURE 1 C.

Protocols

We have studied the effect of various interventions on Ca^{2+} waves, which were induced by stimulus trains (2.5 Hz for 7.5 sec, repeated every 15 sec; $[Ca^{2+}]_o = 2.0$ mmol/L; $23.5°C^{43}$). Ca^{2+} overload was induced using 0.5 Hz pacing at varied $[Ca^{2+}]_o$ of 0.2–10 mM and the effect of the HC jet by measurement of regional SL during 0.5Hz pacing (25°C, $[Ca^{2+}]_o = 0.7$ mM) and quantification of Ca^{2+} waves following the stimulus trains $[Ca^{2+}]_{BATH} = 2.0$ mM.

The effects of SL on F and regional SL inside the jet containing caffeine or BDM were tested during 0.5 Hz regular stimulus at room temperature ($24.4 \pm 0.4°C$). The muscle length was set at 1.9, 2.0, or 2.1 µM of SL_0 before the jet exposure. In 12 trabeculae, we studied the effects of length changes on initiation and propagation of Ca^{2+} waves induced by exposing of the muscle to the jet containing caffeine or BDM. During exposure to the jet solutions Ca^{2+} waves were induced by the rapid stimulus train at SL 2.0 µM. When stimulated twitches and Ca^{2+} waves became steady, the SL was changed from 2.0 to 2.1 µM or to 1.9 µM and the $[Ca^{2+}]_i$ was measured using IIC before and less than 1 min after the length changes.

Data Analysis

Data were expressed as mean $\pm$ SEM. Statistical analysis was performed using unpaired t-test or (analysis of variance) ANOVA followed by a *post hoc* test. Differences were considered as significant when $P < 0.05$.

RESULTS

Ca^{2+} Waves Initiated in a Muscle Region Exposed to High $[Ca^2]_o$

As we have shown before, sarcomeres shortened (~12%) uniformly in these trabeculae during superfusion with normal HEPES solution. Muscle-twitch force decreased and the sarcomeres in the exposed segment were stretched by shortening the normal regions outside the jet when the jet contained caffeine, BDM, or low-$[Ca^{2+}]$.[2,33] During relaxation, the sarcomeres in the exposed segment shortened rapidly. Short trains of stimulation at 2.5 Hz reproducibly caused Ca^{2+} waves to arise from the borders exposed to the jet. These Ca^{2+} waves started during force relaxation of the last stimulated twitch and propagated into segments both inside and outside of the jet. Arrhythmias, in the form of nondriven rhythmic activity, were triggered when the amplitude of the Ca^{2+} wave was increased by raising $[Ca^{2+}]_o$. The arrhythmias disappeared when the muscle uniformity was restored by turning the jet off.[33]

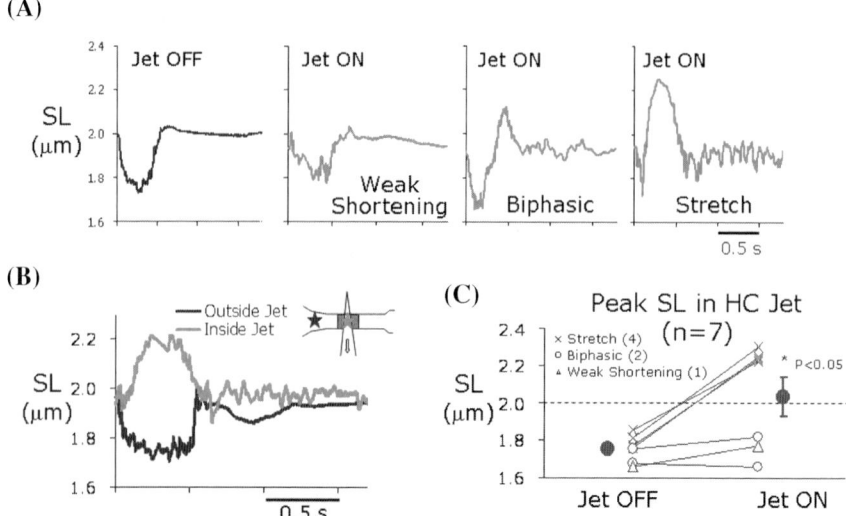

FIGURE 2. Panel **A**. Regional SL recordings in a jet with a high $[Ca^{2+}]_o$ (see text) show reduced shortening, biphasic, and stretch patterns with fluctuating resting SL during jet exposure (Jet ON). Panel **B**. Simultaneous SL recordings inside and outside the HC jet, showing nonuniform sarcomere shortening in the trabecula. Panel **C**. Summary of peak SL in the HC jet before (off) and during (on) the jet exposure. 0.5 Hz pacing, $[Ca^{2+}]_o = 0.7$ mM.

Exposure of the trabeculae to high $[Ca^{2+}]_o$ quite clearly caused Ca^{2+} overload of the SR because spontaneous contractile waves inside myocytes of the muscle were generated in the diastolic intervals between twitches. This spontaneous activity increased with external $[Ca^{2+}]_o$ and reduced force of the twitch following electrical stimuli in proportion to the probability of occurrence of spontaneous contractile events[24] (data not shown).

Similarly, exposure of the muscle segment in the jet to a high $[Ca^{2+}]_o$ in the medium consistently reduced force of the electrically stimulated (see e.g., FIG. 4). Exposure of the muscle segment in the jet to a high $[Ca^{2+}]_o$ in the medium reduced sarcomere shortening or turned the monophasic shortening pattern during the twitch into a pattern in which initial shortening was followed by stretch during the twitch, or into frank stretch during the whole twitch (FIG. 2). This sarcomere stretch occurred despite the fact that the $[Ca^{2+}]_i$ transient during the electrically stimulated twitch was increased (by ~ 25 %) (FIG. 3).

The high $[Ca^{2+}]_o$ jet caused local $[Ca^{2+}]_i$ transients that started 500–600 msec after onset of the electrically evoked $[Ca^{2+}]_i$ transient when the muscle was stimulated at a relatively low stimulus rate (FIG. 3; 1 Hz). This interval was comparable to the interval between the Ca^{2+} surge that we have observed in muscle exposed to CF, BDM, or low $[Ca^{2+}]_o$ jets. When we exposed the

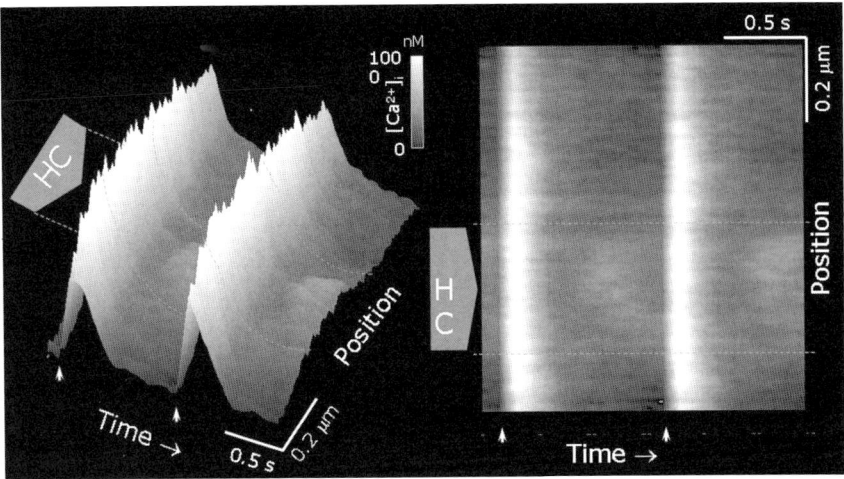

FIGURE 3. Ca^{2+} transients that are initiated in the region exposed to a high $[Ca^{2+}]$ jet. Three- (*left*) and corresponding two-dimensional (*right*) representations show regional $[Ca^{2+}]_i$ changes along the muscle during exposure to a high $[Ca^{2+}]$ jet (HC; *dotted lines*). Diastolic $[Ca^{2+}]_i$ rises in the jet region following Ca^{2+} transients are observed. Arrowhead indicates the moment of electrical stimulation (1Hz Pacing, $[Ca^{2+}]_o = 0.7$ mM calibrations as indicated).

muscles to stimulus trains, Ca^{2+} waves were generated; these Ca^{2+} waves now started in the center of the jet with high $[Ca^{2+}]_o$; this contrasts the behavior in muscle exposed to CF, BDM, or low $[Ca^{2+}]_o$ jets, where the Ca^{2+} waves invariably start in the border zone of the jet-exposed region.[33] Ca^{2+} waves starting in the high $[Ca^{2+}]_o$ jet region propagated with a similar V_{prop} (0.6–4.0 mm/sec) to the V_{prop} that we have described before for damaged muscle and for muscle in muscle exposed to CF, BDM, or low $[Ca^{2+}]_o$ jets.[33] It was striking in these experiments that the combination of a HC jet and repetitive stimulation with stimulus trains causes multiple nondriven $[Ca^{2+}]_i$ transients (FIG. 4).

It is likely that the oscillatory Ca^{2+} release that must have caused these transients may have been caused in part by Ca^{2+} overload of the SR.[44] It is not clear, therefore, what the contribution has been of a Ca^{2+} surge from the myofilaments compared to oscillatory Ca^{2+} release by the overloaded SR. We explored the contribution of oscillatory Ca^{2+} release by an overloaded SR compared to a Ca^{2+} surge from the myofilaments by suppressing cross-bridge activity using a jet solution in which the high $[Ca^{2+}]_o$ was combined with BDM. FIGURE 5 shows an example of the effects of this paradigm: oscillatory Ca^{2+} transients were still prominent, but the origin of the Ca^{2+} waves was now found (see start of the arrow in FIG. 5 B) in the border zone between the segment exposed to the jet and the segment of muscle remote from the jet. The wave initiation in HC+BDM occurred earlier than that in HC.

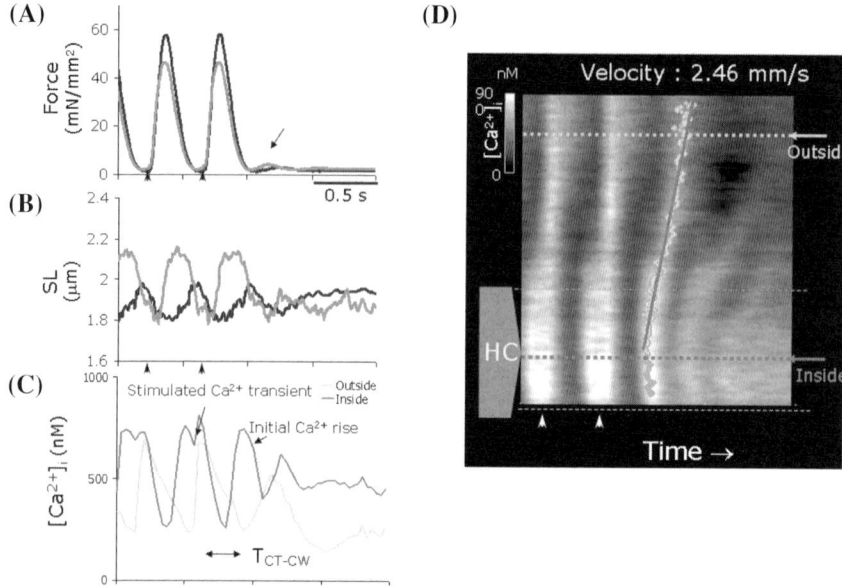

FIGURE 4. Ca^{2+} waves start in the region exposed to the HC jet. Panel **A.** Force (upper) and SL (lower) tracings showing that, during exposure of the HC jet, sarcomeres in the jet became stretched and a TPC (arrow) occurred, although the peak force of the twitches decreased. Panel **B.** Ca^{2+} waves were induced inside the HC jet region and propagated into the normal region. Panel **C.** Tracings of regional $[Ca^{2+}]_i$ inside and outside the HC jet region (shown in online version along red and green lines in panel C) during initiation of Ca^{2+} waves. Inside the HC jet, a large initial Ca^{2+} rise of the wave was observed ($C_W = 743$ nM), which reached 92% of the peak of the last Ca^{2+} transient (CT). Panel **D.** V_{prop} (2.46 mm/sec) was calculated by linear regression of displacement of the peaks of the Ca^{2+} wave. (2.5 Hz pacing, $[Ca^{2+}]_o = 2.0$ mM).

Ca^{2+} waves starting in the high $[Ca^{2+}]_o$ jet region tended to be faster than those in HC+BDM (1.2 ± 0.2; 0.5–1.8 mm/sec). The initial Ca^{2+} rise (CW) was large in both groups and corresponded to ≈90% of the peak stimulated Ca^{2+} transients (CT). A decrease of the initial Ca^{2+} rise (CW) may explain slower wave propagation in HC+BDM.

Arrhythmias could be induced in 4 of 10 muscles exposed to the jet of HC or HC + BDM by raising the frequency of the 7.5 sec stimulus train to 3 or 3.3 Hz-stimulus train. No arrhythmias could be induced in the absence of the jet.

Effects of Muscle Length on Force and Regional SL

If the requirement for the initiation of arrhythmogenic Ca^{2+} waves is that the region from where the Ca^{2+} waves start has a Ca^{2+}-loaded SR and exhibits active contraction owing to TnC activation of cross-bridges, albeit weaker than

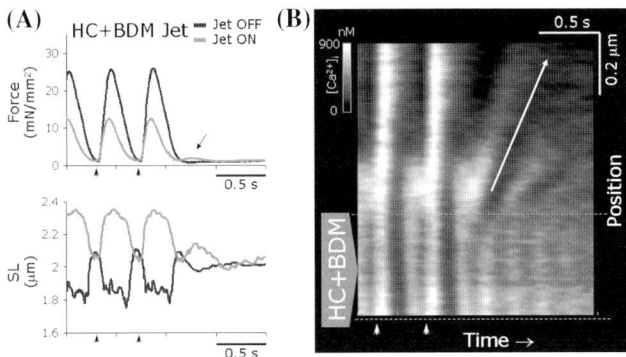

FIGURE 5. Ca^{2+} waves start in the border of the HC jet if contraction is eliminated by the addition of BDM to the jet solution. Panel **A.** Combination of HC and BDM in the jet reduced the peak force of twitches further and caused sarcomere stretch (lower) in the jet region. HC+BDM in the jet accelerated the TPC (arrow) and Ca^{2+} waves (Panel **B**), which now started in the region bordering the jet-exposed region where a large initial Ca^{2+} rise was observed. (2.5 Hz pacing, $[Ca^{2+}]_o = 2.0$ mM)

that of the neighboring muscle, one would expect that enhancing the amount of Ca^{2+} bound to TnC, for example, by stretch of the sarcomeres, would increase the Ca^{2+} surge during the relaxation phase and would accelerate Ca^{2+} waves. We tested this prediction in muscles exposed both to caffeine-containing jets and to BDM-containing jets.

Stretch (1.9–2.1 μM) increases force of the electrically stimulated twitches substantially without a noticeable change in the $[Ca^{2+}]_i$ transient.[45] The $[Ca^{2+}]_i$ transients in the jet as well as in the border zone and in the remote segments of the muscle were similar at 1.9, 2.0, and 2.1 μM (data not shown). Stretch increased the rate of decline of force during relaxation (FIG. 6) both in muscles that were uniformly superfused with HEPES solution and in muscles that were exposed to the caffeine and BDM jets.

The jet with caffeine or BDM reversibly decreased regional activation of sarcomeres in and around the jet, resulting in decrease in the peak force (∼50 % both using caffeine and BDM; FIG. 6 B) and sarcomere stretch in the jet-exposed region at each SL tested (1.9, 2.0, and 2.1 μM). During the jet exposure (with both BDM and caffeine), sarcomeres in the jet were stretched by stronger sarcomeres located outside the jet as reported previously.[2,33,46,47] As twitch force increased by lengthening of the muscle, the peak of sarcomere stretch in the jet-exposed region also increased up to ≈ 0.3 μM.

Effect of Length Changes on Ca^{2+} Waves

Ca^{2+} waves arose in the border zone at the edge of the segments exposed to the caffeine or BDM jets after the last-stimulated Ca^{2+} transient, and then

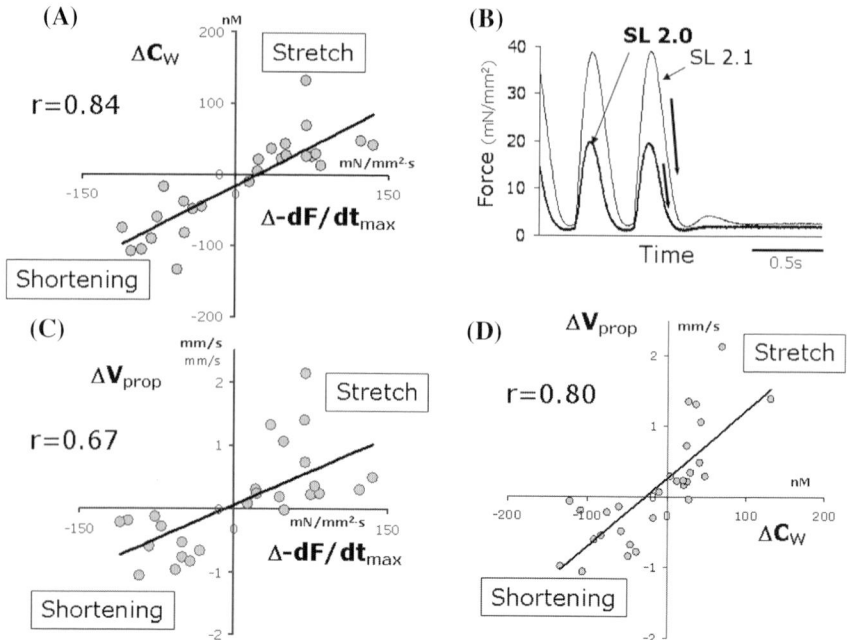

FIGURE 6. Accelerated force relaxation accelerates Ca^{2+}: Panel **B** shows that SL increase increases both twitch force and the rate of decline of twitch force. Panels **A** and **C** show that both amplitude of the initial $[Ca^{2+}]_i$ transient (ΔCw) in the border zone and V_{prop} of Ca^{2+} waves of BDM-exposed muscles are proportional to the rate of decline of the twitch at varied SL_o (range 1.9–2.1 µM; see text for details). Panel **D** shows that V_{prop} correlates tightly with ΔCw.

propagated into the normal muscle outside the jet as well as into the segment exposed to the BDM jet but not into the segment exposed to the caffeine jet.[33] Initiation of the Ca^{2+} waves occurred late during relaxation of the last stimulated twitch (see FIG. 6 A), corresponding to $26 \pm 5\%$ (caffeine; $n = 16$) and $23 \pm 5\%$ (BDM; $n = 11$) of peak force development at SL_0 2.0 µM, were similar to our previous data.[33] Lengthening the sarcomeres from 1.9 to 2.1 µM increased the propagation velocities (V_{prop}) of Ca^{2+} waves (0.98 to 2.00 mm/sec) in caffeine and from 1.14 to 2.66 mm/sec in BDM, together with an increase in the amplitude of the $[Ca^{2+}]_i$ transients during the waves.

We have studied the effect of length changes on initiation and propagation of Ca^{2+} waves separately. We calculated V_{prop} as well as the initial $[Ca^{2+}]_i$ rise (C_W) during initiation of Ca^{2+} waves. Muscle stretch (SL: 1.9–2.1 µm) significantly increased V_{prop} (0.54 ± 0.20 to 1.19 ± 0.17 mm/sec in caffeine and 0.53 ± 0.17 to 1.99 ± 0.62 mm/sec in BDM) and C_W (327 ± 25 to 351 ± 28 nmol/L in caffeine and from 312 ± 65 to 385 ± 38 nmol/L in BDM). SL did not affect SR Ca^{2+} loading (reflected by the peak of the last stimulated Ca^{2+} transient)[45] in the region of the wave initiation (i.e., border zone) and in the region where the Ca^{2+} wave propagated (i.e., outside the jet), suggesting that changes in C_W and V_{prop} were independent of those in regional Ca^{2+} loading. In contrast, V_{prop} correlated strongly and linearly with ΔC_W ($r = 0.8$, $P < 0.001$), independent of the composition of the jet solution, suggesting that changes in V_{prop} by the length changes depend on those in C_W, that is, the magnitude of the initial $[Ca^{2+}]$ rise during the wave initiation.

Effect of Force Development and Relaxation on Ca^{2+} Waves

We have further explored the dependence of wave generation and propagation on the factors that dictate the initial rise of $[Ca^{2+}]_i$ at the initiation site. Our previous work has indicated that the initial $[Ca^{2+}]$ rise during the wave initiation is probably caused by Ca^{2+} dissociation from myofilaments as a result of quick release of active sarcomeres.[48] The amount of Ca^{2+} binding and dissociation from myofilaments by length changes has been shown to be correlated with those in the number of Ca^{2+}-activated cross-bridges; that is, force development of the myocardium.[49] Therefore, we compared the peak of force development (F_T) and the maximum rate of force relaxation ($-dF/dt_{max}$) during the last stimulated twitch with subsequent initiation and propagation of Ca^{2+} waves. F_T increased with stretch both and during exposure to jets with caffeine (4.6-fold) and BDM (3.1-fold) while $-dF/dt_{max}$ also showed similar changes (2.5- and 2.2-fold, respectively). Changes in ΔC_W and ΔV_{prop} of the Ca^{2+} waves correlated clearly with F_T induced by stretch as well as those in $-dF/dt_{max}$ (FIG. 6 A, C). These results strongly suggested that force development and relaxation of the twitch determine the initiation and subsequent propagation of Ca^{2+} waves.

Effect of Dynamic Stretch of the Muscle during Relaxation on Ca^{2+} Waves

The existence cooperativity of force and Ca^{2+} binding by TnC[1] predicts that the initial Ca^{2+} surge is proportional to the amount of Ca^{2+} bound to TnC and to the rate of force decline during relaxation. The rate of force decline is determined in the experiments by the interplay between the strong and weakened segments of the muscle. This interplay leads to rapid shortening of the weak but still contracting sarcomeres exposed to the jet. We tested whether the Ca^{2+} waves are modified by maintaining SL in the weakened segment at the length that was reached during the stretch during the twitch. Evidently, stretch early during the twitch enhances force owing to the positive slope of the F–SL relationship.

We have used exponential stretches ($< 10\%$ ML) to measure the amplitude of the TPC at the new SL; we corrected for length dependence force development of the TPC following the dynamic stretch by expressing the amplitude of the

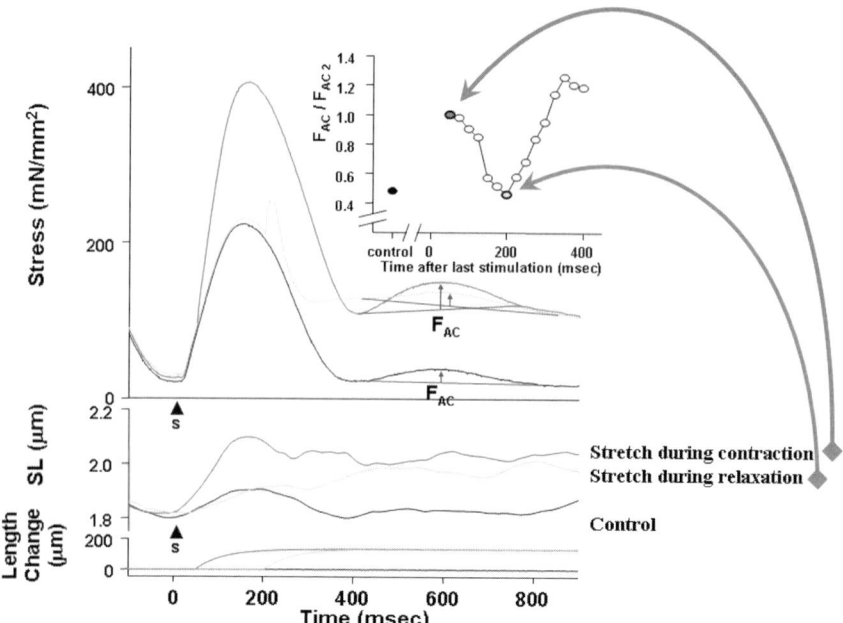

FIGURE 7. Elimination of sarcomere shortening in the border zone of the segment exposed to a BDM jet reduces but does not eliminate the TPC. The upper tracing shows three twitches: (1) the lower tracing at control SLo (1.8 µM; see bottom panel) when sarcomeres in the border zone are stretched by the stronger segments in the muscle [and shorten in the border zone during relaxation;] (2) the middle tracing in the top panel shows force when SL in the border zone is kept constant during relaxation by muscle stretch (starting at 200 msec; bottom panel); (3) a large twitch, which occurs when SL in the border zone is increased by a stretch at the beginning of the twitch. The force of the TPC (F_{AC}) of the control at short SL (1) is similar to the F_{AC} after stretch during relaxation (2) and reduced compared to (3) when the stretch was applied in the beginning of the twitch. The latter reduction (see inset) depended on the moment of the stretch and was proportional to the difference in twitch force between (2) and (3) (see inset).

force of the TPC as a fraction of the amplitude of the TPC following a twitch in which sarcomeres had been stretched at the onset of the twitch. FIGURE 7 top panel shows that the stretches indeed eliminated sarcomere shortening during relaxation. The stretches enhanced force transiently in proportion to the rate of SL increase. Still, maximal force during twitches remained similar to force at the short SL (1.8 µm) and never exceeded 60% of peak force at the greater SL. Accordingly, the amplitude of the TPC induced by elimination of shortening during the relaxation remained similar to TPC-amplitude at short SL 1.8 µM and was 50% of the amplitude of the TPC at SL 2.0 µM (FIG. 7 inset). The TPC following dynamic stretch during relaxation was smaller and started later than the TPC at the SL 2.0 µM following the early dynamic stretch.

DISCUSSION

These findings are consistent with previous observations in muscles exposed to a jet that renders the segment in the jet weaker than the neighboring muscle segments.[2,33] In those studies, we concluded that the requirements for the initiation of arrhythmogenic Ca^{2+} waves is that the region from where the Ca^{2+} waves start has a Ca^{2+}-loaded SR and exhibits active contraction, albeit weaker than that of the neighboring muscle. Exposure of the muscle to a high $[Ca^{2+}]_o$ reduces contractile force in proportion to an increase of spontaneous Ca^{2+} release by the overloaded SR, as has been shown both in normal cardiac muscle[50] and in muscle from failing rat heart.[51] Consistent with these previous studies we observed here that in muscle exposed to a HC jet indeed spontaneous diastolic Ca^{2+} release occurred and sarcomere shortening turned locally into stretch when the muscle was exposed to a jet of HC solution. Similar to the findings in muscles locally exposed to a jet that weakens contraction, it appeared that the cycle of stretch followed by shortening of the sarcomeres during relaxation of the normal segments of the muscle Ca^{2+} waves were initiated in the stretched region. Different from the findings in muscles locally exposed to a jet that weakens contraction, it was clear now that the Ca^{2+} waves started in the segment exposed to the HC jet and not in the border of the jet-exposed region. It is possible that the segment exposed to the HC jet generated such large SR Ca^{2+} overload-induced Ca^{2+} release that this spontaneous diastolic Ca^{2+} release alone was sufficiently large to account for the initiation of Ca^{2+} waves. This is unlikely, however, because inhibition of cross-bridge activity by HC+BDM in the jet shifted the site of origin of the Ca^{2+} waves to the border zone of the jet. Hence, the experiments using HC and HC+ BDM jets are consistent with the hypothesis that initiation of arrhythmogenic Ca^{2+} waves requires that the region from where the Ca^{2+} waves start has a Ca^{2+}-loaded SR and exhibits active contraction, albeit weaker than that of the neighboring muscle. Our experiments also suggest that SR Ca^{2+} overload facilitates the generation of Ca^{2+} waves.

We have previously proposed that the molecular mechanism underlying SL dependence of Ca^{2+} binding to TnC is that cross-bridge force exerted on the actin filament deforms the TnC molecule thus retarding the dissociation of Ca^{2+} from TnC.[2] This effect is bound to be SL-dependent since the number of myosin cross-bridges attaching to actin increases with SL over the range of operation of cardiac muscle. This hypothesis predicts that removal of an external load on a muscle during the twitch will cause a robust additional $[Ca^{2+}]_i$ transient as has been shown experimentally.[52] It is well known that a large amount of Ca^{2+} is bound to TnC during contraction and that the amount of Ca^{2+} bound to the TnC increases with sarcomere stretch owing to the increased number of cross-bridges that interact with actin in the stretched sarcomere. The increased binding of Ca^{2+} to TnC with stretch accelerates the decline of the $[Ca^{2+}]_i$ transient without a change in its amplitude; our data (not shown here[45]) confirm this prediction. It follows that Ca^{2+} release from TnC upon rapid unloading will increase at greater SL. The above hypothesis predicts, therefore, that the Ca^{2+} surge in the nonuniform muscle increases when the muscle operates at greater length; the increased Ca^{2+} surge may in turn increase SR Ca^{2+} release and accelerate propagation of the Ca^{2+} waves. Our findings illustrated in FIGURE 6 indeed show that stretch increases the initial $[Ca^{2+}]_i$ transient ΔCw and Ca^{2+} waves accelerated in proportion to the increase of the initial $[Ca^{2+}]_i$ transient.

The Ca^{2+} surge and ensuing Ca^{2+} waves start during the rapid decline of force during the twitch, while the sarcomeres in the strong muscle segments relax and lengthen; this rapid force decline also coincides with rapid shortening of the sarcomeres in the stretched segment. We tested the contribution of the rapid shortening to the induction of TPCs by eliminating shortening in the weakened segment by stretch at varied time during relaxation of the muscle. We measured SL in the border zone (diameter ~ 100 μM) of the segment exposed to a BDM-containing jet, which precluded simultaneous $[Ca^{2+}]_i$ measurement. Hence, conclusions about the behavior of $[Ca^{2+}]_i$ had to be derived from the observed force and must be considered with caution. The stretches indeed eliminated sarcomere shortening during relaxation (FIG. 7 middle trace of SL panel), but did not enhance twitch force significantly. Elimination of shortening during relaxation of the sarcomeres in the weak segment did not abolish TPCs as is illustrated in FIGURE 7. F_{TPC} was unaffected when compared to F_{TPC} of F_{TPC} without the stretch and reduced by 50% compared to the F_{TPC} when the muscle had been stretched early during the twitch; the latter reduction of F_{TPC} was proportional to the difference in twitch force at short SL compared to long SL. These observations suggest that the shortening of sarcomeres in the weakened segment of muscle does not affect the induction of the Ca^{2+} wave and are consistent with the assumption that the Ca^{2+} wave is initiated by a Ca^{2+} surge that originates from the myofilaments as a result of the rapid decline of force.

ACKNOWLEDGMENTS

This work was supported by grants from Alberta Heart and Stroke Foundation CIHR and NIH (HL 58860-06A2). H.E.D.J. ter Keurs is a Medical Scientist of the Alberta Heritage Foundation for Medical Research (AHFMR).

REFERENCES

1. HUNTER, P.J., A.D. MCCULLOCH & H.E.D.J. TER KEURS. 1998. Modelling the mechanical properties of cardiac muscle. Prog. Biophys. Mol. Biol. **69:** 289–331.

2. TER KEURS, H.E.D.J., Y. WAKAYAMA, et al. 2005. Role of sarcomere mechanics and Ca2+ overload in Ca2+ waves and arrhythmias in rat cardiac muscle. Ann. N. Y. Acad. Sci. **1047:** 345–365.
3. HOUSMANS, P.R., N.K.M. LEE & J.R. BLINKS. 1983. Active shortening retards the decline of the intracellular calcium transient in mammalian heart muscle. Science **221:** 159–161.
4. DANIEL, S.M.C.G., D. FEDIDA, C. LAMONT & H.E.D.J. TER KEURS. 1991. Role of the sarcolemma in triggered propagated contractions in rat cardiac trabeculae. Circ. Res. **68:** 1408–1421.
5. MULDER, B.J.M., P.P. DE TOMBE & H.E.D.J. TER KEURS. 1989. Spontaneous and propagated contractions in rat cardiac trabeculae. J. Gen. Physiol. **93:** 943–961.
6. DANIELS, M.C.G. & H.E.D.J. TER KEURS. 1990. Spontaneous contractions in rat cardiac trabeculae: trigger mechanism and propagation velocity. J. Gen. Physiol. **95:** 1123–1137.
7. DANIELS, M.C.G. & H.E.D.J. TER KEURS. 1990. Propagated contractions in rat cardiac trabeculae: effects of caffeine, ryanodine, Bay K 8644, and D-600 [abstract]. Biophys. J. **57:** 170a.
8. MIURA, M., P.A. BOYDEN & H.E.D.J. TER KEURS. 1999. Ca2+ waves during triggered propagated contractions in intact trabeculae. Determinants of the velocity of propagation. Circ. Res. **84:** 1459–1468.
9. CHENG, H., W.J. LEDERER & M.B. CANNELL. 1993. Calcium sparks: elementary events underlying excitation-contraction coupling in heart muscle. Science **262:** 740–744.
10. CANNELL, M.B., H. CHENG & W.J. LEDERER. 1994. Spatial nonuniformities in Cai during excitation contraction coupling in cardiac myocytes. Biophys. J. **67:** 1942–1956.
11. LOPEZ-LOPEZ, J.R., P.S. SHACKLOCK & W.G. WIER. 1994. Local stochastic release of Ca2+ in voltage clamped rat heart cells: visualization with confocal microscopy. J. Physiol. **480:** 21–29.
12. LOPEZ-LOPEZ, J.R., P.S. SHACKLOCK & W.G. WIER. 1995. Local Ca2+ transients triggered by single L type Ca2+ channel currents in cardiac cells. Science **268:** 1042–1045.
13. CANNELL, M.B., H. CHENG & W.J. LEDERER. 1995. The control of calcium release in heart muscle. Science **268:** 1045–1049.
14. WANG, S.-Q., L.-S. SONG, E.G. LAKATTA & H. CHENG. 2001. Ca2+ signalling between single L type Ca2+ channels and ryanodine receptors in heart cells. Nature **410:** 592–596.
15. CHENG, H., M.R. LEDERER, W.J. LEDERER & M.B. CANNELL. 1996. Calcium sparks and [Ca++]i waves in cardiac myocytes. Am. J. Physiol. **270:** C148–C159.
16. WIER, W.G., T.M. EGAN & J.R. LOPEZ-LOPEZ. 1994. Local control of excitation contraction coupling in rat heart cells. J. Physiol. **474:** 463–471.
17. STERN, M.D., A.A. KORT, G.M. BHATNAGAR & E.G. LAKATTA. 1983. Scattered light intensity fluctuations in diastolic rat cardiac muscle caused by spontaneous calcium dependent cellular mechanical oscillations. J. Gen. Physiol. **82:** 119–153.
18. WIER, W.G., M.B. CANNELL, J.R. BERLIN, et al. 1987. Cellular and subcellular heterogeneity of intracellular calcium concentration in single heart cells revealed by fura-2. Science **235:** 325–328.
19. TAKAMATSU, T. & W.G. WIER. 1990. Calcium waves in mammalian heart: quantification of origin magnitude waveform and velocity. FASEB J. **4:** 1519–1525.

20. FABIATO, A. & F. FABIATO. 1978. Calcium-induced release of calcium from the sarcoplasmic reticulum of skinned cells from adult human, dog, cat, rabbit, rat, and frog hearts and from fetal and new-born rat ventricles. Ann. N. Y. Acad. Sci. **307:** 491–522.
21. FABIATO, A. 1985. Spontaneous versus triggered contractions of "calcium-tolerant" cardiac cells from the adult rat ventricle. Basic Res. Cardiol. **80:** 83–88.
22. CAPOGROSSI, M.C. & E.G. LAKATTA. 1985. Frequency modulation and synchronization of spontaneous oscillations in cardiac cells. Am. J. Physiol. **248:** H412–H418.
23. KORT, A.A. & E.G. LAKATTA. 1984. Calcium-dependent mechanical oscillations occur spontaneously in unstimulated mammalian cardiac tissues. Circ. Res. **54:** 396–404.
24. OBAYASHI, M., B. XIAO, B.D. STUYVERS, et al. 2006. Spontaneous diastolic contractions and phosphorylation of the cardiac ryanodine receptor at serine-2808 in congestive heart failure in rat. Cardiovasc. Res. **69:** 140–151.
25. ORCHARD, C.H., D.A. EISNER & D.G. ALLEN. 1983. Oscillations of intracellular calcium in mammalian cardiac muscle. Nature **304:** 735–738.
26. WIER, W.G., M.B. CANNELL, et al. 1987. Cellular and subcellular heterogeneity of intracellular calcium concentration in single heart cells revealed by fura-2. Science **235:** 325–328.
27. KASS, R.S., W.J. LEDERER, R.W. TSIEN & R. WEINGART. 1978. Role of calcium ions in transient inward currents and aftercontractions induced by strophanthidin in cardiac Purkinje fibres. J. Physiol. **281:** 187–208.
28. ALLEN, D.G., D.A. EISNER & C.H. ORCHARD. 1984. Characterization of oscillations of intracellular calcium concentration in ferret ventricular muscle. J. Physiol. **352:** 113–128.
29. MATSUDA, H., A. NOMA, Y. KURACHI & H. IRISAWA. 1982. Transient depolarization and spontaneous voltage fluctuations in isolated single cells from guinea-pig ventricles. Circ. Res. **51:** 142–151.
30. BOYDEN, P.A., C. BARBHAYA, T. LEE & H.E.D.J. TER KEURS. 2003. Nonuniform Ca2+ transients and arrhythmogenic Purkinje cells that survive in the infarcted canine heart. Cardiovasc. Res. **57:** 681–693.
31. BOYDEN, P.A., J. PU, J. PINTO & H.E.D.J. TER KEURS. 2000. Ca2+ transients and Ca2+ waves in purkinje cells: role in action potential initiation. Circ. Res. **86:** 448–455.
32. MIURA, M., P.A. BOYDEN & H.E.D.J. TER KEURS. 1998. Ca^{2+} waves during triggered propagated contractions in intact trabeculae. Am. J. Physiol. 274: H266–H276.
33. WAKAYAMA, Y., M. MIURA, B.D. STUYVERS, et al. 2005. Spatial nonuniformity of excitation-contraction coupling causes arrhythmogenic Ca2+ waves in rat cardiac muscle. Circ. Res. **96:** 1266–1273.
34. TER KEURS, H.E.D.J., W.H. RIJNSBURGER, et al. 1980. Tension development and sarcomere length in rat cardiac trabeculae. Evidence of length-dependent activation. Circ. Res. **46:** 703–714.
35. KONISHI, M., S. KURIHARA & T. SAKAI. 1984. The effects of caffeine on tension development and intracellular calcium transients in rat ventricular muscle. J. Physiol. **355:** 605–618.
36. SITSAPESAN, R. & A.J. WILLIAMS. 1990. Mechanisms of caffeine activation of single calcium-release channels of sheep cardiac sarcoplasmic reticulum. J. Physiol. **423:** 425–439.

37. SELLIN, L.C. & J.J. MCARDLE. 1994. Multiple effects of 2,3-butanedione monoxime. Pharmacol. Toxicol. **74:** 305–313.
38. HERRMANN, C., J. WRAY, F. Travers & T. BARMAN. 1992. Effect of 2,3-butanedione monoxime on sarcoplasmic reticulum of saponin-treated rat cardiac muscle. Biochemistry **31:** 12227–12232.
39. PHILLIPS, R.M. & R.A. ALTSCHULD. 1996. 2,3-butanedione 2-monoxime (BDM) induces calcium release from canine cardiac sarcoplasmic reticulum. Biochem. Biophys. Res. Commun. **229:** 154–157.
40. BACKX, P.H.M., W.D. GAO, M.D. AZAN-BACKX & E. MARBAN. 1994. Mechanism of force inhibition by 2,3-butanedione monoxime in rat cardiac muscle: roles of [Ca++]i and cross-bridge kinetics. J. Physiol. **476:** 487–500.
41. BACKX, P.H.M. & H.E.D.J. TER KEURS. 1993. Fluorescent properties of rat cardiac trabecule microinjected with fura-2 salt. Am. J. Physiol. **264:** H1098–H1110.
42. GROUSELLE, M., B. STUYVERS, et al. 1991. Digital imaging microscopy analysis of calcium release from sarcoplasmic reticulum in single rat cardiac myocytes. Eur. J. Physiol. **418:** 109–119.
43. MIURA, M., Y. WAKAYAMA, Y. SUGAI, et al. 2001. Effect of transient stretch on intracellular Ca2+ during triggered propagated contractions in intact trabeculae. Can. J. Physiol. Pharmacol. **79:** 68–72.
44. JIANG, D., R. WANG, et al. 2005. Enhanced store overload-induced Ca2+ release and channel sensitivity to luminal Ca2+ activation are common defects of RyR2 mutations linked to ventricular tachycardia and sudden death. Circ. Res. **97:** 1173–1181.
45. BACKX, P.H. & H.E.D.J. TER KEURS. 1993. Fluorescent properties of rat cardiac trabeculae microinjected with fura-2 salt. Am. J. Physiol. **264:** H1098–H1110.
46. TER KEURS, H.E.D.J., Y. WAKAYAMA, M. MIURA, et al. 2006. Arrhythmogenic Ca(2+) release from cardiac myofilaments. Prog. Biophys. Mol. Biol. **90:** 151–171.
47. Ter KEURS, H.E.D.J., Y. WAKAYAMA, M. MIURA, et al. 2005. Spatial nonuniformity of contraction causes arrhythmogenic Ca2+ waves in rat cardiac muscle. Ann. N. Y. Acad. Sci. **1047:** 345–365.
48. WAKAYAMA, Y., Y. SUGAI, Y. KAGAYA, et al. 2001. Stretch and quick release of cardiac trabeculae accelerates Ca2+ waves and triggered propagated contractions. Am. J. Physiol. Circ. Physiol. **281:** H2133–2142.
49. ALLEN, D.G. & J.C. KENTISH. 1985. The cellular basis of the length-tension relation in cardiac muscle. J. Mol. Cell. Cardiol. **17:** 821–840.
50. CAPOGROSSI, M.C., M.D. STERN, H.A. SPURGEON & E.G. LAKATTA. 1988. Spontaneous calcium release from the sarcoplasmic reticulum limits calcium-dependent twitch potentiation in individual cardiac myocytes. J. Gen. Physiol. **91:** 133–155.
51. DAVIDOFF, A.W., P.A. BOYDEN, et al. 2004. Spontaneous sarcomere activity in rat cardiac muscle: implications for force and rhythm of the failing heart. Ann. N. Y. Acad. Sci. **1015:** 84–95.
52. ALLEN, D.G. & S. KURIHARA. 1982. The effects of muscle length on intracellular calcium transients in mammalian cardiac muscle. J. Physiol. **327:** 79–94.

Cellular Basis for the Repolarization Waves of the ECG

CHARLES ANTZELEVITCH

Masonic Medical Research Laboratory, Utica, New York 13501, USA

ABSTRACT: One hundred years after Willem Einthoven first recorded the electrocardiogram (ECG), physicians and scientists are still debating the cellular basis for the various waves of the ECG. In this review, our focus is on the cellular basis for the J, T, and U waves of the ECG. The J wave and T wave are thought to arise as a consequence of voltage gradients that develop as a result of the electrical heterogeneities that exist within the ventricular myocardium. The presence of a prominent action potential notch in epicardium but not endocardium gives rise to a voltage gradient during ventricular activation that inscribes the J wave. Transmural and apico-basal voltage gradients developing as a result of difference in the time course of repolarization of the epicardial, M, and endocardial cell action potentials, and the more positive plateau potential of the M cell contribute to inscription of the T wave. Amplification of these heterogeneities results in abnormalities of the J wave and T wave, leading to the development of the Brugada, long QT, and short QT syndromes. The basis for the U wave has long been a matter of debate. One theory attributes the U wave to mechanoelectrical feedback. A second theory ascribes it to voltage gradients within ventricular myocardium and a third to voltage gradients between the ventricular myocardium and the His–Purkinje system. Although direct evidence in support of any of these three hypotheses is lacking, recent studies involving the short QT syndrome have generated renewed interest in the mechanoelectrical hypothesis.

KEYWORDS: heterogeneity; arrhythmias; electrophysiology; long QT; short QT; Brugada syndrome

INTRODUCTION TO THE ECG

Despite the span of more than 100 years since Willem Einthoven first recorded the electrocardiogram (ECG),[1,2] physicians and scientists are still debating the cellular basis for the various waves of the ECG. Our focus in this review will be on the J, T, and U waves, the cellular basis for repolarization waves of the ECG. The J wave and T wave are thought to arise as a consequence

Address for correspondence: Prof. Charles Antzelevitch, Ph.D., Masonic Medical Research Laboratory, Utica, NY 13501, USA. Voice: 315-735-2217 ext. 117; fax: 315-735-5648.
 e-mail: ca@mmrl.edu

of voltage gradients that develop as a result of the electrical heterogeneities that exist within the ventricular myocardium. The basis for the U wave has long been a matter of debate. We will explore the three prevailing theories that the U wave is (i) caused by mechanoelectrical feedback, (ii) due to voltage gradients within ventricular myocardium, or (iii) due to voltage gradients between the ventricular myocardium and the His–Purkinje system.

Electrical Heterogeneity of Ventricular Myocardium

Studies from our and other laboratories have demonstrated that ventricular myocardium is not homogeneous as previously thought, but is comprised of three electrically and functionally distinct cell types. A number of studies have highlighted regional differences in electrical properties of ventricular cells as well as differences in the response of the different cell types to pharmacological agents and pathophysiological states.[3,4] Among the heterogeneities uncovered are electrical and pharmacologic distinctions between endocardium and epicardium of the canine, feline, rabbit, rat. and human heart as well as differences in the electrophysiologic characteristics and pharmacologic responsiveness of M cells located in the deep structures of the ventricles of the heart.

Ventricular epicardial and M, but not endocardial action potentials display a prominent phase 1 due to a large transient outward current (Ito), giving rise to a spike-and-dome or notched configuration. Regional differences in Ito have been demonstrated in canine, feline, rabbit, rat, and human ventricular myocytes.[4] Important differences also exist in the magnitude of Ito and action potential notch between right and left ventricular epicardial and M cells with right ventricular cells (RV) displaying a much greater Ito.[5,6]

The hallmark of the M cell is the ability of its action potential to prolong more than that of epicardial or endocardial cells in response to a slowing of rate and/or in response to drugs with QT-prolonging actions.[7] The ionic basis for these features includes the presence of a smaller, slowly activating, delayed rectifier current (IKs), a larger, late sodium current (late INa), and a larger electrogenic sodium–calcium exchange current (INa-Ca). Cells with M cell characteristics have been reported in the canine, guinea pig, rabbit, pig, and human ventricles.[8]

The Electrocardiographic J Wave

The presence of a prominent action potential notch in epicardium but not endocardium gives rise to a transmural voltage gradient during ventricular activation that manifests as a late delta wave following the QRS or what more commonly is referred to as a J wave[9] or Osborn wave. A distinct J wave is often observed under baseline conditions in the ECG of some animal species,

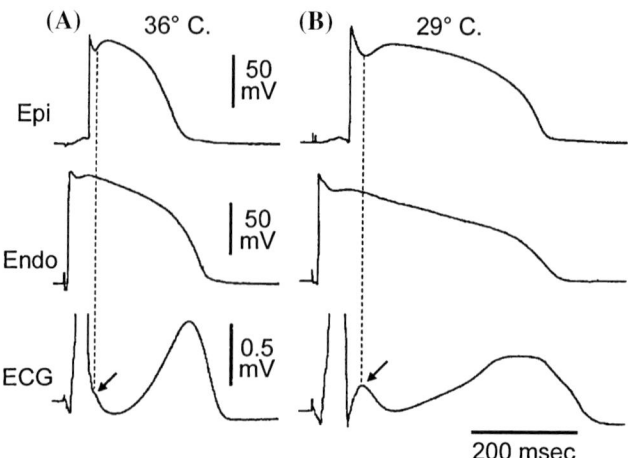

FIGURE 1. Hypothermia-induced J wave. Each panel shows transmembrane action potentials from the epicardial (Epi) and endocardial (Endo) regions of an arterially perfused canine left ventricular wedge and a transmural ECG simultaneously recorded. (**A**): A small but distinct action potential notch in epicardium but not in endocardium is associated with an elevated J point at the R-ST junction (arrow) at 36°C. (**B**): A decrease in the temperature of the perfusate to 29°C results in an increase in the amplitude and width of the action potential notch in epicardium but not endocardium, leading to the development of a transmural voltage gradient that manifests as a prominent J wave on the ECG (arrow). (Modified from Ref. 67 with permission.)

including dogs and baboons. Humans more commonly display a J point elevation rather than a distinct J wave. A prominent J wave in the human ECG is considered pathognomonic of hypothermia[10–12] or hypercalcemia.[13,14]

A transmural gradient in the distribution of Ito is responsible for the transmural gradient in the magnitude of phase 1 and action potential notch, which in turn gives rise to a voltage gradient across the ventricular wall responsible for the inscription of the J wave or J point elevation in the ECG.[15–17] Direct evidence in support of the hypothesis that the J wave is caused by a transmural gradient in the magnitude of the Ito-mediated action potential notch derives from experiments conducted in the arterially perfused right ventricular wedge preparation showing a correlation between the amplitude of the epicardial action potential notch and that of the J wave recorded during interventions that alter the appearance of the electrocardiographic J wave, including hypothermia, premature stimulation (restitution), and block of Ito by 4-aminopyridine (4-AP)[9] (FIG. 1).

The molecular basis for the transmural distribution of Ito has long been a subject of debate. The transmural gradient of Ito in the dog has been ascribed to a transmural distribution of (i) KCND3 gene (Kv4.3), which encodes the α subunit of the Ito channel,[18] (ii) KChIP2, a β subunit that coassembles with Kv4.3,[19] and (iii) IRX5, a transcriptional factor regulating KCND3.[20]

Transmural activation within the thin wall of the RV is relatively rapid causing the J wave to be buried inside the QRS. Thus, although the action potential notch is most prominent in right ventricular epicardium, right ventricular myocardium would be expected to contribute relatively little to the manifestation of the J wave under normal conditions. These observations are consistent with the manifestation of the J wave in ECG leads in which the mean vector axis is transmurally oriented across the left ventricle and septum. Accordingly, the J wave in the dog is most prominent in leads II, III, aVR, aVF, and mid to left precordial leads V_3 through V_6. A similar picture is seen in the human ECG.[14,21] In addition, vectorcardiography indicates that the J wave forms an extra loop that occurs at the junction of the QRS and T loops.[22] It is directed leftward and anteriorly, which explains its prominence in leads associated with the left ventricle.

The first description of the J wave appeared in the 1920s in animal experiments involving hypercalcemia.[13] The first extensive description and characterization appeared 30 years later by Osborn in a study involving experimental hypothermia in dogs.[23] The appearance of a prominent J wave in the clinic is typically associated with pathophysiological conditions, including hypothermia[10,21] and hypercalcemia.[13,14] The prominent J wave induced by hypothermia is the result of a marked accentuation of the spike-and-dome morphology of the action potential of M and epicardial cells (i.e., an increase in both width and magnitude of the notch) (FIG. 1). In addition to inducing a more prominent notch, hypothermia produces a slowing of conduction, which permits the epicardial notch to clear the QRS to manifest a distinct J wave. Hypercalcemia-induced accentuation of the J wave[13,14,24] may also be explained on the basis of an accentuation of the epicardial action potential notch, possibly as a result of an augmentation of the calcium-activated chloride current and a decrease in I_{Ca}.[25]

A prominent action potential notch predisposes canine ventricular epicardium to all-or-none repolarization and phase 2 reentry. Under ischemic conditions and in response to sodium channel blockers, parasympathetic agonists, potassium channel blockers, and a variety of other drugs, canine ventricular epicardium exhibits an all-or-none repolarization at the end of phase 1 of the action potential, leading to a marked abbreviation of the action potential. Failure of the action potential dome to develop at some epicardial sites but not others gives rise to a marked dispersion of repolarization. Propagation of the action potential dome from sites at which it is maintained to sites at which it is abolished can cause local reexcitation of the preparation. This mechanism, called phase 2 reentry, produces a very closely coupled extrasystole, which can in turn initiate one or more cycles of circus movement reentry.[4,26] The amplitude and width of the J wave provides an index of the prominence of the spike-and-dome morphology of the epicardial response, and thus may be of diagnostic value in identifying subjects predisposed to phase 2 reentry or individuals who may be inclined to develop life-threatening arrhythmias such as the Brugada syndrome or other forms of idiopathic ventricular fibrillation.[27,28]

Evidence in support of a role for phase 2 reentry in the initiation of polymorphic ventricular tachycardia (VT) in humans has recently been provided by Thomsen and coworkers.[29] The accentuation of epicardial action potential and eventual loss of the dome underlies the ST segment elevation and arrhythmogenic substrate associated with the Brugada syndrome.[30,31]

The Electrocardiographic T Wave

Transmural and apico-basal heterogeneities of final repolarization of the action potential within ventricular myocardium are thought to be responsible for inscription of the T wave.[32,33] Studies involving the arterially perfused wedge have shown that currents flowing down voltage gradients on either side of the M region are in large part responsible for the T wave.[32]

Under baseline conditions (FIG. 2 A), the T wave begins when the plateau of epicardial action potential separates from that of the M cell. As epicardium repolarizes, the voltage gradient between epicardium and the M region continues to grow giving rise to the ascending limb of the T wave. The voltage gradient between the M region and epicardium (ΔV_{M-Epi}) reaches a peak when the epicardium is fully repolarized—this marks the peak of the T wave. On the other end of the ventricular wall, the endocardial plateau deviates from that of the M cell, generating an opposing voltage gradient (ΔV_{Endo-M}) and corresponding current that limits the amplitude of the T wave and contributes to the initial part of the descending limb of the T wave. The voltage gradient between the endocardium and the M region reaches a peak when the endocardium is fully repolarized. The gradient continues to decline as the M cells repolarize. All gradients are extinguished when the longest M cells are fully repolarized. Under hypokalemic conditions ($[K^+]_o = 1.5$ mM) combined with an IKr blocker dl-sotalol (100 uM) (FIG. 2 B), the QT interval prolongs and a bifurcation of the T wave is apparent. The rate of repolarization of phase 3 of the action potential is slowed giving rise to smaller opposing transmural currents that cross over producing a low amplitude bifid T wave. Initially, the voltage gradient between the epicardium and M regions (M-Epi) is greater than that between endocardium and M region (Endo-M). When endocardium pulls away from the M cell, the opposing gradient (Endo-M) increases, interrupting the ascending limb of the T wave. Predominance of the M-Epi gradient is restored as the epicardial response continues to repolarize and the Epi-M gradient increases, thus resuming the ascending limb of the T wave. Full repolarization of epicardium marks the peak of the T wave. Repolarization of both endocardium and the M region contribute importantly to the descending limb.

Thus the interplay between these opposing forces across the ventricular wall establishes the height and width of the T wave as well as the degree to which

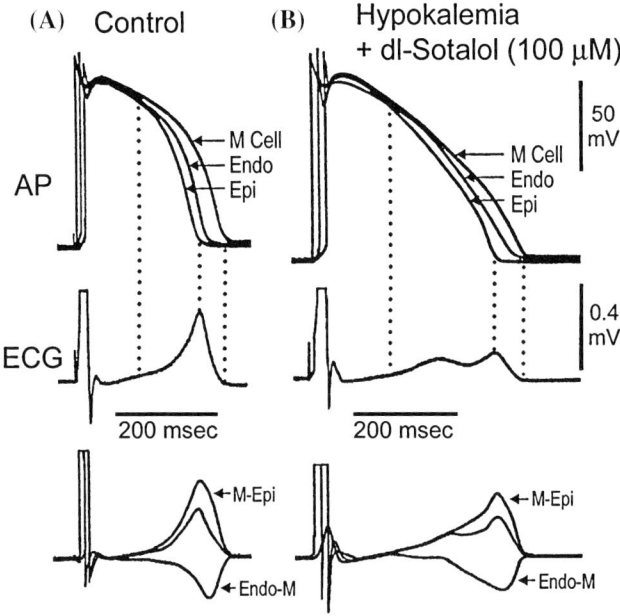

FIGURE 2. Voltage gradients on either side of the M region and the inscription of the T wave. Top: Action potentials simultaneously recorded from endocardial, epicardial, and M region sites of an arterially perfused canine left ventricular wedge preparation. Middle: ECG recorded across the wedge. Bottom: Computed voltage differences between the M-Epi action potentials (ΔV_{M-Epi}) and between the M region and endocardium responses (ΔV_{Endo-M}). If these traces are representative of the opposing voltage gradients on either side of the M region, responsible for inscription of the T wave, then the weighted sum of the two traces should yield a trace (middle trace in bottom grouping) resembling the ECG, which it does. (**A**): Control. (**B**): Hypokalemic conditions ($[K^+]_o = 1.5$ mM) + dl-sotalol (100 uM). Basic cycle length (BCL) = 1,000 msec. (Modified from Ref. 32 with permission.)

either the ascending or descending limb of the T wave is interrupted, leading to a bifurcated or notched appearance of the T wave.[32] The voltage gradients result from a more positive plateau potential in the M region than in epicardium or endocardium as well as from differences in the time course of phase 3 of the action potential of the three predominant ventricular cell types.

Under normal and most long QT conditions, the epicardial response is the earliest to repolarize and the M cell action potential is often the last. Full repolarization of the epicardial action potential is coincident with peak of the T wave and repolarization of the M cells coincides with the end of the T wave. Under these conditions, the Tpeak–Tend (Tp–Te) interval provides an index of transmural dispersion of repolarization, which may prove to be a valuable prognostic tool.[32,34]

Recent studies support Tp–Te interval as an index of transmural dispersion and vulnerability, while others do not.[35] Lubinski et al.[36] demonstrated that this interval is increased in patients with congenital long QT syndrome (LQTS). Other studies suggest that Tp–Te interval may be a useful index of transmural dispersion and thus may be prognostic of arrhythmic risk under a variety of conditions.[37–43] Direct evidence in support of Tp–Te as a valuable index to predict Torsade de Pointes (TdP) in patients with LQTS was provided by Yamaguchi and coworkers.[44] These authors concluded that Tp–Te is more valuable than QTc and QT dispersion as a predictor of TdP in patients with acquired LQTS. Shimizu et al. demonstrated that Tp–Te, but not QTc, predicts sudden cardiac death in patients with hypertrophic cardiomyopathy.[40] Most recently, Watanabe et al. demonstrated that prolonged Tp–Te is associated with inducibility as well as spontaneous development of VT in high-risk patients with organic heart disease[42] and Hevia et al. linked augmented Tp–Te intervals to arrhythmogenesis in the Brugada syndrome.[43] Although further studies are needed to evaluate the utility of these noninvasive indices of electrical heterogeneity and their prognostic value in the assignment of arrhythmic risk, evidence is accumulating in support of the hypothesis that transmural dispersion repolarization (TDR) rather than QT prolongation underlies the substrate responsible for the development of ventricular tachyarrhythmias.[43,45–49] Transmural dispersion of repolarization should not be confused with QT dispersion of repolarization, another proposed risk factor, which remains somewhat controversial.[50–52]

Apico-basal repolarization gradients measured along the epicardial surface have been suggested to play a role in the registration of the T wave.[33,53] In contrast, studies involving the perfused wedge suggest little or no contribution.[32]

The Electrocardiographic U Wave

Since Einthoven's initial description of the U wave,[2] a number of theories have been advanced to explain its origin, including (i) ventricular septum,[54] (ii) papillary muscles,[55] (iii) negative afterpotentials,[56,57] (iv) Purkinje system,[58,59] (v) early or delayed afterdepolarizations,[57] or (vi) mechanoelectrical feedback.[60,61]

Although the most popular hypothesis ascribes the U wave to delayed repolarization of the His–Purkinje system,[58,59] the small mass of the specialized conduction system is difficult to reconcile with the sometimes very large U wave deflections reported in the literature. In 1996 we suggested that the M cells, more abundant in mass and possessing delayed repolarization characteristics similar to those of Purkinje fibers, may be responsible for the inscription of the pathophysiologic U wave.[62] More recent findings employing the perfused wedge clearly indicate that what many clinicians refer to as an accentuated or inverted U wave is not a U wave, but rather a second component of the T wave whose descending or ascending limb (especially during hypokalemia) is interrupted (FIG. 3).[63,64] While delayed repolarization of the M cells contributes to the inscription of the second component of the T2 (pathophysiologic U wave), it is unlikely that it is responsible for the normal U wave.

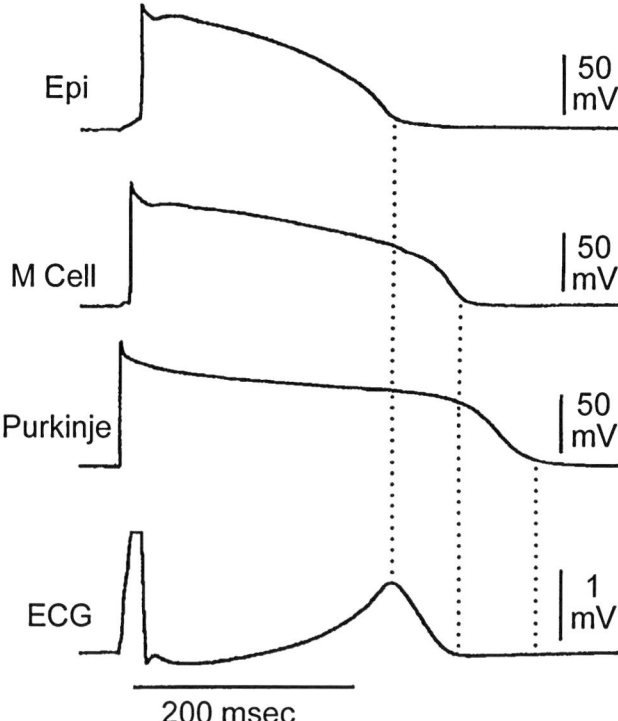

FIGURE 3. Correlation of transmembrane and electrocardiographic activity. Action potentials from epicardium (Epi), midmyocardium (M), and subendocardial Purkinje were recorded simultaneously with a transmural ECG from a canine arterially perfused left ventricular wedge preparation. Note that although repolarization of the subendocardial Purkinje fiber occurs after that of the M cell, it does not register on the ECG. BCL = 2,000 msec. (Modified from Ref. 32 with permission.)

Repolarization of the His–Purkinje system as the basis for the U wave was suggested by Hoffman, Cranefield, and Lepeshkin[58] and by Watanabe and coworkers.[59] In support of this hypothesis, repolarization of the Purkinje system is temporally aligned with the expected appearance of the U wave in the perfused wedge preparation (FIG. 3).[64] The lack of a U wave in the wedge is likely related to a low density of the Purkinje system in the dog. A test of this hypothesis awaits the availability of an experimental model displaying a prominent U wave (most animal species do not manifest a U wave).

Another hypothesis that endures despite lack of direct experimental and clinical evidence is that the normal U wave is associated with the mechanical activity of the heart (mechanoelectrical feedback). This hypothesis, first proposed by Lepeshkin[57] and more recently highlighted by Surawicz,[65] emphasizes the coincidence between the start of the U wave and the second heart sound, suggesting that stretch of the myocardium by rapid ventricular filling following

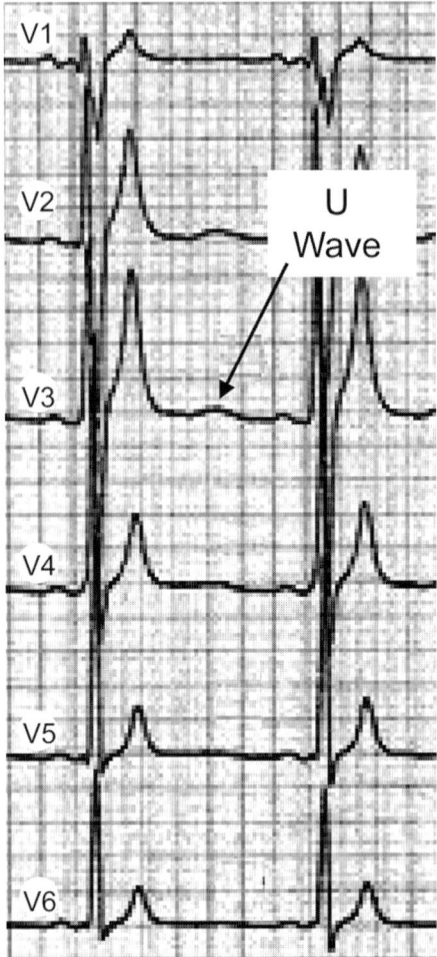

FIGURE 4. Precordial ECG leads recorded from a patient with the short QT syndrome showing a prominent separation of the T and U waves. (Modified from Ref. 68 with permission.)

opening of the atrioventricular (AV) valves generates delayed afterpotentials that are responsible for the inscription of the normal electrocardiographic U wave.

Indirect evidence in support of this hypothesis derives from the dramatic separation of the T and U waves in the short QT syndrome (FIG. 4).[66] The patient whose ECG is pictured in FIGURE 4 was linked to a mutation in hERG, leading to a prominent gain of function in IKr. The increase in IKr is responsible for the abbreviation of the ventricular myocardial action potential and thus the QT interval. Because IKr is also a major repolarizing current in Purkinje fibers, one would expect a comparable abbreviation of the Purkinje action potential. If the Purkinje system is responsible for inscription of the U wave, one would expect the U wave to abbreviate in parallel with the T wave. Its failure to do so suggests an alternative hypothesis, namely the possibility of a mechanoelectrical mechanism. Studies are under way to characterize the mechanical function of the heart in patients with the short QT syndrome. If temporal relationships for the opening of the aortic and atrioventricular valves remain largely unchanged, the U wave would be expected to retain its position and separate from the T wave. Such findings would provide further support for the mechanoelectrical hypothesis, which maintains that the U wave is due to stretch-induced delayed afterdepolarization caused by distension of the ventricular wall during rapid ventricular filling.

SUMMARY

Available data suggest that transmural heterogeneities in the early phases of the action potential inscribe the J wave, and transmural and apico-basal heterogeneities in final repolarization of the action potential inscribe the T wave of the ECG. Amplification of these heterogeneities of repolarization underlies the development of life-threatening cardiac arrhythmias. Although the basis for the U wave is still evolving, recent data have renewed interest in a mechanoelectrical mechanism, which maintains that the U wave is due to stretch-induced delayed afterdepolarizations caused by distension of the ventricular wall during rapid filling.

ACKNOWLEDGMENTS

This study was supported by NIH Grant HL 47678 and the Masons of New York State and Florida.

REFERENCES

1. EINTHOVEN, W. 1903. The galvanometric registration of the human electrocardiogram, likewise a review of the use of the capillary electrometer in physiology. Pflügers Arch. **99:** 472–480.
2. EINTHOVEN, W. 1912. Ueber die Deutung des Electrokardiogramms. Pflügers Arch. **149:** 65–86.
3. ANTZELEVITCH, C., W. SHIMIZU, G.X. YAN, et al. 1999. The M cell: its contribution to the ECG and to normal and abnormal electrical function of the heart. J. Cardiovasc. Electrophysiol. **10:** 1124–1152.
4. ANTZELEVITCH, C. & R. DUMAINE. 2002. Electrical heterogeneity in the heart: physiological, pharmacological and clinical implications. *In* Handbook of Phys-

iology. The Heart. E. Page, H.A. Fozzard & R.J. Solaro, Eds.: 654–692. Oxford University Press. New York.
5. DI DIEGO, J.M., Z.Q. SUN & C. ANTZELEVITCH. 1996. I_{to} and action potential notch are smaller in left vs. right canine ventricular epicardium. Am. J. Physiol. **271:** H548–H561.
6. VOLDERS, P.G., K.R. SIPIDO, E. CARMELIET, *et al.* 1999. Repolarizing K+ currents ITO1 and IKs are larger in right than left canine ventricular midmyocardium. Circulation **99:** 206–210.
7. SICOURI, S. & C. ANTZELEVITCH. 1991. A subpopulation of cells with unique electrophysiological properties in the deep subepicardium of the canine ventricle: the M cell. Circ. Res. **68:** 1729–1741.
8. ANTZELEVITCH, C. & W. SHIMIZU. 2002. Cellular mechanisms underlying the Long QT syndrome. Curr. Opin. Cardiol. **17:** 43–51.
9. YAN, G.X. & C. ANTZELEVITCH. 1996. Cellular basis for the electrocardiographic J wave. Circulation **93:** 372–379.
10. CLEMENTS, S.D. & J.W. HURST. 1972. Diagnostic value of ECG abnormalities observed in subjects accidentally exposed to cold. Am. J. Cardiol. **29:** 729–734.
11. THOMPSON, R., J. RICH, F. CHMELIK & W.L. NELSON. 1977. Evolutionary changes in the electrocardiogram of severe progressive hypothermia. J. Electrocardiol. **10:** 67–70.
12. RUDUSKY, B.M. 2004. The electrocardiogram in hypothermia—the J wave and the Brugada syndrome. Am. J. Cardiol. **93:** 671–672.
13. KRAUS, F. 1920. Ueber die wirkung des kalziums auf den kreislauf. Dtsch Med Wochenschr. **46:** 201–203.
14. SRIDHARAN, M.R. & L.G. HORAN. 1984. Electrocardiographic J wave of hypercalcemia. Am. J. Cardiol. **54:** 672–673.
15. ANTZELEVITCH, C., S. SICOURI, A. LUKAS, *et al.* 1995. Regional differences in the electrophysiology of ventricular cells: physiological and clinical implications. *In* Cardiac Electrophysiology: From Cell to Bedside, 2nd edition. D.P. Zipes & J. Jalife, Eds.: 228–245. W.B. Saunders Co. Philadelphia.
16. LITOVSKY, S.H. & C. ANTZELEVITCH. 1988. Transient outward current prominent in canine ventricular epicardium but not endocardium. Circ. Res. **62:** 116–126.
17. LIU, D.W., G.A. GINTANT & C. ANTZELEVITCH. 1993. Ionic bases for electrophysiological distinctions among epicardial, midmyocardial, and endocardial myocytes from the free wall of the canine left ventricle. Circ. Res. **72:** 671–687.
18. ZICHA, S., L. XIAO, S. STAFFORD, *et al.* 2004. Transmural expression of transient outward potassium current subunits in normal and failing canine and human hearts. J. Physiol. **561:** 735–748.
19. ROSATI, B., Z. PAN, S. LYPEN, *et al.* 2001. Regulation of KChIP2 potassium channel beta subunit gene expression underlies the gradient of transient outward current in canine and human ventricle. J. Physiol. **533:** 119–125.
20. COSTANTINI, D.L., E.P. ARRUDA, P. AGARWAL, *et al.* 2005. The homeodomain transcription factor Irx5 establishes the mouse cardiac ventricular repolarization gradient. Cell **123:** 347–358.
21. EAGLE, K. 1994. Images in clinical medicine. Osborn waves of hypothermia. N. Engl. J. Med. **10:** 680.
22. EMSLIE-SMITH, D., G.E. SLADDEN & G.R. STIRLING. 1959. The significance of changes in the electrocardiogram in hypothermia. Br. Heart J. **21:** 343–351.
23. OSBORN, J.J. 1953. Experimental hypothermia: respiratory and blood pH changes in relation to cardiac function. Am. J. Physiol. **175:** 389–398.

24. SRIDHARAN, M.R., J.C. JOHNSON, L.G. HORAN, et al. 1983. Monophasic action potentials in hypercalcemic and hypothermic "J" waves—a comparative study. Am. Fed. Clin. Res. **31:** 219.
25. DI DIEGO, J.M. & C. ANTZELEVITCH. 1994. High $[Ca^{2+}]$-induced electrical heterogeneity and extrasystolic activity in isolated canine ventricular epicardium: phase 2 reentry. Circulation **89:** 1839–1850.
26. ANTZELEVITCH, C. 2005. *In vivo* human demonstration of phase 2 reentry. Heart Rhythm **2:** 804–806.
27. YAN, G.X. & C. ANTZELEVITCH. 1999. Cellular basis for the Brugada Syndrome and other mechanisms of arrhythmogenesis associated with ST segment elevation. Circulation **100:** 1660–1666.
28. SHU, J., T. ZHU, L. YANG, et al. 2005. ST-segment elevation in the early repolarization syndrome, idiopathic ventricular fibrillation, and the Brugada syndrome: cellular and clinical linkage. J. Electrocardiol. **38**(Suppl.): 26–32.
29. THOMSEN, P.E., R.M. JOERGENSEN, J.K. KANTERS, et al. 2005. Phase 2 reentry in man. Heart Rhythm **2:** 797–803.
30. ANTZELEVITCH, C., P. BRUGADA, J. BRUGADA, et al. 2002. Brugada Syndrome. A decade of progress. Circ. Res. **91:** 1114–1119.
31. ANTZELEVITCH, C., P. BRUGADA, J. BRUGADA, et al. 2005. The Brugada Syndrome: from bench to bedside. Blackwell Futura. Oxford.
32. YAN, G.X. & C. ANTZELEVITCH. 1998. Cellular basis for the normal T wave and the electrocardiographic manifestations of the long QT syndrome. Circulation **98:** 1928–1936.
33. JANSE, M.J., E.A. SOSUNOV, R. CORONEL, et al. 2005. Repolarization gradients in the canine left ventricle before and after induction of short-term cardiac memory. Circulation **112:** 1711–1718.
34. ANTZELEVITCH, C. 1997. The M cell. Invited editorial comment. J. Cardiovasc. Pharmacol. Ther. **2:** 73–76.
35. VAN HUYSDUYNEN, B.H., C.A. SWENNE, J.J. BAX, et al. 2005. Dispersion of repolarization in cardiac resynchronization therapy. Heart Rhythm **2:** 1286–1293.
36. LUBINSKI, A., E. LEWICKA-NOWAK, M. KEMPA, et al. 1998. New insight into repolarization abnormalities in patients with congenital long QT syndrome: the increased transmural dispersion of repolarization. Pacing Clin. Electrophysiol. **21:** 172–175.
37. WOLK, R., S. STEC & P. KULAKOWSKI. 2001. Extrasystolic beats affect transmural electrical dispersion during programmed electrical stimulation. Eur. J. Clin. Invest. **31:** 293–301.
38. TANABE, Y., M. INAGAKI, T. KURITA, et al. 2001. Sympathetic stimulation produces a greater increase in both transmural and spatial dispersion of repolarization in LQT1 than LQT2 forms of congenital long QT syndrome. J. Am. Coll. Cardiol. **37:** 911–919.
39. FREDERIKS, J., C.A. SWENNE, J.A. KORS, et al. 2001. Within-subject electrocardiographic differences at equal heart rates: role of the autonomic nervous system. Pflügers Arch. **441:** 717–724.
40. SHIMIZU, M., H. INO, K. OKEIE, et al. 2002. T-peak to T-end interval may be a better predictor of high-risk patients with hypertrophic cardiomyopathy associated with a cardiac troponin I mutation than QT dispersion. Clin. Cardiol. **25:** 335–339.
41. TAKENAKA, K., T. A.I. SHIMIZU, et al. 2003. Exercise stress test amplifies genotype-phenotype correlation in the LQT1 and LQT2 forms of the long-QT syndrome. Circulation **107:** 838–844.

42. WATANABE, N., Y. KOBAYASHI, K. TANNO, et al. 2004. Transmural dispersion of repolarization and ventricular tachyarrhythmias. J. Electrocardiol. **37:** 191–200.
43. CASTRO, H.J., C. ANTZELEVITCH, B.F. TORNES, et al. 2006. T peak–T end and T peak–T end dispersion as risk factors for ventricular techycardia/ventricular fibrillation in patients with the Brugada syndrome. J. Am. Coll. Cardiol **47(9):** 1828–1834.
44. YAMAGUCHI, M., M. SHIMIZU, H. INO, et al. 2003. T wave peak-to-end interval and QT dispersion in acquired long QT syndrome: a new index for arrhythmogenicity. Clin. Sci. (Lond.) **105:** 671–676.
45. ANTZELEVITCH, C., L. BELARDINELLI, A.C. ZYGMUNT, et al. 2004. Electrophysiologic effects of ranolazine: a novel anti-anginal agent with antiarrhythmic properties. Circulation **110:** 904–910.
46. DI DIEGO, J.M., L. BELARDINELLI & C. ANTZELEVITCH. 2003. Cisapride-induced transmural dispersion of repolarization and torsade de pointes in the canine left ventricular wedge preparation during epicardial stimulation. Circulation **108:** 1027–1033.
47. ANTZELEVITCH, C. 2004. Drug-induced Channelopathies. *In* Cardiac Electrophysiology. From Cell to Bedside, 4th edition. D.P. Zipes & J. Jalife, Eds.: 151–157. W.B. Saunders. New York.
48. BELARDINELLI, L., C. ANTZELEVITCH & M.A. VOS. 2003. Assessing predictors of drug-induced Torsade de Pointes. Trends Pharmacol. Sci. **24:** 619–625.
49. FENICHEL, R.R., M. MALIK, C. ANTZELEVITCH, et al. 2004. Drug-induced Torsade de Pointes and implications for drug development. J. Cardiovasc. Electrophysiol. **15:** 475–495.
50. BATCHVAROV, V. & M. MALIK. 2000. Measurement and interpretation of QT dispersion. Prog. Cardiovasc. Dis. **42:** 325–344.
51. ANTZELEVITCH, C., W. SHIMIZU, G.X. YAN & S. SICOURI. 1998. Cellular basis for QT dispersion. J. Electrocardiol. **30**(Suppl.): 168–175.
52. MALIK, M., B. ACAR, Y. GANG, et al. 2000. QT dispersion does not represent electrocardiographic interlead heterogeneity of ventricular repolarization. J. Cardiovasc. Electrophysiol. **11:** 835–843.
53. COHEN, I.S., W.R. GILES & D. NOBLE. 1976. Cellular basis for the T wave of the electrocardiogram. Nature **262:** 657–661.
54. ZUCKERMAN, R. & E. CABRERA-COSIO. 1947. La ondu U. Arch. Inst. Cardiol. Mex. **17:** 521–532.
55. FURBETTA, D., A. BUFALARI, F. SANTUCCI & P. SOLINAS. 1956. Abnormality of the U wave and the T-U segment of the electrocardiogram: the syndrome of the papillary muscles. Circulation **14:** 1129–1137.
56. NAHUM, L.H. & H.E. HOFF. 1939. The interpretation of the U wave of the electrocardiogram. Am. Heart J. **17:** 585–598.
57. LEPESCHKIN, E. 1957. Genesis of the U wave. Circulation **15:** 77–81.
58. HOFFMAN, B.F. & P.F. CRANEFIELD. 1960. Electrophysiology of the Heart. McGraw-Hill. New York.
59. WATANABE, Y. 1975. Purkinje repolarization as a possible cause of the U wave in the electrocardiogram. Circulation **51:** 1030–1037.
60. LAB, M.J. 1982. Contraction-excitation feedback in myocardium: physiologic basis and clinical revelance. Circ. Res. **50:** 757–766.
61. CHOO, M.H. & D.G. GIBSON. 1986. U waves in ventricular hypertrophy: possible demonstration of mechano-electrical feedback. Br. Heart J. **55:** 428–433.

62. ANTZELEVITCH, C., V.V. NESTERENKO & G.X. YAN. 1996. The role of M cells in acquired long QT syndrome, U waves and torsade de pointes. J. Electrocardiol. **28**(Suppl.): 131–138.
63. SHIMIZU, W. & C. ANTZELEVITCH. 1997. Sodium channel block with mexiletine is effective in reducing dispersion of repolarization and preventing Torsade de Pointes in LQT2 and LQT3 models of the long-QT syndrome. Circulation **96**: 2038–2047.
64. YAN, G.X. & C. ANTZELEVITCH. 1998. Cellular basis for the normal T wave and the electrocardiographic manifestations of the long QT syndrome. Circulation **98**: 1928–1936.
65. SURAWICZ, B. 1998. U wave: facts, hypotheses, misconceptions, and misnomers. J. Cardiovasc. Electrophysiol. **9**: 1117–1128.
66. BRUGADA, R., K. HONG, R. DUMAINE, *et al.* 2004. Sudden death associated with short-QT syndrome linked to mutations in HERG. Circulation **109**: 30–35.
67. YAN, G.X. & C. ANTZELEVITCH. 1995. Cellular basis for the electrocardiographic J wave. [Abstract]. Circulation **92**: I-71.
68. GAITA, F., C. GIUSTETTO, F. BIANCHI, *et al.* 2003. Short QT Syndrome: a familial cause of sudden death. Circulation **108**: 965–970.

Mechanosensitive-Mediated Interaction, Integration, and Cardiac Control

MAX J. LAB

National Heart and Lung Institute, and Imperial College, London, United Kingdom

ABSTRACT: This review covers aspects of the cardiac mechanotransduction field at different levels, and advocates the possibility that mechanoelectro-chemical transduction forms part of a network of mechanically linked integration in heart—mechanically mediated integration (MMI). It assembles evidence and observations in the literature to promote this hypothesis. Mechanical components can provide the bond between interactions at molecular, cellular, and macro levels to enable the integration. Stretch-activated channels (SACs) exist in the heart, but stresses and strains can affect other membrane channels or receptors. A cellular mechanical change can thus promote several ionic or downstream changes. Cell signal cascades have been implicated and can affect membrane electrophysiology. MMI could shape intracellular and downstream signals using the cytoskeleton and intracellular Ca^{2+}. MMI also spans other regulatory systems and processes such as the autonomic nervous system (ANS) and operates throughout the whole heart as an integrative system. Finally, supporting the hypothesis, if elements of the normal integration become deranged it contributes to cardiovascular disease and, potentially, lethal arrhythmia.

KEYWORDS: mechanotransduction; mechanically mediated integration (MMI); mechanical bonding; contribution to disease

INTRODUCTION

This review advocates the possibility that mechanoelectrochemical transduction forms part of a network in heart, and introduces the concept of the network mechanically mediated integration (MMI). In support of this hypothesis it addresses disparate inputs in the cardiac mechanotransduction field at different levels. Taking a little license, the article characterizes "integration" as having mechanical constituents, which provide a common link between the various interactions at molecular, cellular, and macro levels. In searching the

Address for correspondence: Max J. Lab, Imperial College, National Heart and Lung Institute (Charing Cross Campus), and CRC Medical Research Council (Hammersmith Campus) London W6 8RF, United Kingdom.
  e-mail: m.lab@imperial.ac.uk

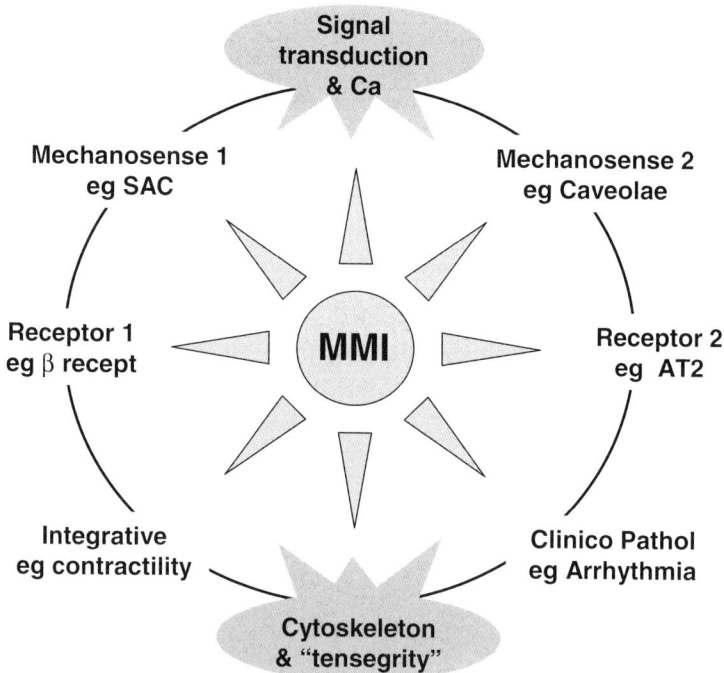

FIGURE 1. Broad interactions involving MMI. Integration is mediated between mechanosensitive channels 1 & 2 (Northwest and Northeast) SAC and caveolae with their signalsomes as well as receptors 1 and 2 (e.g., [equator] β receptor & angiotensin receptor [AT]). MMI acting at membrane and cell signal level can also globally affect the heart, influencing physiology and clinico pathology (Southwest and Southeast). Cytoskeletal and cell signal changes are invoked during MMI.

literature to sustain the MMI hypothesis, we track integration along a path from mechanosensor to the whole heart within an integrative system. MMI spans other regulatory systems and processes. Finally, if elements of normal MMI derange, and the hypothesis holds, it contributes to cardiovascular disease.

MMI AT THE CHANNEL LEVEL

Passive, Mechanically Activated, and Stretch-Activated Channels

Passive mechanically activated channels are shown in FIGURE 1 (at 10 o'clock) and stretch-activated channels (SACs) in FIGURE 2 (at 12 o'clock).

The regulatory integrative chain at the membrane starts here with mechanogated, mechanosensitive channels (SACs). As their definitive

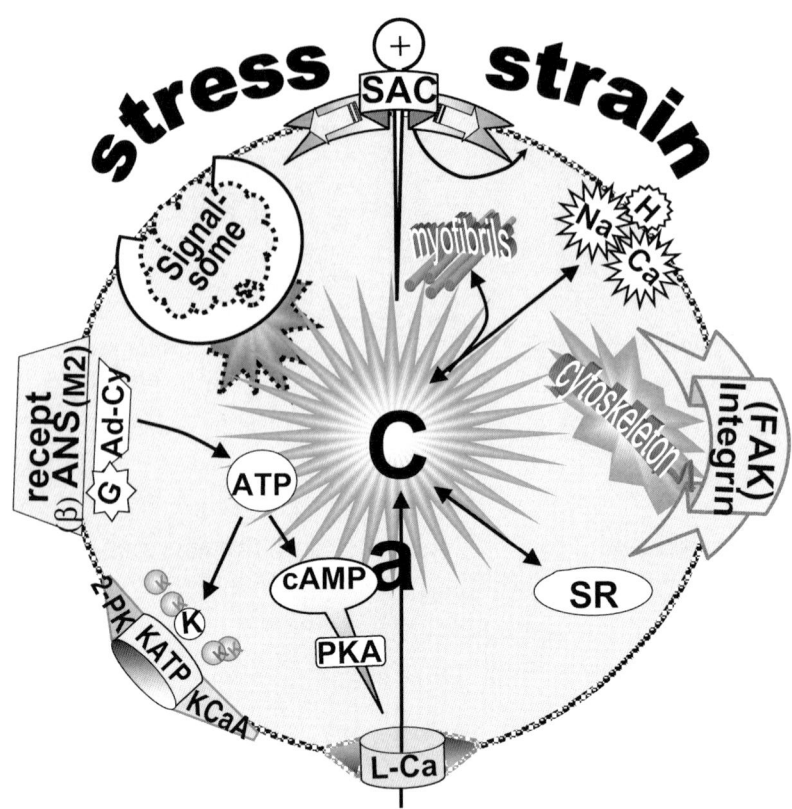

FIGURE 2. Conjectural diagram of MMI at cellular level. "Stress–strain" represents intra- and extracellular mechanical input activating, diagrammatically, all the moieties on the figurative cell membrane. This is indicated roughly clockwise from SAC at 12 o'clock. 1 o'clock—ion exchangers. 3 o'clock—integrin & associated FAK. 6 o'clock—LCa channel. 8 o'clock—KATP channel, which, diagrammatically, incorporates other K-related channels; 2 pore (tandem pore) forming K channels (2-PK), KCaA. 9 o'clock—ANS; including the M2 receptor, and β receptors with their respective G proteins (G). 11 o'clock—caveolae with lipid rafts and signalsomes eliciting downstream signals. This also represents other mechanosensitive signalsomes. (Ad Cy = Adenyl cyclase; cAMP = cyclic adenosine monophosphate; PKA = phosphokinase A; SR = sarcoplasmic reticulum.)

description,[1] SACs have been described in many tissues[2–5] including the heart.[6] Membrane stretch opens the channels to admit charge-carrying ions, for example, calcium and sodium, which can influence the membrane potential directly and indirectly, for example, via calcium-activated currents and ion exchangers such as Na–Ca (FIG. 2: curved arrow from SAC to exchanger at 2 o'clock, which also incorporates the Na/H exchanger). In this way, sodium can influence intracellular calcium (FIG. 2: diagonal two-way arrow between Ca and exchanger). Although the myocardium is actively contracting here, in the current context the resultant geometric shape changes are regarded as being passively transmitted.

Interpretations of stretch effects here could be hazardous. Multicellular preparations experience more tension than isolated cells.[7] However, the characteristics of the channel electrophysiology have found equivalence in intact heart where monophasic action potentials (MAPs) can be used to gain qualitative insights into cellular electrophysiology; for example, isolated perfused heart of frog[8] and mammals.[9–11] Notably, there is a type of reversal potential[8,12] where a stretch early in the action potential produces a repolarizing tendency, whereas if late, it produces depolarization. There is no change at the "reversal potential." There are other examples of the equivalence, in different guises, in intact heart *in situ* in experimental preparations[13] and in man.[14] SACs can thus explain load-induced reductions in action potential duration in these examples. Another example is that compounds such as gadolinium and streptomycin used in cells to block stretch-induced electrophysiological changes also operate in intact preparations. However, the results may have to be carefully interpreted. Streptomycin's effects as a blocker appear heterogeneous in intact atrium.[15] It looks so far as if SACs may well operate in intact heart, suggesting roles from membrane to intact organ.

MMI, other Channels, and Signalsomes

The hypothesis requires that the integration applies to other channels apart from SACs. The adenosine 5′-triphosphate (ATP)-activated potassium (KATP) channel subunits (Kir6.1, Kir6.2, SUR1A, SUR1B, SUR2A, and SUR2B)[16] have been found in atria from neonatal rats. The KATP channel (FIG. 2 at 8 o'clock) is attached to the cytoskeleton and it has been suggested to be mechanosensitive.[17] Several other channels appear to be mechanosensitive, including the L-type calcium (LCa) channel,[18] (FIG. 2 at 6 o'clock) sodium channels,[19] and the tandem pore potassium channels (indicated as 2-PK in FIG. 2 at 8 o'clock) such as TREK-1 [20] (the K channels 2-PK are still controversial as to the extent they exist in myocardium) and K current, arachidonic acid sensitive (IKAA),[21] ion exchangers (FIG. 2 at 2 o'clock).[22]

Interest is increasing for a role for caveolae (FIG. 2 at 11 o'clock). These membrane invaginations contain signalsomes, which are involved in mechanotransduction.[23,24]

MMI and Metabolism

In cultured chick ventricular myocytes, a stretch-activated ion channel [25] was identified as a Ca^{2+}-activated K^+ (KcaA) channel type, reversibly activated by ATP on the intracellular surface. That is, a stretch-activated KCa, ATP channel.

Low intracellular pH as well as intracellular ATP[26] activates the large (111 ± 3.0 pS) mechanosensitive K^+ channels, TREK-1, from the tandem pore family (FIG. 2 at 8 o'clock), which have been found in adult rat ventricular myocytes. It does seem that there is integration with metabolism, albeit vestigial.

MMI and the Neuro-Humoral System

The autonomic nervous system (ANS) and the endocrine system are integrative regulatory systems, and they interact with each other. If the current hypothesis holds as a fully integrated system, the question arises as to whether MMI interplays with these other regulatory systems.

ANS—β Receptor

Mechanosensitive autonomic receptors (FIG. 2 at 9 o'clock) include the acetyl choline (M2) receptor and β receptors with their respective G proteins (G). Here mechanosensitivity in second messengers seems likely, including parts of the cascade in which adenyl cyclase (Ad Cy) splits ATP giving cyclic adenosine monophosphate (cAMP) involving G protein to affect the LCa channel via phosphokinase A (PKA).

β receptor agonists can modulate mechanically induced electrophysiological changes including the electrical restitution curve.[27] Mechanical load accentuates the supernormal period making its initial rising phase steeper, and β receptor agonism exacerbates these arrhythmogenic changes. Conversely, β receptor antagonism curtails mechanically induced arrhythmia.[28] Moreover, raised intraventricular pressure releases catecholamines from the ventricle[29] and this could promote mechanically induced arrhythmia.

In support of this signal chain, catecholamine store depletion curtails mechanoarrhythmia whether the depletion is pharmacological[30] or by chronic sympathetic denervation in the intact preparation.[31] This notion has been supported by a further study in the intact preparation.[32]

ANS—M2 Receptors

ANS—M2 receptors (FIG. 2 at 10 o'clock) via G protein-regulated inward-rectifier potassium channels (GIRK) are part of a superfamily of inward-rectifier K^+ channels. GIRK1 and 4 are found in atrium and sinoatrial node.[33] G proteins and mechanical stretch (FIG. 2 at 11 o'clock) modulates GIRK1–4 (also designated Kir3.1–4). Rabbit atrial muscarinic potassium channels are rapidly and reversibly inhibited by membrane stretch, possibly serving as part of the mechanoelectrical feedback interaction. Hypo-osmolar stress inactivates the heteromeric Kir3.4 channel expressed in Xenopus oocytes.[34] Stretch activates the cardiac G protein (GK)-gated, muscarinic K^+ acetylcholine (KACh) channel if ACh is present and this appears to be independent of receptor/G protein, probably via a direct effect on the channel protein/lipid bilayer.[35]

ACTIVE MYOFIBRILLAR INTERACTION, CALCIUM, AND MECHANOELECTRIC TRANSDUCTION

Consider the myofibrils (FIG. 2, upper right segment). Active myocardial contraction provides an intracellular generator of stress and strain. Stretched or isometric muscle has a short action potential duration compared with the shortening muscle.[36,37] Moreover, isotonic (shortening) muscle, with the reduced force production, has the longer duration calcium transient. This is counterintuitive, for sarcoplasmic reticulum (SR) calcium release (FIG. 2 diagonal two-way arrow in 4 o'clock direction); but a reasonable explanatory mechanism is that the reduced force with the shortening muscle reduces the affinity of troponin C for calcium[37–41]. This reduced calcium buffering allows intracellular calcium to rise in the face of a reduced force production. The raised calcium would influence transmembrane currents to prolong the action potential duration; for example, via electrogenic Na/Ca exchange (FIG. 2 bidirectional arrow in 1 o'clock direction). These calcium aspects, also important in arrhythmogenesis (see below), have been reviewed 40 and include mechanical influences on SR calcium cycling.[42–45]

FACILITATORS OF MMI

MMI, if a tenable hypothesis, will need systems to facilitate its integrative functions. If some of these could be identified, it could strengthen the tenant.

Calcium and Cell Signal Cascades and/or Signalsomes

Calcium (FIG. 2 center) often forms an interlink in mechanochemical processes. A mechanical perturbation can induce a Ca rise.[40,46] However, mechanical stimulation releases a multitude of other second messengers,[47,48] some as signalsomes (represented in FIG. 2 at 11 o'clock) that includes tyrosine kinase,[49] cAMP,[50,51] inositol trisphosphate,[52] and arachidonic acid.[53–55] It also activates mechanisms involving G protein[56,57] and phospholipase C. PKC (bio)physically translocates from the cytosol, under the influence first of diacylglycerol (DAG) and then of receptors for activated C-kinase (RACK) in the membrane, to bring it to its target protein, allowing mitogen-activated protein kinase (MAPK) to switch on immediately early genes (IEGs). More detailed individual mechanochemo sensitivity, including ionic currents carried by channels other than stretch-activated ones, has been reviewed.[5]

Integration could also be provided by AT2 and ET1 receptors,[58] which would affect phospholipuse C (PLC) via Gq. This can alter intracellular Ca first via IP3 and SR Ca release, and second, through PLC to facilitate membrane translocation (DAG/RACK/PKC) to influence Na/H exchange, and therefore intracellular Ca via Na/Ca exchange (FIG. 2 at 2 o'clock).

Cytoskeleton, "Tensegrity:" an MMI Vehicle?

Mechanotransduction appears to involve, or to be modulated by, the intracellular cytoskeleton and its insertions into the surrounding cell membrane via focal adherence complexes. Here (FIG. 1 at 6 o'clock and FIG. 2 at 3 o'clock) the role of the intracellular cytoskeleton appears to be crucial. It can form the mechanical engineering and biochemical basis for intracellular and intercellular integration. Any membrane channel associated with the cytoskeleton could provide a candidate for integration. Stress–strain could be transmitted to the channel via the cytoskeleton to activate it or the cytoskeleton could somehow shield the channel from the mechanical transmission of strain via other paths. The KATP channel, which is mechanosensitive, is attached to the cytoskeleton.[17] Several ion channels are regionally fixed in the membrane,[59] and their modulation by the cytoskeleton is also possible. From the electrophysiological aspect the cytoskeleton may be important because physiologically and geometrically parts of the cytoskeleton are associated with ion channel function.[5,60–62] Many stimuli (FIG. 2) share intracellular signal pathways with mechanoelectrochemical ones, and this can produce composite responses.

Under physiological conditions, the mechanical interconnecting system is prestressed, conferring mechanical balance and stability. This has been described as "tensegrity,"[63] and there is thus a clear line of force communication from the extracellular matrix to intracellular cytoplasmic structures.[64] Mechanical stimuli can provoke changes in adhesions between the cell and the extracellular matrix via the fibronectin and collagen networks. In this way, mechanically distorting one cell can raise the intracellular Ca^{2+} of its neighboring cell.[46]

The elaborate adhesion complex[65,66] also contains focal adhesion kinase (FAK) (FIG. 2 at 3 o'clock). This kinase can be the initiator or modulator of many downstream cell signals and kinases, including tyrosine kinase[67] and the renin angiotensin system.[68] These are possible/probable mechanisms whereby chronic stretch can produce remodeling and hypertrophy.

MMI IN THE INTACT HEART—REGULATION OF CARDIAC FUNCTION

So far, the observations above at the cellular and intracellular level are in keeping with the presented MMI concept. If so, they should find expression at "higher" levels. Spatially, the integrative stress/strain system transmits to the whole heart. This would be by cell attachment through the adherence proteins to the extracellular matrix, which connects cells to each other. Forces at one end of a group of cells are thus transmitted throughout the organ, invoking tensegrity. This provides a clear mechanism by which a mechanically induced functional integration can occur in the intact heart. Additionally, the heart is part of a hydrodynamic system: a mechanical, hydraulically mediated mechanism for MMI, using pressure–volume changes in a system containing incompressible blood provides the MMI. Systemic arterial pressure and/or venous volume changes can influence cardiac electrophysiology and function.[5,69–74] This would invoke the variety of cellular mechanisms covered above.

We also know that sinoatrial stretch can raise heart rate neurologically, but it can also be direct,[75,76] probably by a mechanoelectric mechanism[77] working through SAC and increasing the slope of the diastolic depolarization. Thus, in addition to nervous reflex mechanisms, cellular mechanoelectric transduction provides integrative control mechanisms for raising heart rate in response to an increased venous return to the heart.

On a marginally different track, the prevailing dogma for the familiar Starling's Law of the Heart is a length/force sensitivity of the contractile proteins—perhaps related to calcium.[78,79] A membrane mechanosensitivity probably also makes a contribution in the intact ventricle by mechanotransduction, possibly via SAC.[30] Studies at the membrane level corroborate this, showing that stretch can raise intracellular calcium by affecting mechanosensitive channels,[40,46,80,81] and so increase force.

MMI AND INTEGRATION BY FEEDBACK CONTROL

As both neural and endocrine integrative systems are well described by negative (and sometimes positive) feedback control loops, these can describe mechanically related feedback situations. For example, the interaction between electrical and mechanical events in heart operates within boundaries, and this relationship may have to be maintained for reasonable physiological and integrative function. Any disturbance in the system, for example, altered loop gain, could destabilize matters, if not mitigated, to produce pathology (see below). A highly simplified application of control theory (FIG. 3) demonstrates that the interaction between the electrical and mechanical events can be depicted as a feedback control system. This keeps cellular electromechanical relationships (globally manifest in the ECG and pressure/volume) within normal boundaries.

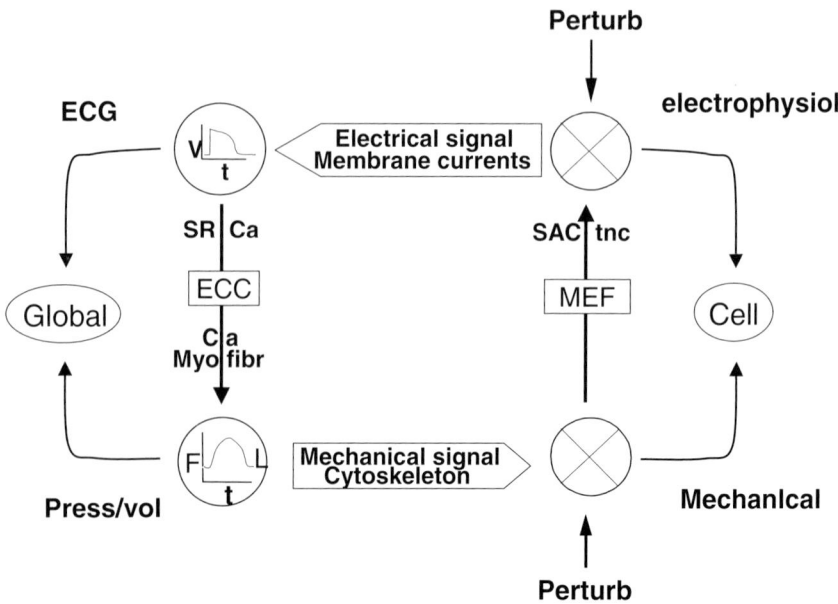

FIGURE 3. Simple engineering portrayal of MEF as a feedback control loop. V versus t = voltage versus time (action potential); SR = sarcoplasmic reticulum; Myofibr = myofibrillar proteins; F/L versus t = force or length against time; SACs = stretch-activated channels; tn-C = troponin C; ECC = excitation-contraction coupling; crossed circles = comparators.

However, it is difficult to precisely identify some of the components in FIGURE 3 (controlled variables, "comparator" [error detector], "error signal," "controller," and transfer functions). In this figure, top left is the action potential electrophysiologically expressed globally (*top left arrow*) as the electrocardiogram (ECG). It also releases Ca^+ (direction down) from the SR for excitation-contraction coupling. Ca interacts with myofibrillar proteins, produces contraction, in bottom left, which is force or length against time. This produces (*lower left arrow*) the global mechanical and haemodynamic changes, for example, pressure/volume changes. The mechanical signals (via the cytoskeleton) feed in to a comparator (*bottom right crossed circle*) including normal mechanical contraction (*lower right arrow*). Any mechanical perturbation would also go to this comparator for summing. The signal out (direction up) then invokes mechanoelectric feedback (MEF) via mechanoelectric transducers; for example, SAC or the troponin C mechanism. The mechanically activated currents feed another comparator (*top right crossed circle*) summing with normal electrophysiological signals and any electrophysiological perturbation. This produces a membrane voltage signal to affect the action potential (returning to top left).

MMI AND PATHOPHYSIOLOGY

As with other physiological integrative regulatory systems in heart, if MMI functions similarly, derangements in function should produce pathophysiological situations (FIG. 1 at 5 o'clock). MEF and its integration, perhaps acting as a homeostatic feedback control system in the normal situation,[58] is amplified in cardiac pathology.[82–88] The feedback is now a destabilizing mechanism, because the integration interactions have altered their interactive "gains." The tentative argument is that it is this derangement in cross-talk in arrhythmic death that provides the lethal expression of MMI.

Intracellular calcium changes have a pivotal role in integration between intracellular signals and the generation of arrhythmia.[89–92] Sustained [Ca]i increases promote [Ca]i oscillations [93] and electrophysiological oscillations are conducive to arrhythmia. Calcium is heavily involved in MEF as alluded above and as reviewed by Calaghan and White.[40] Calcium changes could be pivotal in mechanically linked integration during electrophysiological derangement in myocardial pathology

MMI AND MECHANICAL COMPONENTS IN ARRHYTHMIA

MEF/transduction is increasingly being highlighted as a possible cause of sudden cardiac arrhythmic death in humans, and there are clear correlations with ventricular ejection fraction, which is a purely mechanical rather than electrophysiological predictor.[94–96]

Many clinical correlates with lethal arrhythmia have their equivalent in MEF in pathological mechanical changes, which produce electrical changes. At one extreme, this would be ischemically induced dyskinesia or infarction with localized stretch in the affected part of the ventricular wall. Mechanoelectric dispersion, and thus arrhythmogenic electrical dispersion, would be gross. At the other end, remodeling would produce less mechanoelectric dispersion, but nonetheless a potentially grave one, perhaps because of its patchy nature.

MMI and the Neuro-Humoral Component in Arrhythmia—β Blockade

One of the few therapeutic agents reducing mortality from sudden (arrhythmic) death in many subsets of patients and in related experimental situations are the β blockers (FIG. 2 at 9/10 o'clock). Study in this area is already voluminous, rising exponentially and a few recent reviews and studies are included here.[97–104] The clinical situations covered include infarction, hypertension, subaortic stenosis, cardiomyopathy, mitral valve prolapse, and congestive cardiac failure. Moreover, depleting endogenous catecholamines by bretylium tosylate is one method for treating clinical arrhythmia.[105–110]

Although the mechanism of the therapeutic efficacy may well be due to a combination of direct anti-ischemic effects and preservation of vagal tone, all the above observations have elements of MMI. First, many of the clinical conditions associated with the ANS and arrhythmia are associated with abnormal mechanical loads or wall motion. Second, the clinically related observations are in keeping with the mechanoelectric studies illustrated above. That is, electrophysiology can be modified by autonomic agonists/antagonists.[27,28] Moreover, bretylium tosylate, analogous to its therapeutic effects in abating clinical arrhythmia, curtails stretch arrhythmia.[30] We need a note of caution, for the action of bretylium may be directly electrophysiological.[111]

MMI and the Renin-Angiotensin System

It is likely that the renin-angiotensin system displays cross-talk with mechanotransduction, either by its action as a load-reducing peripheral vasodilator or at the cell signal transduction level.[112] Either integration mechanism could affect arrhythmia. Clinical trials have suggested that the reduction in sudden arrhythmic death observed with angiotensin converting enzyme (ACE) inhibitors may be related to its load reducing actions on electrophysiology;[69,113,114] that is, by its action in reducing wall stress/strain.[115] However, cell signal integration can also explain this effect, and this could be related to the ACE inhibitor's slowing of cardiac remodeling. Cardiovascular drugs such as the ACE inhibitors and carvedilol (possessing β blocker activity), which interact with the remodeling of heart, have proved their efficacy in term of cardiovascular mortality, antiarrhythmic action, and prevention of sudden deaths.

MMI and Hypokalaemia

Diuretic therapy in patients can reduce serum potassium, which can be arrhythmogenic,[116–118] although interaction with other factors may be important.[119] Electrolyte depletion has been considered a risk factor.[120] Hypokalaemia can be related to experimental mechanotransduction.[73,121,122] For example, arrhythmia was generated in isolated heart, normally perfused, by increasing ventricular load. Perfusion with low potassium solutions increased the incidence/severity of this mechanically induced arrhythmia.

LONGER TERM MECHANOELECTRIC CHANGES

The foregoing perusal of observations supporting the existence of some sort of MMI focus mainly on the acute short term. The question arises as to whether there are longer term manifestations.

REMODELING AND CARDIAC FAILURE

Chronic increase in load produces cascades leading to hypertrophy and remodeling. Intracellular calcium, cell signals, and the cytoskeleton could be contenders in the cascades, integration,[123] and genes.

Myocardial failure with a dilated, stretched heart is associated with sudden arrhythmic death. In keeping with the above altered interactive (pathological) gains, studies at the membrane level show that SACs are persistently activated in heart failure.[124] Moreover, mechanosensors are thought to be responsible for the downstream molecular changes[68] in remodeling ventricular structure and function in heart failure (e.g., MAPK, tyrosine kinase). This remodeling involves integration between several cellular mechanisms, which may also be conducive to arrhythmia as early onset genes are turned on in parallel with changes in electrophysiology.[125] It appears that in the longer term, load-induced remodeling in global myocardial failure can produce subtler but significant mechanical heterogeneity, integration, and thus electrophysiological heterogeneity, which is arrhythmogenic.

SUMMARY

The existence of some type of MMI in heart has no shortage of observations supporting it as a hypothesis. Mechanosensitivity (MEF or transduction) has several putative paths for integration. The MMI embraces a plethora of channels, exchangers, and cell "signalsomes"—with pivotal roles for calcium and the cytoskeleton via tensegrity. This can all occur at a molecular, cellular, micro, and macro level. The integration can be spatiotemporal. It has the possibility of becoming deranged with this derangement contributing to mortality. But within MMI there is a deluge of potential therapeutic targets to curtail any derangements.

REFERENCES

1. GUHARAY, F. & F. SACHS. 1984. Stretch-activated single ion channel currents in tissue-cultured embryonic chick skeletal muscle. J. Physiol. **352**: 685–701.
2. MORRIS, C.E. 1990. Mechanosensitive ion channels. J. Memb. Biol. **113**: 93–107.
3. FRENCH, A.S. 1992. Mechanotransduction. Annu. Rev. Physiol. **54**: 135–152.
4. SACKIN, H. 1995. Mechanosensitive channels. Annu. Rev. Physiol. **57**: 333–353.
5. CAZORLA, O., C. PASCAREL, F. BRETTE & J.Y. LE GUENNEC. 1999. Modulation of ion channels and membrane receptor activity by stretch in cardiomyocytes. Possible mechanisms for mechanosensitivity. Prog. Bioph. Molec. Biol. **71**: 29–58.
6. CRAELIUS, W., V. CHEN & N. EL SHERIF. 1988. Stretch activated ion channels in ventricular myocytes. Biosci. Rep. **8**: 407–414.
7. BRADY, A.J. 1991. Mechanical properties of isolated cardiac myocytes. Physiol. Rev. **71**: 413–428.

8. LAB, M.J.. 1978. Mechanically dependent changes in action potentials recorded from the intact frog ventricle. Circ. Res. **42:** 519–528.
9. HANSEN, D.E., C.S. CRAIG & L.M. HONDEGHEM. 1990. Stretch-induced arrhythmias in the isolated canine ventricle: evidence for the importance of mechanoelectrical feedback. Circulation **81:** 1094–1105.
10. DICK, D.J., F.G. HARRISON, P.D. O'KANE, et al. 1993. "Preconditioning" of mechanically induced premature ventricular beats in the isolated rabbit heart. J. Physiol. **459:** p509.
11. LERMAN, B.B., D. BURKHOFF, D.T. YUE, et al. 1985. Mechanoelectrical Feedback: independent role of preload and contractility in modulation of canine ventricular excitibility. J. Clin. Invest. **76:** 1843–1850.
12. ZABEL, M., B.S. KOLLER, F. SACHS & M.R. FRANZ. 1996. Stretch-induced voltage changes in the isolated beating heart: importance of the timing of stretch and implications for stretch-activated ion channels. Cardiovasc. Res. **32:** 120–130.
13. DEAN, J.W. & M.J. LAB. 1987. Effects of changes in afterload on the absolute rerfactory period of the pig ventricle. Pacing Clin. Electrophysiol. **10:** 987.
14. TAGGART, P., P.M.I. SUTTON, T. TREASURE, et al. 1988. Contraction excitation feedback in man. Br. Heart J. **59:** 109.
15. BABUTY, D. & M. LAB. 2001. Heterogeneous changes of monophasic action potential induced by sustained stretch in atrium. J. Cardiovasc. Electrophysiol. **12:** 323–329.
16. BARON, A., L. VAN BEVER, D. MONNIER, et al. 1999. A novel K(ATP) current in cultured neonatal rat atrial appendage cardiomyocytes. Circ. Res. **85:** 707–715.
17. VAN WAGONER, D.R. 1993. Mechanosensitive gating of atrial ATP-sensitive potassium channels. Circ. Res. **72:** 973–983.
18. MATSUDA, N., N. HAGIWARA, M. SHODA, et al. 1996. Enhancement of the L-type Ca2+ current by mechanical stimulation in single rabbit cardiac myocytes. Circ. Res. **78:** 650–659.
19. TABAREAN, I.V., P. JURANKA & C.E. MORRIS. 1999. Membrane stretch affects gating modes of a skeletal muscle sodium channel. Biophys. J. **77:** 758–774.
20. MAINGRET, F., A.J. PATEL, F. LESAGE, et al. 1999. Mechano- or acid stimulation, two interactive modes of activation of the TREK-1 potassium channel. J. Biol. Chem. **274:** 26691–26696.
21. KIM, D. 1992. A mechanosensitive K+ channel in heart cells. Activation by arachidonic acid. J. Gen. Physiol. **100:** 1021–1040.
22. PEREZ, N.G., M.C. DE HURTADO & H.E. CINGOLANI. 2001. Reverse mode of the Na+ -Ca2+ exchange after myocardial stretch: underlying mechanism of the slow force response. Circ. Res. **88:** 376–382.
23. KOHL, P., P.J. COOPER & H. HOLLOWAY. 2003. Effects of acute ventricular volume manipulation on *in situ* cardiomyocyte cell membrane configuration. Prog. Biophys. Mol. Biol. **82:** 221–227.
24. GRATTON, J.P., P. BERNATCHEZ & W.C. SESSA. 2004. Caveolae and caveolins in the cardiovascular system. Circ. Res. **94:** 1408–1417.
25. KAWAKUBO, T., K. NARUSE, T. MATSUBARA, et al. 1999. Characterization of a newly found stretch-activated KCa,ATP channel in cultured chick ventricular myocytes. Am. J. Physiol. **276:** H1827–H1838.
26. TAN, J.H., W. LIU & D.A. SAINT. 2002. Trek-like potassium channels in rat cardiac ventricular myocytes are activated by intracellular ATP. J. Membr. Biol. **185:** 201–207.

27. HORNER, S.M., C.F. MURPHY, B. COEN, et al. 1996. Sympathomimetic modulation of load-dependent changes in the action potential duration in the *in situ* porcine heart. Cardiovasc. Res. **32:** 148–157.
28. LAB, M.J., D. DICK & F.G. HARRISON. 1992. Propranolol reduces stretch arrhythmia in isolated rabbit heart. J. Physiol. (Lond.) **446:** p539.
29. LA FARGE, C.G., R.G. MONROE, W.J. GAMBLE, et al. 1970. Left ventricular pressure and norepinephrine efflux from the dennervated heart. Am. J. Physiol. **219:** 519–524.
30. DICK, D.J., M.J. LAB, F.G. HARRISON, et al. 1994. A possible role of endogeneous catecholamines in stretch induced premature ventricular beats in the isolated rabbit heart. J. Physiol. **479:** p133.
31. DRAKE-HOLLAND, A.J., M.I. NOBLE & M.J. LAB. 2001. Acute pressure overload cardiac arrhythmias are dependent on the presence of myocardial tissue catecholamines. Heart **85:** 576.
32. LERMAN, B.B., E.D. ENGELSTEIN & D. BURKHOFF. 2001. Mechanoelectrical feedback: role of beta-adrenergic receptor activation in mediating load-dependent shortening of ventricular action potential and refractoriness. Circulation **104:** 486–490.
33. MARK, M.D. & S. HERLITZE. 2000. G-protein mediated gating of inward-rectifier K+ channels. Eur. J. Biochem. **267:** 5830–5836.
34. JI, S., S.A. JOHN, Y. LU & J.N. WEISS. 1998. Mechanosensitivity of the cardiac muscarinic potassium channel. A novel property conferred by Kir3.4 subunit. J. Biol. Chem. **273:** 1324–1328.
35. PLEUMSAMRAN, A. & D. KIM. 1995. Membrane stretch augments the cardiac muscarinic K+ channel activity. J. Membr. Biol. **148:** 287–297.
36. KAUFMANN, R.L., M.J. LAB, R. HENNEKES & H. KRAUSE. 1971. Feedback interaction of mechanical and electrical events in the isolated mammalian ventricular myocardium (cat papillary muscle). Pflugers Arch. **324:** 100–123.
37. LAB, M.J., D.G. ALLEN & C.H. ORCHARD. 1984. The effects of shortening on myoplasmic calcium concentration and on the action potential in mammalian ventricular muscle. Circ. Res. **55:** 825–829.
38. BREMEL, R.D. & A. WEBER. 1972. Cooperation within actin filament in vertebrate skeletal muscle. Nat. New Biol. **238:** 97–101.
39. ZHANG, Y. & H.E. TER KEURS. 1996. Effects of gadolinium on twitch force and triggered propagated contractions in rat cardiac trabeculae. Cardiovasc. Res. **32:** 180–188.
40. CALAGHAN, S.C. & E. WHITE. 1999. The role of calcium in the response of cardiac muscle to stretch. Prog. Biophys. Mol. Biol. **71:** 59–90.
41. TAVI, P., C. HAN & M. WECKSTROM. 1998. Mechanisms of stretch-induced changes in [Ca2+]i in rat atrial myocytes: role of increased troponin C affinity and stretch-activated ion channels. Circ. Res. **83:** 1165–1177.
42. GAMBLE, J., P.B. TAYLOR & K.A. KENNO. 1992. Myocardial stretch alters twitch characteristics and Ca2+ loading of sarcoplasmic reticulum in rat ventricular muscle. Cardiovasc. Res. **26:** 865–870.
43. LAB, M.J., B.Y. ZHOU, C.I. SPENCER & W.A. SEED. 1993. Length dependent changes of mechanical restitution in isolated superfused guinea pig papiallry muscle. J. Physiol. **459:** p506.
44. SLINKER, B.K. 1991. Cardiac cycle length modulates cardiovascular regulation that is dependent on previos beat contraction history. Circ. Res. **69:** 2–11.

45. SLINKER, B.K. & K.B. CAMPBELL. 1994. Previous beat contraction history alters mechanical restitution in the isolated left ventricle. Cardiovasc. Res. **28:** 535–541.
46. SIGURDSON, W., A. RUKNUDIN & F. SACHS. 1992. Calcium imaging of mechanically induced fluxes in tissue-cultured chick heart: role of stretch-activated ion channels. Am. J. Physiol. **262:** H1110–H1115.
47. LUNA, E.J. & A.L. HITT. 1992. Cytoskeleton–plasma membrane interactions. Science **258:** 955–964.
48. SADOSHIMA, J. & S. IZUMO. 1997. The cellular and molecular response of cardiac myocytes to mechanical stress. Annu. Rev. Physiol. **59:** 551–571.
49. SADOSHIMA, J. & S. IZUMO. 1993. Mechanical stretch rapidly activates multiple signal transduction pathways in cardiac myocytes: potential involvement of an autocrine/paracrine mechanism. EMBO J. **12:** 1681–1692.
50. WATSON, P.A., T. HANEDA & H.E. MORGAN. 1989. Effect of higher aortic pressure on ribosome formation and cAMP content in rat heart. Am. J. Physiol. **256:** C1257–C1261.
51. HE, Y. & F. GRINNELL. 1995. Role of phospholipase D in the cAMP signal transduction pathway activated during fibroblast contraction of collagen matrices. J. Cell Biol. **130:** 1197–1205.
52. PRASAD, A.R., S.A. LOGAN, R.M. NEREM, *et al.* 1993. Flow-related responses of intracellular inositol phosphate levels in cultured aortic endothelial cells. Circ. Res. **72:** 827–836.
53. KIRBER, M.T., R.W. ORDWAY, L.H. CLAPP, *et al.* 1992. Both membrane stretch and fatty acids directly activate large conductance Ca(2+)-activated K+ channels in vascular smooth muscle cells. FEBS Lett. **297:** 24–28.
54. KIM, D., C.D. SLADEK, C. AGUADO-VELASCO & J.R. MATHIASEN. 1995. Arachidonic acid activation of a new family of K+ channels in cultured rat neuronal cells. J. Physiol. **484:** 643–660.
55. PETROU, S., R.W. ORDWAY, M.T. KIRBER, *et al.* 1995. Direct effects of fatty acids and other charged lipids on ion channel activity in smooth muscle cells. Prostaglandins Leukot Essent Fatty Acids **52:** 173–178.
56. KUCHAN, M.J. & J.A. FRANGOS. 1993. Shear stress regulates endothelin-1 release via protein kinase C and cGMP in cultured endothelial cells. Am. J. Physiol. **264:** H150–H156.
57. BASDRA, E.K., A.G. PAPAVASSILIOU & L.A. HUBER. 1995. Rab and rho GTPases are involved in specific response of periodontal ligament fibroblasts to mechanical stretching. Biochim. Biophys. Acta **1268:** 209–213.
58. LAB, M.J. 1999. Mechanosensitivity as an integrative system in the heart: an audit. Prog. Biophys. Mol. Biol. **71:** 7–27.
59. GU, Y., J. GORELIK, H.A. SPOHR, *et al.* 2002. High-resolution scanning patch-clamp: new insights into cell function. FASEB J. **16:** 748–750.
60. CANTIELLO, H.F., J.L. STOW, A.G. PRAT & D.A. AUSIELLO. 1991. Actin filaments regulate epithelial Na+ channel activity. Am. J. Physiol. **261:** C882–C888.
61. CANTIELLO, H.F. 1995. Role of the actin cytoskeleton on epithelial Na+ channel regulation. Kidney Int. **48:** 970–984.
62. PRAT, A.G. & H.F. CANTIELLO. 1996. Nuclear ion channel activity is regulated by actin filaments. Am. J. Physiol. **270:** C1532–C1543.
63. INGBER, D.E. 1997. Tensegrity: the architectural basis of cellular mechanotransduction. Annu. Rev. Physiol. **59:** 575–599.

64. WANG, N. & D.E. INGBER. 1995. Probing transmembrane mechanical coupling and cytomechanics using magnetic twisting cytometry. Biochem. Cell Biol. **73:** 327–335.
65. YAMADA, K.M. & B. GEIGER. 1997. Molecular interactions in cell adhesion complexes. Curr. Opin. Cell Biol. **9:** 76–85.
66. GUMBINER, B.M. 1993. Proteins associated with the cytoplasmic surface of adhesion molecules. Neuron **11:** 551–564.
67. PLOPPER, G.E., H.P. MCNAMEE, L.E. DIKE, et al. 1995. Convergence of integrin and growth factor receptor signaling pathways within the focal adhesion complex. Mol. Biol. Cell **6:** 1349–1365.
68. SADOSHIMA, J. & S. IZUMO. 1997. The cellular and molecular response of cardiac myocytes to mechanical stress. Annu. Rev. Physiol. **59:** 551–571.
69. DEAN, J.W. & M.J. LAB. 1989. Arrhythmia in heart failure: role of mechanically induced changes in electrophysiology. Lancet **1:** 1309–1312.
70. FRANZ, M.R. 1996. Mechano-electrical feedback in ventricular myocardium. Cardiovasc. Res. **32:** 15–24.
71. LAB, M.J. 1996. Mechanoelectric feedback (transduction) in heart: concepts and implications. Cardiovasc. Res. **32:** 3–14.
72. DALTON, G.R., J.V. JONES, S.J. EVANS & A.J. LEVI. 1997. Wall stress-induced arrhythmias in the working rat heart as left ventricular hypertrophy regresses during captopril treatment. Cardiovasc. Res. **33:** 561–572.
73. EVANS, S.J., A.J. LEVI, J.A. LEE & J.V. JONES. 1995. EMD 57033 enhances arrhythmias associated with increased wall-stress in the working rat heart. Clin. Sci. Colch. **89:** 59–67.
74. SIDERIS, D.A., S. PAPPAS, K. SIONGAS, et al. 1995. Effect of preload and afterload on ventricular arrhythmogenesis. J. Electrocardiol. **28:** 147–152.
75. BAINBRIDGE, F.A. 1915. The influence of venous filling upon the rate of the heart. J. Physiol. **50:** 65–84.
76. BLINKS, J. 1956. Positive chronotropic effect of increasing right atrial pressure in the isolated mammalian heart. Am. J. Physiol. **186:** 299–303.
77. PATHAK, C.L. 1958. Effect of stretch on formation and conduction of electrical impulses in the isolated sinoauricular chamber of the frog's heart. Am. J. Physiol. **192:** 111–113.
78. ALLEN, D.G. & J.C. KENTISH. 1985. The cellular basis of the length-tension relation in cardiac muscle. J. Mol. Cell Caridiol. **17:** 821–840.
79. KENTISH, J.C. & A. WRZOSEK. 1998. Changes in force and cytosolic Ca concentration after length changes in isolated rat ventricular trabeculae. J. Physiol. **506:** 431–444.
80. LE GUENNEC, J.Y., E. WHITE, F. GANNIER, et al. 1991. Stretch-induced increase in resting intracellular calcium concentration in single guinea-pig ventricular myocytes. Exp. Physiol. **76:** 975–978.
81. WHITE, E., J.Y. LE GUENNEC, J.M. NIGRETTO, et al. 1993. The effects of increasing cell length on auxotonic contractions: membrane potential and intracellular calcium transients in single guinea-pig ventricular myocytes. Exp. Physiol. **78:** 65–78.
82. HORNER, S.M., M.J. LAB, C.F. MURPHY, et al. 1994. Mechanically induced changes in action potential duration and left ventricular segment length in acute regional ischaemia in the *in situ* porcine heart. Cardiovasc. Res. **28:** 528–534.
83. CALKINS, H., W.L. MAUGHAN, D.A. KASS, et al. 1989. Electrophysiological effect of volume load in isolated canine hearts. Am. J. Physiol. **256:** H1697–H1706.

84. WANG, Z., L.K. TAYLOR, W.D. DENNEY & D.E. HANSEN. 1994. Initiation of ventricular extrasystoles by myocardial stretch in chronically dilated and failing canine left ventricle. Circulation **90:** 2022–2031.
85. TOBLER, H.G., C.C. GORNIC, R.W. ANDERSON & D.G. BENDITT. 1986. Electrophysiologic properties of the myocardial infarction border zone: effects of transient aortic occlusion. Surgery **100:** 150–156.
86. ZHOU, B.Y., F.G. HARRISON, D.J. DICK, et al. 1993. Ventricular arrhythmogenesis is enhanced by mechanelectric feedback in regional ischaemic heart of the anaesthetised pig. J. Physiol. **473:** p184.
87. PYE, M.P., M. BLACK & S.M. COBBE. 1996. Comparison of *in vivo* and *in vitro* haemodynamic function in experimental heart failure: use of echocardiography. Cardiovasc. Res. **31:** 873–881.
88. MURPHY, C.F. & M.J. LAB. 1994. Ischaemia induced alternans in action potential duration. Eur. J. Cardiol. **15:** 580–581.
89. OPIE, L.H. 1991. Calcium antagonists, ventricular arrhythmias, and sudden cardiac death: a major challenge for the future. J. Cardiovasc. Pharmacol. **18**(Suppl. 10): S81–S86.
90. OPIE, L.H. 1997. Mechanisms whereby calcium channel antagonists may protect patients with coronary artery disease. Eur. Heart J **18**(Suppl. A): A92–A104.
91. LEVY, M.N. & M.N. WISEMAN. 1991. Electrophysiologic mechanisms for ventricular arrhythmias in left ventricular dysfunction: electrolytes, catecholamines and drugs. J. Clin. Pharmacol. **31:** 1053–1060.
92. DI DIEGO, J.M. & C. ANTZELEVITCH. 1994. High [Ca2+]o-induced electrical heterogeneity and extrasystolic activity in isolated canine ventricular epicardium. Phase 2 reentry. Circulation **89:** 1839–1850.
93. ALLEN, D.G., D.A. EISNER & C.H. ORCHARD. 1984. Characterization of oscillations of intracellular calcium concentration in ferret ventricular muscle. J. Physiol. **352:** 113–128.
94. KELLY, M., P. THOMPSON & M. QUINLAN. 1985. Prognostic significance of left ventricular ejection fraction after acute myocardial infarction. Br. Heart J. **53:** 16–24.
95. COPIE, X., K. HNATKOVA, I. BLANKOFF, et al. 1996. Risk of mortality after myocardial infarction: value of heart rate, its variability and left ventricular ejection fraction. Arch. Mal. Coeur. Vaiss. **89:** 865–871.
96. ODEMUYIWA, O., M. MALIK, T. FARRELL, et al. 1991. Multifactorial prediction of arrhythmic events after myocardial infarction. Combination of heart rate variability and left ventricular ejection fraction with other variables. Pacing Clin. Electrophysiol. **14:** 1986–1991.
97. REITER, M.J. & J.A. REIFFEL. 1998. Importance of beta blockade in the therapy of serious ventricular arrhythmias. Am. J. Cardiol. **82:** 9I–19I.
98. SAGER, P.T. 1998. Modulation of antiarrhythmic drug effects by beta-adrenergic sympathetic stimulation. Am. J. Cardiol. **82:** 20I–30I.
99. CAMPBELL, R.W. 1996. ACE inhibitors and arrhythmias. Heart **76**(Suppl. 3): 79–82.
100. WIESFELD, A.C., H.J. CRIJNS, Y.S. TUININGA & K.I. LIE. 1996. Beta adrenergic blockade in the treatment of sustained ventricular tachycardia or ventricular fibrillation. Pacing Clin. Electrophysiol. **19:** 1026–1035.
101. VAN GELDER, I.C., J. BRUGEMANN & H.J. CRIJNS. 1998. Current treatment recommendations in antiarrhythmic therapy. Drugs **55:** 331–346.

102. SINGH, B.N. 1998. Antiarrhythmic drugs: a reorientation in light of recent developments in the control of disorders of rhythm. Am. J. Cardiol. **81:** 3D–13D.
103. HJALMARSON, A. 1997. Effects of beta blockade on sudden cardiac death during acute myocardial infarction and the postinfarction period. Am. J. Cardiol. **80:** 35J–39J.
104. KENNEDY, H.L. 1997. Beta blockade, ventricular arrhythmias, and sudden cardiac death. Am. J. Cardiol. **80:** 29J–34J.
105. KOWEY, P.R. 1996. An overview of antiarrhythmic drug management of electrical storm. Can. J. Cardiol. **12**(Suppl. B): 3B–8B.
106. VON PLANTA, M. & D. CHAMBERLAIN. 1992. Drug treatment of arrhythmias during cardiopulmonary resuscitation. A statement for the advanced life support working party of the European Resuscitation Council. Resuscitation **24:** 227–232.
107. WALLER, D.G. 1991. Treatment and prevention of ventricular fibrillation: are there better agents? Resuscitation **22:** 159–166.
108. CHAMBERLAIN, D.A. 1991. Lignocaine and bretylium as adjuncts to electrical defibrillation. Resuscitation **22:** 153–157.
109. ANDERSON, J.L. 1985. Bretylium tosylate: profile of the only available class III antiarrhythmic agent. Clin. Ther. **7:** 205–224.
110. DUFF, H.J., D.M. RODEN, A. YACOBI, et al. 1985. Bretylium: relations between plasma concentrations and pharmacologic actions in high-frequency ventricular arrhythmias. Am. J. Cardiol. **55:** 395–401.
111. ORTS, A., C. ALCARAZ, K.A. DELANEY, et al. 1992. Bretylium tosylate and electrically induced cardiac arrhythmias during hypothermia in dogs. Am. J. Emerg. Med. **10:** 311–316.
112. ERIKSSON, S.V., P. ENEROTH, J. KJEKSHUS, et al. 1994. Neuroendocrine activation in relation to left ventricular function in chronic severe congestive heart failure: a subgroup analysis from the Cooperative North Scandinavian Enalapril Survival Study (CONSENSUS). Clin. Cardiol. **17:** 603–606.
113. PYE, P. & S.M. COBBE. 1992. Mechanisms of ventricular arrhythmias in cardiac failure and hypertrophy. Cardiovasc. Res. **26:** 740–750.
114. REITER, M.J. 1996. Effects of mechano-electric feedback: potential arrhythmogenic influence in patients with congestive heart failure. Cardiovasc.Res. **32:** 44–51.
115. COHN, J.N., D.G. ARCHIBALD, S. ZIESCHE, et al. 1986. Effect of vasodilator therapy on mortality in chronic congestive heart failure. Results of a Veterans Administration Cooperative Study. N. Engl. J. Med. **314:** 1547–1552.
116. STEWART, D.E., H. IKRAM, E.A. ESPINER & M.G. NICHOLLS. 1985. Arrhythmogenic potential of diuretic induced hypokalaemia in patients with mild hypertension and ischaemic heart disease. Br. Heart J. **54:** 290–297.
117. GULKER, H., W. HAVERKAMP & G. HINDRICKS. 1989. Ion regulation disorders and cardiac arrhythmia. The relevance of sodium, potassium, calcium, and magnesium. Arzneimittelforschung **39:** 130–134.
118. PODRID, P.J. 1990. Potassium and ventricular arrhythmias. Am. J. Cardiol. **65:** 33E–44E.
119. DARGIE, H.J., J.G. CLELAND, B.J. LECKIE, et al. 1987. Relation of arrhythmias and electrolyte abnormalities to survival in patients with severe chronic heart failure. Circulation **75:** IV98–IV107.

120. PACKER, M., S.S. GOTTLIEB & M.A. BLUM. 1987. Immediate and long-term pathophysiologic mechanisms underlying the genesis of sudden cardiac death in patients with congestive heart failure. Am. J. Med. **82:** 4–10.
121. JAMES, M.A. & J.V. JONES. 1992. The paradoxical role of left ventricular hypertrophy in wall stress-related arrhythmia. J. Hypertens. **10:** 167–172.
122. DICK, D.J. & M.J. LAB. 1995. Effect of manipulation of potassium concentration on stretch-induced arrhythmia in the isolated Langendorff rabbit heart. J. Physiol. **487:** p140.
123. BUSTAMANTE, J.O., A. RUKNUDIN & F. SACHS. 1991. Stretch-activated channels in heart cells: relevance to cardiac hypertrophy. J. Cardiovasc. Pharmacol. **17**(Suppl 2): S110–S113.
124. CLEMO, H.F., B.S. STAMBLER & C.M. BAUMGARTEN. 1999. Swelling-activated chloride current is persistently activated in ventricular myocytes from dogs with tachycardia-induced congestive heart failure. Circ. Res. **84:** 157–165.
125. MEGHJI, P., S.A. NAZIR, D.J. DICK, *et al.* 1997. Regional workload induced changes in electrophysiology and immediate early gene expression in intact *in situ* porcine heart. J. Mol. Cell Cardiol. **29:** 3147–3155.

Three-Dimensional Models of Individual Cardiac Histoanatomy: Tools and Challenges

REBECCA A.B. BURTON,[a]* GERNOT PLANK,[b]* JÜRGEN E. SCHNEIDER,[c]* VICENTE GRAU,[d] HELMUT AHAMMER,[b] STEPHEN L. KEELING,[e] JACK LEE,[f,g] NICOLAS P. SMITH,[f,g] DAVID GAVAGHAN,[g] NATALIA TRAYANOVA,[h] AND PETER KOHL[a]

[a]*Department of Physiology, Anatomy and Genetics, University of Oxford, Oxford OX1 3PT, UK*

[b]*Institute of Biophysics, Centre for Physiological Medicine, Medical University Graz, 8010 Graz, Austria*

[c]*Department of Cardiovascular Medicine, University of Oxford, Oxford OX3 7BN, UK*

[d]*Department of Engineering Science, University of Oxford, Parks Road, Oxford OX1 3PJ, UK*

[e]*Institut für Mathematik, Karl Franzens Universität Graz, 8010 Graz, Austria*

[f]*Bioengineering Institute, University of Auckland, Private Bag 92019, Auckland, New Zealand*

[g]*Oxford University Computing Laboratory, Parks Road, Oxford OX1 3QD, UK*

[h]*Department of Biomedical Engineering, Johns Hopkins University, Baltimore, Maryland 21201*

*Equal contribution first authors

ABSTRACT: There is a need for, and utility in, the acquisition of data sets of cardiac histoanatomy, with the vision of reconstructing individual hearts on the basis of noninvasive imaging, such as MRI, enriched by reference to detailed atlases of serial histology obtained from representative samples. These data sets would be useful not only as a repository of knowledge regarding the specifics of cardiac histoanatomy, but could form the basis for generation of individualized high-resolution cardiac structure–function models. The current article presents a step in this general direction: it illustrates how whole-heart noninvasive imaging can be combined with whole-heart histology in an approach to achieve automated construction of histoanatomically detailed models of cardiac 3D

Address for correspondence: Peter Kohl, M.D., Ph.D., Department of Physiology, Anatomy and Genetics, University of Oxford, Oxford OX1 3PT, UK. Voice: 44-01865-272500; fax: 44-01865-272554.
e-mail: peter.kohl@physiol.ox.ac.uk

structure and function at hitherto unprecedented resolution and accuracy (based on 26.4 × 26.4 × 24.4 μm MRI voxel size, and enriched by histological detail). It provides an overview of the tools used in this quest and outlines challenges posed by the approach in the light of applications that may benefit from the availability of such data and tools.

KEYWORDS: noninvasive imaging; MRI; serial histology; three-dimensional histoanatomy; cardiac modeling; personalized medicine

INTRODUCTION

The heart is a highly heterogeneous structure, with intrinsic differences in cell type distribution, complex electromechanical properties, and an organized activation sequence. It appears that properly integrated function at the whole organ level arises from, and necessarily requires, the concerted interplay of intrinsic structure–function gradients.[1] Any change in this well-orchestrated heterogeneity (be it an increase, or indeed a decrease)[2] may have detrimental effects on cardiac function.

In terms of major cell populations, the largest volume of cardiac tissue is occupied by myocytes, while fibroblasts dominate in terms of cell numbers.[3] We have recently shown that these heterogeneous cells are able to communicate directly via gap junctions.[4] In addition, both cardiac myocytes and nonmyocytes are stretch-sensitive, thereby contributing to the functional interaction of cardiac mechanics, electrophysiology, and structure.[5] Finally, relative cell content, distribution, and coupling change significantly during both physiological and pathological remodeling of myocardium, which makes the (ideally noninvasive) identification of cardiac histoanatomical features an important target for fundamental research and clinical application.[6]

Nonetheless, even after more than a century of studies into ventricular tissue architecture,[7,8] there is still controversy about apparently basic issues, such as whether or not there is a "unique band" arrangement of myocardial fibers throughout the heart.[9,10] This seems surprising since cardiac fiber orientation plays crucial roles in physiologically and clinically relevant functions affecting electrical conduction,[11,12] inducibility of arrhythmias,[13,14] electrical defibrillation,[15,16] contraction and relaxation,[17,18] and coronary perfusion.[19,20] The lack of definite insight may be explained by the fact that traditional histological techniques are very time consuming and, hence, often conducted on tissue fragments only. This, in combination with their "destructive" nature (in terms of tissue preparation and sectioning), has thus far made routine reconstruction of individual hearts impossible.

With the improvement of both spatial and temporal resolution of novel imaging techniques, issues such as the one outlined above have begun to be addressed via nondestructive assessment of cardiac anatomy and tissue architecture.[6,21] Magnetic resonance imaging (MRI), and diffusion tensor MRI

(DTMRI) in particular, have demonstrated significant promise in providing reliable data on both cardiac fiber and sheet architecture with a resolution that allows computational reintegration into anatomically based models of mammalian ventricles.[18,22] MRI investigations can be conducted in a fraction of the time required for traditional serial sectioning-based histology. In addition, nondestructive imaging is ultimately aimed at *in situ* assessment of living tissue (even though method development is often conducted *ex vivo*, in fixed samples), where a combination of advanced scanning protocols and computational postprocessing[23–25] makes it increasingly possible to address challenges posed by motion, and to extract functional, rather than "merely" structural, data.

Drawbacks of MR-based cardiac tissue reconstruction include the still limited spatial resolution which, in recent studies, has been 156 μm × 312 μm × 2 mm (DTMRI, rabbit),[26] 350 μm × 350 μm × 800 μm (DTMRI, canine),[27] 1 mm × 1 mm × 4 mm (DTMRI, pig heart),[10] and 800 μm × 800 μm × 2 mm (spin-echo MRI, man)[28] (the first two numbers describe resolution in-plane, the third number relates to interplane distance/out-of-plane resolution). Also, there are still significant challenges in how these data are processed in terms of segmentation, calculation of fiber direction, and computational grid generation.[27,29,30]

Furthermore, histological validation of MRI and DTMRI data has remained incomplete, as previous work focused on using discrete tissue plugs extracted from various cardiac locations and subsequently related back to approximately matching volumes in the MRI data.[18,26,31] Consequently, current cardiac data sets, obtained using the above techniques, do not tend to include the atria, papillary muscles, trabeculae, or segmentation of tissue for different cell populations. Furthermore, while previous efforts to identify the topology of vascular networks,[32] including the coronary vessel trees, have provided morphometric information to define connectivities, radii, and segment lengths,[33–36] data on the spatial distribution of vessels within a tissue (recently characterized for the renal circulation)[37] are still missing.

Clearly, there is a great need for, and utility in, the acquisition of detailed data sets of cardiac histoanatomy. Individual hearts could be reconstructed on the basis of MRI, and enriched by reference to serial histology-based information, to thereby provide high-detail validated information on cardiac geometry, fiber and sheet orientation, cell populations, and a wealth of cardiac microstructural detail. Combining MRI and traditional histological sectioning to achieve this would combine "the best of both worlds": (i) MRI to generate three-dimensional (3D) histoanatomical organ features that guide image stack alignment and compensate nonlinear distortions; and (ii) histology to increase spatial resolution and discriminate cell populations and a-cellular connective tissue.

The acquired data sets will be useful not only as a repository of knowledge regarding the specifics of cardiac histoanatomy, but as the basis for the generation of high-resolution cardiac structure–function models. Indeed,

TABLE 1. Listing of solutions used in this investigation. All solutions were at controlled pH (7.4), osmolality (300±5), and temperature (37°C).

	NaCl [mM]	LiCl [mM]	KCl [mM]	MgCl$_2$ [mM]	CaCl$_2$ [mM]	Glucose [mM]	HEPES [mM]	gassed with
NT	140.0		5.4	1.0	1.8	11.0	5.0	O$_2$
Li		140.0	5.4	1.0	1.8	11.0	5.0	O$_2$
HiK	125.0		20.0	1.0	1.8	11.0	5.0	O$_2$

NT: normal Tyrode solution; Li: sodium-free lithium-containing solution; HiK: high potassium solution.

computational meshes could be generated from these data sets, and functional characteristics of various cell types could be incorporated in the models, providing an unprecedented opportunity to elucidate previously unresolved issues related to cardiac mechanics, electrical behavior, or hemodynamics.

The current article presents a step in this general direction: it illustrates how whole-heart noninvasive imaging can be combined with whole-heart histology in an approach to achieve automated construction of detailed histoanatomical models of individualized cardiac 3D structure and function. It provides an overview of the current tools used in this quest, outlines the challenges posed by the approach, and discusses the broad applications that will benefit from the availability of such data sets and tools.

TOOLS

Wet-Lab

All investigations conformed to the UK Home Office guidance on the Operation of Animals (Scientific Procedures) Act of 1986. Hearts were isolated from 3 female rabbits (~1.2 kg) after induction of terminal anesthesia (100 mg kg^{-1} sodium pentobarbitone; Rhône Merieux, Harlow UK) and swiftly connected, via the aorta, to a constant flow (7–8 mL min^{-1}) Langendorff perfusion system. An incision in the pulmonary artery was made to avoid buildup of hydrostatic pressure. Initial perfusion (2 min) with normal tyrode style solution (NT) containing heparin (5IU mL^{-1}) was conducted to wash the tissue before exposure to any intervention (see TABLE 1 for composition of solutions).

Hearts were fixed with minimal delay either (i) after introduction of contracture (sodium-replacement by lithium, Li solution), (ii) during cardioplegic arrest (using high potassium, HiK), or (iii) in cardioplegic arrest combined with ventricular volume overload. Tissue fixation was by coronary perfusion with 50 mL of the fast-acting Karnovsky's fixative (2% formaldehyde, 2.5% glutaraldehyde mix),[38] containing 2 mM gadodiamide (contrast agent). During the entire procedure, hearts were positioned in a glass container filled with matching solutions to maintain the preparation bubble free. Fixed whole hearts were stored in Karnovsky's for up to 2 days before wax embedding.

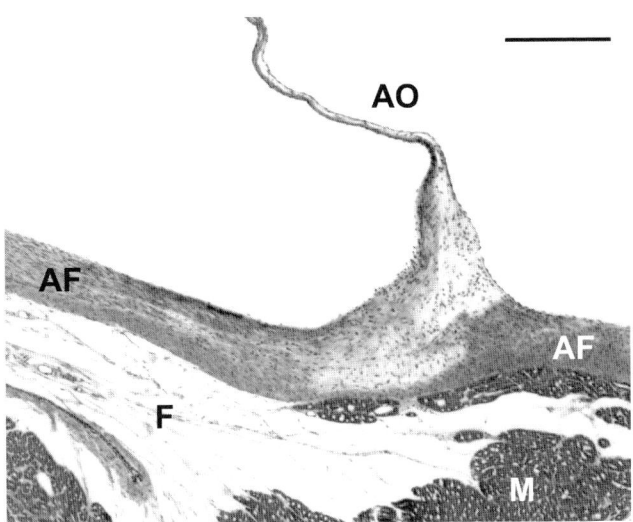

FIGURE 1. Histological appearance of left ventricular tissue (Trichrome stained, 5 × objective), revealing extensive detail on structures such as aortic valve (AO), myocardium (M), and fibrous tissue (F) adjacent to the annulus fibrosus (AF). Scale bar: 250 μm. (see online version for color image.)

For MRI of fixed tissue, hearts were stabilized in an NMR tube, using low melting 1% agar with 2 mM paramagnetic gadodiamide contrast agent. For subsequent histological follow-up, hearts were rinsed in cacodylate buffer (3×) and then dehydrated by exposure to rising alcohol concentrations (8 h each in 20/30/50/70% alcohol, 48 h in 90%, 4 × 6 h in 100% alcohol). The alcohol was then replaced by Xylene (five changes over 48 h) and finally the tissue was gradually infiltrated with wax (48 h 25%; 12 h 50%; 12 h 75%; 1–2 weeks in 100%, depending on the size of the heart).

Histology

Whole hearts were serially sectioned (10 μm thickness) and every section collected on APES (3-aminoproplytriethoxysilane 99%, Acros Organics, Fisher Scientific, UK)-coated slides. Every fifth section was Trichrome stained to identify collagen (bluish green), myocytes (pink), cytoplasm (orange, highlighting nonmyocytes), and nuclei (blue–black; FIG. 1; see online version for color illustration).

Stained sections were mounted in DPX (a mixture of distyrene, plasticiser, and xylene, RA Lamb, UK), and imaged using a Leica QWin workstation and QGO software (Leica, Wetzlar, Germany) to obtain whole cardiac cross-section mosaic images using a 5 × objective, yielding a final image resolution of 1.1 μm (FIG. 2 A). Remaining sections were stored for back up or subsequent

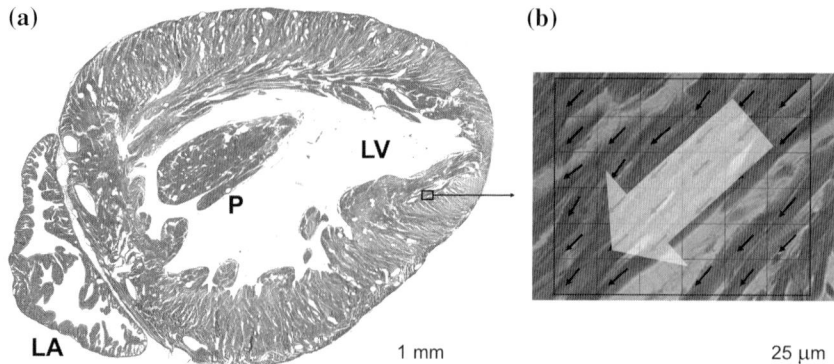

FIGURE 2. (**A**) Mosaic montage image of a longitudinal cardiac section (Trichrome stained), consisting of ~250 individual frames. LA: left auricular appendage; LV: left ventricle; P: papillary muscle. Fiber orientation, cleavage planes, myocardial sheets (or laminae), coronary vasculature, and myocyte/nonmyocyte distribution can be clearly identified. (**B**) Schematic representation of regional fiber orientation extraction (see text for detail). (See online version for color image.)

additional analysis using other imaging modalities and/or staining protocols such as immunohistochemistry for functional studies.

One whole heart histological reconstruction, from fixation to completed two-dimensional (2D) serial imaging of every fifth section, took just under 6 weeks (compared to an unattended overnight run for 3D anatomical MRI, see next section).

MRI

Although MRI provides inferior spatial resolution compared to histology, the noninvasiveness, intrinsic contrast, and true 3D capability of this technique make it attractive for the study of intact organs, both *ex vivo* and *in vivo*.

Imaging experiments were carried out on an 11.7 T (500 MHz) MR system comprising a vertical magnet (bore size 123 mm; Magnex Scientific, Oxon, UK), a Bruker Avance console (Bruker Medical, Ettlingen, Germany), and a shielded gradient system (548 mT m^{-1}, rise time 160 µsec; Magnex Scientific, Oxon, UK). Quadrature-driven birdcage coils with an inner diameter of 28 mm and 40 mm (Rapid Biomedical, Würzburg, Germany) were used to transmit/receive the NMR signals.

Using an established fast gradient echo technique (TE/TR = 7.5/30 msec) for high-resolution gap-free 3D MRI,[39–41] fixed hearts were scanned with an in-plane resolution of 26.4 µm × 26.4 µm, and an out-of-plane resolution of 24.4 µm. Reconstruction of the MR data was performed as described elsewhere.[41] FIGURE 3 shows cross-sections obtained from three hearts, fixed in different mechanical conditions. Two-dimensional image planes were collated

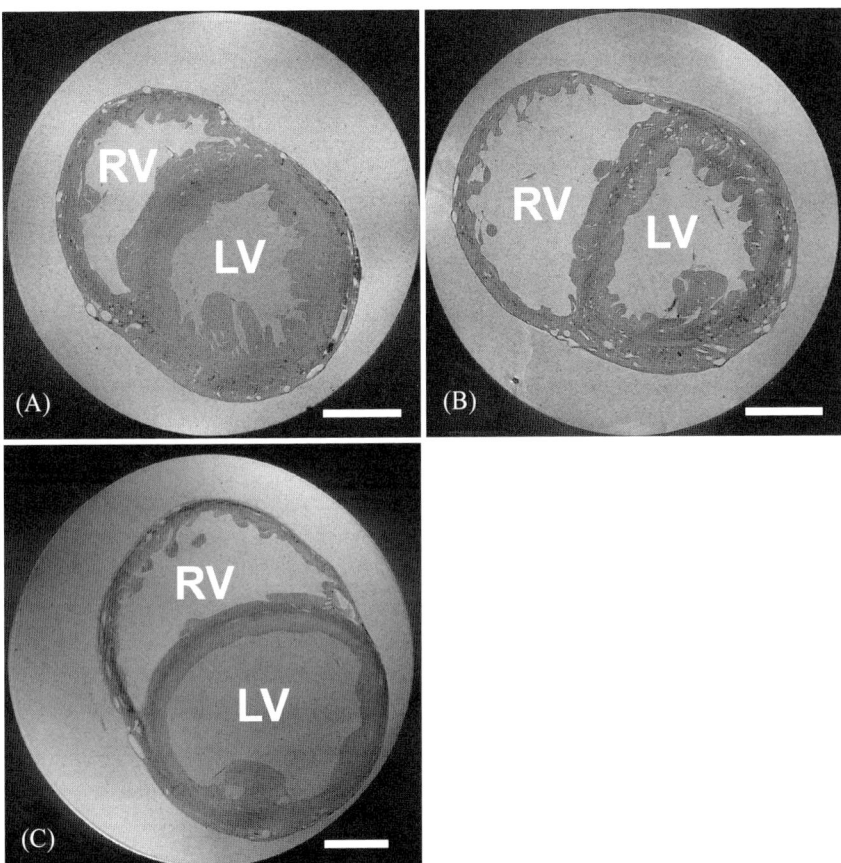

FIGURE 3. MR image planes obtained from contractured (**A**), slack (**B**), and volume-loaded (**C**) hearts (scale bar: 5 mm). In (**A**) and (**B**), voxel size is $26.5 \times 26.5 \times 24.5$ μm, and in (**C**) $32 \times 32 \times 44$ μm (a larger bore NMR tube was required for the volume-loaded heart). RV: right ventricle; LV: left ventricle. A full movie of the data in FIGURE 3B, progressing through transversal MRI sections from aorta to apex, can be downloaded from: http://mef.physiol.ox.ac.uk/MRI/Aorta_to_apex.avi.

and used to generate a 3D MRI-based data set, which could subsequently be sectioned at any desired angle for visualization and analysis (FIG. 4).

Image Alignment

Histological techniques are superior to MRI in spatial resolution and discrimination of cell types, but they are limited by their destructive nature. Thus, tissue slice alignment is lost during mounting and 2D imaging. In addition, histological images are flawed by artifacts from nonlinear deformations, caused

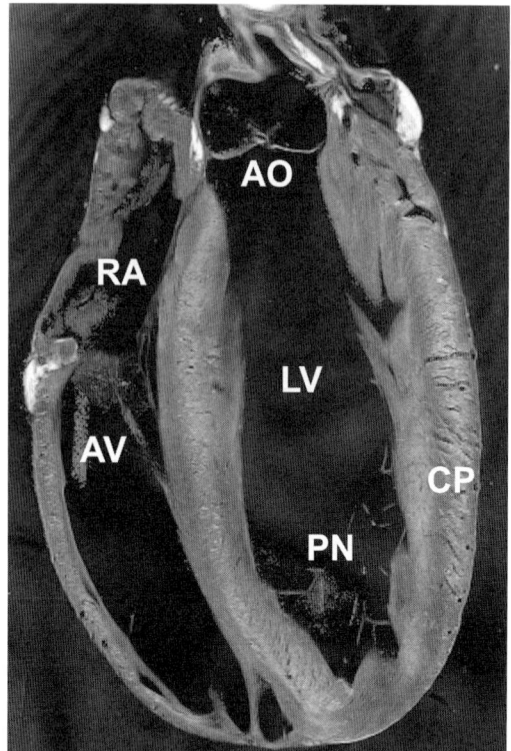

FIGURE 4. Longitudinal section of the data set in FIGURE 3B, reconstructed from multiple transverse 2D MR images showing structural detail such as aortic (AO) and right atrioventricular (AV) valves, free-running Purkinje network (PN), and ventricular cleavage planes (CP). LV: left ventricle, RA: right atrium.

by tissue shrinkage during processing, by mechanical forces during microtome slicing, and by potentially inhomogeneous relaxation of sections before mounting. These drawbacks may be overcome by guiding image alignment using anatomical MRI data obtained from the same preparation prior to sectioning.

Several deformable registration algorithms have been developed to correct distortion in histological images,[42–46] where distortion is compensated for by calculating the deformation that minimizes the difference between two adjacent slices. This may cause loss of real (or gain of artificial) structural data points.

In our approach, alignment is carried out in two steps. An initial coarse alignment step aims to minimize the difference between adjacent slices by applying rigid transformations only; that is, translation and rotation to ensure a good starting point for the subsequent registration procedure (FIG. 5 B, D). In a second step, a partial differential equation-based approach is applied for mapping corresponding points between adjacent slices (FIG. 5 C, E).[45] In this

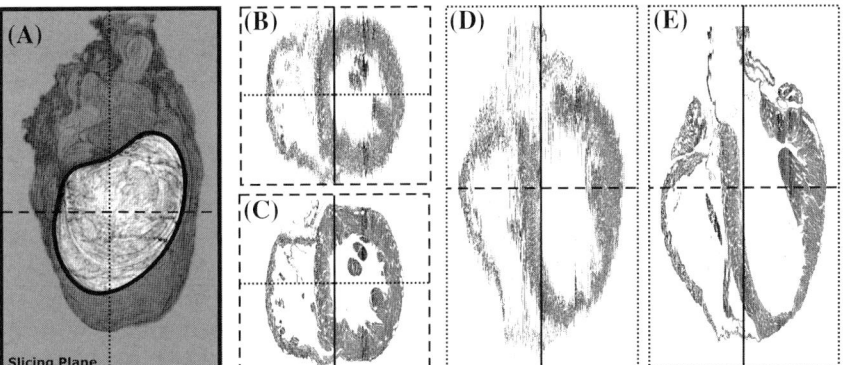

FIGURE 5. Three-dimensional reconstruction of a rabbit heart from serial histological sections that were performed approximately along the mediolateral axis of the heart (i.e., roughly parallel to the ventricular septum, see outline in (**A**). Slices were registered using an elastic registration with maximum rigidity, and results are visualized in two planes that are perpendicular to the original slicing plane, before (**B** and **D**) and after (**C** and **E**) registration. (See online version for color image.)

approach, pixel trajectories between adjacent slices are computed based on a variational formulation in which departure from rigidity in an optical flow is penalized. The approach is "generalized rigid" in the sense that a rigid registration, indeed an interpolation, is obtained when one matches the given data. Otherwise, the registration is more elastic depending upon the strength of regularization. Furthermore, such regularization provides a true measure of elastic energy in relation to the more common linear elastic potential energy of displacements.[45] The associated variational problem is solved by a pyramidal and geometric multigrid scheme.[47]

Results in FIGURE. 5 show the improvement achieved with these two transformations of the histological data sets. However, in the process of correcting geometrical distortion, valuable anatomical information arising from differences between adjacent slices may be lost, potentially compromising the accuracy of models generated. To overcome this drawback, we are working toward the addition of gross anatomical information from MR images to ensure that the slices are not overaligned in the deformation correction process.

Data Extraction

Segmentation

Using histological data, it is straightforward to discriminate different tissue types and the extracellular space. Most importantly, myocardial tissue, which underlies key electromechanical functioning of the heart, can be segmented automatically from Trichrome-stained sections using color thresholding.

Segmentation of the MRI stack is computationally more expensive and requires several processing steps. Typically, due to inevitable spatial variations in coil sensitivity, segmentation cannot be achieved simply by gray-level thresholding since in areas of decreased coil sensitivity an overlap in gray levels between object and background may occur. To circumvent this problem, in the present study thresholding was combined with probe-specific background subtraction and a set of morphological operations to facilitate segmentation. Briefly, two tissue-free slices from the MRI stack, one below the apex and another one above the atria, were selected, interpolated over the stack volume containing the tissue, and subtracted from the MRI stack to remove background gray levels. Subsequently, the entire stack was segmented slice by slice, starting at the apex. In each slice, a gray-level thresholding step was implemented and a binary mask was created, which allowed elimination of all pixels outside the heart. The binary mask was further improved by a set of morphological operations, including hole filling, and closing and removal of connected objects that are of a size below a certain (user-defined) number of voxels. For each slice, the mask from the previous slice was taken into account to avoid abrupt variations, which could possibly occur along low-contrast regions of the heart. Finally, the mask was applied to the entire MRI stack to discriminate the heart's volume, excluding surrounding volume and cavities. Within the heart volume, differences in gray levels were sufficient to allow a direct segmentation between tissue and extracellular cleft space or vessels.

Fiber Orientation

The predominant fiber orientation in 2D images can be determined via filtered magnitude and direction assessment of intensity gradients (FIG. 2 B).[48] For calculating the principal orientation in 3D gray-level data sets, we used the gradient structure tensor.[49] To calculate the structure tensor, the gradient of the image was calculated at each voxel of the histological 3D data sets, previously corrected for deformation as explained above. The tensor product of the gradient vector with itself was calculated, providing a 3×3 matrix for each voxel. The structure tensor is the result of filtering the matrix components using a Gaussian kernel. For "beam-like" structures such as cardiac fibers with a clear spatial orientation, this direction corresponds to the matrix eigenvector of the smallest eigenvalue. User-defined adjustment of the variance of the Gaussian kernel allows focusing on structures of a desired size such as fibers in 3D image stacks.

Coronary Vasculature

The present high-resolution MR image stacks also provide unique spatial information on coronary vascular networks within individual whole hearts. Although no vessel-specific stain was applied during the tissue preparation, the global structure of the vasculature can be segmented from the myocardium, as illustrated in FIGURE 6. This is achieved by isolating the voxels within the myocardium, which have a gray-level intensity range similar to that of the background. Starting from the segmented image stack of the myocardium, generated as described above, an intensity-based connected region-growing technique was combined with nonlinear edge detecting filters to isolate and segment the vasculature, while reducing noise, down to radii of approximately 30 µm. FIGURE 6 A, B show horizontal and frontal views and rendering of the segmented vasculature produced via this process.

The reconstruction of the vascular network into a model description was conducted by reducing the voxel-based graphical elements of the images to a skeletal structure and associating specific radii with each location along this structure (FIG. 6 C, D). The local vessel radius is estimated from lumen boundaries identified by active contours, which supports resolution of irregularly shaped cross-sections. Once all vessel segments are tracked, they are assembled into networks. This compact model description can then be used to characterize the coronary structure and to serve as a mesh for numerical simulations of hemodynamic function.

Mesh Generation

To assemble models of cardiac structure and function, computational meshes have to be extracted from the generated data. These meshes will be used to calculate the origin and spread of electrical signals in the heart, compute active and passive deformation of myocardium, assess coronary flow and, ultimately, combine electrical and mechanical activity in the heart with fluid dynamics and valve movements. With such a broad range of applications in mind, mesh generation needs to address a wide range of demands in terms of accuracy, resolution, and implementation.

The simplest approach to mesh generation uses hexahedral finite elements to discretize domains on a regular structured grid. In this case, meshes can be generated efficiently from segmented image stacks, where each voxel is treated either as a myocardial element or a nonmyocardial element.

Generation of unstructured grids is a more complex operation, but offers several advantages over structured grids such as: (i) unstructured grids are better suited for defibrillation studies as they lack jagged boundaries that are typical for structured grids (which introduce spurious currents due to tip effects) and (ii) unstructured grids can be generated adaptively such that the spatial resolution varies (using a fine mesh with little adaptivity to model the myocardium and representing other tissue by coarser elements that grow in size with distance from myocardial surfaces).

An example of this approach is shown in FIGURE 7, where a mesh for calculating action potential propagation is extracted from the segmented data (FIG. 7 A).

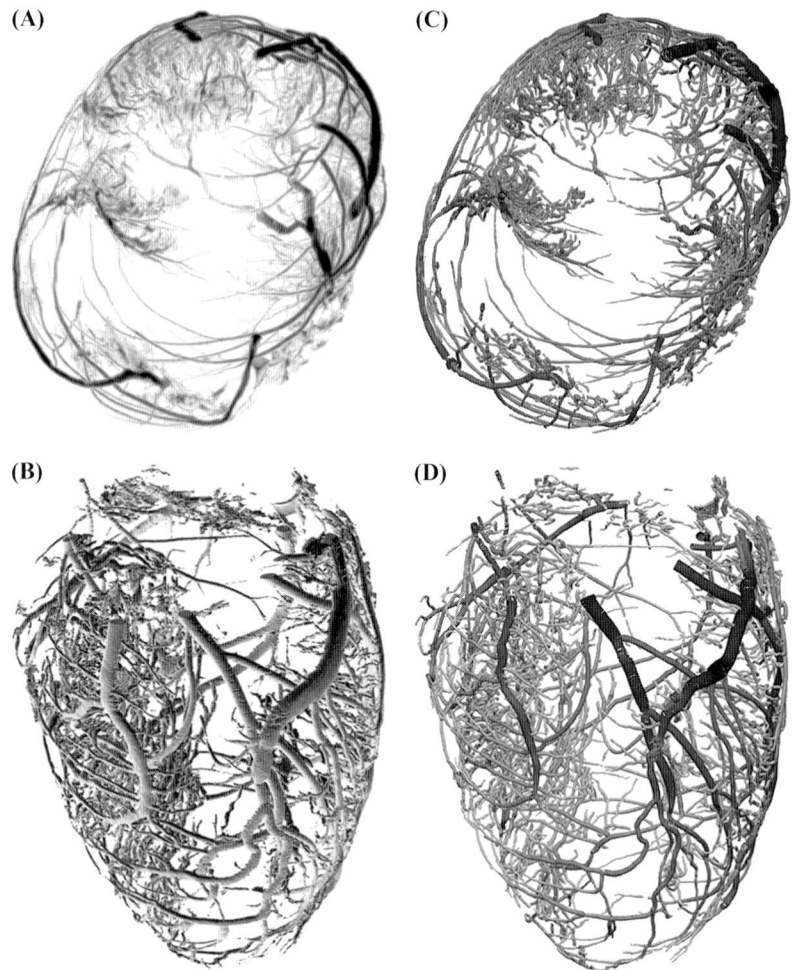

FIGURE 6. Results of vascular segmentation from the data set shown in FIGURE 3B. (**A**) Inverted maximum intensity projection. (**B**) Volume rendering of segmented voxels representing the coronary tree. (**C** and **D**) Gray-level coded vessel radius distribution of coronary vasculature from 340 μm (dark) to 30 μm (light). (**A** and **C**) horizontal projections; (**B** and **D**) lateral projections.

We considered three different mesh generation approaches (Octree, Delaunay, and Advancing Front Techniques),[50] and eventually applied an Octree-based meshing technique to produce boundary-fitted, locally refined, and conformal multielement meshes (FIG. 7 B) that included microheterogeneities (FIG. 7 C). The actual solution to the electrical problem is illustrated in FIGURE 7D.

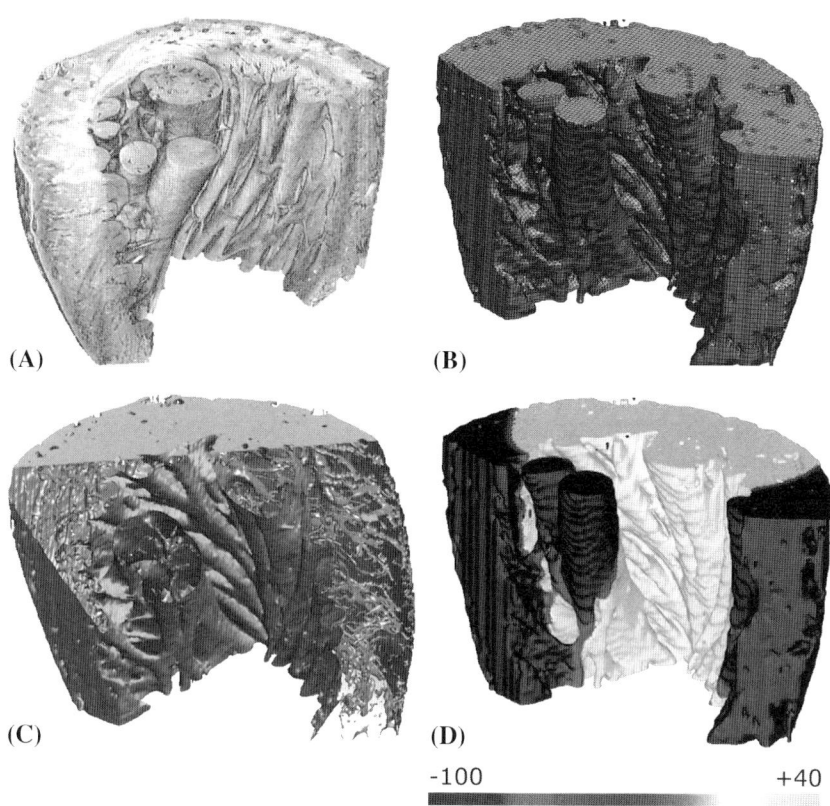

FIGURE 7. Left-ventricular wedge with papillaries and trabeculae. (**A**) 3D visualization of segmented tissue sub-stack. (**B**) adaptive FEM mesh. (**C**) partially cut wedge exposing histology-based microstructural detail. (**D**) bidomain simulation of effects of fiber direction on electrical impulse propagation. Scale bar illustrates voltage distribution in mV. (See online version for color figure.)

CHALLENGES

As outlined in the "Introduction," the long-term objective of the proposed approach is to build individualized whole-heart reconstructions of cardiac structure and function, which are based on noninvasive imaging, enriched with histological data, and used for computational modeling of individual pathophysiological behavior and prediction of responses to experimental or clinical interventions.

This vision crucially hinges on automated construction of histoanatomically detailed computational meshes to support quantitative assessment of individual cardiac 3D structure and function. This requires advanced techniques for mesh generation, which will be aided by atlases and computationally efficient techniques for visualization and modeling to reintegrate the vast data sets in-

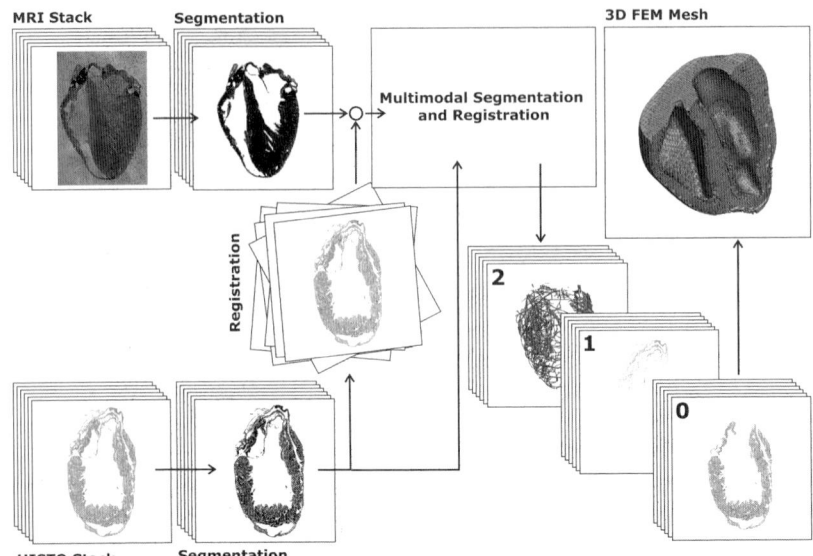

FIGURE 8. Generation of individualized high-resolution computational meshes from combined MRI and histological image data. Segmentation of MRI data results in a contiguous 3D data set. Segmented histological images have to be registered, slice by slice, and transformed to create a 3D histological stack. Both 3D data sets are then fused together. Such a histoanatomical global data set will enable the detailed segmentation of myocardial fibers, interstitial clefts, vessels, and connective tissue. In the process of segmentation, each voxel is classified and indexed (for instance 0 = myocardium, 1 = connective tissue, 2 = vessel, etc.), to account for the different properties of cells and regions that comprise the computational mesh. On this basis, provided the registration of histological data is sufficiently accurate, fiber orientation can be computed even without resorting to DTMRI.

volved in describing an individual heart. A schematic summary of this process is presented in FIGURE 8, illustrating the workflow from MRI- and histology-based segmentation, to registration of histological sections, coregistration of data sets, and finite element mesh generation.

Coregistration will make use of probabilistic atlases, an approach that is successfully used in clinical brain imaging, to complement the limited noninvasively obtained information about any individual patient with more detailed knowledge about generic histoanatomical features.[51] This approach is emerging in the field of cardiac MRI,[52] where template geometries have been successfully used for predictive computational modeling of cardiac anatomy.[27] However, there is a lack of detailed whole-heart histoanatomical data sets to be integrated with these MRI templates; this deficiency is being addressed as described above.

Further challenges include the efficient integration of individual processing steps, suitable user-interfacing, and visualization of the various processing steps and corresponding data levels involved in the generation of individualized 3D representations of the heart.

On the applications side, linking cardiac histoanatomy to electromechanical function represents a major challenge as spatiotemporal heterogeneities in cell properties, coupling, or activation timing are not self-evident from cardiac structure information. Clearly, this is an area where further experimental species-defined research into cardiac electromechanics needs to be interrelated to structural insight to inform model development. This is particularly important for the modeling of pathologically disturbed behavior, which often involves complex structure–function remodeling.

More imminent progress will arise from the successful segmentation and tracking of anatomically based structures such as the Purkinje network or of the individual coronary trees. Thus, knowledge of exit and entry locations of free-running conduction pathways will guide the assignment of tissue properties relevant for simulation of proper sinus node activation patterns of the heart. Vascular structure–function relationships will benefit from the first direct calculation of branch angles and quantification of the relationship between microstructural fiber sheet arrangement and vessel orientation as well as from solving Navier–Stokes[53] and finite deformation equations[54] for functional simulation of the spatiotemporal distribution of coronary flow during the cardiac cycle.

It is evident from this short (and necessarily incomplete) list of challenges that constructing individual 3D histoanatomically detailed hearts requires a wide range of skills and expertise, and is highly collaborative in nature. Projects like this require a suitable backbone structure for curation of a wide variety of data commodities (such as images, executables, spreadsheets, or text) and tools for exchange. Furthermore, computational speed and short processing time are essential aspects of this process since the clinical utility of integrated individual 3D heart modeling crucially depends on its ability to provide results in time frames that are suitable to support data visualization, interpretation, diagnosis, and potentially, prediction of interventions. As a first step in using a broader computational base, the present project made extensive use of the integrative biology infrastructure set up at Oxford (which is open to interested users in the scientific community);[55] other infrastructures will likely become available as progress is made toward the vision outlined in this article.

The authors would like to view the present article as the first step of a long journey. Much remains to be learned along the way to a truly exciting destination.

ACKNOWLEDGMENTS

We thank Dr. Judith Sheldon and Barry Martin at Oxford Brookes University for expert histological advice, and Professor Kieran Clarke at Oxford

University for access to the MR system of her laboratory. Individual facets of this collaborative study were supported by the UK Biotechnology and Biological Sciences Research Council (PK), UK Medical Research Council (RABB), the Austrian Science Fund (GP), the British Heart Foundation (JES; PK), the Royal Society of New Zealand (JL, NPS), and the U.S. National Institutes of Health (NPS; NT [HL63195]). The project is part of the *Integrative Biology* Initiative at Oxford University: http://www.integrativebiology.ox.ac.uk/.

REFERENCES

1. KATZ, A.M. & P.B. KATZ. 1989. Homogeneity out of heterogeneity. Circulation **79:** 712–717.
2. KOHL, P. 2004. Cardiac cellular heterogeneity and remodelling. Cardiovasc. Res. **64:** 195–197.
3. KOHL, P. 2003. Heterogeneous cell coupling in the heart. Circ. Res. **93:** 381–383.
4. CAMELLITI, P., C.R. GREEN, I. LEGRICE & P. KOHL. 2004. Fibroblast network in rabbit sino-atrial node: structural and functional identification of homo- and heterologous cell coupling. Circ. Res. **94:** 828–835.
5. KOHL, P., P. HUNTER & D. NOBLE. 1999. Stretch-induced changes in heart rate and rhythm: clinical observations, experiments and mathematical models. Prog. Biophys. Mol. Biol. **71:** 91–138.
6. HELM, P.A., L. YOURNES, M.F. BEG, *et al.* 2006. Evidence of structural remodeling in the dyssynchronous failing heart. Circ. Res. **98:** 125–132.
7. MACCALLUM, J.B. 1900. On the muscular architecture and growth of the ventricles of the heart. Johns Hopkins Hosp. Rep. **9:** 307–335.
8. MALL, F.P. 1911. On the muscular architecture of the ventricles of the human heart. Am. J. Anat. **11:** 211–266.
9. BUCKBERG, G.D. 2005. New technology and old responsibilities. Euro. J. Cardiothorac. Surg. **27:** 472–474.
10. SCHMID, P., T. JAERMANN, P. BOESIGER, *et al.* 2005. Ventricular myocardial architecture as visualized in postmortem swine hearts using magnetic resonance diffusion tensor imaging. Euro. J. Cardiothorac. Surg. **27:** 468–474.
11. KANAI, A. & G. SALAMA. 1995. Optical mapping reveals that repolarization spreads anisotropically and is guided by fiber orientation in guinea pig hearts. Circ. Res. **77:** 784–802.
12. VETTER, F.J., S.B. SIMONS, S. MIRONOV, *et al.* 2005. Epicardial fiber organization in swine right ventricle and its impact on propagation. Circ. Res. **96:** 244–251.
13. CHEN, P.S., Y.M. CHA, B.B. PETERS & L.S. CHEN. 1993. Effects of myocardial fiber orientation on the electrical induction of ventricular fibrillation. Am. J. Physiol. **264:** H1760–H1773.
14. DE BAKKER, J.M., M. STEIN & H.V. VAN RIJEN. 2005. Three-dimensional anatomic structure as substrate for ventricular tachycardia/ventricular fibrillation. Heart Rhythm **2:** 777–779.
15. EASON, J., J. SCHMIDT, A. DABASINSKAS, *et al.* 1998. Influence of anisotropy on local and global measures of potential gradient in computer models of defibrillation. Ann. Biomed. Eng. **26:** 840–849.

16. HOOKS, D.A., K.A. TOMLINSON, S.G. MARSDEN, et al. 2002. Cardiac microstructure: implications for electrical propagation and defibrillation in the heart. Circ. Res. **91:** 331–338.
17. WALDMAN, L.K., D. NOSAN, F. VILLARREAL & J.W. COVELL. 1988. Relation between transmural deformation and local myofiber direction in canine left ventricle. Circ. Res. **63:** 550–562.
18. CHEN, J., W. LIU, H. ZHANG, et al. 2005. Regional ventricular wall thickening reflects changes in cardiac fiber and sheet structure during contraction: quantification with diffusion tensor MRI. Am. J. Physiol. **289:** H1898–H1907.
19. DELHAAS, T., T. ARTS, P.H. BOVENDEERD, et al. 1993. Subepicardial fiber strain and stress as related to left ventricular pressure and volume. Am. J. Physiol. **264:** H1548–H1559.
20. MAZHARI, R., J.H. OMENS, J.W. COVELL & A.D. MCCULLOCH. 2000. Structural basis of regional dysfunction in acutely ischemic myocardium. Cardiovasc. Res. **47:** 284–293.
21. TSENG, W.Y., J. DOU, T.G. REESE & V.J. WEDEEN. 2006. Imaging myocardial fiber disarray and intramural strain hypokinesis in hypertrophic cardiomyopathy with MRI. J. Magn. Reson. Imag. **23:** 1–8.
22. HELM, P., M.F. BEG, M.I. MILLER & R.L. WINSLOW. 2005. Measuring and mapping cardiac fiber and laminar architecture using diffusion tensor imaging. Ann. N. Y. Acad. Sci. **1047:** 296–307.
23. ABLITT, N.A., J. GAO, J. KEEGAN, et al. 2004. Predictive cardiac motion modeling and correction with partial least squares regression. IEEE Transac. Med Imag. **23:** 1315–1324.
24. LARSON, A.C., P. KELLMAN, A. ARAI, et al. 2005. Preliminary investigation of respiratory self-gating for free-breathing segmented cine MRI. Magn. Resonan. Med. **53:** 159–168.
25. LOTJONEN, J., M. POLLARI, S. KIVISTO & K. LAUERMA. 2005. Correction of motion artifacts from cardiac cine magnetic resonance images. Acad. Radiol. **12:** 1273–1284.
26. SCOLLAN, D.F., A. HOLMES, R.L. WINSLOW & J. FORDER. 1998. Histological validation of myocardial microstructure obtained from diffusion tensor magnetic resonance imaging. Am. J. Physiol. **275:** H2308–H2318.
27. BEG, M.F., P.A. HELM, E. MCVEIGH, et al. 2004. Computational cardiac anatomy using MRI. Magn. Resonan. Med. **52:** 1167–1174.
28. MIQUEL, M.E., D.L.G. HILL, E.J. BAKER, et al. 2003. Three- and four-dimensional reconstruction of intra-cardiac anatomy from two-dimensional magnetic resonance images. Intl. J. Cardiovasc. Imag. **19:** 239–254.
29. ANGELIE, E., P.J. DE KONING, M.G. DANILOUCHKINE, et al. 2005. Optimizing the automatic segmentation of the left ventricle in magnetic resonance imaging. Med. Phys. **32:** 369–375.
30. PLUEMPITIWIRIYAWEJ, C., J.M. MOURA, Y.J. WU & C. HO. 2005. STACS: new active contour scheme for cardiac MR image segmentation. IEEE Transac. Med. Imag. **24:** 593–603.
31. HOLMES, A.A., D.F. SCOLLAN & R.L. WINSLOW. 2000. Direct histological validation of diffusion tensor MRI in formaldehyde-fixed myocardium. Magn. Resonan. Med. **44:** 157–161.
32. CUMMING, G., R. HENDERSON, K. HORSFIELD & S. SINGHAL. 1969. The functional morphology of the pulmonary circulation. *In* The Pulmonary Circulation and Interstitial Space: 327–338. University of Chicago Press. Chicago.

33. VANBAVEL, E. & J. SPAAN. 1992. Branching patterns in the porcine coronary arterial tree. Circ. Res. **71:** 1200–1212.
34. KASSAB, G.S. 2000. The coronary vasculature and its reconstruction. Ann. Biomed. Eng. **28:** 903–915.
35. KASSAB, G.S., C.A. RIDER, N.J. TANG & Y.C. FUNG. 1993. Morphometry of pig coronary arterial trees. Am. J. Physiol. **265:** H350–H365.
36. DHAWAN, S., K.C. DHARMASHANKAR & T. TAK. 2004. Role of magnetic resonance imaging in visualizing coronary arteries. Clin. Med. Res. **2:** 173–179.
37. NORDSLETTEN, D.A., S. BLACKETT, M.D. BENTLEY, et al. 2006. Structural morphology of renal vasculature. Am. J. Physiol. **291:** H296–H309.
38. KARNOVSKY, M.J. 1965. A formaldehyde-glutaraldehyde fixative of high osmolarity for use in electron microscopy. J. Cell Biol. **27:** 137A–138A.
39. SCHNEIDER, J.E., S.D. BAMFORTH, C.R. FARTHING, et al. 2003. Rapid identification and 3D reconstruction of complex cardiac malformations in transgenic mouse embryos using fast gradient echo sequence magnetic resonance imaging. J. Mol. Cell Cardiol. **35:** 217–222.
40. SCHNEIDER, J.E., S.D. BAMFORTH, S.M. GRIEVE, et al. 2003. High-resolution, high-throughput magnetic resonance imaging of mouse embryonic anatomy using a fast gradient-echo sequence. Magma **16:** 43–51.
41. SCHNEIDER, J.E., J. BOSE, S.D. BAMFORTH, et al. 2004. Identification of cardiac malformations in mice lacking PTDSR using a novel high-throughput magnetic resonance imaging technique. Biomed. Central Develop. Biol. **4:** 16.
42. SORZANO, C.O., P. THEVENAZ & M. UNSER. 2005. Elastic registration of biological images using vector-spline regularization. IEEE Transac. Biomed. Eng. **52:** 652–663.
43. MAKELA, T., P. CLARYSSE, O. SIPILA, et al. 2002. A review of cardiac image registration methods. IEEE Transac. Med. Imag. **21:** 1011–1021.
44. WIRTZ, S., N. PAPENBERG, B. FISCHER & O. SCHMITT. 2005. Robust and staining-invariant elastic registration of a series of images from histologic slices. Medical imaging 2005: physiology, function, and structure from Medical Images. 1256–1262.
45. KEELING, S. & W. RING. 2005. Medical image registration and interpolation by optical flow with maximal rigidity. J. Math. Imag. Vision. **23:** 47–65.
46. PITIOT, A., E. BARDINET, P.M. THOMPSON & G. MALANDAIN. 2006. Piecewise affine registration of biological images for volume reconstruction. Med. Image Anal. **10(3):** 465–483.
47. KEELING, S.L. 2006. Geometric multigrid for generalized affine and generalized rigid image registration. J. Math. Imag. Vision. In press.
48. KARLON, W., J.W. COVELL, A.D. MCCULLOCH & J.H. OMENS. 1998. Automated measurement of myofiber disarray in transgenic mice with ventricular expression of Ras. Anat. Rec. **252:** 612–625.
49. WEICKERT, J. 1999. Coherence-enhancing diffusion filtering. Intl J. Comp. Vision **31:** 111–127.
50. OWEN, S. 2004. A survey of unstructured mesh generation technology. http://www.andrew.cmu.edu/user/sowen/survey/index.html.
51. THOMPSON, P.M., M.S. MEGA, K.L. NARR, et al. 2000. Brain image analysis and atlas construction. In SPIE Handbook of Medical Image, Processing and Analysis. M. Fitzpatrick & T M. Sonka, Eds. SPIE Press. In press.

52. LORENZO-VALDES, M., G.I. SANCHEZ-ORTIZ, A.G. ELKINGTON, *et al.* 2004. Segmentation of 4D cardiac MR images using a probabilistic atlas and the EM algorithm. Med. Image Anal. **8:** 255–265.
53. SMITH, N.P., A.J. PULLAN & P.J. HUNTER. 2002. An anatomically based model of coronary blood flow and myocardial mechanics. SIAM J. App. Math. **62:** 990–1018.
54. NASH, M.P. & P.J. HUNTER. 2000. Computational mechanics of the heart. J. Elast. **61:** 121–141.
55. PITT-FRANCIS, J., A. GARNY & D. GAVAGHAN. 2006. Enabling computer models of the heart for high-performance computers and the grid. Phil. Transac. Roy. Soc. **364:** 1501–1516.

Cardiac Defibrillation and the Role of Mechanoelectric Feedback in Postshock Arrhythmogenesis

VIATCHESLAV GUREV, MARY M. MALECKAR, AND NATALIA A. TRAYANOVA

Department of Biomedical Engineering, Tulane University, New Orleans, Louisiana 70118, USA

ABSTRACT: Ventricular dilatation increases the defibrillation threshold (DFT). In order to elucidate the mechanisms responsible for this increase, the present article investigates changes in the postshock behavior of the myocardium upon stretch. A two-dimensional electro-mechanical model of cardiac tissue incorporating heterogeneous fiber orientation was used to explore the effect of sustained stretch on postshock behavior via (*a*) recruitment of mechanosensitive channels (MSC) and (*b*) tissue deformation and concomitant changes in tissue conductivities. Recruitment of MSC had no influence on vulnerability to electric shocks as compared to control, but increased the complexity of postshock VF patterns. Stretch-induced deformation and changes in tissue conductivities resulted in a decrease in vulnerability to electric shocks.

KEYWORDS: defibrillation; mechanoelectric feedback; reentry; myocardial stretch; bidomain model

INTRODUCTION

Strong electrical shocks are commonly used to terminate ventricular fibrillation (VF). The understanding of defibrillation mechanisms and factors influencing defibrillation efficacy is essential to the improvement of existing and development of new defibrillation techniques. Together with other factors influencing defibrillation efficacy, such as electrophysiological properties of the myocardium,[1–3] geometry of the heart,[4] and blood volume,[5] the mechanical conditions of the ventricles and atrial contraction can play an important role in postshock activity via mechanisms of mechanoelectrical feedback (MEF).[6–8] Experimental evidence demonstrates that ventricular dilatation, due to increase in ventricular preload[9] or intracavitary balloon placement,[10] elevates the

Address for correspondence: Natalia Trayanova, Department of Biomedical Engineering, Johns Hopkins University, 3400 N. Charles Street, Clark Hall 201, Baltimore, MD 21218. Voice: 410-516-4116; fax: 410-516-5294.
e-mail: ntrayan1@jhu.edu

defibrillation threshold (DFT). It has been speculated that an increase in DFT is due to changes in refractoriness of cardiac tissue. Changes in refractoriness that take place during ventricular dilatation accelerate VF, increase complexity of the VF activation pattern,[11] and decrease the current threshold for VF onset.[12] Alterations in preshock state have been shown to change the DFT.[13]

During ventricular dilatation, tissue stretch evokes MEF mechanisms, including activation of mechanosensitive channels (MSC).[14–18] Heterogeneous fiber structure within the ventricular wall creates regional strain gradients and subsequent inhomogeneous activation of MSC, which may explain stretch-induced heterogeneities in tissue refractoriness.[12,19–21] Stretch of the myocardium also results in changes in the orientation of myocardial fibers with respect to the defibrillation electrodes, which may affect postshock behavior. Fiber geometry influences the location and magnitude of shock-induced virtual electrodes[22,23] and thus shock outcome.

We hypothesize that increased propensity of postshock arrhythmias following stretch of the ventricular wall is due to heterogeneous fiber structure, which results in

(1) inhomogeneous activation of MSC, leading to a dispersion of refractoriness and a more complex preshock state, and
(2) change in the myocardial fiber angle with respect to defibrillation electrodes, influencing shock-induced virtual electrodes.

The current article investigates changes in postshock electrical activity caused by stretch of cardiac tissue using a two-dimensional electro-mechanical model incorporating heterogeneous fiber structure. The model allowed us to simulate both the recruitment of MSC and the tissue deformation with corresponding changes in conductivities that occur upon stretch.

METHODS

Tissue Geometry

Simulations were performed using a two-dimensional sheet of cardiac tissue (55 × 55 mm). The fiber structure (FIG. 1 A) was identical to the formulation of Beaudoin and Roth,[24] with the angle a between x-axis and fiber direction given by:

$$\alpha(x, y) = \frac{\pi}{2} \cos^2\left(\frac{\pi x}{D}\right) \cos^2\left(\frac{\pi y}{D}\right), \quad (1)$$

where D is the edge length of the tissue square, with the coordinate system origin located in the center of the sheet.

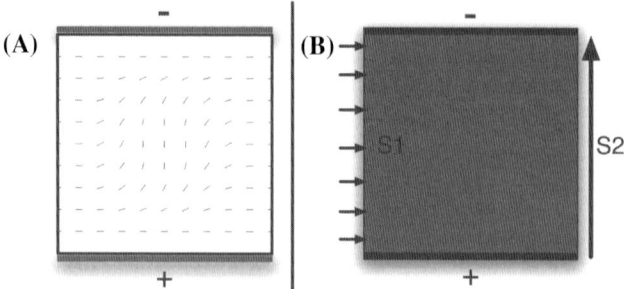

FIGURE 1. Geometry of the model (**A**) and shock protocol (**B**).

Mechanics

The tissue mechanics were based on finite element elasticity theory. This approach to modeling cardiac tissue mechanics has been described in detail elsewhere.[25–27] We considered only the passive mechanical properties of the tissue, as active mechanical properties play a limited role during rapid activation in VF. The central equation of the mechanical problem, solved for the components of the second Piola-Kirchhoff tensor and deformation gradient tensor with respect to the fiber coordinate system (consisting of fiber [f], and cross-fiber [c] directions), is based on the conservation of linear momentum in the absence of body forces.

Stress was formulated as a derivative of the strain energy function. The model incorporated anisotropic mechanical properties using an exponential strain energy function,[28] ignoring radial deformations:

$$W = \frac{1}{2} M(e^Q - 1), \quad Q = b_1 E_{ff}^2 + b_2 E_{cc}^2 + 2b_3 E_{fc}^2 . \quad (2)$$

Here E_{ff}, E_{cc}, and E_{fc} are components of the Lagrangian strain tensor. This equation has four material parameters: M scales the stress, b_1 and b_2 scale the material stiffness in fiber and cross-fiber directions, respectively, and b_3 scales the material rigidity under shear in the fiber–cross-fiber plane. We used $M = 1.76$ kPa, $b_1 = 18.5$, $b_2 = 3.58$, and $b_3 = 1.63$.

Electrical Behavior

Electrical interaction between cells was based on the bidomain model.[29] In bidomain theory, cardiac tissue is considered, at each point, as both an intracellular and an extracellular continuum separated by a membrane. The transmembrane potential, V_m, is governed by the following set of equations:

$$\nabla \sigma_e \nabla \Phi_e = -\beta_m \left(C_m \frac{dV_m}{dt} + I_{ion} \right), \quad \nabla \sigma_i \nabla \Phi_i = \beta_m \left(C_m \frac{dV_m}{dt} + I_{ion} \right), \quad (3)$$

where σ_e and σ_i are extracellular and intracellular conductivity tensors, respectively, Φ_e and Φ_i are the corresponding electrical potentials, C_m is specific membrane capacitance, I_{ion} is transmembrane current density, and β_m is the membrane surface to cell volume ratio. Dirichlet and no-flux Neumann boundary conditions were applied in the extracellular and intracellular spaces, respectively.

We considered three cases: (*a*) unstretched tissue, (*b*) stretched tissue with MSC recruitment, and (*c*) stretched tissue with changes in conductivities and nodal coordinates. In the second case, to simulate the effect of stretch, I_{ion} in Equation (3) included a putative stretch-activated current which depends on the local strain of the tissue; Equation (3) was solved on the unstretched computational grid. In the third case, we altered the spatial coordinates of the nodes in the computational grid according to tissue deformation. We also changed the conductivity tensors in the intracellular space and applied transformations to the conductivity tensors to represent fiber rotation during stretch.[30] From this point forward, this collective set of alterations to the nodal coordinates and conductivities upon stretch is referred to as "changes in fiber angle."

Ionic Model and Electroporation

To describe the membrane kinetics, we used the Luo-Rudy dynamic model.[31–33] The model includes detailed descriptions of the main sarcolemmal ionic currents such as Na^+, K^+, and Ca^{2+}, as well as electrogenic pumps and exchangers, Ca^{2+} induced Ca^{2+} release, and Ca^{2+} buffering. As we are examining the response of the tissue to electric shocks, we also included an electroporation current, as formulated by DeBruin and Krassowska.[34]

MSC

As a basis for representing MSC, we used the formulation of the nonselective current from Zabel *et al.*[35] We modified this formulation by substituting sarcomere length with the stretch ratio λ that corresponds to the strain in the fiber direction, $\lambda = \sqrt{2E_{ff} + 1}$, to obtain the following expression for the current density:

$$I_{\text{ns,stretch}} = -L(\lambda) \times [\gamma \rho (V_m - V_r)], \tag{4}$$

in which the dependence of current magnitude on stretch is as follows:

$$L(\lambda) = \frac{1}{1 + K e^{-\alpha(\lambda - 1)}}. \tag{5}$$

In Equations (4) and (5), γ is the single channel conductance, ρ is the channel density, V_r is the reversal potential, K and α are parameters controlling the amount of current at tissue reference length and the sensitivity to stretch. Values of γ and ρ were taken from the original formulation, and their product

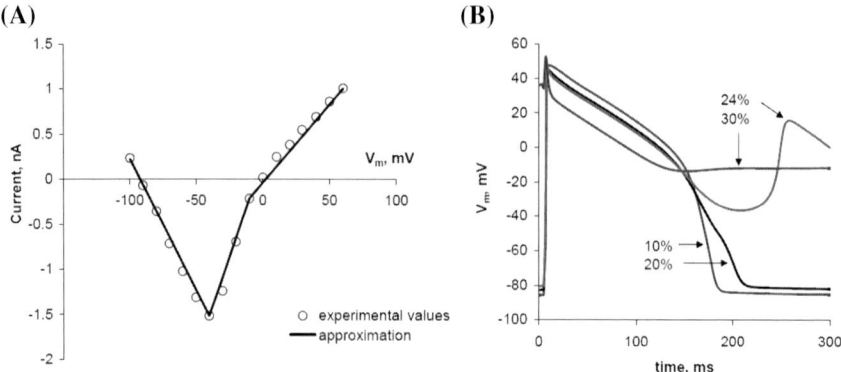

FIGURE 2. Current-voltage relationship of the differential potassium current ΔI_{k+} (see text for detail) (**A**) and action potentials of a single cell at different degrees of stretch (**B**).

being equal to 0.75 mS/cm². The reversal potential V_r was taken as -10 mV. The values of K and α were 110 and 14.7, respectively.

In addition, the change in the inwardly rectifying K⁺ current (I_{K1}) and the outwardly rectifying K⁺ current (I_{Ko}) due to their mechanosensitivity were also incorporated in the model. Assuming the same stretch ratio dependence $L(\lambda)$, it was formulated as:

$$\Delta I_{K^+} = 5.25 \times L(\lambda)$$
$$\times [I_{K1(\text{stretched})} + I_{Ko(\text{stretched})} - I_{K1(\text{unstretched})} - I_{Ko(\text{unstretched})}]. \quad (6)$$

In Equation (6), $I_{K1(\text{stretched})}$ is the inwardly rectifying K⁺ current and $I_{Ko(\text{stretched})}$ is the outwardly rectifying K⁺ whole cell current measured at 22% local stretch of the cell.[16] The term in brackets in Equation (6) is modeled via a piecewise linear function, which depends on membrane potential (FIG. 2 A). The scaling factor 5.25 ensures that the product $5.25 \times L(\lambda)$ equals 1 at $\lambda = 1.22$ (22% stretch). This formulation reproduces experimental results,[16] such as action potential duration shortening at early plateau levels, after depolarization at 22% stretch, delayed repolarization, and depolarization of the resting potential by approximately 10 mV (FIG. 2 B). A large degree of stretch (close to 30%) depolarizes the membrane to approximately -16 mV and prevents the repolarization of the action potential.[16]

Computation

Numerical solutions for the bidomain model employed the explicit finite-element method with a spatial discretization of 100 μm. Dynamic time stepping was used for ionic model solution. The finite element method was used to solve the mechanical formulation. We used bilinear interpolation with square finite elements of edge length 0.37 mm.

Simulation Protocol

In a series of simulations, we compared the postshock behavior of unstretched tissue with tissue stretched in the horizontal direction at 0, 10, 15, or 20% of its reference length. The stretched tissue included introduction of either MSC or changes in the fiber angle distribution.

We used an S1–S2 protocol consisting of a train of 10 S1 transmembrane stimuli applied from the left edge of the sheet at a basic cycle length of 300 ms and S2 monophasic shocks of 8 ms duration and of strengths 10–50 V/cm delivered at various coupling intervals (100–240 ms) via line electrodes at the top and bottom sides of the sheet (FIG. 1 B).

Analysis

As part of the analysis of the simulation results, we constructed vulnerability areas. A vulnerability area encompasses episodes of reentry induction for various coupling intervals and shock strengths.[36] Vulnerability areas were constructed for unstretched tissue, tissue with activated MSC, and tissue with changes in the fiber angles. In addition, we examined the locations of phase singularities of the reentrant circuits using the algorithm employed by Eason and Trayanova.[37]

For visualization purposes, data from stretched tissue, such as transmembrane potential and strain, were mapped from the deformed computational grid onto the undeformed grid.

RESULTS

Tissue Stretch

FIGURE 3 A shows the stretch ratio (corresponding to strain in the fiber direction) for 20% stretch. The smallest strain was observed in the middle of the sheet, because fibers in this region are oriented close to the vertical direction, and horizontal stretch of the sheet increases strain mostly in the cross-fiber direction. In the middle of the left and right edges of the sheet strain was also small, despite the horizontal orientation of the fibers. This is due to the fact that tissue compliance is larger in the cross-fiber direction as compared to the fiber direction, and stretch in the middle of the sheet prevented stretch of the tissue close to the edges.

Typically, fibers in the sheet rotated in a clockwise direction upon stretch, aligning themselves in the horizontal direction as shown in FIGURE 3 B. In

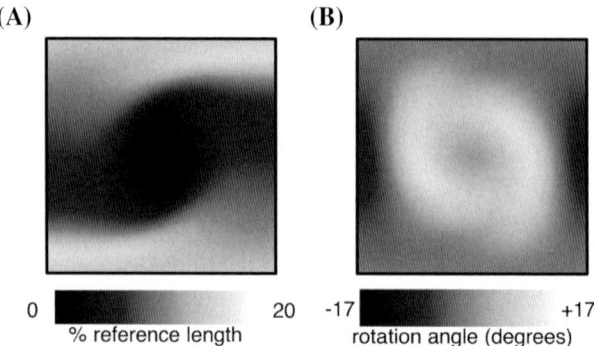

FIGURE 3. Stretch ratio for a horizontal stretch of 20% of the reference length (**A**). Rotation angle between the pre- and poststretch fiber direction (**B**). Clockwise angles of rotation are positive.

the middle of the left and right edges, fibers rotated in a counterclockwise direction. The largest magnitude of rotation was approximately 17°.

Virtual Electrodes and Vulnerability of the Tissue to Electric Shocks

FIGURE 4 shows the transmembrane potential during and after the shock in unstretched tissue (FIG. 4 A), tissue with recruited MSC due to a stretch of 20% (FIG. 4 B), and tissue with changes in the fiber angle directions as the result of 20% stretch (FIG. 4 C). Stretch changes the amplitude (FIG. 4, top panels) of the virtual electrodes. The greatest effect is observed for tissue with changes in the fiber angle, where a significant decrease in shock-induced positive and negative polarization takes place.

In FIGURE 5, the transmembrane potential at shock end along the length of the white arrow depicted in FIGURE 4 A, top panel, is shown. The horizontal axis shows the distance along the arrow starting at the lower left corner of the sheet. The transmembrane potentials for unstretched tissue and tissue with inclusion of MSC were similar. However, the virtual cathode in the tissue incorporating changes in fiber angle revealed different behavior: the transmembrane potential decreased by more than 30 mV, and the spatial transition between the virtual anode and the virtual cathode shifted toward the top edge of the sheet.

Shocks created virtual electrodes with an interlocking spiral morphology. Virtual electrode polarization prolonged repolarization in regions where tissue had not recovered before the shock (FIG. 4). For coupling intervals in the range 100–160 ms, no reentrant circuits were formed. For coupling intervals in the range 160–180 ms, cathode-break excitation was observed, which led to reentry. When the coupling interval was increased to 180–220 ms, the virtual cathodes excited recovered regions, resulting in immediate propagation and

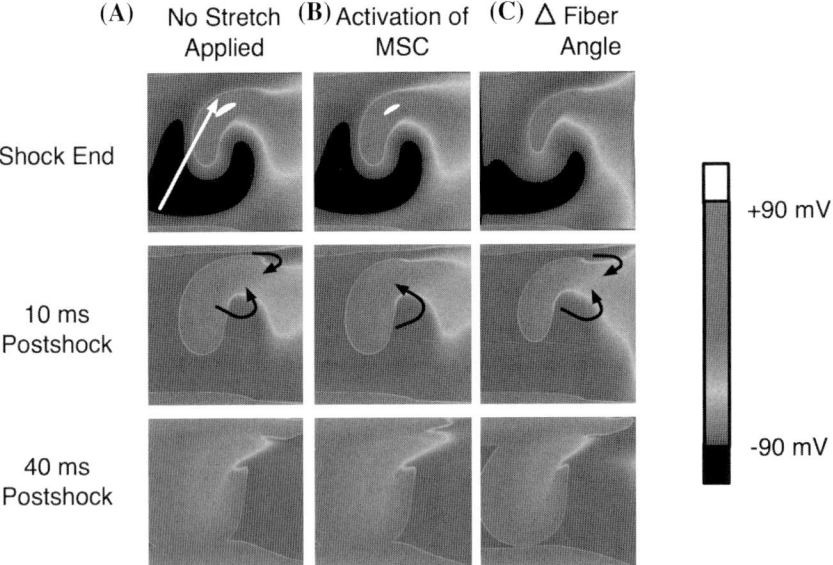

FIGURE 4. Virtual electrode polarization in unstretched tissue (**A**), tissue with recruitment of MSC due to 20% stretch (**B**), and tissue with changes, Δ, in the fiber angle (**C**). The top panel shows the transmembrane potential distribution at shock end. The middle and bottom panels show transmembrane potential maps at 10 ms and 40 ms postshock, respectively. Coupling interval is 200 ms and shock strength is 50 V/cm.

reentry. In FIGURE 4, behavior of the tissue is shown at 10 and 40 ms postshock. In unstretched tissue and stretched tissue with changes in fiber angles, shocks produced a figure-of-eight reentry, as depicted with black arrows. In tissue incorporating MSC, a prolonged refractory period in the top right corner of the sheet prevented activation near that edge, and the shock produced a single spiral wave. As the coupling interval increased beyond 240 ms, the virtual cathode closest to the right edge of the sheet increased in magnitude, resulting in an activation which led to collision of propagation fronts and failure to induce reentry.

We did not find a difference in the vulnerability areas between unstretched tissue and tissue with involvement of MSC. However, change in the fiber angles due to stretch decreased vulnerability significantly (FIG. 6, gray area); for instance, the shock strength required to induce reentry increased from 20 V/cm to 28 V/cm at a coupling interval of 180 ms. At a coupling interval of 160 ms, we did not succeed in inducing reentry in the deformed tissue even for a shock strength of 100 V/cm, while in unstretched tissue the 28 V/cm shock was sufficient to produce reentry.

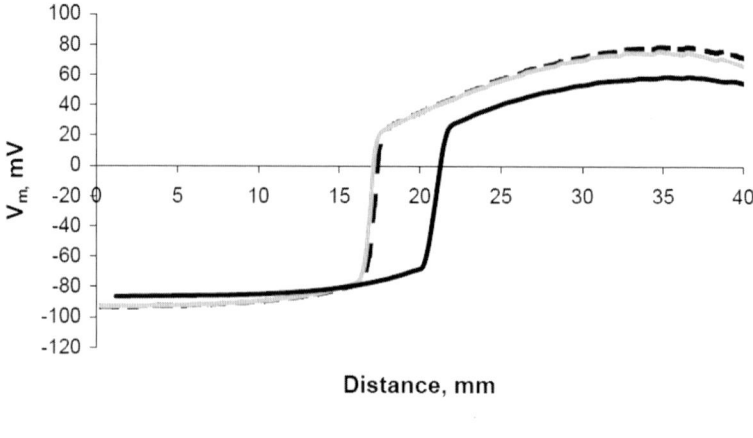

FIGURE 5. Transmembrane potential along the length of the arrow shown in FIGURE 4.

Postshock Spiral Wave Breakup Due to Stretch

In unstretched tissue, reentrant circuits were characterized by figure-of-eight morphology with a rotation period of approximately 100 ms. In stretched tissue incorporating changes in fiber angle, postshock behavior was qualitatively the same. However, in stretched tissue with MSC recruitment, spiral wave breakup and onset of VF were observed. An example is shown in FIGURE 7 A; reentrant circuit phase singularities, as shown in FIGURE 7 B, occur at locations of a large strain gradient. FIGURE 8 depicts action potentials at the location of spiral wave breakup (FIG. 8 A) and in regions with large and small strains (FIG. 8 B). Wave breakup occurred on the fifth rotation of the spiral wave for any shock strength (FIG. 8 A). In the area with large strain, the effective refractory period (ERP) was increased, and was approximately 130 ms long, as compared to 100 ms in the region of small strain. Also evident is an increase of about 5 mV in

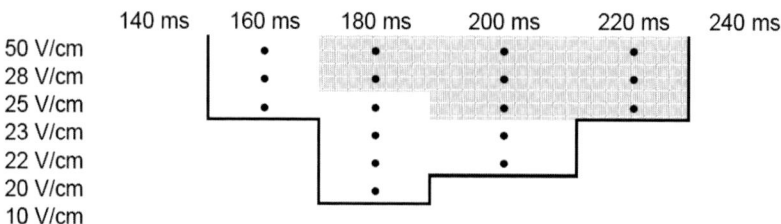

FIGURE 6. Vulnerability areas for unstretched tissue and tissue including MSC recruitment (white area bordered by black line; vulnerability areas are identical). Vulnerability area for tissue with change in the fiber angles is shown in gray. Dots correspond to episodes of stable reentry.

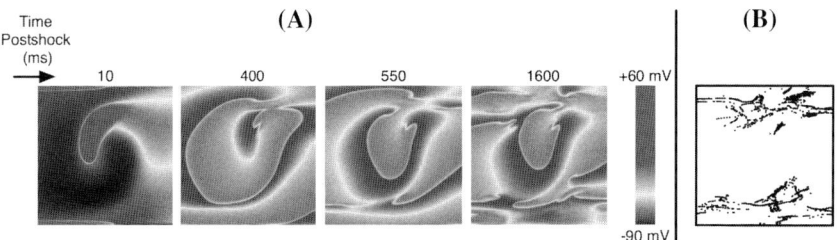

FIGURE 7. Postshock reentry for tissue incorporating MSC (**A**) and locations of the phase singularities from 10 to 1600 ms postshock (**B**). Coupling interval is 200 ms and shock strength is 10 V/cm.

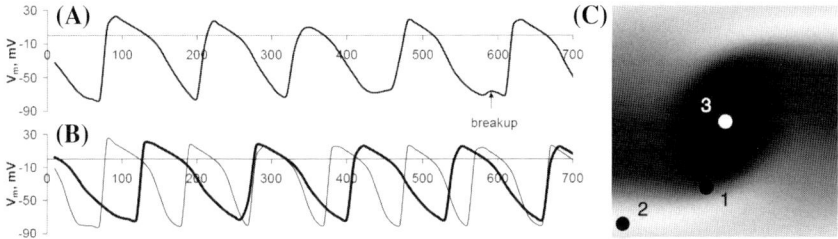

FIGURE 8. (**A**) Action potentials at the location of spiral wave breakup in the tissue with involvement of MSC shown in FIGURE 7. The location of the spiral wave breakup corresponds to a location of high strain gradient (point 1 in panel C). (**B**) Action potentials in an area of large strain (thick line, point 2 in panel C) and in an area of small strain (thin line, point 3 in panel C).

the transmembrane potential at the end of the ERP in areas with a large strain magnitude.

Spiral wave breakup did not depend on shock strength or coupling interval. Breakup also occurred at smaller degrees of stretch (10% and 15% of reference length), but at the sixth or seventh rotation of the spiral wave, and phase singularities shifted closer to the top and bottom borders of the sheet.

DISCUSSION

The current study used a two-dimensional electro-mechanical model of cardiac tissue to investigate how stretch applied to a substrate with heterogeneous fiber structure influences postshock activity. A previous theoretical study has shown that a possible mechanism of decreased efficacy of defibrillation shocks is activation of MSC.[38] However, it involved homogeneous recruitment of MSC throughout the tissue, ignoring heterogeneous loading conditions in the ventricular wall. This limitation constituted the basis of the current study, in which a highly heterogeneous fiber structure determined a strain gradient and resulting dispersion in electrophysiological properties due to incorporation of MSC in the tissue. In addition to the effects of MSC recruitment, the current study examined the influence of tissue deformation and corresponding changes in tissue conductivities on postshock behavior.

The study mentioned above[38] found that stretch leading to homogeneous recruitment of MSC resulted in a small increase in vulnerability to monophasic shocks. The current study did not find such an increase in the case of heterogeneous recruitment of MSC. While heterogeneous MSC recruitment following stretch did not alter the vulnerability of cardiac tissue to electric shocks, it increased dispersion of refractoriness, thus altering the complexity of induced arrhythmias. In contrast, we found that the vulnerability of the tissue incorporating stretch-induced changes in the fiber angle was decreased. This decrease in vulnerability can be explained by the alignment of the fibers in the horizontal direction with stretch, which decreases the fiber curvature. Large fiber curvature results in the development of high magnitude shock-induced virtual electrodes[39] that may result in the establishment of postshock reentry.

The difference in the compliance of the tissue in the fiber and cross-fiber directions results in anisotropic strain of the tissue upon stretch. Differences in strain between the fiber and cross-fiber directions result in a change in the intracellular anisotropy ratio.[30] Changes in the anisotropy ratio in the intracellular versus extracellular space affect virtual electrode polarization[40] and can influence tissue vulnerability to electrical shocks.

Chorro *et al.* have shown an increased complexity of VF due to ventricular dilatation,[11] which occurred due to the modulation of electrophysiological properties, such as ERP, by stretch. In our study, sustained stretch resulted in an increase in ERP. Other studies have shown that ventricular dilatation may cause either a decrease or an increase in ERP. Most experiments with porcine or rabbit ventricles show a consistent decrease of ERP.[19,20,41] However, data on canine ventricles show contrary results,[42,43] which suggests that the effect of stretch on ERP is species-dependent. Despite these contradictory findings, all studies have shown an increased dispersion of ERP with applied stretch.[19–21] One cause of increased dispersion of repolarization may be regional differences in strain, as demonstrated in this study. Indeed, as shown here, dispersion of refractoriness resulted in postshock conduction block and induction of VF at the location of a high strain gradient. To our knowledge, this is the first theoretical study which investigates the relationship between heterogeneous fiber structure and stretch-induced arrhythmias in cardiac tissue.

Chattipakorn *et al.*[44] have shown that biphasic defibrillation shocks near the DFT produce focal activity near the apex. In failed defibrillation episodes, the onset of VF was observed after five postshock cycles of the focal activity. Attempts to explain this phenomenon focus on the origin of the postshock activations near the apex,[45] with little investigation into the transition to fibrillation following these activations. In the porcine heart, the effect of stretch is larger at the apex than at the base of the left ventricle,[21] creating a dispersion of repolarization. Based on our findings, we suggest that rapid activation of the left ventricle apical region leads to reentry at the locations of high strain gradient. Interestingly, we observed the same number of postshock reentrant cycles (5) preceding wave breakup as was observed in the experiments of Chattipakorn *et al.*

Limitations

This study assumed that activation of MSC was a function of strain in the fiber direction only. However, it is possible that MSC recruitment could depend on cross-fiber strain. This might be related to the fact that ventricular dilatation has a larger effect on refractoriness at the endocardial as compared to the epicardial surface,[41] while the transmural distribution of diastolic and systolic strain is more uniform in the fiber as compared to the cross-fiber direction during normal conditions.

ACKNOWLEDGMENTS

This work was supported by NIH, Awards No. RO1-HL63195 and RO1 HL-67322.

REFERENCES

1. IDEKER, R., T. CHATTIPAKORN & R. GRAY. 2000. Defibrillation mechanisms: the parable of the blind men and the elephant. J. Cardiovasc. Electrophysiol. **11:** 1008–1013.
2. EFIMOV, I., Y. CHENG, D. VAN WAGONER, *et al.* 1998. Virtual electrode-induced phase singularity: a basic mechanism of defibrillation failure. Circ. Res. **82:** 918–925.
3. CHATTIPAKORN, S. & N. CHATTIPAKORN. 2004. Electrophysiological concept of ventricular defibrillation mechanism. J. Med. Assoc. Thai. **87:** 1394–1401.
4. HUANG, J., J. ROGERS, C. KILLINGSWORTH, *et al.* 2001. Improvement of defibrillation efficacy and quantification of activation patterns during ventricular fibrillation in a canine heart failure model. Circulation **103:** 1473–1478.
5. LUCY, S., D. JONES & G. KLEIN. 1994. Pronounced increase in defibrillation threshold associated with pacing-induced cardiomyopathy in the dog. Am. Heart J. **127:** 366–376.
6. LAB, M.J. 1982. Contraction-excitation feedback in myocardium. Physiological basis and clinical relevance. Circ. Res. **50:** 757–766.
7. LAB, M.J. 1996. Mechanoelectric feedback (transduction) in heart: concepts and implications. Cardiovasc. Res. **32:** 3–14.
8. FRANZ, M.R. 1996. Mechano-electrical feedback in ventricular myocardium. Cardiovasc. Res. **32:** 15–24.
9. STROBEL, J., G. KAY, G. WALCOTT, *et al.* 1997. Defibrillation efficacy with endocardial electrodes is influenced by reductions in cardiac preload. J. Interv. Card. Electrophysiol. **1:** 95–102.

10. OTT, P. & M. REITER. 1997. Effect of ventricular dilatation on defibrillation threshold in the isolated perfused rabbit heart. J. Cardiovasc. Electrophysiol. **8:** 1013–1019.
11. CHORRO, F.J., J. CANOVES, J. GUERRERO, et al. 2000. Opposite effects of myocardial stretch and verapamil on the complexity of the ventricular fibrillatory pattern: an experimental study. Pacing Clin. Electrophysiol. **23:** 1594–1603.
12. BURTON, F. & S. COBBE. 1998. Effect of sustained stretch on dispersion of ventricular fibrillation intervals in normal rabbit hearts. Cardiovasc. Res. **39:** 351–359.
13. HILLEBRENNER, M., J. EASON & N. TRAYANOVA. 2004. Mechanistic inquiry into decrease in probability of defibrillation success with increase in complexity of preshock reentrant activity. Am. J. Physiol. Heart Circ. Physiol. **286:** H909–H917.
14. SACKIN, H. 1995. Mechanosensitive channels. Annu. Rev. Physiol. **57:** 333–353.
15. MORRIS, C.E. 1990. Mechanosensitive ion channels. J. Membr. Biol. **113:** 93–107.
16. ISENBERG, G., V. KAZANSKI, D. KONDRATEV, et al. 2003. Differential effects of stretch and compression on membrane currents and [Na+]c in ventricular myocytes. Prog. Biophys. Mol. Biol. **82:** 43–56.
17. HU, H. & F. SACHS. 1997. Stretch-activated ion channels in the heart. J. Mol. Cell Cardiol. **29:** 1511–1523.
18. KOHL, P., P. HUNTER & D. NOBLE. 1999. Stretch-induced changes in heart rate and rhythm: clinical observations, experiments and mathematical models. Prog. Biophys. Mol. Biol. **71:** 91–138.
19. ZABEL, M., S. PORTNOY & M. FRANZ. 1996. Effect of sustained load on dispersion of ventricular repolarization and conduction time in the isolated intact rabbit heart. J. Cardiovasc. Electrophysiol. **7:** 9–16.
20. REITER, M., M. LANDERS, Z. ZETELAKI, et al. 1997. Electrophysiological effects of acute dilatation in the isolated rabbit heart: cycle length-dependent effects on ventricular refractoriness and conduction velocity. Circulation **96:** 4050–4056.
21. DEAN, J. & M. LAB. 1990. Regional changes in ventricular excitability during load manipulation of the in situ pig heart. J. Physiol. **429:** 387–400.
22. TUNG, L. & A. KLEBER. 2000. Virtual sources associated with linear and curved strands of cardiac cells. Am. J. Physiol. Heart Circ. Physiol. **279:** H1579–H1590.
23. ASHIHARA, T., T. NAMBA, T. YAO, et al. 2003. Vortex cordis as a mechanism of postshock activation: arrhythmia induction study using a bidomain model. J. Cardiovasc Electrophysiol. **14:** 295–302.
24. BEAUDOIN, D. & B. ROTH. 2005. How the spatial frequency of polarization influences the induction of reentry in cardiac tissue. J. Cardiovasc. Electrophysiol. **16:** 748–752.
25. PANFILOV, A.V. & A.V. HOLDEN, Eds. 1997. Computational Biology of the Heart. p. 428. John Wiley & Sons, Ltd. Chichester.
26. NASH, M.P. & P.J. HUNTER. 2000. Computational mechanics of the heart: from tissue structure to ventricular function. J. Elasticity **61:** 113–141.
27. NASH, M.P. & A.V. PANFILOV. 2004. Electromechanical model of excitable tissue to study reentrant cardiac arrhythmias. Prog. Biophys. Mol. Biol. **85:** 501–522.
28. VETTER, F.J. & A.D. MCCULLOCH. 2000. Three-dimensional stress and strain in passive rabbit left ventricle: a model study. Ann. Biomed. Eng. **28:** 781–792.
29. HENRIQUEZ, C.S. 1993. Simulating the electrical behavior of cardiac tissue using the bidomain model. Crit. Rev. Biomed. Eng. **21:** 1–77.
30. SACHSE, F., G. SEEMANN, C. RIEDEL, et al. 2000. Modeling of the cardiac mechano-electrical feedback. Int. J. Bioelectromagn. **2**(2).

31. Luo, C.H. & Y. Rudy. 1994. A dynamic model of the cardiac ventricular action potential. I. Simulations of ionic currents and concentration changes. Circ. Res. **74:** 1071–1096.
32. Zeng, J., K.R. Laurita, D.S. Rosenbaum & Y. Rudy. 1995. Two components of the delayed rectifier K+ current in ventricular myocytes of the guinea pig type. Theoretical formulation and their role in repolarization. Circ Res. **77:** 140–152.
33. Ashihara, T. & N. Trayanova. 2004. Asymmetry in membrane responses to electric shocks: insights from bidomain simulations. Biophys. J. **87:** 2271–2282.
34. DeBruin, K. & W. Krassowska. 1998. Electroporation and shock-induced transmembrane potential in a cardiac fiber during defibrillation strength shocks. Ann. Biomed. Eng. **26:** 584–596.
35. Zabel, M., B.S. Koller, F. Sachs & M.R. Franz. 1996. Stretch-induced voltage changes in the isolated beating heart: importance of the timing of stretch and implications for stretch-activated ion channels. Cardiovasc. Res. **32:** 120–130.
36. Rodriguez, B., L. Li, J. Eason, et al. 2005. Differences between left and right ventricular chamber geometry affect cardiac vulnerability to electric shocks. Circ. Res. **97:** 168–175.
37. Eason, J. & N. Trayanova. 2002. Phase singularities and termination of spiral wave reentry. J. Cardiovasc. Electrophysiol. **13:** 672–679.
38. Trayanova, N., W. Li, J. Eason & P. Kohl. 2004. Effect of stretch-activated channels on defibrillation efficacy. Heart Rhythm. **1:** 67–77.
39. Trayanova, N., K. Skouibine & F. Aguel. 1998. The role of cardiac tissue structure in defibrillation. Chaos **8:** 221–233.
40. Wikswo, J., S. Lin & R. Abbas. 1995. Virtual electrodes in cardiac tissue: a common mechanism for anodal and cathodal stimulation. Biophys. J. **69:** 2195–2210.
41. Eckardt, L., P. Kirchhof, G. Monnig, et al. 2000. Modification of stretch-induced shortening of repolarization by streptomycin in the isolated rabbit heart. J. Cardiovasc. Pharmacol. **36:** 711–721.
42. Benditt, D., J. Kriett, H. Tobler, et al. 1985. Electrophysiological effects of transient aortic occlusion in intact canine heart. Am. J. Physiol. **249:** H1017–1023.
43. Zhu, W., S. Johnson, R. Brandt, et al. 1997. Impact of volume loading and load reduction on ventricular refractoriness and conduction properties in canine congestive heart failure. J. Am. Coll. Cardiol. **30:** 825–833.
44. Chattipakorn, N., P. Fotuhi, S. Chattipakorn & R. Ideker. 2003. Three-dimensional mapping of earliest activation after near-threshold ventricular defibrillation shocks. J. Cardiovasc. Electrophysiol. **14:** 65–69.
45. Roth, B. 2005. The puzzle of defibrillation: putting the pieces together. J. Cardiovasc. Electrophysiol. **16:** 1206–1208.

Modeling Cardiac Electrical Activity at the Cell and Tissue Levels

TRAVIS M. AUSTIN,[a] DARREN A. HOOKS,[a] PETER J. HUNTER,[a] DAVID P. NICKERSON,[a] ANDREW J. PULLAN,[a,b] GREGORY B. SANDS,[a] BRUCE H. SMAILL,[a,c] AND MARK L. TREW[a]

[a]*Bioengineering Institute, The University of Auckland, New Zealand*
[b]*Department of Engineering Science, The University of Auckland, New Zealand*
[c]*Department of Physiology, The University of Auckland, New Zealand*

ABSTRACT: Significant tissue structures exist in cardiac ventricular tissue, which are of supracellular dimension. It is hypothesized that these tissue structures contribute to the discontinuous spread of electrical activation, may contribute to arrhythmogenesis, and also provide a substrate for effective cardioversion. However, the influences of these mesoscale tissue structures in intact ventricular tissue are difficult to understand solely on the basis of experimental measurement. Current measurement technology is able to record at both the macroscale tissue level and the microscale cellular or subcellular level, but to date it has not been possible to obtain large volume, direct measurements at the mesoscales. To bridge this scale gap in experimental measurements, we use tissue-specific structure and mathematical modeling. Our models, which can incorporate ion channel models at the cell level into the reaction–diffusion equations at the tissue level, have enabled us to consider key hypotheses regarding discontinuous activation.

KEYWORDS: cardiac tissue; electrical activation; ion channels; mathematical modeling

INTRODUCTION

The pathological breakdown of the normal sequence of cardiac electrical activation into life-threatening cardiac arrhythmias depends on biophysical events at many spatial scales[1,2] (see FIG. 1). The various contributing roles of gene mutations, drug binding, and other subcellular level factors are discussed in other sections of this book. Here we focus on the role of larger scale tissue structure, using a new microstructural imaging device to yield structural detail at a submicron scale across several millimeters of tissue and bidomain electrical activation equations to examine wavefront propagation through these

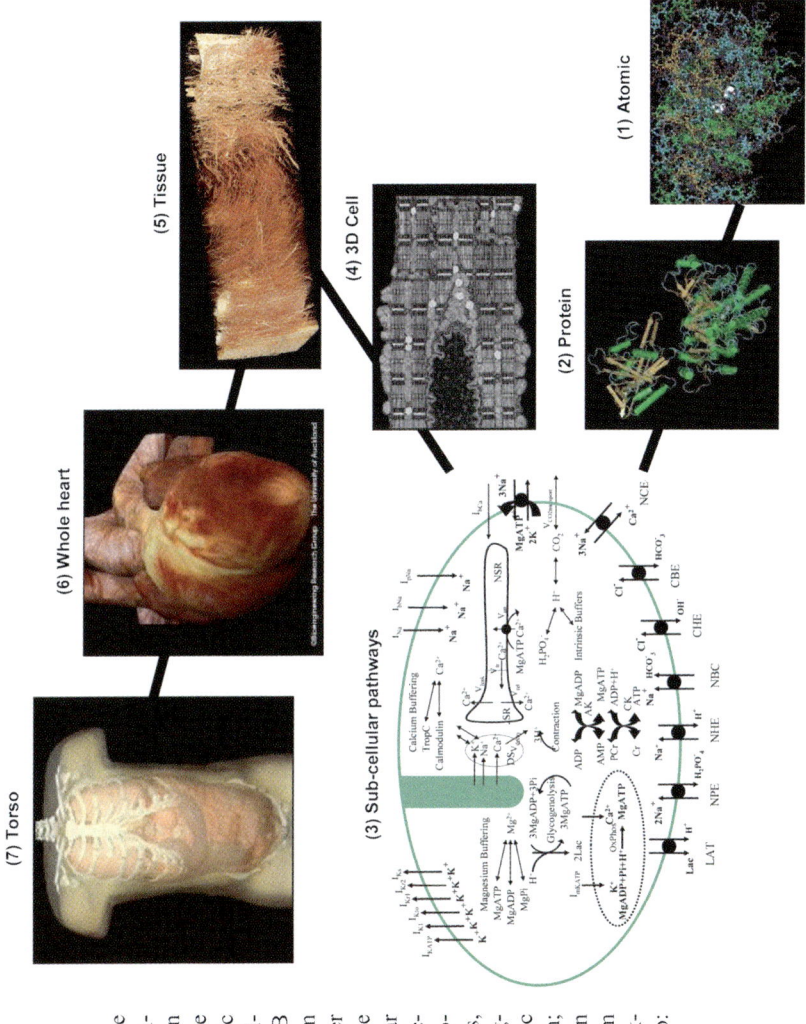

FIGURE 1. An illustration of the hierarchy of spatial scales used in understanding cardiac function (shown in color in online version). The levels are (1) Atomic: Shown here by the atomic coordinates for the sarcoplasmic calcium ATPase (SERCA) from the PDB database (note the two bound calcium atoms in white); (2) Protein: A coarser grained model of structure for the same protein as in (i); (3) Subcellular pathways: these include the cell electrophysiology, calcium transport, proton transport, myofilament mechanics, metabolic pathways, and some cell signaling pathways; (4) 3D cell: cardiac muscle cell from electron micrograph; (5) Tissue: organization of collagen fibers in a transmural tissue block from a rat heart; (6) Whole heart: the Auckland textured virtual heart; (7) Torso: the Auckland human torso model.

measured structures. We examine normal activation processes, arrhythmogenic processes, and possible mechanisms of cardioversion.

TISSUE-SPECIFIC CARDIAC VENTRICULAR STRUCTURAL MODELS

The mechanical function of the heart is heavily dependent on its muscular architecture and this structure also contributes to the anisotropic electrical properties of cardiac tissue. Detailed measurements of transmural myofiber orientation from both dog[3,4,5] and pig[6,7] have shown that there can be significant local variation of fiber orientation. Studies using scanning electron microscopy and confocal microscopy indicate that ventricular myocytes are arranged in layers 4 to 5 cells thick, separated by cleavage planes or collagenous septas.[4,8,9] Muscle layers regularly branch and interconnect, but the clefts between adjacent layers may be relatively extensive, particularly in the deep ventricular myocardium.

There is now a significant body of work in the cardiac mechanics literature, which addresses the role of laminar structure in ventricular myocardium.[10–14] In contrast, the extent to which the laminar architecture of ventricular myocardium affects the spread of electrical activation in the heart is less clear. On a structural basis, it may be argued that electrical activation spreads between adjacent muscle layers via muscle branches and that interlaminar clefts present a barrier to electrical propagation.[4,15,16] Propagation will be least rapid between neighboring layers normal to the cleavage planes that separate them. This view is at variance with the widely held assumption that ventricular myocardium is a uniformly coupled syncytium in which electrical properties are transversely isotropic with respect to the fiber direction.

Obtaining experimental evidence of direct links between structural form and electrical function is an ongoing challenge. Although electric potentials can be recorded with moderately high spatial and temporal resolution on the heart surface,[17,18] and on the transmural surfaces of wedge preparations,[19] and with high spatial resolution in cultured myocyte preparations,[20] it is often difficult to relate these data to intramural electrical activity. Techniques for gathering intramural data[21–24] to date lack the spatial resolution to reconstruct fully all aspects of the three-dimensional spread of electrical activation.

Computer models that incorporate detailed tissue-specific structural information provide a means of investigating the possible effects of myocardial architecture on electrical activation.[16,25–28] However, acquisition and reconstruction of the necessary structural data can be a laborious process. For example, assembly of the high resolution, extended volume images of the rat LV wall presented by Young *et al.*[9] required weeks of imaging and image registration. Similarly, an anatomically detailed three-dimensional reconstruction of the rabbit sinoatrial node[29] took 18 months of painstaking work.

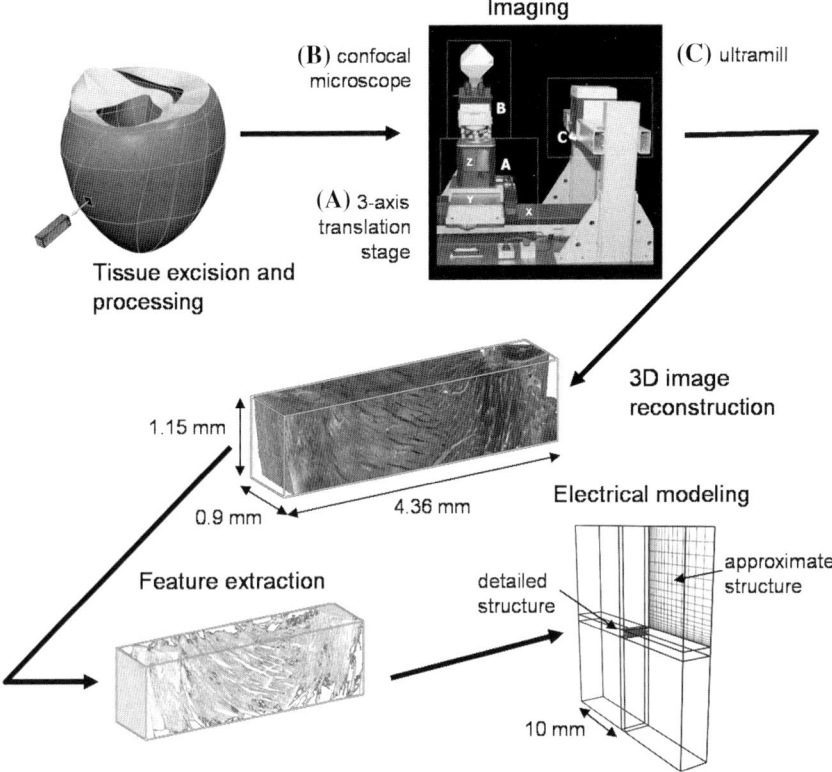

FIGURE 2. The process of building tissue-specific cardiac ventricular structural models. Details on the connection between the cell level equations and the tissue level equations are given in FIGURE 3 (shown in color in online version).

An automated system has recently been developed to enable extended volume images to be acquired more efficiently.[8] Key aspects of the system and the process through to computer modeling are presented in FIGURE 2. The system consists of a confocal microscope (or digital camera), a high-precision three-axis translation stage, and an ultramill, all of which are controlled by a computer using custom-written software. Digital reslicing, segmentation, and volume-rendering methods can be applied to the reconstructed volumes to provide quantitative information about the three-dimensional organization of myocytes, extracellular collagen matrix, and the blood vessel network in the heart that has previously been difficult to attain.

Significant features of the myocardial organization are extracted from the reconstructed volume images using a variety of techniques.[25,30] Local myofiber orientation is identified, while cleavage planes between muscle layers, blood vessels, and other tissue discontinuities are segmented to create detailed representations of specific tissue structures that are used to interpret experimental data and to model electrical activation. The result is detailed structural models with discontinuous myocardial domains. For electrical activation modeling, these detailed structural models are embedded in a region of approximate structure (FIG. 2) to better approximate the behavior of larger tissue samples.

MODELING TISSUE ELECTRICAL ACTIVATION USING DETAILED TISSUE-SPECIFIC STRUCTURE

Computer modeling is used to test the hypothesis that electrical discontinuities arising from myocardial discontinuities (especially cleavage planes) have both local and global effects on the spread of activation. The models allow this hypothesis to be studied more directly than is currently possible given the current scale limitations of intramural experimental recordings.

The electrical behavior of cardiac tissue can be represented by the bidomain model in which intracellular (myocardial) and extracellular domains communicate through the membrane ionic current, I_{ion}. Under certain assumptions, a simplified monodomain model of cardiac electrical activation can be used, which is computationally advantageous. However, a single-domain model is unable to capture the complexities of dynamic current redistributions between the intracellular and extracellular spaces driven by the structural features of the tissue-specific models.

The solution parameters for the bidomain model are the space and time varying transmembrane potential, V_m, and the extracellular potential, ϕ_e, both experimentally measurable quantities. The bidomain conservation of current expressions is

$$A_m C_m \frac{\partial V_m}{\partial t} - \nabla \cdot (\sigma_i \nabla V_m) = \nabla \cdot (\sigma_i \nabla \phi_e) - A_m I_{ion}$$

$$\nabla \cdot ((\sigma_e + \sigma_i)\nabla \phi_e) = -\nabla \cdot (\sigma_i \nabla V_m) - i_e.$$

Here A_m is the surface to volume ratio of the representative cell membrane between the domains, C_m is the specific capacitance of the membrane, σ_i and σ_e are the intra- and extracellular conductivity tensors, and i_e is a current injection per unit volume into the extracellular space. The ionic current, I_{ion}, can be determined by using the appropriate models in the CellML repository, as described elsewhere.[31,32] The modeling results described in this article determine the ionic current using a cubic activation model[33] or a defibrillation modified Beeler–Reuter model.[34] Assuming isolated tissue, these equations are subject to no-flux current boundary conditions on far-field external boundaries and at a set of internal boundaries in the intracellular domain; that is, cleavage planes. Further details can be found in Trew et al.[26]

Initial modeling of electrical activation on detailed tissue structure used a finite element method,[16] however, recent modeling has also used a new, efficient finite volume method[26] that takes advantage of the regular geometry of the tissue samples being considered (refer to FIG. 3 B, C). Simulating electrical activation on tissue-specific geometries is a computationally intensive process, as it requires spatial resolutions of 10 to 20 μM. These resolutions are an order of magnitude smaller than the 100 μM resolution (based on adequately resolving a tissue space-constant of 700–1,200 μm) that is usually required for simulations in continuous tissue (e.g., Poelzing et al.[35]). The studies described in this article have simultaneously solved between 8 and 16 million equations, describing intra- and extracellular current conservation, at a set of instances in time. In general, solutions of up to 20 msec simulated time have been computed in 12 h or less of elapsed real time (using 8–12 Power 5, 1.9 GHz processors on a 210 GB shared memory IBM Regatta). To maintain the viability of solving such large problems, we continue to develop our computer simulation tools (e.g., Austin et al.[36]).

FIGURE 4 shows simulation results from midwall stimuli applied to detailed tissue-specific geometric models. These results illustrate that the initial propagation from a focal activation (a bipolar extracellular current injection in FIG. 4 A–C, and an ectopic stimulus in FIG. 4 D) is significantly impacted by the local laminar tissue structure. Similar results have been obtained for unipolar midwall stimulation.[30] As the activation wavefront becomes more developed, the impact of the laminar structure is reduced—although the anisotropic conductivity remains important. A comparison of simulation results with and without tissue-specific structural features (FIG. 4 A and B) shows similar, fully developed activation patterns. The model without the detailed geometry used a reduced sheet-normal conductivity suggested by Hooks et al.[16] An interesting observation from FIGURE 4 C is the classic "dog-bone" pattern of virtual sources along the midwall fiber orientation arising from the extracellular stimulation. The formation of virtual sources following unipolar extracellular current injection or extraction were predicted using the bidomain model before their existence could be verified experimentally by fluorescence imaging on the epicardium.[37] The influence of the cleavage planes on the midwall formation of the virtual sources is such that although details of early and late activation vary, the principal features remain consistent. These results also highlight that fully anisotropic continuous conductivities are required to match the solutions generated using transversely isotropic conductivities and explicit tissue structures.

Results such as those of FIGURE 4 suggest that the electrical discontinuities arising from cleavage planes have local effects in that the tissue structure most strongly impacts the propagation from a focal activation in its initial development, when the wavefront curvature is greatest. If the desired model output is a map of gross transmembrane potential arising from a focal activation, then a detailed tissue-specific model of transmural laminar geometry may not be necessary and it may be sufficient to rely on a detailed, but continuous, description of the fiber, sheet, and sheet-normal orientations along with the

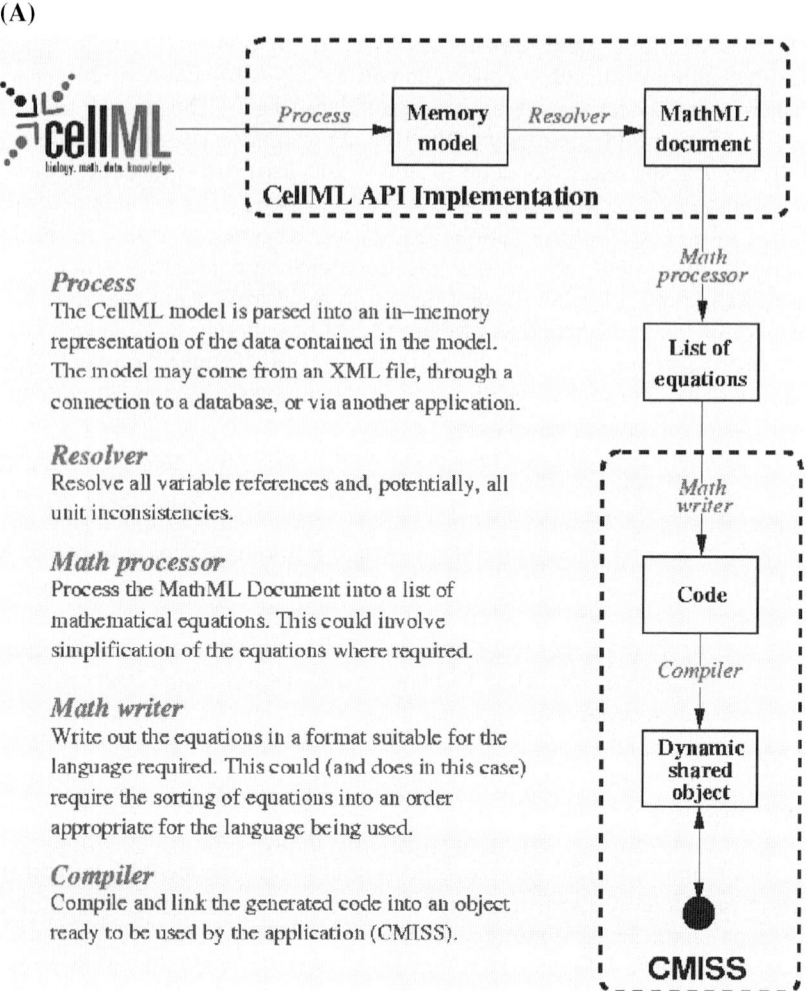

FIGURE 3. (**A**) An illustration of the work flow involved in the generation of computational code in the tissue level modeling package (CMISS) from a CellML source file (CellML is an XML-based markup language for describing cellular models—see www.cellml.org). The upper dashed box encapsulates the processes that are internal to the CellML API implementation, and the lower encapsulates those internal to CMISS. The math processor is independent and external to both of these.

appropriate homogenized effective conductivity values.[16] Slow, nonuniform, or discontinuous activation (such as that shown in FIG. 4) is often associated with myocardial infarctions and ischemia, and is expressed experimentally as electrograms with polyphasic, or fractionated downstrokes.[38] However, there

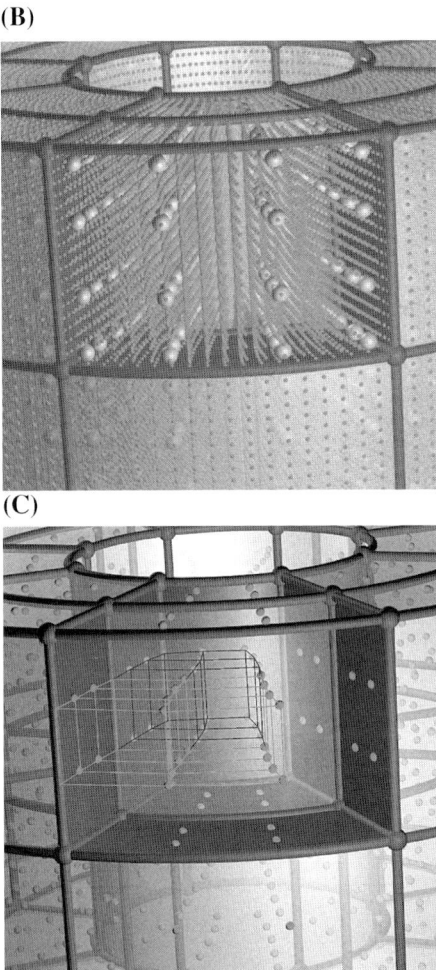

FIGURE 3. (**B**) Finite elements based on tricubic Hermite basis functions are used to define a tissue region in which a large number of material points are generated. The larger gold spheres (shown in color in online version) indicate the Gauss points of a Galerkin finite element mechanics model for coupled electromechanical problems (not used here). (**C**) The material points are used to create finite volume meshes for the solution of the reaction–diffusion bidomain equations using a much lower resolution than (**B**) to aid clarity.

is growing evidence that similar observations can be made for externally stimulated normal myocardium.[39,24]

The results of FIGURE 4 were derived from a near-threshold extracellular current injection or a direct membrane depolarization. When the tissue is

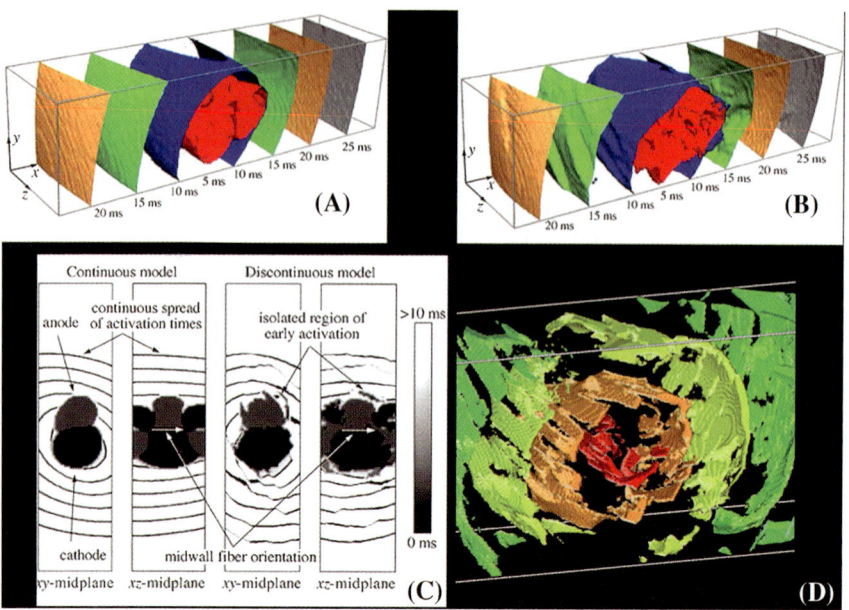

FIGURE 4. The spread of electrical activation following a midwall stimulus in continuous and discontinuous structural models—local effects (shown in color in online version). (**A–C**) Bipolar extracellular stimulus (modified from Trew *et al.* 2005a[26]). (**D**) Ectopic membrane depolarization stimulus. (**A**) Continuous structural model with no explicit cleavage plane geometry, but fully anisotropic conductivities. (**B**) Model with explicit discontinuous geometry and transversely isotropic conductivities. (**C**) Comparison of activation time fields for (**A** and **B**) on transmural cutting planes. (**D**) The discontinuous spread of activation from a midwall stimulus in a geometrically detailed model.

stimulated by a strong electric field (e.g., defibrillation strength shock), myocardial electrical discontinuities produced by the laminar structure play a significant role in total tissue activation. This is illustrated in FIGURE 5 where a 10 V/cm transmural electric field has been placed across a detailed tissue model, with the cathode on the epicardium (left) and the anode on the endocardium (right). The figure shows the three-dimensional development of virtual sources on the anodal (endocardial) side of certain intracellular discontinuities. These results contribute to observations from previous modeling[16] and experimental[19] studies. The significance of such results is that they suggest a mechanism by which a strong electric shock can rapidly activate cardiac tissue and thereby extinguish reentrant behavior. Thus, modeling supports the hypothesis that the application of a sufficiently strong extracellular potential field can result in rapid global activation and that to observe these effects requires the direct explicit modeling of electrically discontinuous tissue features.

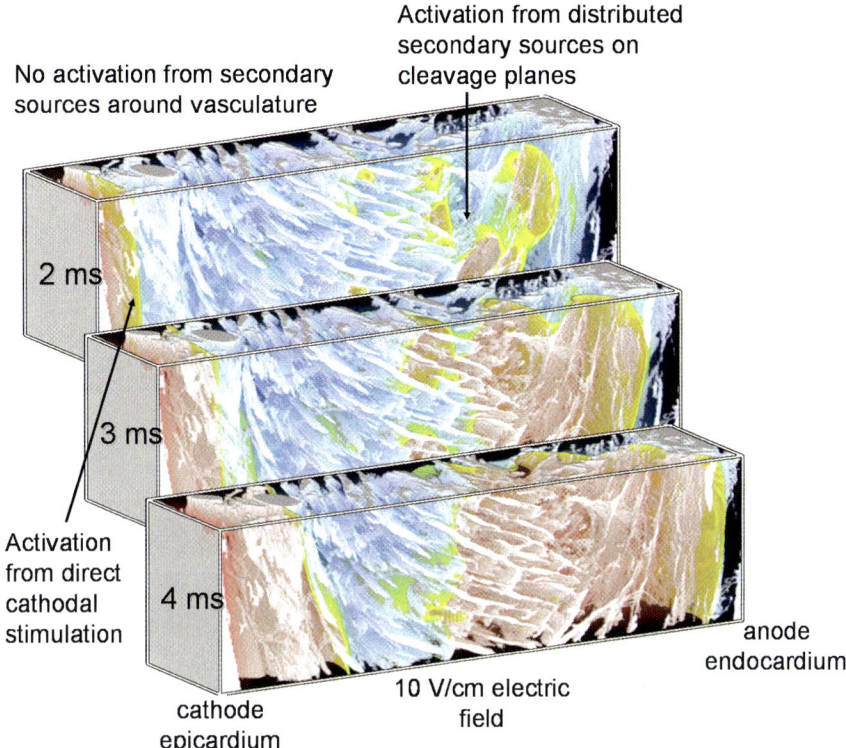

FIGURE 5. The global response of a detailed tissue model to a transmural electrical shock (shown in color in online version). Depolarizations form on the anodal side of significant myocardial voids, resulting in distributed intramural secondary sources and rapid transmural depolarization.

In recent work, Hooks et al.[28] have used computer modeling to support a link between tissue structure and the optimal shock strengths for rapid transmural activation. Key findings from that study are presented in FIGURE 6. That figure shows the detailed tissue model response to varying shock strengths. The shocks are rectangular and of 10 msec duration. The tissue model demonstrates a biphasic response of total activation time (FIG. 6 B) to varying shock strength that has similar characteristics to the response measured experimentally.[19] As the shock strength increases beyond 15 V/cm, the total activation time becomes longer. This is also observed experimentally. At stronger shock strengths, the current supplied by the secondary sources of activation is insufficient to rapidly counter the adjacent strongly polarized regions. This matches experimental findings that during strong shocks, the activation of areas showing negative transmembrane potential changes was delayed until after the termination of the shock.[40]

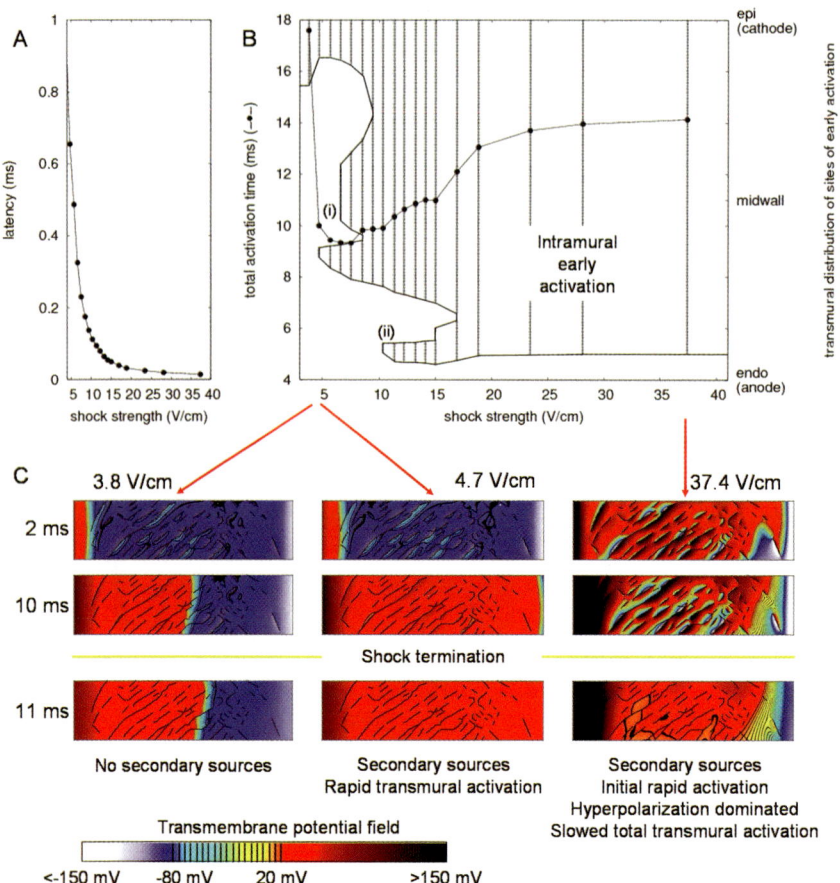

FIGURE 6. The impact of varying shock strengths on tissue response to 10 msec duration rectangular monophasic transmural shocks (shown in color in online version). (**A**) Latency to first recorded activation. (**B**) Total transmural activation times and the spread of early activation; progressive (i) midwall and (ii) subendocardial recruitment of cleavage-plane secondary sources with increasing shock strengths. (**C**) Maps of intramural transmembrane potential distributions on a transmural cutting plane for three representative shock strengths. Modified from Hooks et al.[28]

An interesting feature of the model and experimental comparisons is that the absolute activation times recorded experimentally were significantly shorter.[19] This difference may be explained in terms of the relatively coarse spatial resolution (1.2 mm) of those experimental recordings, which leads to an artificially reduced total activation time. Higher resolution (0.11 mm/pixel) recordings have detected larger activation delays that were not apparent from low resolution recordings of the same tissue.[40] In both the model and the experiments, activation latency (FIG. 6 A) was prolonged below field strengths of about 10 V/cm. The predicted latency was an order of magnitude faster than the measured latency. However, a similar argument to the transmural activation times can be used to explain this. Small areas of depolarization will be obscured by larger areas of resting or hyperpolarized tissue within the early stages of the shock, and consequently the measured activation latency will appear to be prolonged.

SUMMARY

Detailed, tissue-specific modeling of electrical activation of cardiac tissue has shown that electrical discontinuities arising from the cleavage planes have both local and global effects. On the basis of these results, it can be argued that the standard view of the ventricular myocardium as a uniformly coupled electrical continuum, with transversely isotropic conductance normal to the fiber direction, is likely to be incorrect.[16,26] We have also shown that interlaminar clefts could play a significant role in the termination of fibrillation by an applied shock.[16,27,28] These results are supported by experimental observations.

Controlled experimental measurements and computer models should be used as complementary parts of an iterative process toward developing a fuller understanding of cardiac tissue electrophysiology. The sequence of this process is scale dependent. Experimental measurement of electrophysiology at both the cellular microscale and the tissue macroscale is accessible with current technology. Computer modeling of electrical activation enables hypotheses to be tested and insights to be gained at the "in-between" mesoscale, so bridging the scale gap. The key factor in this modeling is the detailed and accurate representation of the geometric tissue structures.

REFERENCES

1. HUNTER, P.J. & T. BORG. 2003. Integration from proteins to organs: the physiome project. Nature Rev. Mol. Cell. Biol. **4:** 237–243.
2. CRAMPIN, E.J., M. HALSTEAD, P.J. HUNTER, et al. 2004. Computational physiology and the physiome project. Exp. Physiol. **89:** 1–26.
3. NIELSEN, P.M.F., I.J. LEGRICE, B.H. SMAILL, et al. 1991. Mathematical model of geometry and fibrous structure of the heart. Am. J. Physiol. Heart C. **260:** 1365–1378.
4. LEGRICE, I.J., B.H. SMAILL, L.Z. CHAI, et al. 1995a. Laminar structure of the heart: ventricular myocyte arrangement and connective tissue architecture of the dog. Am. J. Physiol. Heart C. **269:** 571–582.
5. LEGRICE, I.J., P.J. HUNTER & B.H. SMAILL. 1997. Laminar structure of the heart: a mathematical model. Am. J. Physiol. Heart C. **272:** 2466–2476.
6. STEVENS, C.S., E. REMME, I.J. LEGRICE, et al. 2003. Ventricular mechanics in diastole: material parameter sensitivity. J. Biomech. **36:** 737–748.
7. VETTER, F.J., S.B. SIMONS, S. MIRONOV, et al. 2005. Epicardial fiber organization in swine right ventricle and its impact on propagation. Circ. Res. **96:** 244–251.

8. SANDS, G.B., D.A. GERNEKE, D.A. HOOKS, et al. 2005. Automated imaging of extended tissue volumes using confocal microscopy. Microsc. Res. Techniq. **67**: 227–239.
9. YOUNG, A.A., I.J. LEGRICE, M.A. YOUNG & B.H. SMAILL. 1998. Extended confocal microscopy of myocardial laminae and collagen network. J. Microsc. **192**: 139–150.
10. LEGRICE, I.J., Y. TAKAYAMA & J.W. COVELL. 1995b. Transverse shear along myocardial cleavage planes provides a mechanism for normal systolic wall thickening. Circ. Res. **77**: 182–193.
11. COSTA, K.D., Y. TAKAYAMA, A.D. MCCULLOCH & J.W. COVELL. 1999. Laminar fiber architecture and three-dimensional systolic mechanics in canine ventricular myocardium. Am. J. Physiol. Heart C. **276**: 595–607.
12. DOU, J., W-Y.I. TSENG, T.G. REESE & V.J. WEDEEN. 2003. Combined diffusion and strain MRI reveals structure and function of human myocardial laminar sheets in vivo. Magnet. Reson. Med. **50**: 107–113.
13. HARRINGTON, K.B., F. RODRIGUEZ, A. CHENG, et al. 2005. Direct measurement of transmural laminar architecture in the anterolateral wall of the ovine left ventricle: new implications for wall thickening mechanics. Am. J. Physiol. Heart C. **288**: 1324–1330.
14. HELM, P.A., M.F. BEG, M.I. MILLER & R.L. WINSLOW. 2005. Measuring and mapping cardiac fiber and laminar architecture using diffusion tensor MR imaging. Ann. N. Y. Acad. Sci. **1047**: 296–307.
15. KLÉBER, A.G., V.G. FAST & S. ROHR. 2000. Continuous and discontinuous propagation. In Cardiac Electrophysiology: From Cell to Bedside. Third edition. D.P. Zipes & J. Jalife, Eds.: 205–213. WB Saunders. Philadelphia, PA.
16. HOOKS, D.A., K.A. TOMLINSON, S.G. MARSDEN, et al. 2002. Cardiac microstructure: implications for electrical propagation and defibrillation in the heart. Circ. Res. **91**: 331–338.
17. KNISLEY, S.B.. 1998. Optical mapping of cardiac electrical stimulation. J. Electrocardiol. **30**(Suppl.): 11–18.
18. GRAY, R.A., G. AYERS & J. JALIFÉ. 1997. Video imaging of atrial defibrillation in the sheep heart. Circulation **95**: 1038–1047.
19. SHARIFOV, O.F. & V.G. FAST. 2003. Optical mapping of transmural activation induced by electrical shocks in isolated left ventricular wall wedge preparations. J. Cardiovasc. Electr. **14**: 1215–1222.
20. CHEEK, E.R., O.F. SHARIFOV & V.G. FAST. 2005. Role of microscopic tissue structure in shock-induced activation assessed by optical mapping in myocyte cultures. J. Cardiovasc. Electr. **16**: 991–1000.
21. HOOKS, D.A., I.J. LEGRICE, J.D. HARVEY & B.H. SMAILL. 2001. Intramural multisite recording of transmembrane potential in the heart. Biophys. J. **81**: 2671–2680.
22. ROGERS, J.M., S.B. MELNICK & J. HUANG. 2002. Fiberglass needle electrodes for transmural cardiac mapping. IEEE T Biomed. Eng. **49**: 1639–1641.
23. FRAZIER, D.W., W. KRASSOWSKA, et al. 1988. Transmural activations and stimulus potentials in three-dimensional anisotropic canine myocardium. Circ. Res. **63**: 135–146.
24. CALDWELL, B.J., I.J. LEGRICE, D.A. HOOKS, et al. 2005. Intramural measurement of transmembrane potential in the isolated pig heart: validation of a novel technique. J. Cardiovasc. Electr. **16**: 1001–1010.

25. SANDS, G.B., M.L. TREW, D.A. HOOKS, et al. 2004. Constructing a tissue-specific model of ventricular microstructure. Proceedings of the 26th Annual International Conference of the IEEE EMBS. 3589–3592.
26. TREW, M.L., I.J. LEGRICE, B.H. SMAILL & A.J. PULLAN. 2005a. A finite volume method for modeling discontinuous electrical activation in cardiac tissue. Ann. Biomed. Eng. **33:** 590–602.
27. TREW, M.L. & G.B. SANDS. 2005. Shock-induced transmembrane potential fields in a model of cardiac microstructure. J. Cardiovasc. Electr. 9/1025.
28. HOOKS, D.A., M.L. TREW, B.H. SMAILL & A.J. PULLAN. 2005. Do intramural virtual electrodes facilitate successful defibrillation? Model based analysis of experimental evidence. J. Cardiovasc. Electr. **17:** 305–311.
29. DOBRZYNSKI, H., J. LI, J. TELLEZ, et al. 2005. Computer three-dimensional reconstruction of the sinoatrial node. Circulation **111:** 846–854.
30. TREW, M.L., G.B. SANDS, B.J. CALDWELL, et al. 2005b. Modeling cardiac activation and the impact of a discontinuous myocardium. Proceedings 27th Annual Conference of the IEEE Engineering in Medicine and Biology Society, Shanghi, China, no. 1005.
31. NICKERSON, D.P. & P.J. HUNTER. 2006. The Noble cardiac ventricular electrophysiology models in CellML. Prog. Biophys. Mol. Biol. **90:** 346–359.
32. NICKERSON, D.P., M.P. NASH, P.M.F. NIELSEN, et al. 2006. Computational multiscale modeling in the IUPS Physiome Project: modeling cardiac electromechanics. IBM J. Res. Dev. In press.
33. HUNTER, P.J., P.A. MCNAUGHTON & D. NOBLE. 1975. Analytical models of propagation in excitable cells. Prog. Biophys. Mol. Bio. **30:** 99–144.
34. SKOUIBINE, K.B., N.A. TRAYANOVA & P.K. MOORE. 2000. A numerically efficient model for simulation of defibrillation in an active bidomain sheet of myocardium. Math. Biosci. **166:** 85–100.
35. POELZING, S., B.J. ROTH & D.S. ROSENBAUM. 2005. Optical measurements reveal nature of intercellular coupling across ventricular wall. Am. J. Physiol. Heart C. **289:** 1428–1435.
36. AUSTIN, T.M., M.L. TREW & A.J. PULLAN. 2006. Solving the cardiac bidomain equations for discontinuous conductivities. IEEE T Biomed. Eng. **53(7):** 1265–1272.
37. ROTH, B.J., S.F. LIN, J.P. WIKSWO JR.. 1998. Unipolar stimulation of cardiac tissue. J. Electrocardiol. **31**(Suppl): 6–12.
38. INO, T., M.C. FISHBEIN, W.J. MANDEL, et al. 1995. Cellular mechanisms of ventricular bipolar electrograms showing double and fractionated potentials. J. Am. Coll. Cardiol. **26:** 1080–1089.
39. PUNSKE, B.B., Q. NI, R.L. LUX, et al. 2003. Spatial methods of epicardial activation time determination in normal hearts. Ann. Biomed. Eng. **31:** 781–792.
40. SHARIFOV, O.F., R.E. IDEKER & V.G. FAST. 2004. High-resolution optical mapping of intramural virtual electrodes in porcine left ventricular wall. Cardiovasc. Res. **64:** 448–456.

Cardiac β-Adrenergic Signaling

From Subcellular Microdomains to Heart Failure

JEFFREY J. SAUCERMAN AND ANDREW D. McCULLOCH

Department of Bioengineering, University of California San Diego, La Jolla, California 92093-0412, USA

ABSTRACT: β-adrenergic signaling plays a central role in the neurohumoral regulation of the heart and the progression of heart failure. Initially thought to be a simple linear cascade, this complex network is now recognized to utilize cross-talk with numerous other pathways, spatial compartmentation, and feedback control to coordinate cardiac electrophysiology, contractility, and adaptive remodeling. Here, we review recent basic insights and novel quantitative approaches that are leading to a more comprehensive understanding of β-adrenergic signaling and thus motivate new therapeutic strategies for cardiac disease.

KEYWORDS: heart; cell signaling; cyclic AMP; protein kinase A; compartmentation

INTRODUCTION

β-adrenergic signaling transduces sympathetic stimulation into a cascade of biochemical reactions that coordinate cellular responses. This process is initiated by β-adrenergic receptors (β-ARs), members of a large gene family of seven transmembrane receptors, which activate upon binding the sympathetic neurotransmitter norepinephrine or the hormone epinephrine. β-ARs are expressed in a variety of tissues and are responsible for diverse physiologic regulation, such as relaxation of blood vessels, increases in liver metabolism, and relaxation of the bronchioles. In the heart, β-adrenergic signaling increases heart rate and contractility, key components of the fight-or-flight response. β-AR signaling also plays a fundamental role in heart failure and other cardiac diseases. While β-AR signaling is one of the most well-understood cell signaling networks, recent advances are demonstrating that this network is much

Address for correspondence: Prof. Andrew D. McCulloch, PhD, Department of Bioengineering, University of California San Diego, 9500 Gilman Dr, La Jolla, CA 92093-0412. Voice: 858-534-2547; fax: 858-534-5722.
e-mail: amcculloch@ucsd.edu

more complex than previously believed. Here, we briefly review conventional cardiac β-AR signaling and then expand upon growing research areas that are casting a new light on β-AR signaling and its consequences for the treatment of heart failure.

CONVENTIONAL β-ADRENERGIC SIGNALING IN THE HEART

Cardiac myocytes express two main β-AR isoforms, $β_1$-AR and $β_2$-AR (75%:25%). Norepinephrine or epinephrine-bound β-ARs activate the heterotrimeric G protein G_s, promoting dissociation of its α and βγ subunits. $G_{sα}$-GTP then binds the membrane-bound effector protein adenylyl cyclase (AC), stimulating synthesis of cyclic AMP (cAMP) from ATP. cAMP, a ubiquitous second messenger, causes the dissociation of regulatory and catalytic subunits of protein kinase A (PKA), allowing PKA's catalytic subunits to phosphorylate numerous substrate proteins including ion channels, myofilament proteins, and metabolic enzymes. PKA-dependent phosphorylation mediates many of the physiologic consequences of β-AR signaling. These events are eventually reversed as phosphodiesterases (PDEs) degrade the cAMP and protein phosphatases dephosphorylate PKA substrates.

β-AR signaling has been thought to have four main functional roles in the heart: to increase the heart beating rate (chronotropy), contractility (inotropy), relaxation rate (lusitropy), and to modulate metabolism as required by those increased energetic demands. Heart rate is primarily controlled by the sino-atrial (SA) node, which contains the most effective pacemaker cells. Sympathetic nervous system (SNS) activation increases the pacemaker rate (chronotropy) via voltage-dependent increases in I_f, the pacemaker current, secondary to direct binding of cAMP[1]. Inotropic responses are primarily attributed to PKA-mediated phosphorylation of the L-type calcium channel (I_{Ca}) and phospholamban. β-AR signaling increases I_{Ca}, bringing additional calcium into myocytes for larger contractions.[2,3] Phosphorylation of phospholamban releases its tonic inhibition of the sarcoplasmic reticulum (SR) Ca^{2+} pump, sequestering more Ca^{2+} into the SR for larger subsequent contractions.[4] Phospholamban phosphorylation also contributes to lusitropy, as the increase in Ca^{2+} flux from cytosol to SR accelerates relaxation of the myofilaments. Troponin I is also phosphorylated by PKA and has been thought to increase lusitropy by reducing the Ca^{2+} affinity of its partner protein troponin C.[5] The inotropic response, by increasing myofilament work and ATP-dependent SR Ca^{2+} pump rate, expends additional energy in order to generate stronger contractions. To keep up with these demands, PKA also activates phosphorylase kinase, a metabolic enzyme that increases rates of glycogen breakdown,[6] thereby providing additional glucose and increasing cellular ATP.

Congestive heart failure (CHF), while resulting from a number of causes, involves reduced cardiac output and contractility. Historical and conventional treatments for CHF have aimed at restoring cardiac contractility either indirectly through the use of cardiac glycosides (e.g., digoxin) or more directly by using inotropic agents that act through β-ARs (e.g., dobutamine) or PDEs (e.g., milrinone).[7] While potent inotropic agents have been shown to restore short-term contractility, many have been associated clinically with increased mortality in CHF.[7] In contrast, β-AR blockers are associated with reduced mortality and improved cardiac function in CHF.[8] Such counterintuitive results are forcing a reevaluation of the β-AR signaling network once thought to be so well understood. Does β-AR signaling mediate additional, important cellular functions? Does increased β-AR signaling contribute to the pathophysiology of heart failure, or is it a protective response? Is restoration of cardiac contractility the most appropriate goal in the treatment of heart failure? New findings are revealing surprising answers to some of these questions, with great promise toward future improvements in the treatment of heart failure.

COMPARTMENTATION OF cAMP AND PKA SIGNALING

Initial descriptions of cAMP signaling assumed a linear relationship from hormone-stimulated activation of AC through cAMP, PKA, and functional consequences such as inotropy.[9] However, even 25 years ago, some studies were inconsistent with such a simple relationship, finding that as opposed to β-AR stimulation, activation of prostaglandin E_1 (PGE_1) receptors increased cAMP but did not increase particulate PKA activity or lead to inotropy.[10,11] These findings led to the hypothesis of cAMP compartmentation, that the cell could contain distinct pools of cAMP with varying ability to activate PKA and produce functional responses.[12] However, the cAMP compartmentation hypothesis was unconvincing for many as its molecular basis was unknown and cAMP compartmentation could not be directly measured.

In the last several years, a number of candidate molecular mechanisms for cAMP and PKA compartmentation have emerged. The plasma membrane is now known to be a heterogeneous environment, with lipid rafts and nonhomogeneous distribution of membrane-bound proteins among such microdomains. Caveolae, or "little caves," form membrane invaginations roughly 60 nm in diameter that are thought to play a role in endocytosis in endothelial cells and the formation of T tubules in cardiac myocytes.[13] Caveolae also appear to concentrate signaling proteins involved in β-AR signaling and other cascades. While the precise distribution of components is still unclear, caveolae appear to concentrate β-ARs, ACs, and PKA in both neonatal and adult cardiac myocytes.[14–16] At the same time, a number of receptors that act through cAMP but are not functionally well coupled to PKA and inotropy appear excluded from caveolae, including PGE_2 receptors.[14] Due to the ambiguities involved in the sucrose density fractionation often used to study caveolae, immunofluorescence microscopy and electron microscopy have provided vital information on caveolae organization from intact isolated adult myocytes and myocardium.[17] Functional evidence for the role of caveolae in cAMP/PKA compartmentation is just beginning to emerge. Filipin, a sterol-binding agent that disrupts lipid rafts, prevented β_2- but not β_1-AR increases in the spontaneous beating rate of neonatal cardiac myocytes.[18] While L-type calcium channels have been shown to colocalize with caveolae in skeletal muscle[19] and neonatal cardiac myocytes,[20] regulation of these channels by β_1-AR- or β_2-AR-specific agonists has not been tested with caveolae disruption. Further work is necessary to characterize the extent to which caveolar localization is required for specific β_1-AR or β_2-AR regulation of L-type calcium currents and inotropic responses in adult cardiac myocytes.

Molecular evidence is also growing for the role of protein complexes in the compartmentation of cell signaling. Numerous A-kinase-anchoring proteins (AKAPs) tether the regulatory subunit of PKA, RII, or RI to individual PKA substrates or microdomains. In the context of cAMP/PKA compartmentation, AKAPs may localize PKA near individual pools of cAMP, ensuring that certain PKA substrates are only regulated in response to a subset of cAMP signals. Some AKAPs recruit many other signaling proteins to these scaffolds as well, possibly forming functional signaling modules.[21] In the heart, AKAPs have been shown to target PKA to the L-type calcium channel, the ryanodine receptor complex, the nuclear membrane, β_2-AR, the KNCQ1/KCNE1 K$^+$ channel, mitochondria, and additional sites.[22] While there is insufficient PKA (<1 μmol/L cytosol) to stoichiometrically target high-abundance substrates such as phospholamban ($\sim$100 μmol/L cytosol), AKAPs may serve to maintain a stoichiometric balance between PKA and low abundance substrates to ensure their proper regulation.

Functional roles of AKAPs have been studied using AKAP mutagenesis in cell expression systems and Ht31 peptides, which competitively inhibit PKA's binding site for AKAPs. Ht31 peptides were shown to disrupt β-adrenergic regulation of the L-type calcium channel current in adult mouse cardiac myocytes, providing a clear indication of the functional importance for AKAPs.[23] Unexpectedly, Ht31 peptides expressed in adult rat cardiac myocytes enhanced β-AR-induced increases in contractility and myocyte relaxation rate but not calcium transients.[24] This result may be due to an unidentified myofilament-bound AKAP that facilitates increases in Ca^{2+} sensitivity. However, methodological differences may have also played a role. In the study by Gao et al.,[23] Ht31 peptides were delivered acutely through a patch pipette to freshly isolated mouse cardiac myocytes, while in the study by Fink et al.,[24] Ht31 peptides were expressed using an adenovirus in cultured rat cardiac myocytes. In neonatal cardiac myocytes, mAKAP has been shown to integrate cAMP pathway components and many other proteins at the nuclear membrane, playing a role in both cytokine and β-AR-induced hypertrophy.[25,26]

Caveolae and AKAPs provide intriguing candidate molecular mechanisms to support the cAMP/PKA compartmentation hypothesis. Yet a significant gap has remained between these possible molecular mechanisms and functional or *in vitro* data that appear difficult to explain without a compartmentation hypothesis. Recently developed experimental approaches are now providing much more solid evidence of cAMP/PKA compartmentation in intact cardiac myocytes. A number of these studies have involved creative use of cellular electrophysiology, which has a tradition of quantitative studies. By providing separate perfusion to opposite ends of a single frog ventricular myocyte, Jurevicius and Fischmeister were able to measure both local and distant changes in I_{Ca} in response to locally applied stimuli.[27] Through this technique, they demonstrated that isoproterenol but not forskolin-induced signaling was compartmented, and that PDEs played a direct role in limiting cAMP diffusion. Cyclic nucleotide gated (CNG) channels have been genetically modified and expressed in simple cells, providing real-time measurements of sub-membrane cAMP concentrations through the whole-cell patch clamp.[28,29] Even in simple cells, these CNG channels demonstrated much higher and transient cAMP concentrations at the membrane than seen with average global measurements of cAMP. These constructs have been recently expressed in adult rat ventricular myocytes, allowing characterization of negative feedback involved in PKA-mediated activation of PDEs.[30]

Another exciting innovation in experimental approaches has been the advent of green fluorescent protein (GFP)-based imaging. Numerous recombinant protein biosensors have been designed based on fluorescence resonance energy transfer (FRET) between the cyan (CFP) and yellow (YFP) mutants of GFP, either on different proteins (intermolecular FRET), or in a single protein (intramolecular FRET). These fluorescent indicators have allowed real-time imaging of Ca^{2+}, cAMP, PKA, protein kinase C (PKC), and many other second messengers and kinase activities in live cells.[31] Particularly notable has been the development of cAMP sensors based on dissociation of PKA's regulatory and catalytic subunits.[32] Expression of a GFP-based cAMP sensor in neonatal cardiac myocytes allowed the first direct visualization of cAMP compartmentation in response to β-AR signaling.[33] While these gradients of cAMP aligned with 2 μm periodicity suggestive of T-tubule membranes, cAMP diffusion is likely even more locally restricted given the above-mentioned differential functional responses to specific β-AR agonists, forskolin, and other G-protein coupled receptor agonists. Further work is required to achieve even greater resolution with genetically targeted sensors and to quantitatively characterize the connections between molecular mechanisms, cAMP compartmentation, and its functional consequences. For example, this GFP-based cAMP sensor was recently used to demonstrate a role for $β_3$-ARs in PDE2 activation, which restricts cAMP diffusion during $β_1$-AR stimulation with norepinephrine.[34] Appreciation of cAMP/PKA compartmentation and its functional consequences will help provide a more refined understanding of how β-AR signaling coordinates diverse functions in health and disease.

LONG-TERM β-ADRENERGIC SIGNALING

There is increasing evidence that β-AR signaling cross-talks with other signaling pathways in addition to the conventional steps of β-AR, G_s, AC, cAMP, PKA, and substrates (FIG. 1). These "new" forms of signaling trigger long-term consequences (hours to days) of β-AR action such as cardiac hypertrophy and apoptosis. While organized into classical signaling downstream of PKA and nonclassical (cAMP/PKA-independent) β-AR signaling, numerous cross-talk and feedback mechanisms blur this distinction in some situations.

Classical Long-Term β-Adrenergic Signaling

As discussed above, β-AR signaling acts through PKA-mediated phosphorylation to increase cardiac myocyte calcium and contractility. Increases in cellular calcium due to β-AR signaling can trigger a number of calcium-dependent signaling pathways, one of which is Ca^{2+}–calmodulin-dependent

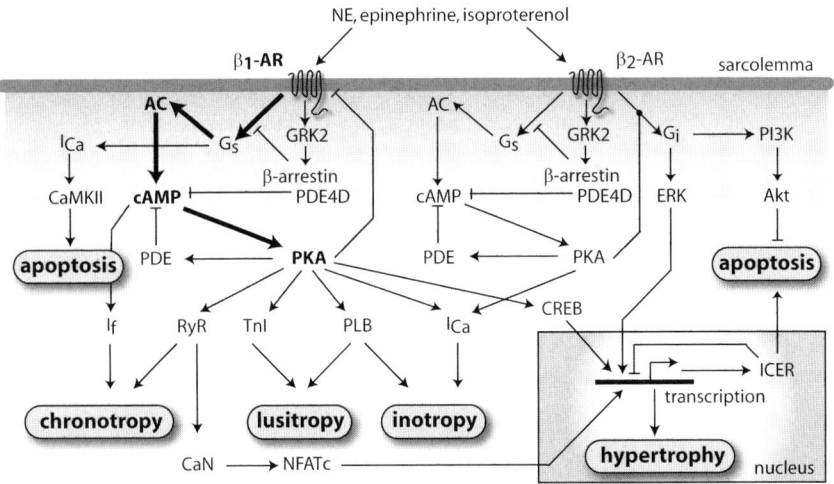

FIGURE 1. Functional consequences of cardiac β-AR signaling. Historically, cardiac β-AR signaling was known only to act through the $β_1$-AR–AC–cAMP–PKA signaling axis (bold arrows) to acutely regulate heart rate (chronotropy), inotropy (contractility), and lusitropy (relaxation rate). Recent evidence additionally demonstrates an important role for $β_2$-AR signaling and long-term cardiac remodeling including regulation of hypertrophy and apoptosis.

kinase II (CaMKII). CaMKII appears to act as a frequency-dependent positive feedback loop. Increased heart rates and calcium levels from β-AR signaling stimulate CaMKII, which further increases calcium influx through I_{Ca} and SR Ca^{2+} pump activity through phosphorylation of phospholamban.[35] Thus some portion of the functional response to β-AR signaling may be attributed to CaMKII-dependent effects.

CaMKII signaling also appears to mediate some of the long-term consequences of β-AR signaling. The appreciation of a role for cardiac myocyte apoptosis in heart failure has been fairly recent.[36] Long-term $β_1$-AR signaling has been shown to induce apoptosis in cardiac myocytes, which appeared dependent upon PKA and increases in I_{Ca}.[37] This led to the finding that CaMKII, activated by increases in calcium influx, was an important intermediate in $β_1$-AR-mediated apoptosis.[38] Unexpectedly, Zhu et al.[38] demonstrated that such signaling may be PKA-independent through the use of multiple PKA inhibitors. H89, used by Communal et al.[37] to inhibit PKA, may not be specific as it has been shown to also act as a β-AR blocker.[39] A subsequent study found that long-term (hours) β-adrenergic responses in excitation–contraction (E–C) coupling may also be due to PKA-independent activation of CaMKII, while short-term (minutes) β-adrenergic regulation of E–C coupling were found to be PKA-mediated and independent of CaMKII.[40]

Together, these studies suggest that $β_1$-AR signaling, long thought to act only through cAMP and PKA, undergoes a functional shift from PKA to CaMKII signaling with long-term stimulation. Responsible mechanisms for PKA-independent activation of CaMKII are unclear. There appear to be some inconsistencies between initial PKA-dependent CaMKII activation,[35] which occurs rather quickly, and PKA-independent CaMKII activation,[38,40] which occurs over 2 h. This apparent discrepancy may turn out to be due to compartmentation of CaMKII signaling. One intriguing possible mechanism is direct stimulation of I_{Ca} by β-AR-activated G_s,[41] shown to contribute only a small portion of the total β-AR response[42] yet may explain a slowly increasing activation of CaMKII.

Regardless of whether or not β-AR activation of CaMKII is downstream of PKA, inhibition of CaMKII may serve as an attractive therapeutic target for heart failure. Such a therapy could prevent CaMKII-dependent apoptosis while retaining responsiveness to β-AR stimuli.[43] This hypothesis was tested *in vivo* with a transgenic mouse expressing the CaMKII inhibitor peptide AC3-I.[44] Remarkably, CaMKII inhibition in this mouse prevented maladaptive remodeling in response to excessive β-AR stimuli and myocardial infarction while retaining responsiveness to physiologic β-AR stimuli.

Some long-term responses to $β_1$-AR stimulation may be the result of more direct transcriptional regulation. Increases in cAMP allow PKA-mediated phosphorylation of cAMP response element (CRE)-binding (CREB) transcription factors that bind to the CRE in promotor regions of several genes.[45] While CRE-induced transcription contributes to a cardiac hypertrophic response, it also increases expression of inducible cAmP early repressor (ICER), an inducible repressor of CRE transcription and an inhibitor of the anti-apoptotic protein Bcl-2.[46] Through these mechanisms, excessive β-AR stimulation may trigger apoptosis through ICER. Recently, Ding *et al.* demonstrated that chronic PDE3 but not PDE4 inhibition triggered apoptosis through an ICER-dependent pathway, while constitutive expression of PDE3 A with an adenovirus prevented isoproterenol-induced apoptosis.[47] Differences between the PDE3 and PDE4 responses suggest that ICER-mediated apoptosis may rely on cAMP compartmentation to respond in a context-dependent manner. Thus PKA-independent CaMKII signaling and PKA-dependent ICER signaling represent two pathways that may underlie β_1-AR-induced cardiac apoptosis. Future studies will be required to determine the relative roles of these pathways, particularly in animal models relevant to human heart failure.

Nonclassical β-Adrenergic Signaling

Unlike traditional β_1-AR signaling, which acts through G_s, β_2-ARs undergo a transition from G_s to G_i signaling mediated by PKA phosphorylation of β_2-AR.[48] This transition has been implicated in enhanced β_2-AR compartmentation of cAMP, allowing functional coupling to I_{Ca} but not to phospholamban or other cytosolic substrates of PKA.[49,50] β_2-AR stimulation of G_i has also been shown to prevent cardiac apoptosis through a pathway involving PI3 K and Akt.[51,52] Thus there appears to be a balance between pro-apoptotic β_1-AR signaling and anti-apoptotic β_2-AR signaling. Such duality is reminiscent of the β-adrenergic inotropy/lusitropy duality, for which Arnold Katz described β-AR signaling as "a man who blows hot and cold air with one breath," a reference to Aesop's fable, "The Man and the Satyr."[53]

Stimulated β-ARs are well recognized to desensitize to prolonged stimulation. Desensitization of β_1-ARs occurs via two pathways: phosphorylation of the activated receptor by G-protein receptor kinase 2 (GRK2) or PKA.[54] β_2-ARs desensitize via the GRK2 pathway, initializing receptor internalization through clathrin-coated pits.[55] PI3 K has been shown to form a complex with GRK2, contributing to downregulation of β-ARs via desensitization[56] but also initiating a hypertrophic response.[57] Inhibiting GRK2 or disrupting PI3 K/GRK2 interaction has prevented β-AR downregulation and prolonged survival in several heart failure models.[55,58,59] Relative roles for β-AR downregulation and consequent reduction in PI3 K-dependent inhibition of apoptosis in the transition to heart failure remain to be determined.

Recent evidence has shown that in addition to its role in GRK-mediated receptor desensitization, β-arrestin serves as a scaffold for many signaling proteins, bringing them to the membrane upon receptor activation.[60] β-arrestin acts as a scaffold for the MAPK cascade, enabling ERK phosphorylation through G_i signaling in response to isoproterenol in cardiac myocytes.[61] PDE4D is bound to β-arrestin as well, causing an increase in membrane PDE4D activity with stimulation of β_2-ARs.[62] PDE recruitment by β-arrestin was shown to form a negative feedback loop by decreasing PKA activity at the membrane, which placed a restraint on the transition from G_s to G_i signaling and downstream ERK phosphorylation.[61] Long-term β_2-AR activation can also recruit β-arrestin in a G-protein-independent manner leading to prolonged ERK activation.[63] ERK phosphorylation is a key component of hypertrophy signaling,[64] raising the intriguing possibility that long-term β_2-AR signaling may lead to cardiac hypertrophy. This would serve as a natural balance to the pro-apoptotic signaling due to β_1-AR stimulation.

Much of nonclassical signaling through β-ARs has been discovered in just the last several years. Over 20 proteins have been shown to be targeted to β-arrestins, with β-arrestin 1 and 2 showing selectivity for binding partners and receptors.[60] It is likely that many more binding proteins will be found. Given the large number of binding partners for β-arrestins, there exists a possibility for further functional differentiation and specificity in receptor targeting based on the set of binding proteins on a given β-arrestin scaffold. While further work is required on the mechanisms of nonclassical signaling by β-arrestins and their functional consequences, it is clear that β-arrestins exemplify an emerging theme of compartmentation by signaling complexes.

CONCLUSIONS AND FUTURE DIRECTIONS

The historical view of β-AR signaling as a linear pathway with a single functional role led to the use of inotropic agents in the treatment of heart failure. Recent advances in our knowledge of β-AR signaling have revealed a much more complex signaling network than previously believed. Live-cell imaging techniques are providing direct evidence of cAMP/PKA compartmentation and numerous molecular mechanisms are being revealed, including caveolae, AKAPs, and β-arrestins. Compartmentation underlies important aspects of signaling specificity, and while only short-term consequences have been studied to date, compartmentation is likely to be crucial in the ordered transitions from "short-term" to "long-term" term signaling in the β-AR network. Further work will be required to quantitatively characterize how molecular mechanisms contribute to cAMP compartmentation in response to both short- and long-term stimuli. Long-term β-AR stimuli are now recognized to facilitate coupling to many additional pathways including CaMKII, PI3 K, and MAP kinases. These pathways contribute to pro-apoptotic, anti-apoptotic, and hypertrophic responses. Further work will be required to understand the relative roles of β-adrenergic regulation of cardiac contractility and these additional pathways in the development and progression of human heart failure.

An appreciation for the roles of compartmentation, dynamics, and combinatorial complexity of signaling networks suggests that we should not expect to reduce the pathophysiology of heart failure to a single underlying mechanism or treat it with a single therapy. Rather, multiple therapeutics may be required simultaneously to prevent maladaptive responses. One approach may, for example, attempt to prevent cardiac apoptosis while restoring β-AR responsiveness. Rational design of therapies will also require a greater basic understanding of the mechanisms of compartmentation and dynamics in signaling to achieve the desired specificity.

Given the complexity of these processes, this will require quantitative experimental approaches such as live-cell imaging, high-throughput genomics and proteomics, and integrative animal studies. Systems approaches and computational models such as those proposed by the Alliance for Cellular Signaling will also be required to integrate and distill understanding from such heterogeneous data.[65] Mechanistic and experimentally validated computational models of cardiac β_1-AR signaling have already been used to predict the relative efficacy of proposed gene therapies and molecular mechanisms of cardiac myocyte inotropy.[66,67] Integrated models of β_1-AR signaling and ventricular electrophysiology predicted a mechanistic link between a gene mutation that disrupts AKAP interactions and a form of long-QT syndrome.[68] Similar approaches may be valuable for exploring which molecular mechanisms can quantitatively explain cAMP/PKA compartmentation or how multiple pathways interact to produce coordinated long-term adaptations to adrenergic stimuli. Despite the challenges ahead, a more mechanistic and comprehensive understanding of cardiac β-AR signaling will have a great impact on our understanding and treatment of heart failure and other cardiac diseases.

ACKNOWLEDGMENTS

This research was supported by the NIH through the National Biomedical Computation Resource (P41 RR08605), the National Science Foundation (BES 0506252), and a Whitaker Foundation Graduate Fellowship (to JJS).

REFERENCES

1. DiFrancesco, D. & P. Tortora. 1991. Direct activation of cardiac pacemaker channels by intracellular cyclic AMP. Nature **351:** 145–147.
2. Tsien, R.W., W. Giles & P. Greengard. 1972. Cyclic AMP mediates the effects of adrenaline on cardiac Purkinje fibres. Nat. New Biol. **240:** 181–183.
3. Reuter, H. 1967. The dependence of slow inward current in Purkinje fibres on the extracellular calcium-concentration. J. Physiol. **192:** 479–492.
4. Tada, M., M.A. Kirchberger & A.M. Katz. 1975. Phosphorylation of a 22,000-Dalton component of the cardiac sarcoplasmic reticulum by adenosine 3′:5′-monophosphate-dependent protein kinase. J. Biol. Chem. **250:** 2640–2647.
5. Solaro, R.J., A.J. Moir & S.V. Perry. 1976. Phosphorylation of troponin I and the inotropic effect of adrenaline in the perfused rabbit heart. Nature **262:** 615–617.

6. Cohen, P. 1973. The subunit structure of rabbit-skeletal-muscle phosphorylase kinase, and the molecular basis of its activation reactions. Eur. J. Biochem. **34:** 1–14.
7. Eichhorn, E.J. & M.R. Bristow. 1996. Medical therapy can improve the biological properties of the chronically failing heart. A new era in the treatment of heart failure. Circulation **94:** 2285–2296.
8. Bristow, M.R. 2000. Beta-adrenergic receptor blockade in chronic heart failure. Circulation **101:** 558–569.
9. Kuo, J.F. & P. Greengard. 1969. Cyclic nucleotide-dependent protein kinases. IV. Widespread occurrence of adenosine 3′,5′-monophosphate-dependent protein kinase in various tissues and phyla of the animal kingdom. Proc. Natl. Acad. Sci. USA **64:** 1349–1355.
10. Hayes, J.S., L.L. Brunton & S.E. Mayer. 1980. Selective activation of particulate cAMP-dependent protein kinase by isoproterenol and prostaglandin E1. J. Biol. Chem. **255:** 5113–5119.
11. Brunton, L.L., J.S. Hayes & S.E. Mayer. 1979. Hormonally specific phosphorylation of cardiac troponin I and activation of glycogen phosphorylase. Nature **280:** 78–80.
12. Brunton, L.L., J.S. Hayes & S.E. Mayer. 1981. Functional compartmentation of cyclic AMP and protein kinase in heart. Adv. Cyclic Nucleotide Res. **14:** 391–397.
13. Cohen, A.W. *et al.* 2004. Role of caveolae and caveolins in health and disease. Physiol. Rev. **84:** 1341–1379.
14. Ostrom, R.S. *et al.* 2001. Receptor number and caveolar co-localization determine receptor coupling efficiency to adenylyl cyclase. J. Biol. Chem. **276:** 42063–42069.
15. Rybin, V.O. *et al.* 2003. Developmental changes in beta2-adrenergic receptor signaling in ventricular myocytes: the role of Gi proteins and caveolae microdomains. Mol Pharmacol. **63:** 1338–13348.
16. Ostrom, R.S., R.A. Bundey & P.A. Insel. 2004. Nitric oxide inhibition of adenylyl cyclase type 6 activity is dependent upon lipid rafts and caveolin signaling complexes. J. Biol. Chem. **279:** 19846–19853.
17. Head, B.P. *et al.* 2005. G-protein-coupled receptor signaling components localize in both sarcolemmal and intracellular caveolin-3-associated microdomains in adult cardiac myocytes. J. Biol. Chem. **280:** 31036–31044.
18. Xiang, Y. *et al.* 2002. Caveolar localization dictates physiologic signaling of beta 2-adrenoceptors in neonatal cardiac myocytes. J. Biol. Chem. **277:** 34280–34286.
19. Jorgensen, A.O. *et al.* 1989. Subcellular distribution of the 1,4-dihydropyridine receptor in rabbit skeletal muscle in situ: an immunofluorescence and immunocolloidal gold-labeling study. J. Cell Biol. **109:** 135–147.
20. Lohn, M. *et al.* 2000. Ignition of calcium sparks in arterial and cardiac muscle through caveolae. Circ. Res. **87:** 1034–1039.
21. Wong, W. & J.D. Scott. 2004. AKAP signalling complexes: focal points in space and time. Nat. Rev. Mol. Cell Biol. **5:** 959–970.
22. Ruehr, M.L., M.A. Russell & M. Bond. 2004. A-kinase anchoring protein targeting of protein kinase A in the heart. J. Mol. Cell Cardiol. **37:** 653–665.
23. Gao, T. *et al.* 1997. cAMP-dependent regulation of cardiac L-type Ca^{2+} channels requires membrane targeting of PKA and phosphorylation of channel subunits. Neuron **19:** 185–196.

24. Fink, M.A. et al. 2001. AKAP-mediated targeting of protein kinase a regulates contractility in cardiac myocytes. Circ. Res. **88:** 291–297.
25. Pare, G.C. et al. 2005. The mAKAP complex participates in the induction of cardiac myocyte hypertrophy by adrenergic receptor signaling. J. Cell Sci. **118:** 5637–5646.
26. Dodge-Kafka, K.L. et al. 2005. The protein kinase A anchoring protein mAKAP coordinates two integrated cAMP effector pathways. Nature **437:** 574–578.
27. Jurevicius, J. & R. Fischmeister. 1996. cAMP compartmentation is responsible for a local activation of cardiac Ca^{2+} channels by beta-adrenergic agonists. Proc. Natl. Acad. Sci. USA. **93:** 295–299.
28. Rich, T.C. et al. 2000. Cyclic nucleotide-gated channels colocalize with adenylyl cyclase in regions of restricted cAMP diffusion. J. Gen. Physiol. **116:** 147–161.
29. Rich, T.C. et al. 2001. A uniform extracellular stimulus triggers distinct cAMP signals in different compartments of a simple cell. Proc. Natl. Acad. Sci. USA **98:** 13049–13054.
30. Rochais, F. et al. 2004. Negative feedback exerted by cAMP-dependent protein kinase and cAMP phosphodiesterase on subsarcolemmal cAMP signals in intact cardiac myocytes: an *in vivo* study using adenovirus-mediated expression of CNG channels. J. Biol. Chem. **279:** 52095–52105.
31. Zhang, J. et al. 2002. Creating new fluorescent probes for cell biology. Nat. Rev. Mol. Cell Biol. **3:** 906–918.
32. Adams, S.R. et al. 1991. Fluorescence ratio imaging of cyclic AMP in single cells. Nature **349:** 694–697.
33. Zaccolo, M. & T. Pozzan. 2002. Discrete microdomains with high concentration of cAMP in stimulated rat neonatal cardiac myocytes. Science **295:** 1711–1715.
34. Mongillo, M. et al. 2005. Compartmentalized phosphodiesterase-2 activity blunts β-adrenergic cardiac inotropy via an NO/cGMP-dependent pathway. Circ. Res **98(2):** 226–234..
35. Maier, L.S. & D.M. Bers. 2002. Calcium, calmodulin, and calcium-calmodulin kinase II: heartbeat to heartbeat and beyond. J. Mol. Cell Cardiol. **34:** 919–939.
36. Colucci, W.S. 1996. Apoptosis in the heart. N. Engl. J. Med. **335:** 1224–1226.
37. Communal, C. et al. 1998. Norepinephrine stimulates apoptosis in adult rat ventricular myocytes by activation of the beta-adrenergic pathway. Circulation **98:** 1329–1334.
38. Zhu, W.Z. et al. 2003. Linkage of beta1-adrenergic stimulation to apoptotic heart cell death through protein kinase A-independent activation of Ca^{2+}/calmodulin kinase II. J. Clin. Invest. **111:** 617–625.
39. Penn, R.B. et al. 1999. Pharmacological inhibition of protein kinases in intact cells: antagonism of beta adrenergic receptor ligand binding by H-89 reveals limitations of usefulness. J. Pharmacol. Exp. Ther. **288:** 428–437.
40. Wang, W. et al. 2004. Sustained beta1-adrenergic stimulation modulates cardiac contractility by Ca^{2+}/calmodulin kinase signaling pathway. Circ. Res. **95:** 798–806.
41. Yatani, A. et al. 1987. A G protein directly regulates mammalian cardiac calcium channels. Science **238:** 1288–1292.
42. McDonald, T.F. et al. 1994. Regulation and modulation of calcium channels in cardiac, skeletal, and smooth muscle cells. Physiol. Rev. **74:** 365–507.
43. Bers, D.M. 2005. Beyond beta blockers. Nat. Med. **11:** 379–380.
44. Zhang, R. et al. 2005. Calmodulin kinase II inhibition protects against structural heart disease. Nat. Med. **11:** 409–417.

45. Muller, F.U., J. Neumann & W. Schmitz. 2000. Transcriptional regulation by cAMP in the heart. Mol. Cell Biochem. **212:** 11–17.
46. Tomita, H. *et al.* 2003. Inducible cAMP early repressor (ICER) is a negative-feedback regulator of cardiac hypertrophy and an important mediator of cardiac myocyte apoptosis in response to beta-adrenergic receptor stimulation. Circ. Res. **93:** 12–22.
47. Ding, B. *et al.* 2005. Functional role of phosphodiesterase 3 in cardiomyocyte apoptosis: implication in heart failure. Circulation **111:** 2469–2476.
48. Daaka, Y., L.M. Luttrell & R.J. Lefkowitz. 1997. Switching of the coupling of the beta2-adrenergic receptor to different G proteins by protein kinase A. Nature **390:** 88–91.
49. Xiao, R.P., X. Ji & E.G. Lakatta. 1995. Functional coupling of the beta 2-adrenoceptor to a pertussis toxin-sensitive G protein in cardiac myocytes. Mol. Pharmacol. **47:** 322–329.
50. Kuschel, M. *et al.* 1999. G(i) protein-mediated functional compartmentalization of cardiac beta(2)-adrenergic signaling. J. Biol. Chem. **274:** 22048–22052.
51. Communal, C. *et al.* 1999. Opposing effects of beta(1)- and beta(2)-adrenergic receptors on cardiac myocyte apoptosis: role of a pertussis toxin-sensitive G protein. Circulation **100:** 2210–2212.
52. Zhu, W.Z. *et al.* 2001. Dual modulation of cell survival and cell death by beta(2)-adrenergic signaling in adult mouse cardiac myocytes. Proc. Natl. Acad. Sci. USA **98:** 1607–1612.
53. Katz, A.M. 1983. Cyclic adenosine monophosphate effects on the myocardium: a man who blows hot and cold with one breath. J. Am. Coll. Cardiol. **2:** 143–149.
54. Rapacciuolo, A. *et al.* 2003. Protein kinase A and G protein-coupled receptor kinase phosphorylation mediates beta-1 adrenergic receptor endocytosis through different pathways. J. Biol. Chem. **278:** 35403–35411.
55. Tachibana, H. *et al.* 2005. Level of beta-adrenergic receptor kinase 1 inhibition determines degree of cardiac dysfunction after chronic pressure overload-induced heart failure. Circulation **111:** 591–597.
56. Naga Prasad, S.V. *et al.* 2001. Agonist-dependent recruitment of phosphoinositide 3-kinase to the membrane by beta-adrenergic receptor kinase 1. A role in receptor sequestration. J. Biol. Chem. **276:** 18953–18959.
57. Naga Prasad, S.V. *et al.* 2000. Gbetagamma-dependent phosphoinositide 3-kinase activation in hearts with *in vivo* pressure overload hypertrophy. J Biol Chem. **275:** 4693–4698.
58. Nienaber, J.J. *et al.* 2003. Inhibition of receptor-localized PI3K preserves cardiac beta-adrenergic receptor function and ameliorates pressure overload heart failure. J. Clin. Invest. **112:** 1067–1079.
59. Perrino, C. *et al.* 2005. Restoration of beta-adrenergic receptor signaling and contractile function in heart failure by disruption of the betaARK1/phosphoinositide 3-kinase complex. Circulation **111:** 2579–2587.
60. Lefkowitz, R.J. & S.K. Shenoy. 2005. Transduction of receptor signals by beta-arrestins. Science **308:** 512–517.
61. Baillie, G.S. *et al.* 2003. beta-Arrestin-mediated PDE4 cAMP phosphodiesterase recruitment regulates beta-adrenoceptor switching from Gs to Gi. Proc. Natl. Acad. Sci. USA **100:** 940–945.
62. Perry, S.J. *et al.* 2002. Targeting of cyclic AMP degradation to beta 2-adrenergic receptors by beta-arrestins. Science **298:** 834–836.

63. Shenoy, S.K. *et al*. 2006. beta-Arrestin-dependent, G protein-independent ERK1/2 activation by the beta2 adrenergic receptor. J. Biol. Chem. **281:** 1261–1273.
64. Molkentin, J.D. & I.G. Dorn, II. 2001. Cytoplasmic signaling pathways that regulate cardiac hypertrophy. Annu. Rev. Physiol. **63:** 391–426.
65. Gilman, A.G. *et al*. 2002. Overview of the alliance for cellular signaling. Nature **420:** 703–706.
66. Saucerman, J.J. *et al*. 2003. Modeling beta-adrenergic control of cardiac myocyte contractility *in silico*. J. Biol. Chem. **278:** 47997–48003.
67. Saucerman, J.J. & A.D. McCulloch. 2004. Mechanistic systems models of cell signaling networks: a case study of myocyte adrenergic regulation. Prog. Biophys. Mol. Biol. **85:** 261–278.
68. Saucerman, J.J. *et al*. 2004. Proarrhythmic consequences of a KCNQ1 AKAP-binding domain mutation: computational models of whole cells and heterogeneous tissue. Circ. Res. **95:** 1216–1224.

Multiscale Modeling of Calcium Signaling in the Cardiac Dyad

RAIMOND L. WINSLOW, ANTTI TANSKANEN, MINDAO CHEN, AND JOSEPH L. GREENSTEIN

Institute for Computational Medicine and The Center for Cardiovascular Bioinformatics & Modeling, The Johns Hopkins University School of Medicine and Whiting School of Engineering, Baltimore, Maryland 21218, USA

ABSTRACT: Calcium (Ca^{2+})-induced Ca^{2+}-release (CICR) takes place in spatially restricted microdomains known as dyads. The length scale over which CICR occurs is on the order of nanometers and relevant time scales range from micro- to milliseconds. Quantitative understanding of CICR therefore requires development of models that are applicable over a range of spatio-temporal scales. We will present several new approaches for multiscale modeling of CICR. First, we present a model of dyad Ca^{2+} dynamics in which the Fokker-Planck equation (FPE) is solved for the probability $P(x, t)$ that a Ca^{2+} ion is located at dyad position x at time t. Using this model, we demonstrate that (a) Ca^{2+} signaling in the dyad is mediated by approximately tens of Ca^{2+} ions; (b) these signaling events are noisy due to the small number of ions involved; and (c) the geometry of the RyR (ryanodine receptors) protein may function to restrict the diffusion of and to "funnel" Ca^{2+} ions to activation-binding sites on the RyR, thus increasing RyR open probability and excitation-contraction (EC) coupling gain. Simplification of this model to one in which the dyadic space is represented using a single compartment yields the stochastic local-control model of CICR developed previously. We have shown that this model captures fundamental properties of CICR, such as graded release and voltage-dependent gain, may be integrated within a model of the myocyte and may be simulated in reasonable times using a combination of efficient numerical methods and parallel computing, but remains too complex for general use in cell simulations. To address this problem, we show how separation of time scales may be used to formulate a model in which nearby L-type Ca^{2+} channels (LCCs) and RyRs gate as a coupled system that may be described using low-dimensional systems of ordinary differential equations, thus reducing computational complexity while capturing fundamentally important properties of CICR. The

Address for correspondence: Raimond L. Winslow, Institute for Computational Medicine and Center for Cardiovascular Bioinformatics & Modeling, The Johns Hopkins University School of Medicine and Whiting School of Engineering, Baltimore, MD 21218. Voice: 410-516-5417; fax: 410-516-5294. e-mail: rwinslow@jhu.edu

Ann. N.Y. Acad. Sci. 1080: 362–375 (2006). © 2006 New York Academy of Sciences.
doi: 10.1196/annals.1380.027

simplified model may be solved many orders of magnitude faster than can either of the more detailed models, thus enabling incorporation into tissue-level simulations.

KEYWORDS: dyad; calcium-induced calcium-release; excitation-contraction coupling; modeling

INTRODUCTION

Contraction of cardiac muscle is initiated when individual L-type calcium (Ca^{2+}) channels (LCCs) open in response to membrane depolarization, producing Ca^{2+} flux into a microdomain known as the dyad. The resulting increase in dyadic Ca^{2+} leads to opening of Ca^{2+}-sensitive Ca^{2+}-release channels (ryanodine receptors [RyR2s]) in the closely apposed junctional sarcoplasmic reticulum (JSR) membrane, producing additional flux of Ca^{2+} from the JSR into the dyad. These two sources of Ca^{2+} flux generate the intracellular Ca^{2+} transient triggering cardiac muscle contraction. Understanding the molecular basis of this Ca^{2+}-induced Ca^{2+}-release (CICR) process is therefore of fundamental importance to understanding cardiac muscle function in both health and disease.

Recent measurements indicate that there are $\sim$20–100 RyR2s per dyad and that dyad diameter and height (i.e., sarcolemmal-JSR membrane spacing) are $\sim$100 nm and $\sim$12 nm, respectively.[1,2] A variety of computational models predict that during an action potential (AP), peak Ca^{2+} concentration in the dyad ranges from 100 to 1,000 μM,[3,4] corresponding to 10–100 free Ca^{2+} ions in the dyad. These calculations indicate that both feed forward and feed back signaling between RyR2s and LCCs in the dyad are mediated by relatively few Ca^{2+} ions. Consequently, conclusions based on models which determine gradients in dyad Ca^{2+} concentration using laws of mass-action may be problematic.[5] Rather, the stochastic motion of Ca^{2+} ions in the dyad may impart a degree of "signaling noise" between LCCs and RyR2s and this signaling noise may in turn affect macroscopic properties of CICR at the cell and tissue level.

A number of large proteins are located within the dyad. The largest is RyR2, composed of four 565-kDa subunits. RyR2 structure has been measured at 3.0 nm resolution,[6] while that of the skeletal muscle isoform RyR1, sharing $\sim$70% sequence identity to RyR2,[7] has been measured at 1.0 nm resolution.[8] The cytoplasmic portion of the protein has dimensions $\sim$27 nm $\times$ 27 nm $\times$ 10 nm,[8,9] where the 10 nm height spans nearly the full distance between JSR and T-tubule membranes.[10] The crystal structure of the cardiac LCC (comprised of α_1, α_2, β, and δ subunits) has also been measured at $\sim$0.4 nm resolution.[11] The LCC is $\sim$19 nm in height and $\sim$14.5 nm in width, protruding from the T-tubule membrane about 2 nm into the dyad.[11] The structure of the Ca^{2+}-binding protein calmodulin (CaM), one molecule of which is tethered to the LCC,[12] has been measured at 0.1 nm resolution.[13] CaM is a dual-lobed protein of dimensions ~4.5 nm × 4.5 nm × 6.5 nm. Given the small dimensions of the dyad, it is likely that the physical location and dimensions of these dyad proteins have considerable influence on motion of Ca^{2+} ions and thus properties of CICR.

In this article, we address the following questions: (*a*) how does "signaling noise" due to the small number of Ca^{2+} ions within the dyad affect the nature of CICR?; and (*b*) how does the physical arrangement of large proteins within the dyad influence CICR? We address these questions by developing a molecularly and structurally detailed computational model of the cardiac dyad describing motions of Ca^{2+} ions, as determined by the Brownian motion in a potential field. While this model is useful for addressing the above questions, it is too complex for describing the process of CICR in more integrative models of the myocyte. We therefore present mathematical methods for generating a hierarchy of models of CICR which retain essential features of the release process, but which lend themselves to incorporation into whole myocyte models.

METHODS

Molecularly and Structurally Detailed Model of the Cardiac Dyad

The dyad is represented using a 100 nm × 100 nm × 12 nm lattice (FIG. 1 B). The lower dyad boundary is formed by the T-tubular membrane and the upper boundary is formed by the JSR membrane (FIG. 1 A). Ca^{2+} can diffuse across the lateral boundary of the dyad between the dyadic volume and the myoplasm (FIG. 1 A). The dyad volume accessible to diffusing Ca^{2+} ions is determined by the shape, and location of dyad proteins. Chief among these are LCCs, RyR2s, and CaM. RyR2s are located in the JSR membrane in quasi-crystalline arrays of tens of RyR2s (FIG. 1 B).[1] We employ a geometric model of the dyadic portion of RyR2 derived from cryo-electron microscopy (cryo-EM) measurements (FIG. 1 C),[9,14] with the pore of the RyR2 complex located in the center of the tetrameric structure.[8] Each model dyad is assumed to contain 20 RyR2s arranged in an asymmetric 4 × 5 quasi-crystal (FIG. 1 B).[15] A 5:1 RyR2:LCC ratio is assumed.[16]

Definitive locations of the Ca^{2+}-binding sites mediating RyR2 activation and inactivation are not yet available. Evidence suggests that the glutamate at position 3987 of physical domain 3 plays an important role in Ca^{2+} activation.[6,17–23] We therefore assume that each of the four RyR2 subunits contains a single activation site in a position corresponding to domain 3 (FIG. 1 C). Locations of RyR2 Ca^{2+}-binding inactivation sites are also uncertain.[21,24,25] Recently, Thomas *et al.*[26] suggested that inactivation-binding sites are localized to the N-terminal and central domains. We therefore positioned the low affinity Ca^{2+}-binding inactivation sites to the cleft regions between domains 10 and 9 on the clamp portions of the RyR2 tetramer (FIG. 1 C), based on

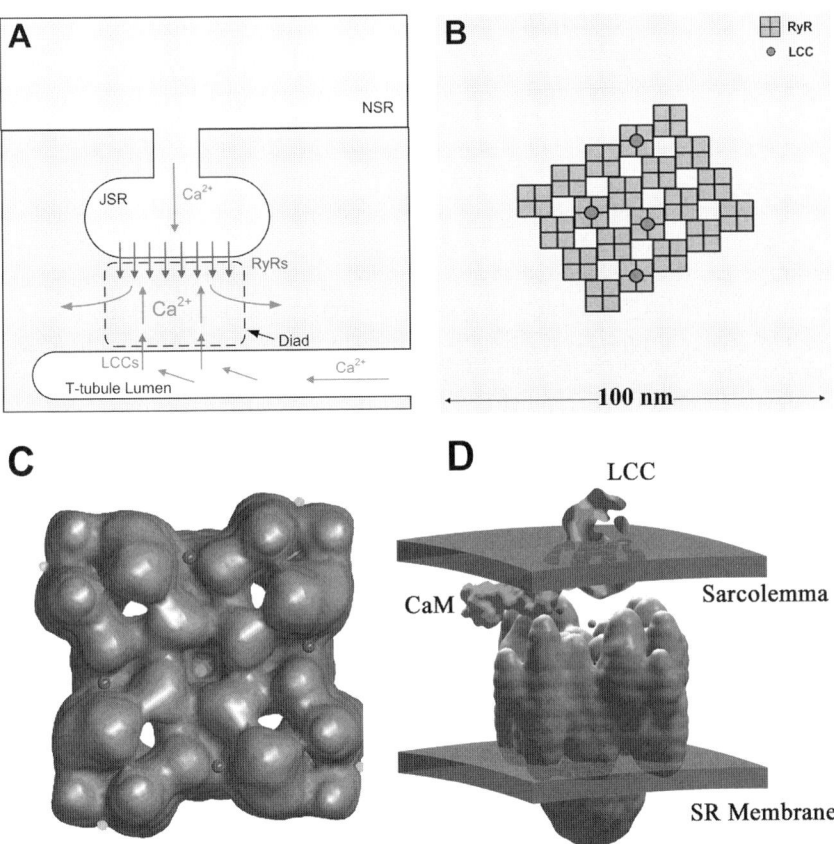

FIGURE 1. (**A**) A dyad cross-section. (**B**) Relative placement of RyR2s (gray boxes) and LCCs (circles) in the dyad. (**C**) Model of the RyR2 derived from experimental data showing the central pore, Ca^{2+}-binding activation (dark shaded circles) and inactivation (light shaded circles) sites. (**D**) Side view of the model dyad showing an RyR2, an LCC, and its associated CaM.

the observation that mutations to either domain inhibit Ca^{2+}-dependent inactivation (CDI).[26] The cytosolic region of each LCC structure occupies an area of width 14.5 nm extending 2 nm from the inner surface of the membrane. The geometry of this surface was modeled using LCC crystal structure data.[11] A constitutively tethered CaM acts as the Ca^{2+} sensor for CDI of LCCs.[27,28] A single CaM molecule is both necessary and sufficient to produce CDI of the associated LCC[12] (FIG. 1 D). CaM geometry (FIG. 1 D) was modeled by representing its surface structure (identified as 1CFD in Protein Data Bank).[29] A single CaM molecule contains four Ca^{2+}-binding sites. Two sites located on the carboxyl-tail have been shown to be responsible for CDI of the associated LCC.[27,28] Thus, in our model, CDI can proceed when both of the carboxyl-tail binding sites are occupied.

The kinetic model of the LCC was an eleven-state continuous time Markov chain model developed previously.[30–32] The kinetics of RyR2 gating were described using a four-state Markov model originally developed by Stern et al.[33,34] Based on the fourfold symmetry of the RyR2 protein, the original model of Stern et al.[33,34] was modified to incorporate the assumption that channel opening requires Ca^{2+} binding to all four activation sites.[35] In order for a Ca^{2+}-dependent state transition to occur in both these models, the required Ca^{2+}-binding sites must first be occupied by Ca^{2+} ions. We therefore assumed that when a freely diffusing Ca^{2+} ion enters a lattice position adjacent to an available Ca^{2+}-binding site, that Ca^{2+} ion may then bind to the site. Ion channel transition rates were therefore defined as functions depending on the occupancy of the Ca^{2+}-binding sites (rather than Ca^{2+} concentration).

Membrane phospholipid head groups act as fixed Ca^{2+} buffers. Binding-site density and Ca^{2+}-binding/unbinding rates in this model were based on the work of Langer and Peskoff[3] and Soeller and Cannell.[4] Both low-affinity and high-affinity Ca^{2+}-binding sites were assumed to be present on the SR and sarcolemmal membranes. Ca^{2+} binding to buffer sites is implemented in the same manner as described above for Ca^{2+} binding to ion channel proteins.

The motion of a Ca^{2+} ion in the dyad is influenced by the Brownian random force from the surrounding solvent and the electrostatic potential stemming from proteins, membranes, and other ions, including other Ca^{2+} ions. We model the joint positions $(\mathbf{r}_1, \ldots, \mathbf{r}_N)$ of N Ca^{2+} ions present in the dyad as a three N-dimensional Brownian motion in a potential field, which describes both interactions of Ca^{2+} ions with other Ca^{2+} ions as well as electrostatic potentials. The time evolution of the joint probability density of these Ca^{2+} ions to be present at positions $(\mathbf{r}_1, \ldots, \mathbf{r}_N)$ in the dyad at time t, $P(\mathbf{r}_1, \ldots, \mathbf{r}_N, t)$, is described by the Fokker-Planck equation (FPE; see, e.g., Ref. 36)

$$\frac{\partial P}{\partial t} = D \sum_{i=1}^{N} \frac{\partial}{\partial \mathbf{r}_i} \left[\frac{1}{k_B T} \frac{\partial V}{\partial \mathbf{r}_i} P(\mathbf{r}_1, \ldots, \mathbf{r}_N, t) + \frac{\partial P}{\partial \mathbf{r}_i} \right], \quad (1)$$

where $\mathbf{r}_i = (r_{i,1}, r_{i,2}, r_{i,3})$ is a vector indicating the position of the i-th ion, D is the diffusion constant, k_B is Boltzmann's constant, T is temperature and the notation $\partial/\partial \mathbf{r}_i$ is defined as

$$\frac{\partial}{\partial \mathbf{r}_i} = \left(\frac{\partial}{\partial r_{i,1}}, \frac{\partial}{\partial r_{i,2}}, \frac{\partial}{\partial r_{i,3}} \right).$$

V is the total potential energy of the system given as a function of the ion positions,

$$V(\mathbf{r}_1, \mathbf{r}_2, \ldots, \mathbf{r}_N) = \sum_{i=1}^{N} [2q\phi(\mathbf{r}_i) + u(\mathbf{r}_i)] + U(\mathbf{r}_1, \ldots, \mathbf{r}_N), \quad (2)$$

where q is the elementary charge. The total potential V has several contributions: (*a*) $\phi(\mathbf{r}_i)$ is the electrostatic potential of the i-th ion due to charges on the surrounding lipids and proteins (e.g., φ contains the potential due to surface charge density, ρ, from the negatively charged phospholipid head groups); (b) $u(\mathbf{r}_i)$ is known as a hard-core potential which becomes nonzero at the location of impenetrable structures, such as proteins within the dyad. This potential defines the space accessible for the mobile ions and is ultimately determined by the structural model of the dyad; and (c) $U(\mathbf{r}_1, \ldots, \mathbf{r}_N)$ is the mutual interaction potential between the Ca^{2+} ions. This potential is determined by the physical size (hard-core repulsion) of the ions, and the dielectric/buffering conditions in the dyad. For two ions, U depends on the ionic separation and the range of U is determined by the Debye length, κ, within the dyad. As the cytosolic fluid, including buffers, typically has a very high dielectric constant, κ is approximately 1 nm.[4] In effect, the ions feel a strong repulsion if they are within distance κ and no interaction otherwise. Therefore κ serves as a natural correlation length between the ions.

The electrostatic potential, φ, is dominated by membrane surface charges in the dyad. We use the Debye-Hückel model of charge–charge interaction, in which φ is given by

$$\phi(\mathbf{r}) = -\phi_0 \int_S \rho(\mathbf{r}') \frac{e^{-|\mathbf{r}-\mathbf{r}'|/\kappa}}{|\mathbf{r}-\mathbf{r}'|} d\mathbf{r}', \tag{3}$$

where the integral is taken over the surface S of the membrane, ρ is the membrane surface charge density, and κ is again the Debye length. The constant ϕ_0 depends on the dielectric constant and ionic conditions in the dyad. We follow Soeller and Cannell[4] and approximate φ as a sum of monoexponential functions

$$\phi(\mathbf{r}) = -\phi_{SL} e^{-z/\kappa} - \phi_{SR} e^{-(h-z)/\kappa}, \tag{4}$$

where h is the height of the dyad, z is the vertical distance from the sarcolemma at point $\mathbf{r}$, and h-z is the vertical distance from the SR membrane at point $\mathbf{r}$ (see FIG. 1 of Ref. 4).

The multidimensional FPE describes the evolution of the probability density function for the position of a Brownian particle subject to a potential. Rather than solving the time-dependent joint probability from the FPE (Equation 1), we generate sample paths of Ca^{2+} ion movement in the dyad using the Monte Carlo solution algorithm described by Wang et al.[37] A typical simulation involves an ensemble of 100 dyads, each of which is clamped to test potentials in the range of −40 mV to +50 mV in 10 mV increments where each voltage-clamp step is held for 100 ms.

RESULTS

FIGURE 2 A shows a typical sample of the time evolution of the number of Ca^{2+} ions in a dyad (ordinate) including only a single gating LCC (no RyR2s)

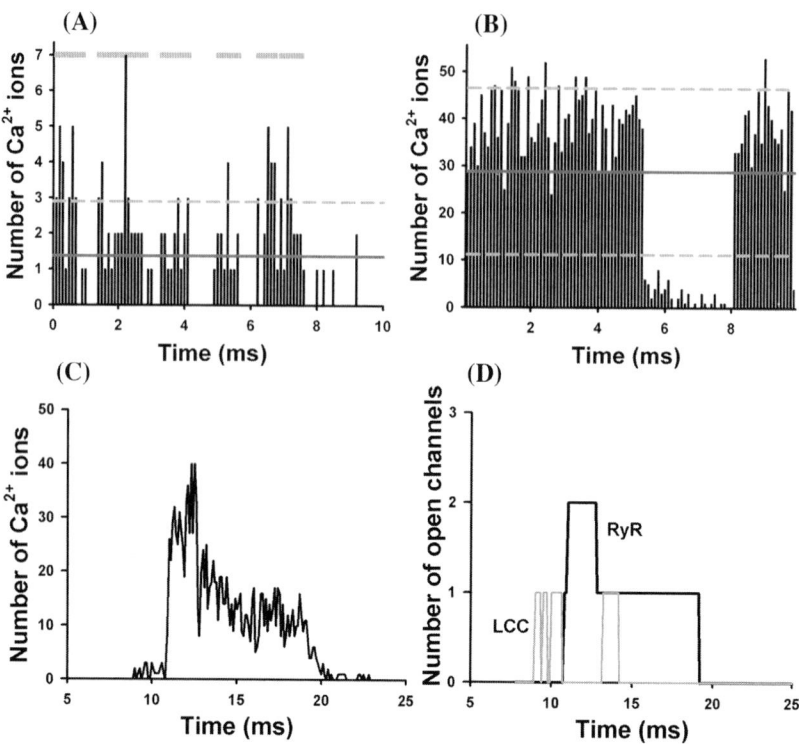

FIGURE 2. Free Ca^{2+} ions in the dyad during gating of a single LCC, clamp potential 0 mV (**A**) and gating of a single RyR2 (**B**). Number of free Ca^{2+} ions (**C**) and open LCCs and RyR2s (**D**) of the full model dyad in response to a voltage-clamp step from -100 to 0 mV.

as a function of time (abscissa; ms) with membrane potential clamped at 0 mV (gray bars indicate when the LCC is open). The average number of Ca^{2+} ions in the dyad is ~ 1, however, the number present at any given time varies widely ($\sigma = 1.53$). In this example, the peak number of Ca^{2+} ions present is seven and at times there are zero Ca^{2+} ions even when the LCC is open. Because each Ca^{2+} ion corresponds to a concentration of 14.1 μmol/L, the equivalent Ca^{2+} concentration changes in large discrete steps as Ca^{2+} ions enter and exit the dyad, reaching a maximum of 98.7 μmol/L for seven Ca^{2+} ions. FIGURE 2 B shows the number of Ca^{2+} ions in the dyad with a single RyR2 allowed to gate with all other channels closed. The RyR2 is initially open, inactivates at ~ 5.5 msec and then recovers and reopens at ~ 8 msec. The average number of Ca^{2+} ions is 28.8 ± 17.7. FIGURE 2 C shows the number of free Ca^{2+} ions in a single model dyad (ordinate) as a function of time (ms; abscissa) in response to a voltage-clamp stimulus with holding potential -100 mV and a step to 0 mV applied at 5 ms. At the peak of the dyad Ca^{2+} transient, there are roughly 40 free Ca^{2+} ions, declining to approximately 10 free Ca^{2+} ions during the late phases of the response. FIGURE 2 D shows the number of RyR2s open (ordinate) as a function of time (ms; abscissa). Following clamp onset, there are three openings of an LCC followed by opening of two RyR2s with a latency of about 2.5 ms. One of the RyR2s inactivates after ~4 ms, whereas the second RyR2 remains open for ~16 ms. Computation of the distribution of duration of 169 Ca^{2+} release events from 500 simulated dyads shows that the average duration is 16 ± 11.5 ms, comparable to a mean duration of 13.6 ms measured experimentally by Wang et al.[34] Approximately 16% of these release events result from the opening of a single RyR2, whereas the most common release event resulted from opening of three RyR2s. These features are qualitatively similar to the recent experimental results of Wang et al.,[34] where it was found that ~12% of Ca^{2+} sparks result from the opening of a single RyR2 and that the typical number of open RyR2s during a spark was 2–3. None of the simulated Ca^{2+} release events were produced by more than eight open RyR2s, in agreement with experiments.[34] These simulations demonstrate that the number of Ca^{2+} ions present in a single dyad is small and that fluctuations in the average number of Ca^{2+} ions are significant, contributing "noise" to LCC–RyR2 signaling.

FIGURE 3 A shows excitation-contraction (EC) coupling gain computed using a model with 400 dyads with (solid lines) and without (dashed lines) the geometric models of protein structures described in the "Methods" section of this article (i.e., the model without protein structure includes stochastic boundary Ca^{2+} fluxes generated by gating of LCCs and RyR2s as well as all other model properties, but does not include the space-filling properties of LCCs, RyR2s, and CaM). In each case, three different independent simulations are run in order to assess variability of EC coupling gain. Gain is plotted on the ordinate as a function of membrane potential (mV; abscissa). Gain is higher at all potentials for models incorporating protein structure. To assess the significance of differences in EC coupling gain, we estimated variance of gain for a population of 12,500 dyads using a bootstrapping procedure. FIGURE 3 B shows the distribution of peak EC coupling gain computed for the full structural model at a clamp potential of 0 mV. Mean and standard deviation of gain at −10, 0 and 10 mVsec are 15.02 ± 1.63, 11.97 ± 1.32, and 9.15 ± 1.02, respectively. These data demonstrate that gain differences with and without structure are significant at depolarized potentials and that variance of gain is relatively low at depolarized membrane potentials. The existence of ~5000 independent dyads in a single ventricular myocyte dramatically reduces the effects of noise that arise from the fact that LCC–RyR2 signaling within the dyad is mediated by tens of Ca^{2+} ions. Computation of the time between opening of the first LCC and opening of the first RyR2 in response to a voltage-clamp step to 0 mV in an ensemble of dyads shows no difference in the presence (latency 0.89 ± 0.51 ms) versus absence (latency 0.90 ± 0.44 ms) of protein structures in the dyad, however, incorporation of protein structure increases

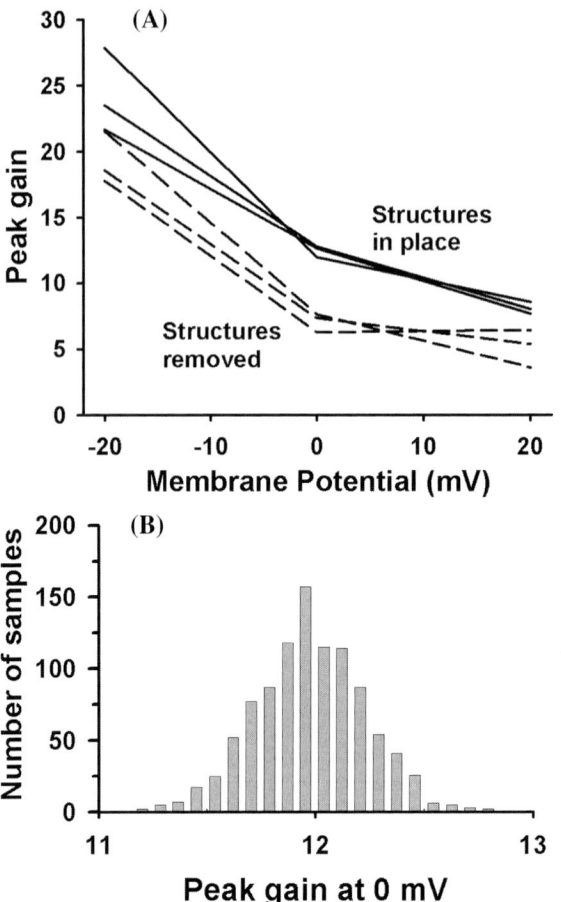

FIGURE 3. (**A**) EC coupling gain at −20, 0, and 20 mV computed for model dyads with (solid lines) and without (dashed lines) protein structure. (**B**) Distribution of gain values at 0 mV computed using a bootstrapping procedure.

open probability from 0.25 (no structures) to 0.36 (with structures)—a 44% increase. Based on these results, we hypothesize that the feet structure of the large RyR2 protein play an important role in acting to "funnel" Ca^{2+} ions to activation-binding sites on the RyR2, thus increasing probability of RyR2 opening and EC coupling gain.

SUMMARY

Simulation results obtained using the molecularly and structurally detailed computational model of the dyad demonstrate the following points. First, the number of free Ca^{2+} ions in the dyad, even at the peak of the Ca^{2+} transient is small, on the order of tens of ions. This in turn contributes noise to LCC–RyR2 signaling within the dyad. This noise is seen in variation of the number of free Ca^{2+} ions in the dyad under voltage-clamp conditions (FIG. 2), by variation of EC coupling gain measured at any given clamp potential (FIG. 3) and by variable latency to first opening of a RyR2 in response to LCC opening. However, the effects of this noise at the cellular level are reduced by the fact that cell behavior reflects the integrated function of a large number (∼5000) of independent dyads. This reduction of variability is demonstrated by the fact that variance of EC coupling gain estimated using the model is low. Second, simulation results suggest that the physical structure of the RyR2, namely a tetrameric protein with large feet structure approaching the LCC pore, may function as a guide by which Ca^{2+} ions are funneled to Ca^{2+} activation sites within the RyR2.

These detailed dyad simulations require ∼10 h of run-time on an IBM BladeCenter with 64 nodes (White Plains, NY), each with 2 Intel Xeon 2.8 Ghz processors (Santa Clara, CA). While this run-time is orders of magnitude faster than a typical molecular dynamics simulation, the computational task of simulating this model is substantial compared to most conventional myocyte models. We have previously described an approach whereby this model can be simplified, yielding a model we refer to as the stochastic local control model.[38] In this model, we represent the dyad using a single compartment. Thus, we abandon the approach of simulating the motion of Ca^{2+} ions as they move between discrete lattice points within the dyad and instead calculate Ca^{2+} fluxes using Ca^{2+} concentrations. The effects of random fluctuation of dyad Ca^{2+} concentration could be accounted for in these models by defining Ca^{2+}-dependent transition rates as functions of random variables representing the number of free Ca^{2+} ions in the dyad, thus changing the governing master equations for the LCC and RyR2 channels from ordinary to stochastic differential equations. However, our initial results show that the effects of noisy signaling produced by small numbers of Ca^{2+} ions in each dyad may be reduced by the fact that there are a large number of approximately independent dyads within the myocyte. The space filling properties of EC coupling proteins appear to play a more significant role in EC coupling, and may be incorporated in the stochastic local control model by reducing dyad volume.

Unlike the molecularly and structurally detailed model of the dyad, the stochastic local control model may be incorporated within integrative models of the myocyte. Using a combination of parallel computing and optimized numerical methods, it is possible to simulate 1 s of cell activity in roughly 10 min. However, this is still prohibitively long for general use and does require access to specialized computing resources. We have recently developed a novel approach by which the stochastic local control model may be simplified and incorporated within integrative models of the myocyte. These models may be simulated roughly five times faster than real time using conventional single

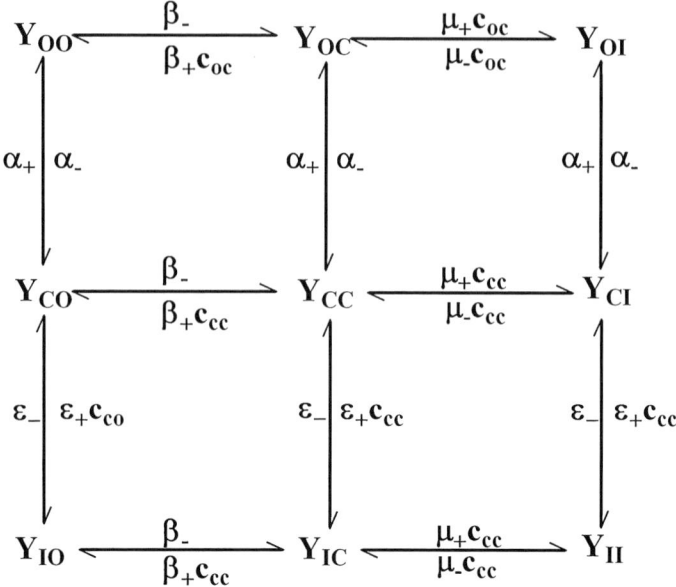

FIGURE 4. The coupled LCC–RyR2 model in which Yij represents the joint behavior of a dyad model in which there is a single LCC and RyR2 communicating via a dyadic space. "i" indexes the state of the LCC and "j" indexes the state of the RyR2. The LCC and RyR2s are represented using three-state models including closed (C), open (O), and inactivated (I) states. See Hinch et al.[40] for more details.

processor desktop systems.[39–41] We first illustrated this general approach by developing a coupled LCC–RyR2 gating model (FIG. 4) from highly simplified, three-state models of both the LCC and RyR2 channels. The key assumption in developing this model was that Ca^{2+} concentration in the dyad changes rapidly with channel opening (time scale of ∼μs) so that it can be assumed to be an algebraic function of LCC and RyR2 channel states as well as cytosolic and SR Ca^{2+} levels (this is known as the "rapid equilibrium approximation"). Under this assumption, Ca^{2+} concentration in the dyad becomes a joint function of LCC and RyR2 states, allowing the formulation of a continuous time Markov chain-state model describing transitions between the nine possible states formed by pairing states of the two, underlying three-state models of the LCC and RyR2. Importantly, we demonstrated it was possible to analytically derive the transition rates for this coupled LCC–RyR2 gating model (FIG. 2) from transition rates of the underlying LCC and RyR2 models. We later showed that this approach could be generalized to LCC and RyR2 models of arbitrary structure and to Ca^{2+} release units comprised of arbitrary numbers of LCC and RyR2 channels.[39] We then showed that use of these CICR models could quantitatively reconstruct the key EC coupling properties of graded release with voltage-dependent gain and that their integration in myocyte models enabled incorporation of data showing that CDI of LCCs is much stronger than voltage-dependent inactivation.

We have, therefore, developed a hierarchy of computational models of CICR. The models share a common structure (i.e., they are built from the same LCC and RyRs channel models and can be simulated with identical LCC:RyR stoichiometries). Key parameters of the simplified models may be derived analytically from parameters of the underlying, more complex models. Finally, the simplest of these models (the coupled LCC–RyR2 gating model) captures fundamental features of CICR and is of sufficiently low complexity that it may be used in cell-, tissue-, and organ-level simulations. These models therefore constitute an integrated computational framework for investigating EC coupling at spatial scales ranging from that of the molecule to that of the cell.

ACKNOWLEDGMENTS

This work was supported by NIH grant HL-60133, the Whitaker Foundation, the Falk Medical Trust, and by IBM Corporation. Model source code is available for download at http://www.ccbm.jhu.edu.

REFERENCES

1. FRANZINI-ARMSTRONG, C., F. PROTASI & V. RAMESH. 1999. Shape, size, and distribution of Ca($^{2+}$) release units and couplons in skeletal and cardiac muscles. Biophys. J. **77**: 1528–1539.
2. BERS, D.M. 1991. Excitation-Contraction Coupling and Cardiac Contractile Force. Kluwers. Boston.
3. LANGER, G.A. & A. PESKOFF. 1996. Calcium concentration and movement in the diadic cleft space of the cardiac ventricular cell. Biophys. J. **70**: 1169–1182.
4. SOELLER, C. & M.B. CANNELL. 1997. Numerical simulation of local calcium movements during L-type calcium channel gating in the cardiac diad. Biophys. J. **73**: 97–111.
5. BHALLA, U.S. 2004. Signaling in small subcellular volumes. I. Stochastic and diffusion effects on individual pathways. Biophys. J. **87**: 733–474.
6. LIU, Z. et al. 2002. Three-dimensional reconstruction of the recombinant type 2 ryanodine receptor and localization of its divergent region 1. J. Biol. Chem. **277**: 46712–46719.
7. DULHUNTY, A.F. & P. POULIQUIN. 2003. What we don't know about the structure of Ryanodine receptor calcium release channels. Clin. Exp. Pharmacol. Physiol. **30**: 713–723.
8. SAMSO, M., T. WAGENKNECHT & P.D. ALLEN. 2005. Internal structure and visualization of transmembrane domains of the RyR1 calcium release channel by cryo-EM. Nat. Struct. Mol. Biol. **12**: 539–544.
9. SERYSHEVA, I.I. et al. 2005. Structure of Ca^{2+} release channel at 14 A resolution. J. Mol. Biol. **345**: 427–431.

10. RADERMACHER, M. et al. 1992. Cryo-EM of the native structure of the calcium release channel/ryanodine receptor from sarcoplasmic reticulum. Biophys. J. **61:** 936–940.
11. WANG, M.C. et al. 2004. The three-dimensional structure of the cardiac l-type voltage-gated calcium channel: comparison with the skeletal muscle form reveals a common architectural motif. J. Biol. Chem. **279:** 7159–7168.
12. MORI, M.X., M.G. ERICKSON & D.T. YUE. 2004. Functional stoichiometry and local enrichment of calmodulin interacting with Ca^{2+} channels. Science **304:** 432–435.
13. WILSON, M.A. & A.T. BRUNGER. 2000. The 1.0 A crystal structure of Ca^{2+}-bound calcmodulin: an analysis of disorder and implications for functionally relevant plasticity. J. Mol. Biol. **301:** 1237–1256.
14. SHARMA, M.R. et al. 2000. Three-dimensional structure of ryanodine receptor isoform three in two conformational states as visualized by cryo-electron microscopy. J. Biol. Chem. **275:** 9485–9491.
15. WAGENKNECHT, T. & M. RADERMACHER. 1997. Ryanodine receptors: structure and macromolecular interactions. Curr. Opin. Struct. Biol. **7:** 258–265.
16. WANG, S.Q. et al. 2001. Ca^{2+} signalling between single L-type Ca^{2+} channels and ryanodine receptors in heart cells. Nature **410:** 592–596.
17. TAKESHIMA, H. et al. 1989. Primary structure and expression from complementary DNA of skeletal muscle ryanodine receptor. Nature **339:** 439–445.
18. CHEN, S.R., L. ZHANG & D.H. MACLENNAN. 1992. Characterization of a Ca^{2+} binding and regulatory site in the Ca^{2+} release channel (ryanodine receptor) of rabbit skeletal muscle sarcoplasmic reticulum. J. Biol. Chem. **267:** 23318–23326.
19. DU, G.G., V.K. KHANNA & D.H. MACLENNAN. 2000. Mutation of divergent region 1 alters caffeine and $Ca^{(2+)}$ sensitivity of the skeletal muscle $Ca^{(2+)}$ release channel (ryanodine receptor). J. Biol. Chem. **275:** 11778–11783.
20. BENACQUISTA, B.L. et al. 2000. Amino acid residues 4425–4621 localized on the three-dimensional structure of the skeletal muscle ryanodine receptor. Biophys. J. **78:** 1349–1358.
21. FESSENDEN, J.D. et al. 2004. Mutational analysis of putative calcium binding motifs within the skeletal ryanodine receptor isoform, RyR1. J. Biol. Chem. **279:** 53028–53035.
22. LI, P. & S.R. CHEN. 2001. Molecular basis of Ca(2)+ activation of the mouse cardiac Ca(2)+ release channel (ryanodine receptor). J. Gen. Physiol. **118:** 33–44.
23. WILLIAMS, A.J., D.J. WEST & R. SITSAPESAN. 2001. Light at the end of the $Ca^{(2+)}$-release channel tunnel: structures and mechanisms involved in ion translocation in ryanodine receptor channels. Q. Rev. Biophys. **34:** 61–104.
24. DU, G.G. & D.H. MACLENNAN. 1999. $Ca^{(2+)}$ inactivation sites are located in the COOH-terminal quarter of recombinant rabbit skeletal muscle $Ca^{(2+)}$ release channels (ryanodine receptors). J. Biol. Chem. **274:** 26120–26126.
25. SHARMA, M.R. & T. WAGENKNECHT. 2004. Cryo-electron microscopy and 3D reconstructions of ryanodine receptors and their interactions with E-C coupling proteins. Basic Appl. Myol. **14:** 299–306.
26. THOMAS, N.L., F.A. LAI & C.H. GEORGE. 2005. Differential Ca^{2+} sensitivity of RyR2 mutations reveals distinct mechanisms of channel dysfunction in sudden cardiac death. Biochem. Biophys. Res. Commun. **331:** 231–238.
27. PETERSON, B.Z et al. 1999. Calmodulin is the Ca^{2+} sensor for Ca^{2+}-dependent inactivation of L-type calcium channels. Neuron **22:** 549–558.

28. PETERSON, B.Z. et al. 2000. Critical determinants of Ca^{2+}-dependent inactivation within an EF-hand motif of L-type Ca^{2+} channels. Biophys. J. **78:** 1906–1920.
29. KUBONIWA, H. et al. 1995. Solution structure of calcium-free calmodulin. Nat. Struct. Biol. **2:** 768.
30. JAFRI, S., J.J. RICE & R.L. WINSLOW. 1998. Cardiac Ca^{2+} dynamics: The roles of ryanodine receptor adaptation and sarcoplasmic reticulum load. Biophys. J. **74:** 1149–1168.
31. RICE, J.J., M.S. JAFRI & R.L. WINSLOW. 1999. Modeling gain and gradedness of $Ca(^{2+})$ release in the functional unit of the cardiac diadic space. Biophys. J. **77:** 1871–1884.
32. GREENSTEIN, J.L. & R.L. WINSLOW. 2002. An integrative model of the cardiac ventricular myocyte incorporating local control of Ca^{2+} release. Biophys. J. **83:** 2918–2945.
33. STERN, M. et al. 1999. Local control models of cardiac excitation-contraction coupling. A possible role for allosteric interactions between ryanodine receptors. J. Gen. Physiol. **113:** 469–489.
34. WANG, S.Q. et al. 2004. The quantal nature of Ca^{2+} sparks and in situ operation of the ryanodine receptor array in cardiac cells. Proc. Natl. Acad. Sci. USA **101:** 3979–3984.
35. ZAHRADNIKOVA, A. et al. 1999. Rapid activation of the cardiac ryanodine receptor by submillisecond calcium stimuli. J. Gen. Physiol. **114:** 787–798.
36. RISKEN, H. 1997. The Fokker-Planck Equation. Springer. Berlin.
37. WANG, H., C.S. PESKIN & T.C. ELSTON. 2003. A robust numerical algorithm for studying biomolecular transport processes. J. Theor. Biol. **221:** 491–511
38. GREENSTEIN, J.L. & R.L. WINSLOW. 2002. An integrative model of the cardiac ventricular myocyte incorporating local control of ca(2+) release. Biophys. J. **83:** 2918–2945.
39. GREENSTEIN, J.L., R. HINCH & R.L. WINSLOW. 2006. Mechanisms of excitation-contraction coupling in an integrative model of the cardiac ventricular myocyte. Biophys. J. **90:** 77–91.
40. HINCH, R. et al. 2004. A simplified local control model of calcium-induced calcium release in cardiac ventricular myocytes. Biophys. J. **87:** 3723–3736.
41. HINCH, R., J.L. GREENSTEIN & R.L. WINSLOW. 2006. Multi-scale models of local control of calcium induced calcium release. Prog. Biophys. Mol. Biol. **90:** 136–150.

Nonlinear Dynamics of Paced Cardiac Cells

YOHANNES SHIFERAW,[a] ZHILIN QU,[a] ALAN GARFINKEL,[a] ALAIN KARMA,[b] AND JAMES N. WEISS[a,c]

[a]*Department of Medicine (Cardiology), David Geffen School of Medicine at UCLA, Los Angeles, California 90095, USA*

[b]*Department of Physics and Center for Interdisciplinary Research on Complex Systems, Northeastern University, Boston, Massachusetts 02115, USA*

[c]*Department of Physiology, David Geffen School of Medicine at UCLA, Los Angeles, California 90095, USA*

ABSTRACT: When a cardiac cell is rapidly paced it can exhibit a beat-to-beat alternation in the action potential duration (APD) and the intracellular calcium transient. This dynamical instability at the cellular level has been shown to correlate with the genesis of cardiac arrhythmias and has motivated the application of nonlinear dynamics in cardiology. In this article, we review mathematical approaches to describe the underlying mechanisms for alternans using beat-to-beat iterated maps. We explain the development and properties of these maps, and show that they provide a fruitful framework to understand dynamical instabilities of voltage and calcium in paced cardiac cells.

KEYWORDS: nonlinear dynamics; alternans; calcium cycling; cardiac arrhythmias

INTRODUCTION

Ventricular fibrillation (VF) occurs when electrical waves in the heart breaks up into multiple wavelets. This breakup has been traditionally attributed to the presence of fixed anatomical and/or electrophysiological heterogeneities in the heart, such as the presence of an infraction or ischemic zone. However, recent experimental and theoretical studies have shown that the dynamical properties of cardiac cells can play an important role in promoting VF.[1,2] In this case, it is argued that the onset and maintenance VF is dictated by the intrinsic dynamics of cardiac cells, such as the gating kinetics of ion channels. From this perspective, it is critical to explore the dynamical behavior of cardiac cells in order to fully understand the genesis and maintenance of VF.

The relationship between the dynamics of cardiac cells and arrhythmogenesis at the whole heart level has been studied extensively in the last decade.[1–4] Much of this work has centered around the experimentally observed phenomenon of "alternans,"[5,6] where the action potential duration (APD) and calcium transient alternate from one beat to the next. Alternans occurs during rapid pacing or pathophysiological conditions, such as ischemia and heart failure. The observation of alternans in a clinical setting has been shown to correlate with sudden cardiac death.[7–10] Alternans has also been studied theoretically as a period doubling instability of rapidly paced cardiac cells which can induce the break up of reentrant activity in the heart.[1,2] These studies and others have highlighted the intimate connection between nonlinear dynamics at the cellular level, and the genesis of cardiac arrhythmias in the heart.

In this article we give an overview of recent experimental and theoretical work on the nonlinear dynamical properties of paced cardiac cells. After reviewing the experimental literature on both calcium transient and APD alternans, we describe theoretical approaches to explain this phenomenon using iterated nonlinear maps and physiologically based ionic models. In particular, we describe recent work on the nonlinear dynamics of calcium cycling in paced cardiac cells, and the rich dynamical behavior that arises due to the bidirectional coupling between membrane voltage dynamics and intracellular calcium.

ALTERNANS IN CARDIAC MYOCYTES: EXPERIMENTAL OBSERVATIONS

APD alternans has been observed in a wide variety of cardiac cell types and experimental conditions (see Refs. 5 and 6 for comprehensive reviews of the experimental literature). Experimentally, APD alternans is typically observed during rapid pacing at fixed pacing frequency, as shown in FIGURE 1 A, so that beyond a critical pacing frequency the normally periodic response is replaced by a sequence of long and short APDs. If the rapid pacing frequency is held fixed, then this alternating pattern is maintained at steady state. This is in contrast to transient alternans which occurs for only several beats immediately after an abrupt change in pacing frequency. APD alternans has also been observed when a cardiac cell is paced after pharmacologic or other interventions. For example, application of tetracaine[11] and pyruvate[12] are known to induce alternans in cardiac cells. Also APD alternans has been observed at low pacing rates under ischemic conditions.[12]

Fluorescence imaging of intracellular calcium reveals that the calcium transient can also alternate from beat to beat.[5,13,14] In this case, the peak of the calcium transient, which measures the amount of calcium released during one beat from the sarcoplasmic reticulum (SR) to the bulk myoplasm, typically alternates in a large-small-large sequence. Again, this pattern can be observed

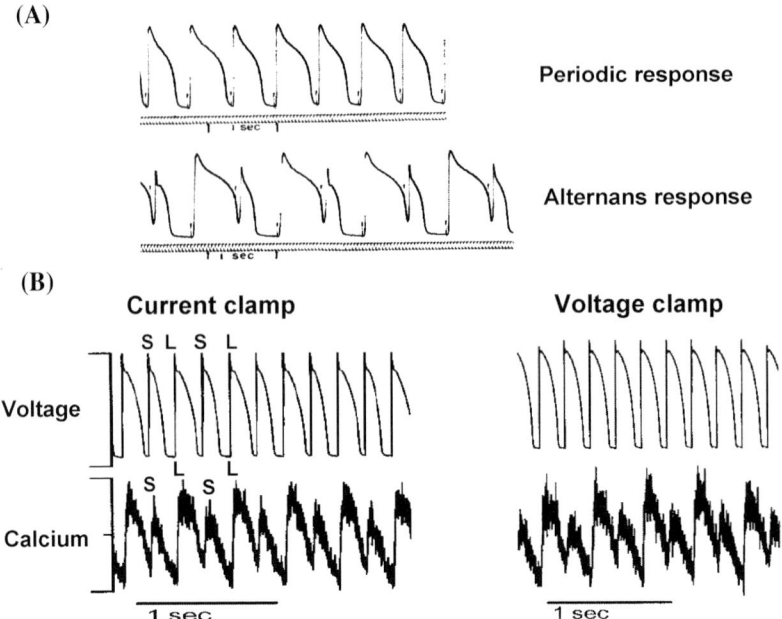

FIGURE 1. Experimental observations of APD and calcium-transient alternans in paced cardiac cells. (**A**) Periodic and alternans response measured in frog ventricular muscle strips, as observed in Nolasco and Dahlen's classic study.[16] (**B**) APD and calcium-transient alternans observed under current and AP clamp conditions in rabbit ventricular myocytes.[14] As shown, alternans in the calcium-transient was still observed when the membrane voltage was clamped using a periodic AP waveform.

at steady state, and also as a transient response to a change in pacing cycle length. Experimentalists have also recorded APD alternans simultaneously with calcium-transient alternans (see FIG. 1 B), or alternatively, cell contraction, which is known to be directly proportional to the peak of the calcium transient. In these measurements, alternans in the calcium transient (contraction) is always associated with alternans of APD. This is not surprising because intracellular calcium and membrane voltage are bidirectionally coupled via calcium-sensitive ion currents that regulate voltage. Moreover, the features of this bidirectional coupling are dependent on species and experimental conditions. For example, in rabbit heart ventricular cells, a large-small-large calcium transient is typically associated with a long-short-long APD[14] (electromechanically in-phase), while in cat atrial cells a large-small-large calcium corresponds to a short-long-short APD[12] (electromechanically out-of-phase). Both of these dynamical modes have been observed in a variety of species and experimental conditions,[5] revealing the underlying complexity of the system.

In critical experiments, Chudin et al.[14] paced a rabbit ventricular cell under both current and AP clamp conditions. As shown in FIGURE 1 B, they found that under current clamp conditions, both the APD and the calcium transient alternated in-phase. However, when the AP was clamped using a periodic waveform, as shown in FIGURE 1 C, they found that calcium-transient alternans still occurred. This result demonstrated convincingly that calcium alternans, at least in the rabbit, can originate from a dynamical instability of calcium cycling, independently of APD alternans. Diaz et al.[15] paced rat ventricular myocytes using a square voltage clamp waveform and showed that they could induce a form of alternans in which every other beat was associated with a propagating intracellular calcium wave. Again, this result showed that alternans originated via a mechanism intrinsic to the calcium cycling machinery, and independently of the dynamics of membrane voltage.

ALTERNANS AND APD RESTITUTION

The first theoretical explanation of APD alternans is attributed to Nolasco and Dahlen[16] who pioneered a geometrical construction, equivalent to iterating a discrete map, to elucidate the mechanism of APD alternans. Their basic assumption was that the APD at any given beat was completely determined by the time spent at full repolarization at the previous beat, that is, the diastolic interval (DI). This assumption was motivated by the basic observation that changes in the APD always correlated with changes in DI, and the intuitive notion that the APD should depend on recovery processes which occur during the previous DI. The corresponding map that describes beat-to-beat changes of APD is given by

$$APD_{n+1} = F(DI_n), \qquad (1)$$

where APD_{n+1} is the APD measured for the $n+1$th beat, and DI_n is the DI at the previous beat. This functional relationship is referred to as the restitution curve. Nolasco and Dahlen showed geometrically that if the cell is paced at a pacing period $T = APD^* + DI^*$, such that

$$\left.\frac{dF}{dDI_n}\right|_{DI_n=DI^*} > 1, \qquad (2)$$

where DI^* denotes the steady state DI, then a beat-to-beat alternation of the APD would ensue. Thus, alternans would arise when the slope of the restitution curve is steep, and small changes in DI lead to large variations of APD during the ensuing beat. Later Guevarra et al.[17,18] cast the Nolasco and Dahlen analysis in the mathematical language of nonlinear dynamics, and identified alternans as a period doubling bifurcation of the nonlinear mapping given by Equation 1.

Beyond the discrete map approach, alternans can also be studied by modeling the dynamics of membrane voltage using the standard equation

$$\frac{dV}{dt} = -\frac{1}{C_m}(I_{ion} + I_{stim}), \qquad (3)$$

where C_m is the cell membrane capacitance, I_{ion} is the current due to Na^+, K^+, Ca^{2+} ions flowing across the membrane, and where I_{stim} is a periodically applied stimulus current. Much work has been devoted to developing physiologically accurate models for I_{ion}, by fitting the kinetic properties of measured ion currents and incorporating these formulations in Hodgkin–Huxley type ordinary differential equations (ODEs).[18–25] Using this approach, alternans can be obtained during steady state pacing if the kinetics of ion currents are adjusted appropriately. For instance Qu et al.[26] used the first generation Luo-Rudy model[27] to show that alternans can be obtained at rapid rates when the time constant of the slow outward current was adjusted to steepen the APD restitution curve. Also, Karma[1,28] analyzed alternans in a model of Purkinje cells due to Noble,[29] and showed that alternans onset was determined by the slope of the restitution curve. Finally, Fenton and Karma[30] obtained APD alternans at high rates using a simplified three-variable ionic model. In all these models the restitution relationship (Equation 1) computed using the ionic model was found to be correct. That is, the APD was essentially determined by the previous DI, and alternans were observed precisely when the slope of the restitution curve exceeded 1.

In an experimental setting, the APD restitution curve has traditionally been measured using the S1-S2 restitution protocol, where the cell is paced to steady state at a pacing interval S1, before applying an extrastimulus at a pacing interval S2, as illustrated in FIGURE 2 A. The APD of the S2 beat is then measured and graphed with respect to the previous DI. Several experimental studies have attempted to uncover the ionic mechanisms that regulate the APD restitution curve. An older study in mammalian myocardial fibers by Gettes and

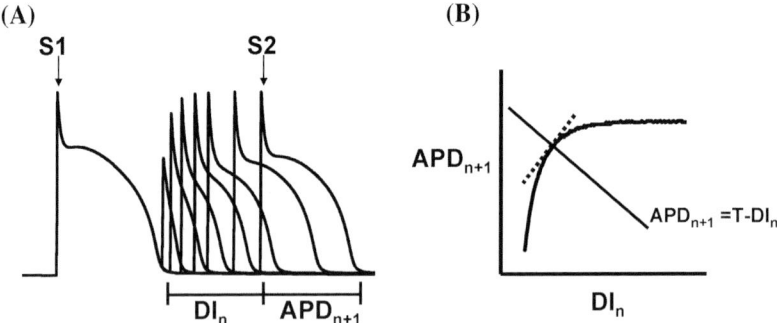

FIGURE 2. The APD restitution curve and alternans. (**A**) Demonstration of the measurement of the APD restitution curve using the S1-S2 protocol. (**B**) APD restitution curve showing intersection with the line $APD_{n+1} = T\text{-}DI_n$ where T is the pacing period. The dashed line represents the slope which controls the onset of steady state APD alternans.

Reuter[31] showed that recovery from inactivation of the L-type calcium current was the dominant factor in dictating the shape of the APD restitution curve. More recently, Goldhaber et al.[32] showed in rabbit ventricular myocytes that the steepness of the restitution curve measured at physiological temperatures was strongly dependent on the time course of recovery of the L-type calcium current. Other studies[33–35] have also shown that incomplete deactivation of K^+ currents can substantially influence the shape of the APD restitution curve. A comprehensive analysis of ion currents in the ferret ventricular cells due to Janvier et al.,[36] showed that the sodium–calcium exchange current (I_{NaCa}) and the fast outward K^+ current (I_{to}) were also critical in shaping the AP. Thus, in general a variety of ionic mechanisms contribute to the shape of the APD restitution curve.

The connection between alternans and the shape of the restitution curve has been investigated experimentally. Saitoh et al.[37] applied different doses of lidocaine to modulate the slope of the APD restitution curve in dog Purkinje muscle fibers. They found that the magnitude of APD alternans, measured after a change in cycle length, increased in proportion to the slope of the APD restitution curve. Further work by Riccio et al.[38] in the canine hearts showed that drugs which selectively flattened the APD restitution curve, such as procainamide and verapamil, abolished alternans. These results showed convincingly that the restitution slope has a major influence on the dynamics of alternans.

LIMITATIONS OF THE RESTITUTION HYPOTHESIS

The APD restitution relationship is an essential tool to understand the dynamics of alternans in paced cardiac cells. However, in many experiments, Equation 2 does not hold precisely. That is, the restitution relationship does not always predict the precise onset of alternans. For example Hall et al.[39] found that alternans was absent even though the slope of the APD restitution curve significantly exceeded 1. Also, in a comprehensive study, Dilly and Lab[40] found that during ischemia, alternans was observed even though the restitution slope was significantly less than 1. More recent work in the guinea pig heart[41] showed that the onset of alternans in the epicardium did not correlate with regions where the APD restitution curve was the steepest. These results indicate that in many cases the APD restitution curve may not give a complete quantitative description of alternans dynamics.

A major shortcoming of the APD restitution relationship is that it assumes that the APD is dependent only on the previous DI. Or rather, in the language of ion current kinetics, that the ionic recovery processes that occur during the DI completely determine the ensuing APD. However, this picture is clearly over simplified. First, ionic recovery processes that occur during times before the previous DI may also influence, to some degree, the APD at a later beat.

Second, the ionic concentrations in the cell can accumulate as a function of pacing rate via the dynamics of the various ion pumps and exchangers which determine the steady state properties. This ion accumulation can occur over many beats and is distinct from gating kinetics which typically have a much shorter time scale. A direct consequence of these factors is that the APD is likely to depend on the pacing history of the cell, an effect referred to in the literature as "cardiac memory" or "APD accommodation."[42–44]

In the experimental setting, this effect is manifested in the fact that the APD restitution curve can only be defined once the pacing history of the cell has been specified. For instance, a dynamic APD restitution curve can also be defined,[38] where the cell is paced to steady state at a fixed pacing interval, and the steady state APD and DI are recorded. A sequence of pacing intervals are scanned and the steady state APDs are then graphed with respect to the steady state DIs. Note that if the restitution relationship given in Equation 1 holds exactly, then the curve measured using the dynamic and S1-S2 protocols should be the same. However, in general these curves can be quite different. For example, Elharrar and Surawicz[45] found that the S1-S2 restitution curve in dog cardiac fibers depended critically on the S1 interval chosen, and was significantly steeper than the dynamic restitution curve at small DIs, while much shallower at larger DIs. On the other hand, measurements in the canine ventricle[38] showed that the S1-S2 restitution was significantly flatter than the dynamic restitution curve. These authors also found that alternans were observed in these hearts when the dynamic restitution slope was greater than 1, while the S1-S2 restitution slope was less than 1. These results suggest that in the canine ventricle the dynamic restitution curve is more predictive of alternans.

In order to model the effect of memory, Tolkacheva et al.[46] have attempted to generalize the restitution relationship in order to obtain a more accurate determinant of the onset of alternans. As a starting point they replaced the restitution relationship given in Equation 1 with

$$APD_{n+1} = F(DI_n, APD_n), \qquad (4)$$

so that the APD depends on both the previous DI and APD. Given this map, they showed that indeed the slope of the dynamic restitution curve (S_{dyn}) was not the same as the S1-S2 restitution slope (S_{S1S2}), and also that the onset of alternans was instead given by the condition,

$$\left|1 - \left(1 + \frac{1}{S_{dyn}}\right) S_{S1S2}\right| > 1. \qquad (5)$$

Given this relation, it is easy to see that simply measuring S_{S1S2} or S_{dyn} alone is not enough to determine the onset of alternans. These authors have also considered more general relationships[47] of the form

$$APD_{n+1} = F(DI_n, APD_n, DI_{n-1}, APD_{n-1}, \ldots), \qquad (6)$$

and have developed a hierarchy of restitution protocols which can be used to more precisely predict the onset of alternans. However, experimental validation of these results has not yet been achieved. These, and other results,[43,44] show that further work is required in order to construct more quantitative discrete maps which can be used to more accurately predict alternans dynamics.

CALCIUM CYCLING AND ALTERNANS

The experimental and theoretical studies mentioned above suggest that the APD restitution relationship given by Equation 1 is too restrictive and that memory effects have to be taken into account for a more complete description of alternans. However, these modifications are still made under the assumption that the APD is completely determined by the history of the membrane voltage of the cell. However, this basic assumption will not be true if voltage is coupled to dynamical processes inside the cell which have their own intrinsic dynamics. This possibility is borne out in the experiments of Chudin et al.[14] who showed that calcium-transient alternans can be observed even though the cell was paced with a periodic voltage clamp. Hence, in order to completely understand the dynamics of alternans in cardiac cells it is crucial to understand the nonlinear dynamics of calcium cycling.

During an AP, calcium is released from intracellular stores and signals cell contraction.[48,49] Several mathematical models have been proposed to describe the dynamics of calcium cycling.[21,22,50–52] However, a fundamental difficulty, often overlooked in modeling studies, is that calcium release is a local process which occurs within several thousand submicron scale junctions distributed throughout the volume of the cell. Within these junctions, localized clusters of calcium release channels called ryanodine receptors (RyR), which gate the flow of calcium from intracellular stores into the cytoplasm, open in response to calcium entry via L-type calcium channels on the surface cell membrane.[48] Signaling within these junctions occurs via a calcium-induced calcium-release (CICR) process which endows the calcium system with a rich dynamical behavior (see FIG. 3 for an illustration of the calcium cycling system). In a classic theoretical study, Stern[53] pointed out that basic features of excitation–contraction (EC) coupling in cardiac cells, such as the roughly linear relation between calcium entry and release, cannot be explained without explicitly accounting for the local nature of calcium signaling in the cell.

In order to resolve these difficulties Shiferaw et al.[52] introduced a phenomenological model of calcium cycling which explicitly accounted for the local nature of calcium release. Using this model, calcium-transient alternans could be induced at rapid pacing rates when the cell was paced with a periodic AP clamp. A mathematical reduction of the ODEs describing calcium cycling revealed that close to the periodic fixed point the beat-to-beat dynamics could

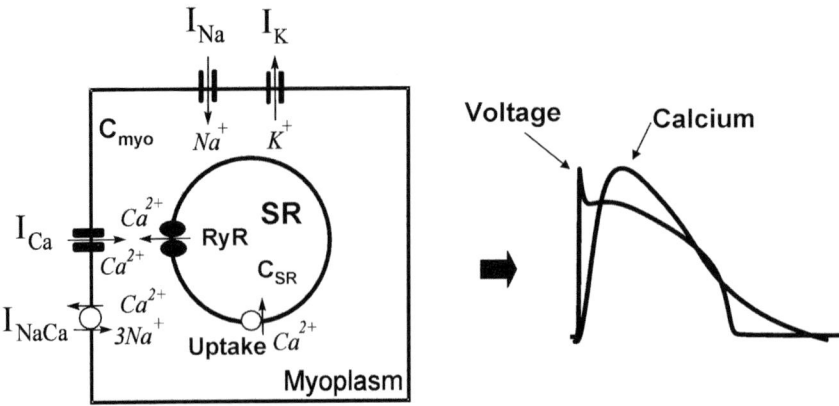

FIGURE 3. Illustration of calcium cycling machinery and membrane voltage currents. During calcium cycling calcium is released from the SR into the myoplasm, and then gets pumped back in to the SR via uptake pumps. Calcium release is triggered by the L-type calcium current via a CICR mechanism. Coupling between membrane voltage and intracellular calcium cycling is mediated by the L-type calcium current and the electrogenic sodium–calcium exchange current.

be reduced to a discrete mapping of calcium concentration variables in the SR and the myoplasm. This discrete mapping can be expressed as

$$c_{myo}^{n+1} = c_{myo}^n + R_n - U_n + \Delta_n, \tag{7}$$

$$c_{SR}^{n+1} = c_{SR}^n - R_n + U_n, \tag{8}$$

where c_{myo}^n and c_{SR}^n are the calcium concentration in the myoplasm and SR at the beginning of beat n (see FIG. 6 A for illustration of variables), R_n is the total amount of calcium released from the SR to the myoplasm during beat n, where U_n is the net amount of calcium pumped back into the SR during this beat (i.e., SR uptake less SR leak), and finally where Δ_n denotes the net calcium influx across the sarcolemma. Here, R_n, U_n, and Δ_n are functions of c_{SR}^n and c_{myo}^n, which can be explicitly computed from the ionic currents in the cell that participate in calcium cycling. Using this two-dimensional nonlinear mapping, which can be further reduced to one dimension by assuming that the total number of calcium ions in the cell is essentially constant from beat to beat, it is straightforward to show that calcium cycling is unstable to alternans when

$$-1 - \frac{\partial G_n}{\partial c_{myo}^n} + \frac{\partial G_n}{\partial c_{SR}^n} > 1, \tag{9}$$

where $G_n = R_n - U_n$. This relation reveals that calcium alternans can arise if the function G varies sufficiently steeply with respect to the SR load and/or the diastolic calcium concentration in the cell. In this sense, the function G_n

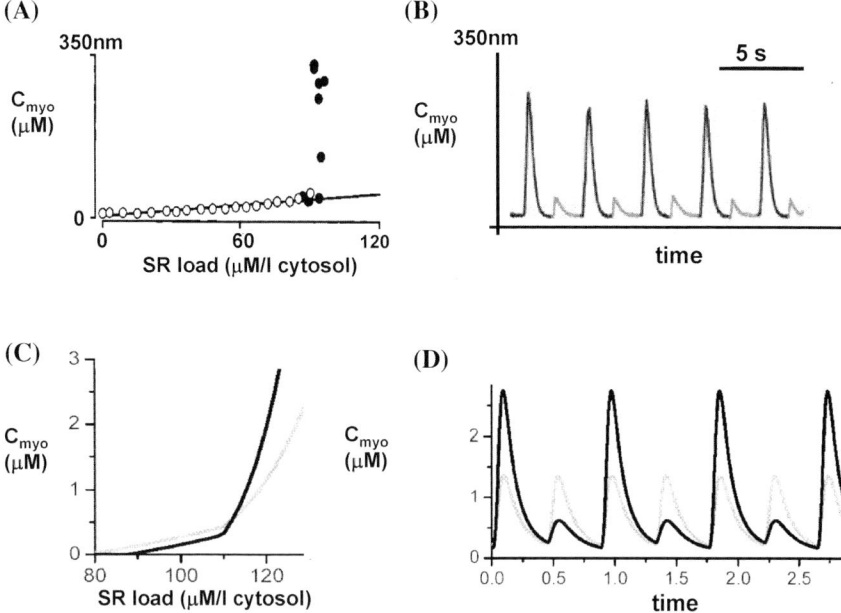

FIGURE 4. Demonstration of calcium-transient alternans in rat ventricular myocytes reproduced from Diaz et al.,[15] and also using a physiologically based mathematical model. (**A**) Experimental demonstration of a steep release-load functional relationship. Here, the peak of the calcium transient is plotted with respect to the SR load, which is estimated by integrating the sodium–calcium exchange current. (**B**) Calcium transients estimated by measuring the mean fluorescence in the cell. (**C**) Plot of peak calcium transient versus SR calcium load using the calcium cycling model of Shiferaw et al.[52] The dark/gray lines corresponds to a steep/shallow dependences of SR calcium release on SR load. (**D**) Alternans are observed when the release function is steep (dark traces), and not when it is shallow (gray traces).

controls the nonlinear dynamical properties of calcium cycling, in much the same way as the APD restitution function describes the dynamics of membrane voltage.

A recent experimental study due to Diaz et al.[15] in the rat ventricular cells measured the SR calcium release as a function of the initial SR load. As shown in FIGURE 4 A and 4 B, which is reproduced from that study, they found that when the cell was paced using a square AP clamp, alternans were observed at high SR loads where the calcium released from the SR depended steeply on the SR load. Similarly, Shiferaw et al.[52] were able to induce alternans in their model by steepening the dependence of calcium release on SR calcium load, as shown in FIGURE 4 C and 4 D. Hence, as predicted by Equation 9, alternans can be induced by letting the calcium release process depend sensitively on the calcium concentration inside the SR. A possible explanation for this steep dependence is that normally localized calcium release events may stimulate neighboring release units when the SR approaches a calcium overloaded state. This property will endow the release process with a nonlinear dependence of release on SR load which may drive alternans. A further analysis of the discrete mapping[52] revealed that the beat-to-beat dynamics can undergo even more complex dynamics, such as period 4, period 8, and chaotic dynamics if calcium released from the SR varied substantially with respect to the calcium concentration variables. These kinds of higher order periodicities have been frequently observed in paced cardiac cells,[43,44,54] and may be manifestations of chaotic properties of calcium cycling.

VOLTAGE AND CALCIUM DYNAMICS: TWO COUPLED NONLINEAR SYSTEMS

In the discussion so far, we have considered the nonlinear dynamics of membrane voltage independently of calcium cycling, and also of calcium cycling when driven with a clamped AP waveform. In general a complete understanding of alternans in cardiac myocytes will involve the coupled dynamics of both of these nonlinear systems. The dynamics of this coupled system is complex because it involves the interaction of ion channel kinetics which regulate the APD, and calcium fluxes which participate in the calcium cycling process. In this setting alternans can be induced via two independent mechanisms: (*a*) a steep dependence of APD on DI due to ionic recovery processes, that is, APD restitution, and (*b*) a steep calcium concentration dependence of calcium release and/or uptake between the SR and the myoplasm. Once alternans ensues by either of these mechanisms, both the APD and the calcium transient will alternate from beat to beat, because membrane voltage is bidirectionally coupled to intracellular calcium. Thus, in general it is difficult to pinpoint the underlying mechanism for alternans, especially in an experimental setting.

The essential feature of the system, which turns out to critically influence the coupled dynamics, is the precise nature of the bidirectional coupling between voltage and calcium. This coupling is mediated by calcium-sensitive ion currents, such as the L-type calcium current and the sodium–calcium exchange current (see FIG. 3), which mediate calcium cycling while also providing a substantial ionic flux across the cell membrane. Shiferaw *et al.*[55] identified several essential features of the bidirectional coupling which are critical to understanding the dynamics of the system. These are:

1. *Graded release coupling*: This involves the effect of the voltage waveform on the amount of calcium released from the SR, as illustrated in FIGURE 5 A. It is determined by the well-established phenomenon of graded SR calcium release,[48,56] where the amount of SR calcium released is graded with respect to the whole cell L-type calcium current. The availability of the L-type calcium current at a given beat depends critically on the previous DI, with larger

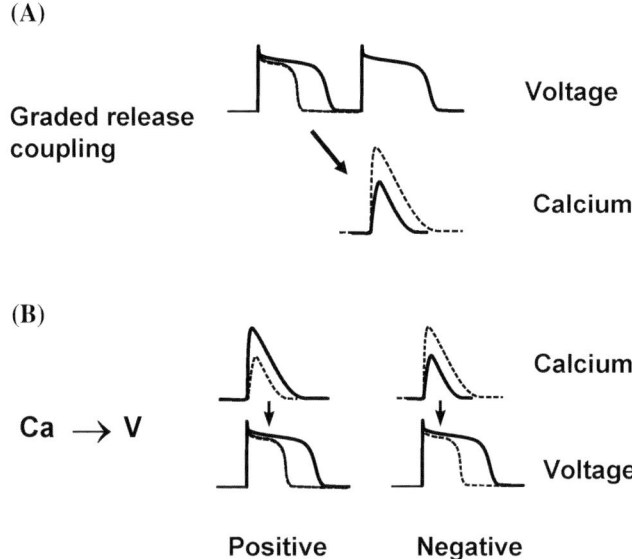

FIGURE 5. Illustration of bidirectional coupling between calcium and membrane voltage. (**A**) Graded release coupling between the APD and the calcium transient on the next beat. (**B**) Coupling between the calcium transient and the APD on the same beat. Positive/negative coupling denotes whether a larger calcium transient lengthens/shortens the APD.

DI giving more time for recovery of L-type calcium channels at the resting membrane potential. Thus, graded release requires that the peak of the calcium transient increases in response to an increase of DI in the previous beat.

2. *Ca → V coupling*: The coupling of the calcium transient on the APD, is illustrated in FIGURE 5 B. There are two parameter regimes which lead to distinct dynamical behaviors. The first, referred to as *positive Ca → V coupling*, corresponds to the case when a large peak calcium transient lengthens the APD of that beat. The second, referred to as *negative Ca → V coupling*, corresponds to the case when a large calcium transient shortens the APD. The sign of the coupling is dictated by the relative contributions of the L-type calcium current and the sodium–calcium exchange current to APD. A larger calcium transient tends to inactivate the whole cell L-type calcium current more rapidly via calcium-induced inactivation, which tends to shorten the APD. However, a large calcium transient also increases inward current from electrogenic sodium–calcium exchange, which tends to prolong APD.

Shiferaw et al.[55] studied the coupled dynamics of the system using a physiologically based ionic model due to Fox et al.[21] which was coupled to the calcium cycling model described earlier. Using this model alternans could be induced by either steepening the dependence of calcium release on SR load, or alternatively, by increasing the time constant of recovery of the L-type calcium current to steepen the dependence of APD on DI. Shiferaw et al.[55] found that the dynamics of voltage and calcium alternans depended critically on both the underlying dynamical instability, and also on the sign of the $Ca \rightarrow V$ coupling. For *positive $Ca \rightarrow V$ coupling* calcium transient and APD alternans were always electromechanically in-phase, that is, a large-small-large calcium transient corresponds to long-short-long APD sequence. However, for *negative $Ca \rightarrow V$ coupling*, a much richer dynamical behavior was observed. In this case, if alternans is induced by unstable calcium cycling, then calcium and APD alternans are electromechanically out-of-phase, that is, a large-small-large calcium transient corresponds to a short-long-short APD sequence. On the other hand, if alternans is due to steep APD restitution, then calcium-transient alternans was in-phase with APD alternans. When both subsystems were unstable, both the calcium transient and APD exhibited quasi-periodic oscillations. Interestingly, the later dynamical mode has been observed experimentally in paced Purkinje fibers[43,44] and more recently in tissue cultures.[57]

In order to understand the qualitative nature of the coupled nonlinear dynamics, Shiferaw et al.[55] reduced their complex ionic model to a set of discrete maps that described the beat-to-beat evolution of voltage and calcium. The motivation was to integrate the classic restitution relationship given in Equation 1, with the nonlinear maps for calcium cycling given by Equations 7 and 8. In this case the beat-to-beat mapping of both calcium and APD can be described by a three-variable mapping of the form

$$APD_{n+1} = F(DI_n, c_{myo}^n, c_{SR}^n)$$
$$c_{myo}^{n+1} = c_{myo}^n + R_n - U_n + \Delta_n, \quad (10)$$
$$c_{SR}^{n+1} = c_{SR}^n - R_n + U_n.$$

Here, the first equation is simply a modification of the standard APD restitution relationship which includes the dependence of the APD on the diastolic calcium concentration c_{myo}^n, and the SR calcium load c_{SR}^n, as illustrated in FIGURE 6 A. Close to the onset of alternans, the total amount of calcium in the cell is roughly the same from beat to beat, so that the three-variable map can be reduced to a two-variable map. The condition for alternans can then be analyzed by computing the eigenvalues of the resulting two-dimensional discrete map. The condition for alternans is then given by the condition

$$\frac{1}{2}\left[\lambda_v + \lambda_c - \sqrt{(\lambda_v - \lambda_c)^2 + 4C}\right] > 1, \quad (11)$$

where

$$\lambda_v = \frac{\partial F}{\partial DI_n}, \quad (12)$$

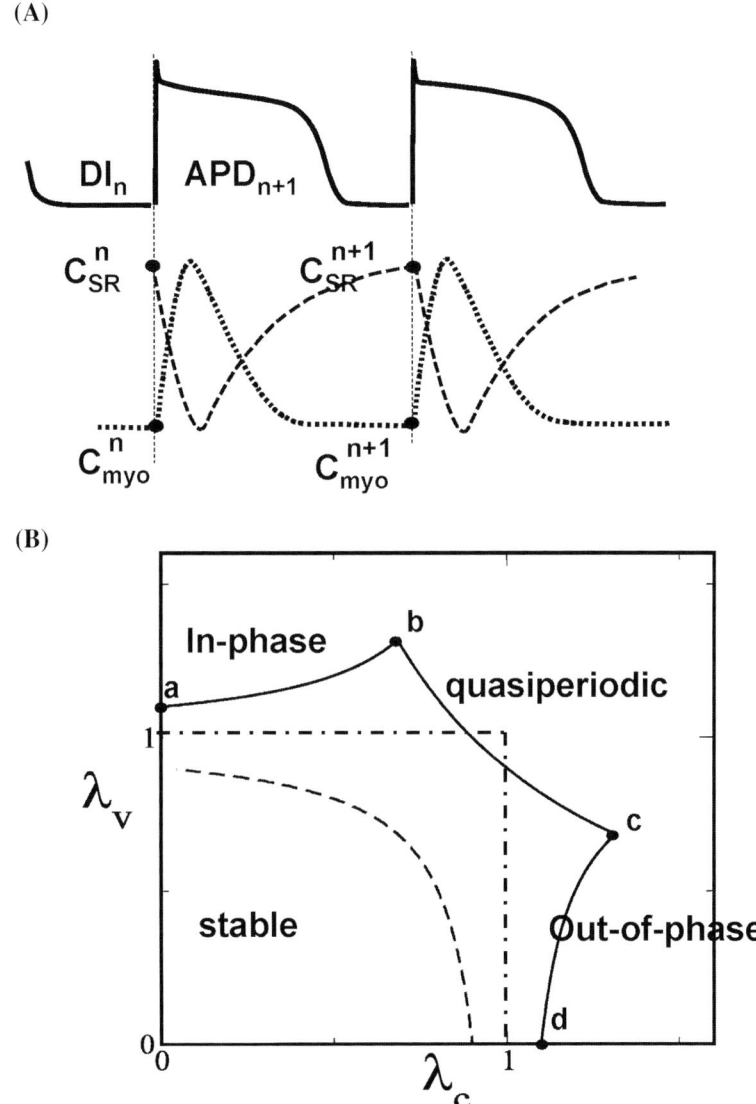

FIGURE 6. (**A**) Definition of discrete map variables describing the beat-to-beat dynamics of voltage and calcium. (**B**) Stability boundaries computed using the discrete map analysis. The dot-dashed lines denotes the stability boundary when voltage and calcium are uncoupled. The dashed line denotes the stability boundary when the $Ca \rightarrow V$ coupling is positive. In this case the periodic fixed point always looses stability to electromechanically in-phase alternans. The solid line denotes the stability boundary in the case of negative $Ca \rightarrow V$ coupling. Three dynamical modes are observed when the cell looses stability along the indicated line segments: electromechanically in-phase alternans (a–b), electromechanically out-of-phase alternans (c–d), and finally quasiperiodicity (b–c).

$$\lambda_c = -1 - \frac{\partial G}{\partial c_{myo}^n} + \frac{\partial G}{\partial c_{SR}^n}, \tag{13}$$

and where C is positive/negative depending on whether the $Ca \to V$ coupling is positive/negative. Here λ_v is simply the standard restitution slope, while λ_c measures the degree of instability of calcium cycling. For the case when voltage and calcium are uncoupled ($C = 0$), then Equation 11 simply reduces to Equation 2 and 9, found earlier by analyzing each system independently. In FIGURE 6 B, we plot Equation 11 to show the boundary separating stable periodic dynamics and unstable alternans or quasiperiodic dynamics. Now, when both systems are positively coupled ($C > 0$), the stability boundary is given by the dashed line. Here, we see that the domain of stability shrinks for positive coupling, showing that the coupled system is more unstable than its constituents, that is, APD alternans enhance calcium alternans and vice versa. On the other hand, when the coupling between calcium on voltage is negative ($C < 0$), then the stability boundary expands, so that the coupled system becomes more stable. In other words alternans in APD tends to stabilize calcium-transient alternans, and vice versa. Moreover, as seen in the ionic model simulations the fixed point can loose stability to electromechanically in-phase, out-of phase, and also a quasi-periodic dynamical mode.

The generalization of the standard APD restitution relationship to include calcium cycling, as given by the three-variable map in Equation 10, serves as a framework to interpret the rich set of dynamical behavior observed experimentally. The advantage of the map analysis is that it allows to interpret experiments in terms of three critical parameters: the APD restitution slope, the degree of instability of calcium cycling as measured by the concentration dependence of the release and uptake from the SR, and the sign of the calcium on voltage coupling. Remarkably, all three dynamical modes predicted by the model have been observed experimentally in different cell types and pharmacologic conditions,[5,6,43,44] and also in tissue cultures.[57] However, up to now these observations have not been explained within a general framework. It is interesting to speculate that perhaps these different cell types and pharmacologic interventions simply correspond to different points in the phase diagram shown in FIGURE 6 B.

SUMMARY

In this article we have reviewed the various mathematical approaches that have been applied to understand the nonlinear dynamics of paced cardiac cells. In particular, we have described the various theoretical approaches to describe alternans using discrete beat-to-beat maps. The main advantage of this approach is that it makes it possible to reduce the complex dynamics of a paced cardiac cell to basic nonlinear relationships between experimentally measured quantities. Hence, this approach can help shed light on the key physiological mechanisms that underlie alternans, and help suggest experiments to uncover these mechanisms.

ACKNOWLEDGMENTS

This study was supported by NIH/NHLBI grant P01 HL078931, the Laubisch and Kawata endowments.

REFERENCES

1. KARMA, A. 1994. Electrical alternans and spiral wave breakup in cardiac tissue. Chaos **4**: 461–472.
2. GARFINKEL, A., Y.H. KIM, O. VOROSHILOVSKY, et al. 2000. Preventing ventricular fibrillation by flattening cardiac restitution. Proc. Natl. Acad. Sci. USA **97**: 6061–6066.
3. QU, Z. & A. GARFINKEL. 1999. An advanced algorithm for solving partial differential equation in cardiac conduction. IEEE Trans. Biomed. Eng. **46**: 1166–1168.
4. QU, Z., J.N. WEISS & A. GARFINKEL. 2000. From local to global spatiotemporal chaos in a cardiac tissue model. Phys. Rev. E Stat. Phys. Plasmas Fluids Relat. Interdiscip. Topics **61**: 727–732.
5. EULER, D.E. 1999. Cardiac alternans: mechanisms and pathophysiological significance. Cardiovasc. Res. **42**: 583–590.
6. WALKER, M.L. & D.S. ROSENBAUM. 2003. Repolarization alternans: implications for the mechanism and prevention of sudden cardiac death. Cardiovasc. Res. **57**: 599–614.
7. PASTORE, J.M., S.D. GIROUARD, K.R. LAURITA, et al. 1999. Mechanism linking T-wave alternans to the genesis of cardiac fibrillation. Circulation **99**: 1385–1394.
8. PRUVOT, E.J. & D.S. ROSENBAUM. 2003. T-wave alternans for risk stratification and prevention of sudden cardiac death. Curr. Cardiol. Rep. **5**: 350–357.
9. ROSENBAUM, D.S., L.E. JACKSON, J.M. SMITH, et al. 1994. Electrical alternans and vulnerability to ventricular arrhythmias. N. Engl. J. Med. **330**: 235–241.
10. ARMOUNDAS, A.A., M. OSAKA, T. MELA, et al. 1998. T-wave alternans and dispersion of the QT interval as risk stratification markers in patients susceptible to sustained ventricular arrhythmias. Am. J. Cardiol. **82**: 1127–1129, A9.
11. DIAZ, M.E., D.A. EISNER & S.C. O'NEILL. 2002. Depressed ryanodine receptor activity increases variability and duration of the systolic Ca2+ transient in rat ventricular myocytes. Circ. Res. **91**: 585–593.
12. HUSER, J., Y.G. WANG, K.A. SHEEHAN, et al. 2000. Functional coupling between glycolysis and excitation-contraction coupling underlies alternans in cat heart cells. J. Physiol. **524**: 795–806.
13. EISNER, D.A., H.S. CHOI, M.E. DIAZ, et al. 2000. Integrative analysis of calcium cycling in cardiac muscle. Circ. Res. **87**: 1087–1094.
14. CHUDIN, E., J. GOLDHABER, A. GARFINKEL, et al. 1999. Intracellular Ca(2+) dynamics and the stability of ventricular tachycardia. Biophys. J. **77**: 2930–2941.

15. DIAZ, M.E., S.C. O'NEILL & D.A. EISNER. 2004. Sarcoplasmic reticulum calcium content fluctuation is the key to cardiac alternans. Circ. Res. **94:** 650–656.
16. NOLASCO, J.B. & R.W. DAHLEN. 1968. A graphic method for the study of alternation in cardiac action potentials. J. Appl. Physiol. **25:** 191–196.
17. GUEVARA, M.R., L. GLASS & A. SHRIER. 1981. Phase locking, period-doubling bifurcations, and irregular dynamics in periodically stimulated cardiac cells. Science **214:** 1350–1353.
18. GUEVARA, M.R., G. WARD, A. SHRIER & L. GLASS. 1984. Electrical alternans and period doubling bifurcations. IEEE Comput. Cardiol. 167–170.
19. BEELER, G.W. & H. REUTER. 1977. Reconstruction of the action potential of ventricular myocardial fibres. J. Physiol. **268:** 177–210.
20. LUO, C.H. & Y. RUDY. 1994. A dynamic model of the cardiac ventricular action potential. I. Simulations of ionic currents and concentration changes. Circ. Res. **74:** 1071–1096.
21. FOX, J.J., J.L. MCHARG & R.F. GILMOUR, JR. 2002. Ionic mechanism of electrical alternans. Am. J. Physiol. Heart Circ. Physiol. **282:** H516–H530.
22. JAFRI, M.S., J.J. RICE & R.L. WINSLOW. 1998. Cardiac Ca2+ dynamics: the roles of ryanodine receptor adaptation and sarcoplasmic reticulum load. Biophys. J. **74:** 1149–1168.
23. RICE, J.J., M.S. JAFRI & R.L. WINSLOW. 1999. Modeling gain and gradedness of Ca2+ release in the functional unit of the cardiac diadic space. Biophys. J. **77:** 1871–1884.
24. BONDARENKO, V.E., G.P. SZIGETI, G.C. BETT, *et al*. 2004. Computer model of action potential of mouse ventricular myocytes. Am. J. Physiol. Heart Circ. Physiol. **287:** H1378–H1403.
25. BONDARENKO, V.E., G.C. BETT & R.L. RASMUSSON. 2004. A model of graded calcium release and L-type Ca2+ channel inactivation in cardiac muscle. Am. J. Physiol. Heart Circ. Physiol. **286:** H1154–H1169.
26. QU, Z., J.N. WEISS & A. GARFINKEL. 1999. Cardiac electrical restitution properties and stability of reentrant spiral waves: a simulation study. Am. J. Physiol. **276:** H269–H283.
27. LUO, C.H. & Y. RUDY. 1991. A model of the ventricular cardiac action potential. Depolarization, repolarization, and their interaction. Circ. Res. **68:** 1501–1526.
28. KARMA, A. 1993. Spiral breakup in model equations of action potential propagation in cardiac tissue. Phys. Rev. Lett. **71:** 1103–1106.
29. NOBLE, D. 1962. A modification of the Hodgkin–Huxley equations applicable to Purkinje fibre action and pace-maker potentials. J. Physiol. **160:** 317–352.
30. FENTON, F. & A. KARMA. 1998. Vortex dynamics in three-dimensional continuous myocardium with fiber rotation: filament instability and fibrillation. Chaos **8:** 20–47.
31. GETTES, L.S. & H. REUTER. 1974. Slow recovery from inactivation of inward currents in mammalian myocardial fibres. J. Physiol. **240:** 703–724.
32. GOLDHABER, J.I., L.H. XIE, T. DUONG, *et al*. 2005. Action potential duration restitution and alternans in rabbit ventricular myocytes: the key role of intracellular calcium cycling. Circ. Res. **96:** 459–466.
33. DE HEMPTINNE, A. 1971. The frequency dependence of outward current in frog auricular fibres. An experimental and theoretical study. Pflugers Arch. **329:** 332–340.

34. HAUSWIRTH, O., D. NOBLE & R.W. TSIEN. 1972. Separation of the pace-maker and plateau components of delayed rectification in cardiac Purkinje fibres. J. Physiol. **225:** 211–235.
35. HUA, F. & R.F. GILMOUR, JR. 2004. Contribution of IKr to rate-dependent action potential dynamics in canine endocardium. Circ. Res. **94:** 810–819.
36. JANVIER, N.C., S.O. MCMORN, S.M. HARRISON, et al. 1997. The role of Na(+)-Ca2+ exchange current in electrical restitution in ferret ventricular cells. J. Physiol. **504:** 301–314.
37. SAITOH, H., J.C. BAILEY & B. SURAWICZ. 1989. Action potential duration alternans in dog Purkinje and ventricular muscle fibers. Further evidence in support of two different mechanisms. Circulation **80:** 1421–1431.
38. RICCIO, M.L., M.L. KOLLER & R.F. GILMOUR, JR. 1999. Electrical restitution and spatiotemporal organization during ventricular fibrillation. Circ. Res. **84:** 955–963.
39. HALL, G.M., S. BAHAR & D.J. GAUTHIER. 1999. Prevalence of rate-dependent behaviors in cardiac muscle. Phys. Rev. Lett. **82:** 2995.
40. DILLY, S.G. & M.J. LAB. 1988. Electrophysiological alternans and restitution during acute regional ischaemia in myocardium of anaesthetized pig. J. Physiol. **402:** 315–333.
41. PRUVOT, E.J., R.P. KATRA, D.S. ROSENBAUM & K.R. LAURITA. 2004. Role of calcium cycling versus restitution in the mechanism of repolarization alternans. Circ. Res. **94:** 1083–1090.
42. WATANABE, M.A. & M.L. KOLLER. 2002. Mathematical analysis of dynamics of cardiac memory and accommodation: theory and experiment. Am. J. Physiol. Heart Circ. Physiol. **282:** H1534–H1547.
43. GILMOUR, R.F., JR., N.F. OTANI & M.A. WATANABE. 1997. Memory and complex dynamics in cardiac Purkinje fibers. Am. J. Physiol. **272:** H1826–H1832.
44. OTANI, N.F. & R.F. GILMOUR, JR. 1997. Memory models for the electrical properties of local cardiac systems. J. Theor. Biol. **187:** 409–436.
45. ELHARRAR, V. & B. SURAWICZ. 1983. Cycle length effect on restitution of action potential duration in dog cardiac fibers. Am. J. Physiol. **244:** H782–H792.
46. TOLKACHEVA, E.G., D.G. SCHAEFFER, D.J. GAUTHIER & W. KRASSOWSKA. 2003. Condition for alternans and stability of the 1:1 response pattern in a "memory" model of paced cardiac dynamics. Phys. Rev. E Stat. Nonlin. Soft Matter Phys. **67:** 031904–031913.
47. KALB, S.S., E.G. TOLKACHEVA, D.G. SCHAEFFER, et al. 2005. Restitution in mapping models with an arbitrary amount of memory. Chaos **15:** 23701.
48. BERS, D.M. 2002. Cardiac excitation-contraction coupling. Nature **415:** 198–205.
49. BERS, D.M. 2001. Excitation-Contraction Coupling and Cardiac Contractile Force. Kluwer. Boston.
50. SHANNON, T.R., F. WANG, J. PUGLISI, et al. 2004. A mathematical treatment of integrated Ca dynamics within the ventricular myocyte. Biophys. J. **87:** 3351–331.
51. WINSLOW, R.L., J. RICE & S. JAFRI. 1998. Modeling the cellular basis of altered excitation-contraction coupling in heart failure. Prog. Biophys. Mol. Biol. **69:** 497–514.
52. SHIFERAW, Y., M.A. WATANABE, A. GARFINKEL, et al. 2003. Model of intracellular calcium cycling in ventricular myocytes. Biophys. J. **85:** 3666–3686.
53. STERN, M.D. 1992. Theory of excitation-contraction coupling in cardiac muscle. Biophys. J. **63:** 497–517.

54. CHIALVO, D.R., R.F. GILMOUR, JR. & J. JALIFE. 1990. Low dimensional chaos in cardiac tissue. Nature **343:** 653–657.
55. SHIFERAW, Y., D. SATO & A. KARMA. 2005. Coupled dynamics of voltage and calcium in paced cardiac cells. Phys. Rev. E Stat. Nonlin. Soft Matter Phys. **71:** 021903–021907.
56. WIER, W.G., T.M. EGAN, J.R. LOPEZ-LOPEZ & C.W. BALKE. 1994. Local control of excitation-contraction coupling in rat heart cells. J. Physiol. **474:** 463–471.
57. BIEN, H., L. YIN & E. ENTCHEVA. 2006. Calcium instabilities in mammalian cardiomyocyte networks. Biophys. J. **90:** 2628–2640.

Modeling Cardiac Ischemia

BLANCA RODRÍGUEZ,[a] NATALIA TRAYANOVA,[c] AND DENIS NOBLE[b]

[a]*Computing Laboratory, University of Oxford, Oxford OX1 3QD, UK*

[b]*Department of Physiology, Anatomy and Genetics, University of Oxford, Oxford OX1 3PT, UK*

[c]*Department of Biomedical Engineering, Johns Hopkins University, Baltimore, Maryland*

> ABSTRACT: Myocardial ischemia is one of the main causes of sudden cardiac death, with 80% of victims suffering from coronary heart disease. In acute myocardial ischemia, the obstruction of coronary flow leads to the interruption of oxygen flow, glucose, and washout in the affected tissue. Cellular metabolism is impaired and severe electrophysiological changes in ionic currents and concentrations ensue, which favor the development of lethal cardiac arrhythmias such as ventricular fibrillation. Due to the burden imposed by ischemia in our societies, a large body of research has attempted to unravel the mechanisms of initiation, sustenance, and termination of cardiac arrhythmias in acute ischemia, but the rapidity and complexity of ischemia-induced changes as well as the limitations in current experimental techniques have hampered evaluation of ischemia-induced alterations in cardiac electrical activity and understanding of the underlying mechanisms. Over the last decade, computer simulations have demonstrated the ability to provide insight, with high spatiotemporal resolution, into ischemic abnormalities in cardiac electrophysiological behavior from the ionic channel to the whole organ. This article aims to review and summarize the results of these studies and to emphasize the role of computer simulations in improving the understanding of ischemia-related arrhythmias and how to efficiently terminate them.
>
> KEYWORDS: myocardial ischemia; computer simulations; cardiac arrhythmias; vulnerability to electric shocks

INTRODUCTION

Ventricular tachycardia and fibrillation are major causes of sudden cardiac death.[1,2] These arrhythmias arise from various clinical conditions, however, the foremost perpetrator among them is ischemic heart disease. Myocardial ischemic injury ensues from deficiencies in both energetic input and waste

Address for correspondence: Dr. Blanca Rodríguez, Oxford University Computing Laboratory, Wolfson Building, Parks Road, Oxford, UK. Voice: +44-1865-283557; fax: +44-1865-273839.
e-mail: blanca@comlab.ox.ac.uk.

removal.[3] The result is progressive deterioration of electrical activity in the region of injury, leading to failure of contraction, and finally, cell death. At the organ level, this chain of events manifests itself ultimately as malignant arrhythmias and pump failure.[4]

The mechanisms underlying potentially lethal ventricular arrhythmias associated with ischemic cardiac disease are difficult to elucidate by clinical studies on patients who develop them; arrhythmias may occur before hospital admission, and even if occurring in the hospital setting, the primary concern is resuscitation and maintaining the patient's life, and not research in arrhythmogenesis. To study the electrophysiological changes associated with myocardial ischemic injury and how they lead to the establishment of ventricular tachycardia and fibrillation, animal models of clinical pathophysiology have been developed,[3,5] overcoming the limitations of clinical studies and playing an invaluable role in advancing mechanistic insight. Animal model studies have provided new ideas and hypotheses that have been tested in clinical studies and have thus increased the level of knowledge regarding arrhythmogenesis in the ischemic milieu.

Experimental models, however, have their own set of limitations that hamper the comprehensive evaluation of arrhythmogenic mechanisms, and thus the development of improved antiarrhythmia therapies to combat the consequences of ischemic cardiac disease. Electrophysiological changes following coronary occlusion are extremely rapid, particularly during the initial acute stage of ischemia (first 10-min postocclusion),[3] making it difficult to thoroughly assess the cause-and-effect relations between metabolic and electrophysiological parameters. In addition, current experimental techniques for recording electrical behavior at the tissue and organ level are limited in their ability to document, with sufficient spatial resolution, events confined within the depths of the ventricular wall.

Over the last decade, analysis of electrophysiological phenomena has been significantly augmented and advanced by the use of mathematical modeling and computer simulations, from the ionic channel to the whole organ. One of the major contributions of computational research in electrophysiology has been the ability of mathematical models to dissect various effects and to tease out important relations between electrophysiological parameters. This effort has been particularly important in ascertaining the role of ischemic abnormalities in cardiac electrophysiological behavior. The purpose of this article is to briefly review some of the computational models, from ionic fluxes to whole-heart behavior, which have been used to elucidate (1) the electrophysiological consequences of ischemic injury, (2) the mechanisms that underlie arrhythmia generation under the conditions of ischemia, and (3) how defibrillation works in the ischemic heart. The review focuses on modeling and simulation representing events during the initial acute phase of ischemic injury, phase 1A, since it constitutes the most rapid and difficult to analyze phase of ischemic cardiac disease.

Alterations in Metabolism and Ionic Concentrations in Ischemia

Membrane ionic transporters are sensitive to intracellular and extracellular ions and metabolites. It is through these interactions that metabolic changes in ischemia exert their electrophysiological effects.[3] Large changes in these parameters in ischemia have been measured experimentally, including increased concentrations of intracellular Na^+ and Ca^{2+}, increased extracellular K^+, decreased extracellular Na^+, and decreased intracellular ATP and pH. Arrhythmias under the conditions of myocardial ischemia are therefore multifactor pathologies. One of the earliest attempts to simulate arrhythmic mechanisms linked to ischemia was made by Ch'en et al.[6] who succeeded in connecting Na^+/Ca^+ overload during ATP depletion and intracellular acidity to oscillations of internal Ca^{2+} that could be the trigger of some forms of arrhythmia. Their modeling of metabolism was, however, limited to ATP depletion and fall in pH. More extensive models now exist.

Zhou et al.[7] have modeled both the transport and metabolism of various chemical species, including blood-interstitial fluid, cytosolic and mitochondrial compartments as well as a glycolytic subdomain in the cytosol. The model successfully simulated the activation of glycogen breakdown and the switch to lactate production induced by reduced blood flow in an *in vivo* experimental system. Cabrera et al.[8] have described a mathematical model of myocardial energy metabolism that was used to investigate the role of cytosolic and mitochondrial redox states in regulating cardiac energetics during reduced myocardial blood flow.

One of the controversial questions in this field is the function of Na^+/Ca^{2+} exchange, with some studies proposing that the exchanger reverses direction in ischemia. That it does so transiently is not in doubt, but long-term reversal seems unlikely, since this would always create precisely those changes in ion concentrations required to revert to forward mode. Computations done with a simplified form of the Ch'en et al. model show that this view is consistent with the experimental data provided that a substantial fall in interstitial Na^+ occurs.[9] Unraveling the impact of Na^+/Ca^{2+} exchange in ischemia is difficult since it plays more than one role. Under normal circumstances, the exchanger is the main route for Ca^{2+} efflux, accounting for up to 90% of this flux.[10] But it also carries ionic current, which in the forward mode is inward, meaning that it is capable of causing ectopic excitations. Despite carrying the great majority of Ca^{2+} efflux in normal electrical activity, knockout of 80–90% of the Na^+/Ca^{2+} exchanger in mice leaves functional cardiac cells.[11] Clearly, other transporter mechanisms, in particular the sarcolemmal Ca^{2+} pump, can take over. The implications of these results for the study of ischemia have yet to be explored. In an important study, Imahashi et al.[12] have shown that cardiac specific ablation of the Na^+/Ca^{2+} exchanger confers protection against ischemia and reperfusion injury, although they also conclude that the rise in intracellular sodium is not itself a major factor determining injury.

Changes in interstitial ion concentrations have been highlighted in the work of Rodríguez et al.,[13] with a focus on the mechanisms of extracellular K^+ accumulation in ischemia. Extracellular K^+ concentration ($[K^+]_o$) is known to increase very quickly following coronary occlusion, reaching a plateau level of 6–11 mmol/L above its normal value at 10–15 min postocclusion.[14–20] The increase in $[K^+]_o$ is one of the major contributors to the genesis and sustenance of ischemia-related cardiac arrhythmias,[4] and thus a large body of research has been devoted to the mechanisms of extracellular K^+ accumulation in ischemia. However, this daunting task requires gathering information on ischemia-induced alterations in all ionic currents and concentrations and in the transmembrane potential simultaneously, which is next to impossible using current experimental techniques. Rodríguez et al.[13] used a computer model of a single cardiomyocyte to dynamically calculate ionic concentrations and fluxes under ischemic conditions with the aim of providing mechanistic insight into the extracellular K^+ accumulation in ischemia. The model considered ionic fluxes between three compartments: the intracellular medium, the interstitial cleft, and the bulk extracellular medium, in which concentrations were assumed to be constant. Membrane kinetics were represented by a modified version of the Luo–Rudy action potential (AP) model[21,22] that includes a formulation of the ATP-sensitive K^+ current ($I_{K(ATP)}$) current by Ferrero et al.[23] and a new ischemia-activated Na^+ current (I_{NaS}). Interruption of coronary flow was simulated by steeply increasing the time constant of diffusion between the bulk extracellular medium and the interstitial clefts from its normoxic value to infinity. Experimental results suggest that three mechanisms, namely inhibition of the Na^+/K^+ pump (I_{NaK}),[24,25] activation of the $I_{K(ATP)}$,[18,26] and activation of an inward Na^+ current[18,27–29] could be responsible for the increase in $[K^+]_o$ in acute ischemia. Rodríguez et al.[13] conducted computer simulations to investigate the role of each of these three mechanisms in extracellular K^+ accumulation during the early phase of ischemia.

FIGURE 1 summarizes the main results of the simulations, which ascertain that the simultaneous participation of the three mechanisms (Trace VII) is necessary to obtain the biphasic (quick rise and then plateau phase) increase in $[K^+]_o$ observed experimentally during the first 10–15 min following interruption of coronary flow. Engagement of only one (Traces I–III) or two (Traces IV–VI) of these mechanisms cannot explain the extracellular K^+ accumulation recorded experimentally: the increase in $[K^+]_o$ is either too low as compared to experimental data or does not replicate the biphasic increase. The simulation results also demonstrate that the rate of activation of the three mechanisms as well as the rate at which the cell is paced determine the level and the time to onset of the $[K^+]_o$ plateau phase, consistent with experimental recordings.[15,17–19,30] Acidosis and ischemic shrinkage of the extracellular space[3,20,31] have a minor effect on the ischemic increase in $[K^+]_o$ and only produce a slight anticipation in time of the $[K^+]_o$ plateau phase. According to the simulation results, the ischemic cellular K^+ loss is mainly due to an

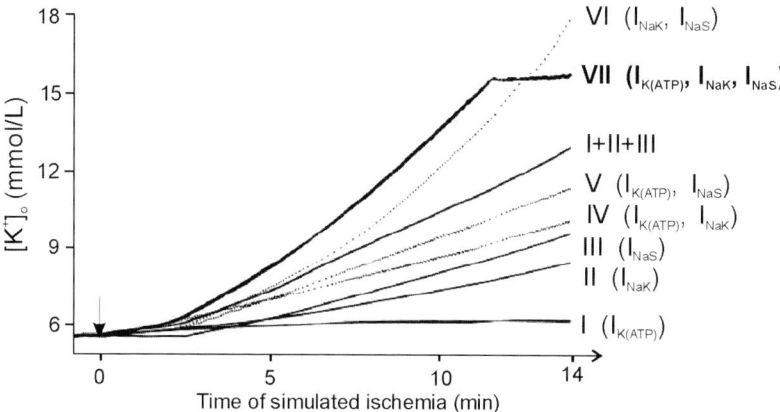

FIGURE 1. Time courses of the extracellular K$^+$ concentration ([K$^+$]$_o$) during 14 min of ischemia obtained for different ischemic mechanisms. Traces I–III represent individual effects on [K+]$_o$ of: change in ATP-sensitive K$^+$ current ($I_{K(ATP)}$); current through the Na$^+$/K$^+$ pump (I_{NaK}); and inclusion of ischemia-activated Na$^+$ inward current (I_{NaS}), respectively. Trace "I + II + III" is the sum of traces I–III. Traces IV–VI correspond to the combined effect of the two mechanisms indicated next to each trace. Trace VII depicts the simultaneous effect of the three mechanisms on [K$^+$]$_o$. In all cases, when $I_{K(ATP)}$ was activated, the final value of the fraction of activated ATP-sensitive K$^+$ (K$_{ATP}$) channels was 0.8%. When I_{NaS} was activated, the final value of I_{NaS} was 1.2 μA/μF, and when an inhibition of the maximum current through the Na$^+$/K$^+$ pump was considered, the final value of the degree of inhibition of the Na$^+$/K$^+$ was 35%. (Modified from reference 13.)

increase in the K$^+$ efflux via the time-independent K$^+$ current and the $I_{K(ATP)}$, rather than to a decrease in K$^+$ influx via the Na$^+$/K$^+$ pump. The insight provided by these simulations is an important stepping stone in understanding the pathophysiology of ischemic injury in the heart.

Ischemia-Induced Changes in Action Potential and Propagation

Over the last four decades, increasing wealth in experimental data on ionic channel behavior has prompted its integration into highly sophisticated data-driven mathematical models of cardiac cell membrane kinetics, including representations of the ischemic milieu. Computer simulations with such models have improved significantly the understanding of the ionic mechanisms underlying ischemia-induced electrophysiological changes at the cellular and tissue level. FIGURE 2 illustrates a simulation of the evolution of ventricular cell AP over the first 12 min following coronary occlusion. Ischemia was simulated by incorporating effects of hyperkalemia, acidosis, and anoxia.[32,33] Specifically, the [K$^+$]$_o$ was increased from its normal value, 5.4 mmol/L, to 12 mmol/L;[15,34] the maximum conductances of the Na$^+$ and L-Type Ca^{2+} channels (currents

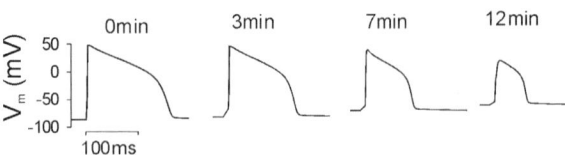

FIGURE 2. Evolution of the action potential during 12 min of simulated ischemia.

I_{Na} and I_{CaL}, respectively) were decreased by 25%, representing inhibition by acidosis;[35–37] and the $I_{K(ATP)}$ was activated by decreasing the intracellular ATP concentration from 6.8 mmol/L to 4.6 mmol/L and increasing the intracellular ADP concentration from 15 μmol/L to 99 μmol/L.[23,34] Shaw and Rudy[38,39] and Ferrero et al.[23] demonstrated using computer simulations that these changes account for the most significant alterations in AP morphology and wave propagation over the course of ischemia. Indeed, FIGURE 2 shows that during the first 12 min of ischemia, resting potential becomes elevated to –60mV from its normal value of –85 mV, action potential duration shortens by almost 50% of its normal value, and the action potential amplitude progressively decreases from 125 mV to 88 mV. These changes are consistent with experimental recordings.[3,15,34,40]

The high degree of electrophysiological detail provided by computer simulations allows examination of the specific contribution of each ischemic change at the ionic level to the electrophysiological alterations in AP and propagation following coronary occlusion. For instance, computer simulation studies have shown that activation of a small portion of the K(ATP) channels is responsible for the significant action potential duration (APD) shortening observed in anoxic cardiomyocytes, while increase in $[K^+]_o$ plays only a secondary role in APD shortening.[23,38] The main effect of $[K^+]_o$ elevation is resting depolarization, which causes decreased availability of Na^+ channels and slow recovery of the Na^+ channel inactivation gates, thus resulting in depressed excitability and prolonged postrepolarization refractoriness in ischemic cardiomyocytes.[38] Excitability of ischemic myocytes is further reduced by acidosis that acts to decrease the maximum conductances of the Na^+ and Ca^{2+} channels.

As demonstrated by computer simulations and experimental studies, ischemia-induced alterations in Na^+ and Ca^{2+} currents have a significant impact on the AP upstroke, thus affecting propagation velocity. During the first minutes of ischemia, mild elevation of resting potential due to an initial increase in $[K^+]_o$ to around 8 mM leads to a decrease in the difference between resting potential and the threshold for activation, resulting in a slight increase in conduction velocity.[39,41,42] With further progression of ischemia, and further increase in $[K^+]_o$ above 8mM, severe depolarization at rest results in reduced availability of Na^+ current and thus in slow AP upstroke and decreased propagation velocity.[39,41,42] While under normal conditions and in mild ischemia the AP upstroke velocity is mainly determined by the Na^+

current, under severe ischemic conditions (10–12-min postocclusion), the AP upstroke becomes biphasic, with the first phase corresponding to the influx of (decreased) Na^+ current and the second component due to the activation of the Ca^{2+} current.[39,43–47] Simulation studies have demonstrated that, under these conditions, Ca^{2+} current plays a critical role in the occurrence of propagation block and the development of alternans in the ischemic region, both phenomena being precursors of reentrant activity in ischemia.[39,47–49]

Ischemia-Induced Changes in the Electrocardiogram (ECG)

ECG ST-segment depression is recognized clinically as a sign of myocardial ischemia,[50,51] but the underlying mechanisms remain controversial. A number of studies have used computer simulations to investigate the role of specific features of the ischemic region, such as its location, in ST-segment displacement, in an attempt to ascertain the diagnostic value of the latter. Li *et al.*[52] investigated the origin of ST depression in the ECG for subendocardial ischemia by mapping the epicardial and endocardial potential distribution in *in vivo* sheep heart and by conducting computer simulations using a geometrically realistic passive model of the human heart. The results showed that ST depression was caused by an "injury current" generated by a spatial gradient in transmembrane potential at the border between ischemic and healthy tissue. As subendocardial ischemia progressed to full-thickness transmural ischemia, epicardial ST depression over the boundary region gradually increased, and ST elevation took place over the ischemic region. However, the location of the ischemic region in the ventricles could not be predicted by the ST depression on the epicardium.

The computer model by Li *et al.*,[52] while anatomically based, did not incorporate anisotropic conductivities. Follow-up work by the same group[53,54] and research by others[55–58] employed passive bidomain models to investigate how the anisotropic myocardial conductivities modulate the ST segment shift resulting from subendocardial ischemia. Results show that fiber rotation and tissue anisotropy play a key role in determining epicardial potential distributions and ST displacements in regional ischemia. However, these studies have an important limitation—the use of steady-state passive models, in which ischemia-induced alterations in membrane kinetics are not represented; such models cannot provide insight into the ionic basis of ischemia-induced alterations in the ECG in its entirety (and not only in ST segment shifts).

Gima and Rudy[59] and later Aslanidi *et al.*[60] adopted an alternative approach to investigate the cellular mechanisms underlying ischemia-induced changes in the ECG. They used a geometrically simple but electrophysiologically detailed 1D model of a virtual ventricular wall to compute the pseudo-ECG in normoxia and under conditions of global and subendocardial ischemia. Consistent with clinical and experimental data, the simulations showed that propagation through the ventricular wall results in an ST-segment at base line

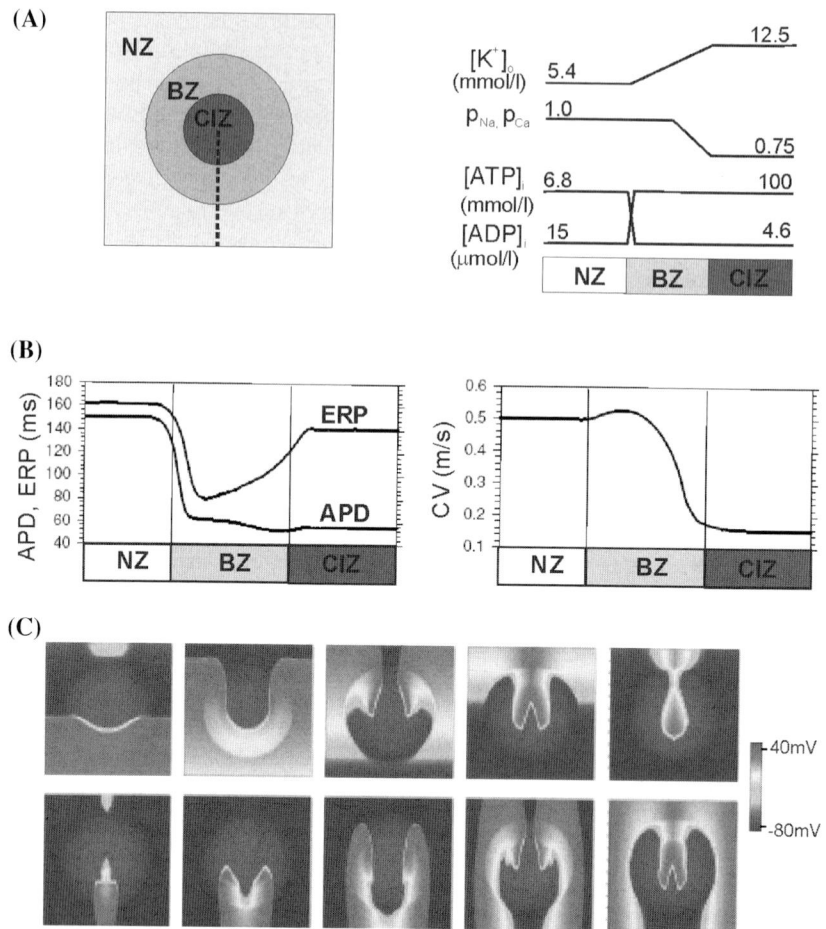

FIGURE 3. Arrhythmogenesis in regional ischemia. Panel **A:** Schematic of the 2D model of regionally ischemic tissue (left) and the spatial variations in extracellular potassium concentration ($[K^+]_o$), intracellular ATP and ADP concentrations ($[ATP]_i$ and $[ADP]_i$), and the degree of inhibition of the maximum conductances of the Na^+ and Ca^{2+} currents in the central ischemic zone (CIZ), border zone (BZ), and normal zone (NZ) (right). Panel **B:** Spatial variation in the effective refractory period and action potential duration (left) and in the longitudinal conduction velocity (right) along the dashed line depicted in panel **A**, left. Panel **C:** Snapshots of transmembrane potential distribution at different instants of time following the delivery of a premature stimulus at CI = 210 msec in the lower part of the 2D sheet illustrated in panel **A**. Snapshots are separated by 50 msec; the first corresponds to 50 msec after the delivery of the premature stimulus. Panel C is shown in color online. (Modified from reference 47.)

in normoxia, ST-segment elevation in global ischemia, and ST-segment depression in subendocardial ischemia caused by the abnormal transmural sequence of repolarization and resting potential elevation in the ischemic tissue.

Ischemia-Related Cardiac Arrhythmias

Ischemic impact on the myocardium is characterized with a high degree of heterogeneity. Electrophysiological properties vary not only with time postocclusion, but also spatially. Due to diffusion of ions and metabolites, the core of the tissue suffering from a lack of flow, that is the central ischemic zone (CIZ), is surrounded by border zones (BZ), which comprise progressive changes in electrophysiological properties between the healthy and ischemic regions. Experimental measurements of $[K^+]_o$, oxygen, and metabolite distribution in the ischemic area[61–65] were used by Ferrero *et al.*[47] to develop the 2D model of regional ischemia depicted in FIGURE 3A, which included the first electrophysiologically detailed model of the BZ. As in previous studies, ischemia was represented by the effects of hyperkalemia, acidosis, and hypoxia on $[K^+]_o$, I_{Na}, I_{CaL}, and $I_{K(ATP)}$, at levels corresponding to 10-min postocclusion. Severity of ischemic changes is most pronounced within the CIZ and decreases progressively in the BZ. The varying levels of $[K^+]_o$, I_{Na}, I_{CaL}, and $I_{K(ATP)}$ in the ischemic region result in a significant dispersion of refractoriness and of conduction velocity by the mechanisms explained in the previous section. FIGURE 3 B shows the spatial variation of conduction velocity, APD, and effective refractory period in the border zone, as quantified by Ferrero *et al.*[47]

Dispersion of refractoriness and of conduction velocity in regional ischemia provides the substrate for the establishment of reentrant circuits, the main mechanism of arrhythmogenesis following coronary occlusion.[45,46,63] FIGURE 3 C illustrates the initiation of a figure-of-eight reentry in the model of regional ischemia described above. Following pacing stimulation, a premature stimulus is applied at the bottom border of the 2D sheet. The premature stimulus elicits a wavefront, which propagates through the healthy region as well as the BZs, but blocks at the CIZ where refractoriness is extended. Meanwhile, tissue in the CIZ recovers allowing reentry of the wavefront from the top, and the establishment of a figure-of-eight reentrant circuit, a pattern similar to the one observed experimentally.[66–69] Simulation results show that the degree of activation of the $I_{K(ATP)}$ plays an important role in vulnerability to reentry in regional ischemia.[47,70]

The occlusion of a coronary artery leads to important electrophysiological heterogeneities, not only intramurally as represented in the model developed by Ferrero *et al.*, but also transmurally, in the depth of the ventricular wall. A thin layer of tissue, approximately 1–2 mm, on both epi- and endocardium, receives nutrients and oxygen from blood in the cavities and the medium surrounding the heart, thus remaining viable over the course of acute ischemia.[71] In addition, the severity of ischemic changes varies transmurally through the core of the ischemic region. Extracellular K^+ accumulation is faster in the subendocardium than in the subepicardium while APD shortening due to $I_{K(ATP)}$ activation is more pronounced in the subepicardium, thus leading to gradients in the electrophysiological properties within the central ischemic region.[72–76]

The contribution of transmural electrophysiological heterogeneities in the ischemic region to arrhythmogenesis in acute ischemia remains unknown due to limitations in current experimental techniques, which prevent the examination of cardiac activity in the depth of the ventricular wall with high spatial and temporal resolution. Recently, Tice et al.[48] developed an anatomically based 2D model of a transmural section of the ischemic rabbit ventricles following LAD occlusion. The model was used to investigate the role of regional ischemia-induced transmural heterogeneities in providing the substrate for reentry over the course of the first 10-min postocclusion. Ischemic substrate was represented by progressive changes in membrane dynamics due to hyperkalemia, acidosis, and hypoxia corresponding to 2–10-min postocclusion. The model, illustrated in FIGURE 4 A, includes realistic CIZ, lateral BZ, endocardial and epicardial BZ (EBZ), and transmural I_{KATP} and $[K^+]_o$ gradients in CIZ. The LV wall was paced at 200 msec basic cycle length and premature stimulation was applied to the RV endocardium at a range of coupling intervals (CIs). The simulation results show that a premature stimulus is more likely to initiate arrhythmia at 7–8-min postocclusion, when refractoriness in normal tissue and CIZ differs the most. Arrhythmia induction is then heralded by alternans in the EBZ, as shown in FIGURE 4 B. Within the vulnerable window (VW), propagation induced by the premature stimulus encounters refractory RV and CIZ, while tissue in the EBZs is already recovered, resulting in reentry (FIG. 4 B). Halving EBZ decreases the safety factor for propagation, resulting in 58.8% decrease in reentry initiation. Omission of transmural CIZ I_{KATP} gradient from the model causes 29.4% increase in probability of arrhythmia initiation due to greater difference in normal versus CIZ refractoriness. These simulation results provide an important mechanistic insight into the role of electrophysiological heterogeneities to arrhythmogenesis in regional ischemia.

Response of Ischemic Tissue to Electric Shocks

The only effective therapy currently available to terminate lethal cardiac arrhythmias arising from ischemic injury is electrical defibrillation by timely application of an electric shock. Due to the strong link between defibrillation threshold and upper limit of vulnerability (ULV),[77–79] numerous studies have investigated the mechanisms of cardiac vulnerability to electric shocks in an attempt to understand defibrillation failure. However, the majority of these studies focused on healthy ventricles[80–89] and rarely on hearts with ischemic disease,[90] thus little is known about the response of ischemic tissue to the application of electric shocks. This is in part due to the fact that experimental evaluation of shock-induced responses of ischemic tissue is hampered by the rapidity and complexity of ischemic changes that follow coronary occlusion.

Bidomain simulations have demonstrated ability to provide insight, based on behavior monitored with high spatiotemporal resolution, into the mechanisms

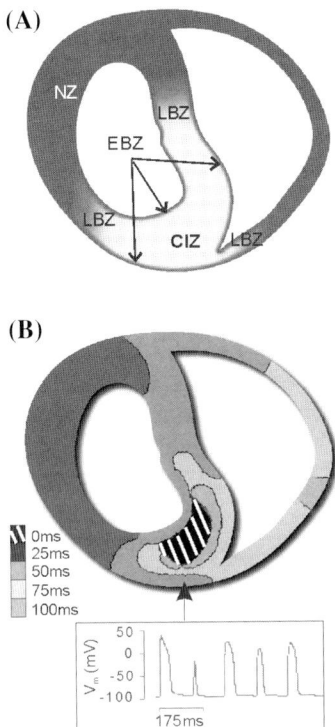

FIGURE 4. Contribution of transmural heterogeneities to arrhythmogenesis in regional ischemia. Panel **A**: 2D anatomically accurate rabbit ventricular model of regional ischemia following LAD occlusion. CIZ is central ischemia zone, NZ–normal zone, EBZ–endo and epicardial border zone, and LBZ–lateral border zone. Panel **B**: Activation time map of a reentrant beat following a premature stimulus (top) and time course of transmembrane potential in the node marked by the arrow (bottom). (Modified from reference.[48])

of cardiac defibrillation in the healthy and ischemic ventricles.[41,42,81,84–86] The bidomain model[87] represents the myocardium as two coupled continuous media, the intracellular and the extracellular spaces, and allows for the study of the macroscopic tissue response to electric stimuli. As shown by experimental[88–93] and bidomain simulation studies,[82,83,94,95] the application of a strong electric field to the myocardium induces positive and negative changes in transmembrane potential, and results in large-scale regions of positive and negative membrane polarization termed virtual electrode polarization (VEP). Regions negatively polarized at shock end represent new excitable areas through which postshock wavefronts will propagate. The positively polarized regions play the dual role of first providing the electrical stimulus necessary for initiation of postshock propagating wavefronts and second being regions of immediate postshock refractoriness that could result in propagation block.

Tissue is vulnerable to an electric shock if postshock propagation results in reentry, which implies the fulfillment of three conditions: (1) new excitations have to be generated at the end of the shock at the borders of oppositely polarized areas; (2) postshock refractoriness in the positively polarized regions has to be long enough to result in propagation block in part of the ventricles; (3) the spatial extent of postshock wavefronts and their propagation velocity has to be such that tissue depolarized by the shock recovers before the postshock excitable areas have been completely consumed by postshock wavefronts.

Bidomain simulations using anatomically based finite element models have shown how these three factors manifest themselves in the 3D volume of the normal and the globally ischemic ventricles.[41,81,85] As in previous studies, changes in membrane dynamics over the course of the first 10 min following occlusion were implemented via the effects of hyperkalemia, acidosis, and hypoxia at the ionic level. To examine vulnerability to electric shocks in global ischemia, in the study by Rodríguez et al.,[41] three representative levels of increasing severity within the first 10-min interval were singled out. Simulations were conducted in normoxia and for each ischemic state to determine changes in cardiac vulnerability to electric shocks over the course of ischemia. To do so, the ventricles were paced at the apex and monophasic shocks of several strengths were applied at different CIs via two planar electrodes located at the boundaries of the perfusing bath to determine the vulnerability grids, that is, 2D grids encompassing the episodes of shock-induced arrhythmogenesis. The ULV was determined in normoxia and over the course of ischemia as the lowest shock strength above which no sustained arrhythmia was induced.

Consistent with experimental results,[81] the simulations showed that the application of an external shock induces two main areas of opposite-in-sign polarization in both the normoxic and the globally ischemic ventricles (see FIG. 5: 0 ms panel). In both normoxia and ischemia, following shocks below the ULV, a new wavefront arises at shock end at the apex, proceeding toward the base through the shock-induced excitable gap in the LV. Meanwhile, shock-induced refractoriness in the RV-free wall causes a transient unidirectional block. Thus, while LV and septal tissue is being depolarized by wavefront propagation, the RV myocardium recovers, providing the return pathway for reentry (FIG. 5).

While the same type of reentrant pattern is induced in normoxia and in global ischemia, important differences in the characteristics of the postshock wavefronts and in their propagation develop over the course of global ischemia phase 1A; these differences result in a decrease in the ULV at around 4–5 min following the interruption of coronary flow. As described above, action potential duration is significantly shorter at 4–5 min of ischemia as compared to normoxia, resulting in shorter repolarization times and in an increase in the amount of tissue repolarized at a given CI (FIG. 5, preshock panel). As a consequence of these changes, the spatial extent of shock-end wavefronts increases in global ischemia as compared to normoxia. Larger wavefronts traverse the

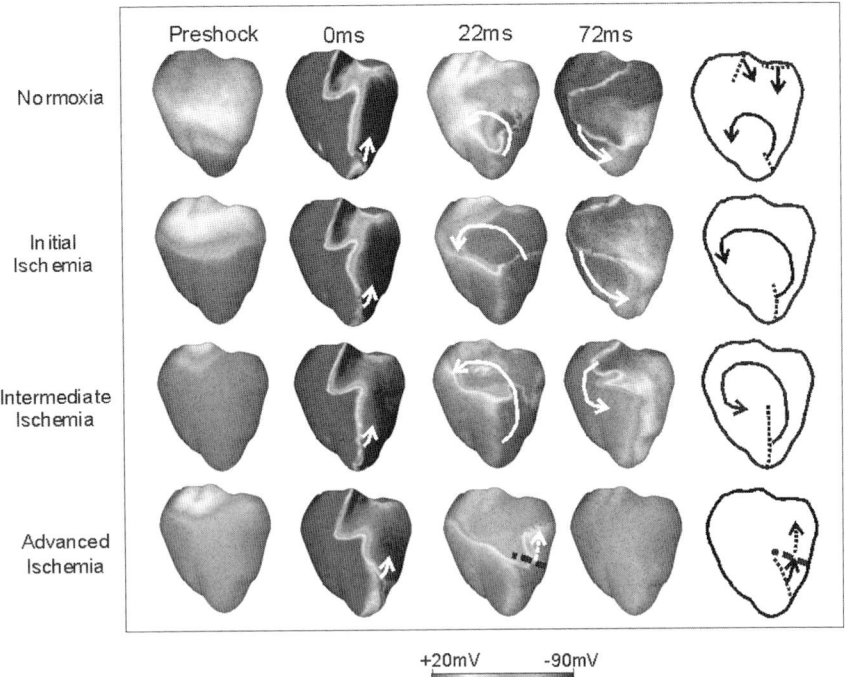

FIGURE 5. Anterior transmembrane potential distribution in normoxia and global ischemia for a 6.4 V/cm shock applied at CI = 160 msec. Times refer to shock end. Color scale is saturated, that is, potentials above +20 mV and below –90 mV appear red and blue, respectively. Diagrams present major features of postshock behavior. Dotted lines indicate spatial extent of wavefronts at shock end. Solid arrows show direction of propagation. Dashed arrows depict direction of decremental conduction. Thick dashed lines mark locations at which conduction becomes decremental. The Figure is shown in color online. (Modified from reference 40.)

postshock excitable gap faster for the same shock strength, thus increasing the likelihood of wavefronts being blocked by the prolonged refractoriness in positively polarized areas immediately after shock end, and resulting in a decrease in ULV from its normal value of 12.75 V/cm to 9.6 V/cm at 4–5 min of global ischemia.

As ischemia progresses, APD shortening continues, however, resting potential elevation becomes more severe, causing prolonged postrepolarization refractoriness. As stated above, the APD shortening in ischemia results in an increase in the amount of tissue repolarized at a given CI. However, in the late stages of ischemia phase 1A, some of the tissue experiences low postshock excitability due to delay in the recovery of the Na inactivation gates caused by resting potential elevation. Since the ventricles are paced at the apex, the apical regions are always more recovered than the rest of the ventricles. Therefore, in the late stages of ischemia, postshock activations manage to traverse the apical regions, only to become decremental and to fail in the less-recovered basal portions (FIG. 5), thus resulting in a further decrease in cardiac vulnerability to electric shocks. At the end of ischemia phase 1A, no arrhythmia or even a single extra beat can be induced, regardless of CI or shock strength.[42] For all combinations of shock strength and CI, propagation initiated at shock end terminates shortly thereafter due to conduction failure. These fascinating results clearly underscore the utility of 3D realistic modeling in providing novel information regarding the electrical behavior of the heart under ischemic conditions as well as its response to antiarrhythmia therapy.

SUMMARY

This article provided a brief review of some of the computational models, from models of ionic fluxes to those of the whole organ, used to assess the electrophysiological effects of acute myocardial ischemia in its most rapid phase, 1A. It focused on alterations in metabolism and ionic fluxes; the changes in the cell AP morphology and its propagation; the manifestation of ischemia in the ECG; the mechanisms of arrhythmia generation; and the responses of the ischemic heart to electric shocks. The selection of topics included here is (necessarily) incomplete, but provides a mosaic of a variety of simulation approaches that have addressed different aspects of the big picture. The review emphasized the fact that computer simulations are capable of providing mechanistic insight at any level of structural complexity. The article also provided an overview of the development of computer models of ever-increasing ionic and structural detail; models are now available from the single channel and cell level to the entire organ. Whole organ models that incorporate detailed ionic representation of the impact of ischemic injury are now becoming state-of-the-art[96] and hold the promise to lead to a breakthrough in understanding the arrhythmogenic mechanisms of myocardial ischemia and ultimately, in advancement of antiarrhythmia therapies.

ACKNOWLEDGMENTS

This work was supported by the EPSRC-funded Integrative Biology e-Science pilot project (ref no: GR/S72023/01), by the EU BioSim Grant (005137) and by AHA Established Investigator Award (N.T.), and the grant HL63195 from NIH (N.T.). The authors would like to thank Drs. Jose María Ferrero, Jr., and Beatriz Trénor (Universidad Politécnica de Valencia), and Mr. Brock Tice (Tulane University) for helpful comments and for material provided for the figures.

REFERENCES

1. ZIPES, D.P. & H.J.J. WELLENS. 1998. Sudden cardiac death. Circulation **98:** 2334–2351.
2. RUBART, M. & D.P. ZIPES. 2005. Mechanisms of sudden cardiac death. J. Clin. Invest. **115:** 2305–2315.
3. CARMELIET, E. 1999. Cardiac ionic currents and acute ischemia: from channels to arrhythmias. Physiol. Rev. **79:** 917–1017.
4. HARRIS, A.S., A. BISTENI, R.A. RUSSELL, et al. 1954. Excitatory factors in ventricular tachycardia resulting from myocardial ischemia. Potassium a major excitant. Science **119:** 200–203.
5. WIT, A.L. & M.J. JANSE. 1992. Experimental models of ventricular tachycardia and fibrillation caused by ischemia and infarction. Circulation **85**(Suppl I): I32–I42.
6. CH'EN, F.F., R.D. VAUGHAN-JONES, K. CLARKE & D. NOBLE. 1998. Modelling myocardial ischaemia and reperfusion. Prog. Biophys. Mol. Biol. **69:** 515–538.
7. ZHOU, L., J.E. SALEM, G.M. SAIDEL, et al. 2005. Mechanistic model of cardiac energy metabolism predicts localization of glycolysis to cytosolic subdomain during ischemia. Am. J. Physiol. Heart Circ. Physiol. **288:** H2400–H2411.
8. CABRERA, M.E., L. ZHOU, W.C. STANLEY & G.M. SAIDEL. 2005. Regulation of cardiac energetics: role of redox state and cellular compartmentation during ischemia. Ann. N. Y. Acad. Sci. **1047:** 259–270.
9. NOBLE, D. 2002. Simulation of Na-Ca exchange activity during ischemia. Ann. N. Y. Acad. Sci. **976:** 431–437.
10. EISNER, D.A. & K.R. SIPIDO. 2004. Sodium calcium exchange in the heart. Necessity or Luxury? Circ. Res. **95:** 549–551.
11. HENDERSON, S.A., J.I. GOLDHABER, J.M. SO, et al. 2004. Functional adult myocardium in the absence of Na^+-Ca^{2+} exchange: cardiac specific knockout of NCX1. Circ. Res. **95:** 604–611.
12. IMAHASHI, K., C. POTT, J. GOLDHABERI, et al. 2005. Cardiac-specific ablation of the Na^+-Ca^{2+} exchanger confers protection against ischemia/reperfusion injury. Circ. Res. **97:** 916–921.
13. RODRÍGUEZ, B., J.M. FERRERO, Jr., & B. TRENOR. 2002. Mechanistic investigation of extracellular K^+ accumulation during acute myocardial ischemia. Am. J. Physiol. **283:** H490–H500.
14. GASSER, R.N.A. & R.D. VAUGHAN-JONES. 1990. Mechanism of potassium efflux and action potential shortening during ischaemia in isolated mammalian cardiac muscle. J. Physiol. **431:** 713–741.
15. WEISS, J.N. & K.I. SHINE. 1982. $[K^+]_o$ accumulation and electrophysiological alterations during early myocardial ischemia. Am. J. Physiol. Heart Circ. Physiol. **243:** H318–H327.
16. WEISS, J.N. & K.I. SHINE. 1982. Extracellular K^+ accumulation during myocardial ischemia in isolated rabbit heart. Am. J. Physiol. Heart Circ. Physiol. **242:** H619–H628.
17. WEISS, J.N. & K.I. SHINE. 1986. Effects of heart rate on extracellular K^+ accumulation during myocardial ischemia. Am. J. Physiol. Heart Circ. Physiol. **250:** H982–H991.
18. WILDE, A.A.M. & G. AKSNES. 1995. Myocardial potassium loss and cell depolarization in ischaemia and hypoxia. Cardiovasc. Res. **29:** 1–15.

19. WILDE, A.A.M., D. ESCANDE, C.A. SCHUMACHER, et al. 1990. Potassium accumulation in the globally ischaemic mammalian heart: a role for the ATP-sensitive K channel. Circ. Res. **67:** 835–843.
20. YAN, G.X., J. CHEN, K.A. YAMADA, et al. 1996. Contribution of shrinkage of extracellular space to extracellular K+ accumulation in myocardial ischemia of the rabbit. J. Physiol. **490:** 215–228.
21. LUO, C.H. & Y. RUDY. 1994. A dynamic model of the cardiac ventricular action potential. I. Simulations of ionic currents and concentration changes. Circ. Res. **74:** 1071–1096.
22. ZENG, J., K.R. LAURITA, D.S. ROSENBAUM & Y. RUDY. 1995. Two components of the delayed rectifier K^+ current in ventricular myocytes of the guinea-pig type: theoretical formulation and their role in repolarization. Circ. Res. **77:** 140–152.
23. FERRERO, J.M., Jr., J. SAIZ, J.M. FERRERO & N.V. THAKOR. 1996. Simulation of action potentials from metabolically impaired cardiac myocytes. Role of ATP-sensitive K^+ current. Circ. Res. **79:** 208–221.
24. WILDE, A.A.M., R.L.G. PETERS & M.J. JANSE. 1988. Catecholamine release and potassium accumulation in the isolated globally ischemic rabbit heart. J. Mol. Cell. Cardiol. **20:** 887–896.
25. BERSOHN, M.M., K.D. PHILIPSON & J.Y. FUKUSHIMA. 1982. Sodium–calcium exchange and sarcolemmal enzymes in ischemic rabbit hearts. Am. J. Physiol. Cell. Physiol. **242:** C288–C295.
26. NOMA, A. 1983. ATP-regulated K^+ channels in cardiac muscle. Nature **305:** 147–149.
27. SHIVKUMAR, K., N.A. DEUTSCH, S.T. LAMP, et al. 1997. Mechanisms of hypoxic K loss in rabbit ventricle. J. Clin. Invest. **100:** 1782–1788.
28. HARTMANN, M., U. DECKING & J. SCHRADER. 1998. Cardioprotective actions of KC 12291. II. Delaying Na+ overload in ischemia improves cardiac function and energy status in reperfusion. Arch. Pharm. (Weinheim) **358:** 554–560.
29. JU, Y.K., D.A. SAINT & P.W. GAGE. 1996. Hypoxia increases persistent sodium current in rat ventricular myocytes. J. Physiol. **497:** 337–347.
30. KANDA, A., I. WATANABE, M.L. WILLIAMS, et al. 1997. Unanticipated lessening of the rise in extracellular potassium during ischemia by pinacidil. Circulation **95:** 1937–1944.
31. KNOPF, H., R. THEISING, C.H. MOON & H.J. HIRCHE. 1990. Continuous determination of extracellular space and changes of K, Na, Ca, and H during global ischaemia in isolated rat hearts. J. Mol. Cell. Cardiol. **22:** 1259–1272.
32. MORENA, H., M.J. JANSE, A.W.T. FIOLET, et al. 1980. Comparison of the effects of regional ischemia, hypoxia, hyperkalemia, and acidosis on intracellular and extracellular potentials and metabolism in the isolated porcine heart. Circ. Res. **46:** 634–646.
33. KODAMA, I., A. WILDE, M.J. JANSE, et al. 1984. Combined effects of hypoxia, hyperkalemia and acidosis on membrane action potential and excitability of guinea-pig ventricular muscle. J. Mol. Cell. Cardiol. **16:** 247–259.
34. WEISS, J.N., N. VENKATESH & S.T. LAMP. 1992. ATP-sensitive K^+ channels and cellular K^+ loss in hypoxic and ischemic mammalian ventricle. J. Physiol(Lond). **447:** 649–673.
35. KAGIYAMA, Y., J.L. HILL & L.S. GETTES. 1982. Interaction of acidosis and increased extracellular potassium on action potential characteristics and conduction. Circ. Res. **51:** 614–623.

36. Sato, R., A. Noma & Y. Kurachi. 1985. Effects of intracellular acidification on membrane currents in ventricular cells of the guinea pig. Circ. Res. **57:** 553–561.
37. Irisawa, H. & R. Sato. 1986. Intra- and extracellular actions of proton on the calcium current of isolated guinea pig ventricular cells. Circ. Res. **59:** 348–355.
38. Shaw, R. & Y. Rudy. 1997. Electrophysiological effects of acute myocardial ischemia: a theoretical study of altered cell excitability and action potential duration. Cardiovasc. Res. **35:** 256–272.
39. Shaw, R. & Y. Rudy. 1997. Electrophysiologic effects of acute myocardial ischemia. A mechanistic investigation of action potential conduction and conduction failure. Circ. Res. **80:** 124–138.
40. Kleber, A.G., C.B. Riegger & M.J. Janse. 1987. Extracellular K^+ and H^+ shifts in early ischemia: mechanisms and relation to changes in impulse propagation. J. Mol. Cell. Cardiol. **19:** 35–44.
41. Rodríguez, B., B. Tice, J. Eason, et al. 2004. Cardiac vulnerability to electric shocks during phase 1A of acute global ischemia. Heart Rhythm **1:** 695–703.
42. Rodríguez, B., B. Tice, J.C. Eason, et al. 2004. Effect of acute global ischemia on the upper limit of vulnerability. Am. J. Physiol. **286:** H2078–H2088.
43. Downar, E., M.J. Janse & D. Durrer. 1977. The effect of 'ischemic' blood on transmembrane potentials of normal porcine ventricular myocardium. Circulation **55:** 455–462.
44. Kleber, A.G., M.J. Janse, F.J. Van Capelle & D. Durrer. 1978. Mechanisms and time course of S-T and T-Q segment changes during acute regional myocardial ischemia in the pig heart determined by extracellular and intracellular recordings. Circ. Res. **42:** 603–613.
45. Pogwizd, S.M. & P.B. Corr. 1987. Electrophysiologic mechanisms underlying arrhythmias due to reperfusion of ischemic myocardium. Circulation **76:** 402–426.
46. Wit, A.L. & M.J. Janse. 1993. The Ventricular Arrhythmias of Ischemia and Infarction: Electrophysiological Mechanisms. Futura Publishing, Mount Kisko.
47. Ferrero, J.M., Jr., B. Trenor, B. Rodríguez & J. Saiz. 2003. Electrical activity and reentry during acute regional myocardial ischemia: insights from simulations. Int. J. Bif. Chaos **13:** 1–13.
48. Tice, B., B. Rodríguez & N. Trayanova. 2005. Arrthythmogenicity of transmural heterogeneities in a realistic model of regional ischemia. Heart Rhythm **2:** S261.
49. Bernus, O., C.W. Zemlin, R.M. Zaritsky, et al. 2005. Alternating conduction in the ischaemic border zone as precursor of reentrant arrhythmias: a simulation study. Europace **7:** 93–104.
50. Wolferth, C.C., S. Bellet, M.M. Livezey & F. Murphy. 1945. Negative displacement of the RS-T segment in the electrocardiogram and its relationships to positive displacement: an experimental study. Am. Heart J. **29:** 220–244.
51. Holland, R.P. & H. Brooks. 1975. Precordial and epicardial surface potentials during myocardial ischemia in the pig: a theoretical and experimental analysis of the TQ and ST segments. Circ. Res. **37:** 471–480.
52. Li, D., C.Y. Li, A.C. Yong & D. Kilpatrick. 1998. Source of electrocardiographic ST changes in subendocardial ischemia. Circ. Res. **82:** 957–970.
53. Johnston, P.R., D. Kilpatrick & C.Y. Li. 2001. The importance of anisotropy in modeling ST segment shift in subendocardial ischaemia. IEEE Trans. Biomed. Eng. **48:** 1366–1376.

54. JOHNSTON, P.R. & D. KILPATRICK. 2003. The effect of conductivity values on ST segment shift in subendocardial ischaemia. IEEE Trans. Biomed. Eng. **50:** 150–158.
55. HOPENFELD, B., J.G. STINSTRA & R.S. MACLEOD. 2004. Mechanism for ST depression associated with contiguous subendocardial ischemia. J. Cardiovasc. Electrophysiol. **15:** 1200–1206.
56. HOPENFELD, B., J.G. STINSTRA & R.S. MACLEOD. 2005. The effect of conductivity on ST-segment epicardial potentials arising from subendocardial ischemia. Ann. Biomed. Eng. **33:** 751–763.
57. MACLEOD, R.S., S. SHOME, J. STINSTRA, *et al*. 2005. Mechanisms of ischemia-induced ST-segment changes. J. Electrocardiol. **38**(4 Suppl): 8–13.
58. MACLACHLAN, M.C., J. SUNDNES & G.T. LINES. 2005. Simulation of ST segment changes during subendocardial ischemia using a realistic 3-D cardiac geometry. IEEE Trans. Biomed. Eng. **52:** 799–807.
59. GIMA, K. & Y. RUDY. 2002. Ionic current basis of electrocardiographic waveforms: a model study. Relates the electrocardiographic waveforms to cellular electrophysiological processes. Several conditions including global ischemia. Circ. Res. **90:** 889–896.
60. ASLANIDI, O.V., R.H. CLAYTON, J.L. LAMBERT & A.V. HOLDEN. 2005. Dynamical and cellular electrophysiological mechanisms of ECG changes during ischaemia. J. Theor. Biol. **237:** 369–381.
61. CORONEL, R. 1988. Distribution of extracellular potassium during myocardial ischemia. Ph.D. Thesis, University of Amsterdam. The Netherlands.
62. CORONEL, R., J.W. FIOLET, *et al*. 1988. Distribution of extracellular potassium and its relation to electrophysiologic changes during acute myocardial ischemia in the isolated perfused porcine heart. Circulation **77:** 1125–1138.
63. CORONEL, R. 1994. Heterogeneity in extracellular potassium concentration during early myocardial ischaemia and reperfusion: implications for arrhythmogenesis. Cardiovasc. Res. **28:** 770–777.
64. JANSE, M.J., J. CINCA, *et al* 1979. The 'border zone' in myocardial ischemia. An electrophysiological, metabolic, and histochemical correlation in the pig heart. Circ. Res. **44:** 576–588.
65. WALFRIDSON, H., S. ODMAN & N. LUND. 1985. Myocardial oxygen pressure across the lateral border zone after acute coronary occlusion in pig heart. Adv. Exp. Med. Biol. **191:** 203–210.
66. JANSE, M.J., F.J.L. VAN CAPELLE, *et al*. 1980. Flow of "injury current" and patterns of excitation during early ventricular arrhythmias in acute regional myocardial ischemia in isolated porcine and canine hearts. Circ. Res. **47:** 151–165.
67. JANSE, M.J. & A.G. KLEBER. 1981. Electrophysiological changes and ventricular arrhythmias in the early phase of regional myocardial ischemia. Circ. Res. **49:** 1069–1081.
68. KLEBER, A.G. 1987. Conduction of the impulse in the ischemia myocardium: implications for malignant ventricular arrhythmias. Experientia **43:** 1056–1061.
69. COSTEAS, C., N.S. PETERS, B. WALDECKER, *et al*. 1997. Mechanisms causing sustained ventricular tachycardia with multiple QRS morphologies. Circulation **96:** 3721–3731.
70. TRENOR, B., J.M. FERRERO, Jr. B. RODRÍGUEZ & F. MONTILLA. 2005. Effect of pinacidil on reentrant arrhythmias generated during acute myocardial ischemia. Ann. Biomed. Eng **33:** 897–906.

71. WILKENSKY, R.L., J. TRANUM-JENSEN, et al. 1986. The subendocardial border zone during acute ischemia of the rabbit heart: an electrophysiologic, metabolic and morphologic correlative study. Circulation **74:** 1137–1146.
72. HILL, J.L. & L.S. GETTES. 1980. Effect of acute coronary artery occlusion on local myocardial extracellular K^+ activity in swine. Circulation **61:** 768–778.
73. GILMOUR, R.F., Jr. & D.P. ZIPES. 1980. Different electrophysiological responses of canine endocardium and epicardium to combined hyperkalemia, hypoxia, and acidosis. Circ. Res. **46:** 814–825.
74. KIMURA, S., A.L. BASSETT, T. KOHYA, et al. 1986. Simultaneous recording of action potentials from endocardium and epicardium during ischemia in the isolated cat ventricle: relation of temporal electrophysiologic heterogeneities to arrhythmias. Circulation **74:** 401–409.
75. SCHAAPHERDER, A.F.M., C.A. SCHUMACHER, R. CORONEL & J.W.T. FIOLET. 1990. Transmural heterogeneity of extracellular $[K^+]$ and pH and myocardial energy metabolism in the isolated rat heart during acute global ischemia; dependence on gaseous environment. Bas. Res. Cardiol. **85:** 33–44.
76. FURUKAWA, T., S. KIMURA, N. FURUKAWA, et al. 1991. Role of cardiac ATP-regulated potassium channels in differential responses of endocardial and epicardial cells to ischemia. Circ Res. **68:** 1693–1702.
77. BEHRENS, S., C. LI & M.R. FRANZ. 1997. Effects of myocardial ischemia on ventricular fibrillation inducibility and defibrillation efficacy. J. Am. Coll. Cardiol. **29:** 817–824.
78. CHEN, P.S., N. SHIBATA, E.G. DIXON, et al. 1986. Comparison of the defibrillation threshold and the upper limit of ventricular vulnerability. Circulation **73:** 1022–1028.
79. HWANG, C., C.D. SWERDLOW, R.M. KASS, et al. 1994. Upper limit of vulnerability reliably predicts the defibrillation threshold in humans. Circulation **90:** 2308–2314.
80. EFIMOV, I.R., Y. CHENG, et al. 1998. Virtual electrode-induced phase singularity: a basic mechanism of defibrillation failure. Circ. Res. **82:** 918–925.
81. RODRÍGUEZ, B., L. LI, J.C. EASON, et al. 2005. Differences between left and right ventricular chamber geometry affect cardiac vulnerability to electric shocks. Circ. Res. **97:** 168–175.
82. TRAYANOVA, N. 2001. Concepts of ventricular defibrillation. Phil. Trans. Roy. Soc. Lond. **359:** 1327–1337.
83. SKOUIBINE, K., N.A. TRAYANOVA & P. MOORE. 2000. Success and failure of the defibrillation shock: insights from a simulation study. J. Cardiovasc. Electrophysiol. **11:** 785–796.
84. TRAYANOVA, N.A., J.C. EASON & F. AGUEL. 2002. Computer simulations of cardiac defibrillation: A look inside the heart. Comput. Visual Sci. **4:** 259–270.
85. RODRÍGUEZ, B. & N. TRAYANOVA. 2003. Upper limit of vulnerability in a defibrillation model of the rabbit ventricles. J. Electrocardiol. **36**(Suppl): 51–56.
86. TRAYANOVA, N., F. AGUEL, C. LARSON & C. HARO. 2004. Modeling cardiac defibrillation: an inquiry into post-shock dynamics. *In* Cardiac Electrophysiology: From Cell to Bedside. D.P. Zipes & J. Jalife, Eds.: 282–291. Fourth edition. W.B. Saunders. Philadelphia.
87. PLONSEY, R. 1989. The use of a bidomain model for the study of excitable media. Lec. Math. Life Sci. **21:** 123–149.

88. WIKSWO, J.P., Jr., S.F. LIN & R.A. ABBAS. 1995. Virtual electrodes in cardiac tissue: a common mechanism for anodal and cathodal stimulation. Biophys. J. **69:** 2195–2210.
89. EFIMOV, I.R., Y. CHENG, D.R. Van WAGONER, *et al.* 1998. Virtual electrode-induced phase singularity: a basic mechanism of defibrillation failure. Circ. Res. **82:** 918–925.
90. CHENG, Y., K.A. MOWREY, *et al.* 2002. Mechanisms of shock-induced arrhythmogenesis during acute global ischemia. Am. J. Physiol. Heart Circ. Physiol. **282:** H2141–H2151.
91. CHENG, Y., K.A. MOWREY, D.R. VAN WAGONER, *et al.* 1999. Virtual electrode-induced reexcitation: a mechanism of defibrillation. Circ. Res. **85:** 1056–1066.
92. EFIMOV, I.R., F. AGUEL Y. CHENG, *et al.* 2000. Virtual electrode polarization in the far field: implications for external defibrillation. Am. J. Physiol. Heart Circ. Physiol. **279:** H1055–H1070.
93. EVANS, F.G., R.E. IDEKER & R.A. GRAY. 2002. Effect of shock-induced changes in transmembrane potential on reentrant waves and outcome during cardioversion of isolated rabbit hearts. J. Cardiovasc. Electrophysiol. **13:** 1118–1127.
94. LINDBLOM, A.E., F. AGUEL & N.A. TRAYANOVA. 2001. Virtual electrode polarization leads to reentry in the far field. J. Cardiovasc. Electrophysiol. **12:** 946–956.
95. ROTH, B.J. 2000. An S1 gradient of refractoriness is not essential for reentry induction by an S2 stimulus. IEEE Trans. Biomed. Eng. **47:** 820–821.
96. RODRÍGUEZ, B., B.M. TICE, R. BLAKE, *et al.* 2006. Vulnerability to electric shocks in regional ischemia. Heart Rhythm Abstract. **3(5):** 5226.

Cardiovascular Therapeutic Aspects of Cell Therapy and Stem Cells

LIOR GEPSTEIN

The Bruce Rappaport Institute in the Medical Sciences, Faculty of Medicine, Technion, Israel Institute of Technology, and the Cardiology Department, Rambam Medical Center, Haifa 31096, Israel

ABSTRACT: The recent advancements in stem cell biology, molecular and cell biology, and tissue engineering have paved the way to the development of a new biomedical discipline: regenerative medicine. The heart represents an attractive candidate for this emerging discipline since these emerging technologies could be used to potentially treat a variety of myocardial disorders. Here we describe our efforts in using stem cell and cell therapy strategies to restore the myocardial electromechanical properties. Specifically, our research has focused on the potential role of human embryonic stem cells (hESC) for myocardial regeneration (for the treatment of heart failure) and on using genetically engineered cell grafts to modify the myocardial electrophysiological properties (for the treatment of cardiac arrhythmias). The recently described hESC lines are unique pluripotent cell lines that can be propagated in the undifferentiated state in culture and coaxed to differentiate into cell derivatives of all three germ layers, including cardiomyocytes. The current article describes this unique cardiomyocyte differentiating system and details the molecular, ultrastructural, and functional properties of the generated hESC-derived cardiomyocytes (hESC-CMs). The ability of the hESC-CMs to integrate structurally and functionally with host cardiomyocytes in both *in vitro* and *in vivo* studies will be described as well as their ability to restore the myocardial electromechanical function in animal models of diseased hearts. We will next present detailed *in vitro, in vivo*, and computer simulation studies performed in our laboratory testing the hypothesis that cell grafts, engineered to express specific ion channels, can be used to modify the myocardial electrophysiological properties of cardiac tissue. The potential and drawbacks of this novel approach for the treatment of both tachyarrhythmias (using cell grafts expressing potassium channels) and bradyarrhythmias (using hESC coaxed to differentiate into pacemaking cells or conducting tissue) will be described.

KEYWORDS: stem cells; tissue engineering; human embryonic stem cells; heart failure; ion channels; arrhythmias

Address for correspondence: Prof. Lior Gepstein, M.D., Ph.D., The Shonis Family Research Laboratory for Cardiac Electrophysiology and Regenerative Medicine. The Bruce Rappaport Institute in the Medical Sciences, Faculty of Medicine, Technion, Israel Institute of Technology, and the Cardiology Department, Rambam Medical Center, Haifa 32000, Israel. Voice: 972-4-8295303; fax: 972-4-852-4758.
  e-mail: gepsteinl@medicine.ucsf.edu

INTRODUCTION

Regenerative medicine is an exciting new biomedicine discipline that attempts to capitalize on the recent developments in stem cell biology, cell therapy, and tissue engineering to devise methods to regenerate or modify the function of diseased tissues and organs. The heart represents an attractive candidate for these emerging technologies due to the magnitude of the clinical problem (with cardiovascular disease being the leading cause for morbidity and mortality in the Western world), the readily accessibility of the heart (using surgery or minimally invasive percutaneous catheterization procedures), and the theoretical ability to target a variety of cardiovascular disorders (such as ischemic heart disease, congestive heart failure, and cardiac arrhythmias). Consequentially, cardiac regenerative medicine has raised significant interest for both the scientist studying the heart as well as the practicing physician.

This review will focus on our experimental efforts in this field with specific emphasis on the electrophysiological implications associated with cardiovascular cell therapies. Specifically, we will discuss our research efforts on using the recently described human embryonic stem cells (hESC) for myocardial regeneration (for the treatment of heart failure) and on using the same cells or genetically engineered cell grafts to modify the myocardial electrophysiological properties (for the treatment of both brady- and tachyarrhythmias).

MYOCARDIAL REGENERATION STRATEGIES USING HESC

The heart is one of the least regenerative organs and only a limited number of species (e.g., newts and zebrafish) is capable of myocardial self-renewal. Unfortunately, we as humans can only venerate on the ability of these organisms since the human heart has only limited regenerative capacity. Consequentially, any significant loss of heart cells is mostly irreversible and may lead to progressive loss of ventricular function and finally to the development of heart failure. Congestive heart failure is a growing epidemic that affects more than 5 million Americans and is associated with significant morbidity and mortality.[1] Despite advances in the pharmacological, interventional, and surgical therapeutic measures, the prognosis for heart failure patients remains poor. With the chronic lack of organ donors limiting the number of patients that could benefit from heart transplantations, the development of new therapeutic strategies for the treatment of heart failure has become imperative.

Cell therapy is emerging as a novel therapeutic paradigm for myocardial repair. The rationale behind the cell replacement approach is based on the assumption that an increase in the number of functional myocytes within the diseased area may potentially improve the mechanical properties of this compromised region.[2–5] Based on this assumption, a number of cell types have been suggested as a potential source for tissue grafting, including skeletal myoblasts,[6,7] fetal cardiomyocytes,[8–11] smooth muscle cells,[12] murine embryonic stem cells,[13] and bone marrow-derived stromal[14,15] and hematopoietic[16,17] stem cells. A major limitation to the clinical application of this approach, however, is the lack of sources for human cardiomyocytes and the limited evidence for functional integration of donor cells to the host network of cardiac tissue.

Most of the cell types discussed above are stem cells and therefore share a number of properties.[18] First, they are capable of self-renewal, giving rise to stem cell progeny with similar properties. Second, stem cells are clonogenic with each stem cell being able to form a colony in which all progeny derived from this single cell have identical genetic constitution. Third, they are capable of differentiation into one or more mature cell types. The different stem cells can be categorized anatomically, functionally, or by different surface markers, transcription factors, and the proteins they express. One clear division of the stem cell family is between those present in adult somatic tissue known as adult stem cells and those isolated from the early-stage embryo known as embryonic stem cells (ESC).

Although adult stem cells have been found to be more versatile than originally believed, they typically can differentiate to a relatively limited number of cell types. HESC, on the other hand, are pluripotent stem cell lines that were derived from human blastocytes.[19,20] These unique cells have the ability to be propagated *in vitro* in the undifferentiated state under special conditions and coaxed to differentiate into cell-derivatives of all three germ layers.[19–21] Recently, using the embryoid body (EB) differentiation system, we were able to establish a reproducible spontaneous cardiomyocyte differentiating system from these unique cells.[22] Briefly, the hESC are cultured in suspension for 7–10 days where they form the three-dimensional differentiating cell aggregates (EBs). During this period, the culture conditions could be manipulated to assess the effects of different growth factors and physical stimuli to augment cardiomyocyte yield. The EBs are then cultured on gelatin-covered plates and in ∼10% of EBs, spontaneously contracting areas could be identified.

The contracting areas within the EBs were demonstrated to display molecular, structural, and functional properties of early-stage cardiomyocytes phenotype.[22] Several lines of evidence confirmed the cardiomyocyte nature of the cells within the beating EBs. RT-PCR studies demonstrated the expression of cardiac-specific transcription factors (such as GATA4 and Nkx2.5) and cardiac-specific structural genes (cTnI, cTnT, ANP, MLC-2V, MLC-2a). Gene expression analysis during the *in vitro* cardiomyocyte differentiation process of the hESC revealed a reproducible developmental temporal pattern.[23] This was manifested initially by a gradual decrease in the expression of undifferentiated stem cell markers such as OCT-4, coupled with an early increase, during the suspension phase, in the expression of known cardiogenic-inducing growth factors such as Wnt11 and BMP-2. This was followed by expression of cardiac-specific transcription factors (Nkx2.5, Mef2c, and GATA4) and finally by the expression of cardiac-specific structural genes, such as ANP and myosin heavy chains (MHC).

Immunostaining studies of cells isolated from the contracting areas within the EBs confirmed the presence of cardiac-specific proteins (MHC, sarcomeric α-actinin, desmin, cTnI, and ANP). These studies also demonstrated the presence of early cardiac morphology with a typical early-striated staining pattern. Transmission electron microscopy of EBs at varying developmental stages showed the progressive ultrastructural maturation from an irregular myofilament distribution to a more mature sarcomeric organization in late-stage EBs.[24] Interestingly, in parallel to this ultrastructural maturation process, we could also observe a reproducible temporal pattern of early cardiomyocyte cell proliferation, cell-cycle withdrawal, and cell hypertrophys and structural maturation.

Several functional assays including extracellular and intracellular electrophysiological recordings, calcium imaging, and pharmacological studies clearly demonstrated that the contracting areas within the EBs display functional properties consistent with an early-stage human cardiac phenotype. These studies also revealed important insights to the mechanism of automaticity, excitability, and repolarization in these developing cardiomyocytes as well as calcium handling and electromechanical coupling. More recently, we have demonstrated that this system is not limited to the differentiation of isolated cardiomyocyte cells. Using a high-resolution microelectrode array (MEA) mapping technique, we demonstrated the presence of a functional cardiomyocyte syncytium with stable pacemaker activity and synchronous action potential propagation within the beating EB.[25]

Optimal functional improvement following cell grafting would require structural, electrophysiological, and mechanical coupling of donor cells to the existing network of host cardiomyocytes. In a recent study, we tested the ability of the hESC-derived cardiomyocytes to integrate structurally and functionally with host cardiac tissue both *in vitro* and *in vivo*.[26] The ability of the hESC cardiomyocytes to form electromechanical connections with primary cardiac cultures was assessed in a high-resolution *in vitro* co-culturing system. Primary cultures were created from neonatal rat ventricular myocytes. The contracting areas within the EBs were then mechanically dissected and added to the co-cultures. Interestingly, within 24-h postgrafting, we could detect synchronous contraction in the co-cultures that persisted for several weeks.

To further elucidate the functional interaction within the co-cultures we used the MEA mapping technique. Detailed activation mapping demonstrated tight, long-term electromechanical coupling with electrical activation propagating between the rat and human cardiomyocyte tissues. Immunostaining studies demonstrated that this coupling results from the generation of gap junctions (the protein structures responsible for intercellular electrical coupling) between the rat and human cardiomyocytes.

Despite the enormous potential demonstrated by the hESC and the fact that their cardiomyocyte derivatives have the potential to fulfill most of the properties of the ideal donor cell, a number of critical obstacles needs to be overcome prior to clinical application. Some of these obstacles are described below.

Directed Differentiation

Although cardiomyocytes can be reproducibly generated from the hESC using the EB differentiating system, these cells typically account for only a minority of the total population within the differentiating EBs. Thus, initially strategies need to be developed for directing and augmenting hESC differentiation into the cardiac lineage. Possible strategies for increasing cardiomyocyte yield may include the use of different growth factors, overexpression of cardiac transcription factors, co-culturing with feeder layers, and mechanical factors.[23]

Cardiomyocyte Selection

Although the strategies described above may result in augmentation of the cardiomyocyte yield, it is unlikely that the degree of purity that will be achieved would be sufficient for clinical purposes. Since the contracting areas derived from hESC comprise a mixed population of cells, selection strategies are crucial not only for increasing cardiomyocyte numbers but also for preventing the presence of other cell derivatives as well as ensuring the absence of pluripotent stem cells carrying the risk of teratomas. An elegant strategy to achieve this goal was demonstrated in the mouse ESC model by Field's group using a genetic selection strategy. Using a cardiac-specific promoter driving the expression of a selection marker (antibiotic resistance), they were able to select the differentiating cardiomyocytes with a purity $> 99\%$. We and others are currently using similar concepts to try and establish similar transgenic hESC lines (unpublished data).

Upscaling

The human left ventricle contains more than 5×10^9 cardiomyocytes. Given the fact that a typical myocardial infarct that results in development of heart failure may result in loss of more than 25% of cardiac cells, cell transplantation strategies aiming to completely regenerate the myocardium would therefore require several hundred million cells. Moreover, transplantation of an even greater number of cells may be required to replace this cell loss because of the relatively low survival rate of the grafted cells. Strategies to increase the number of cardiomyocytes may theoretically be employed at different levels:

by increasing the number of undifferentiated hESC used, by increasing the percentage of hESC differentiating to the cardiac lineage, by increasing the ability of the cardiomyocytes to proliferate, by upscaling the entire process using bioreactors, and by improving the long-term survival of the cells following cell grafting.

Prevention of Immune Rejection

Although initial studies suggested that hESC-derived tissue may be less immunogenic than adult tissue,[27,28] it is still believed that they will be rejected. Strategies aiming at achieving immune tolerance of these cells include establishment of "banks" of major histocompatibility complex (MHC) antigen typed hESC lines, establishment of hematopoeitic chimerism by using hESC-derived hematopoeitic tissues, nuclear transfer technology to establish isogenic lines tailored specifically for each patient, and the generation of universal donor hESC lines.[29] The latter could be achieved by silencing genes associated with the assembly or transcriptional regulation of the MHCs or by inserting or deleting other genes that can modulate the immune response.

HESC-DERIVED CARDIOMYOCYTES AS BIOLOGICAL PACEMAKERS

Abnormalities in cardiac impulse formation or conduction may result in the appearance of abnormally slow heart rate, circulatory failure, and even death. Traditionally, these bradyarrhythmias have been treated by implantation of electronic pacemakers. Despite their proven efficacy and safety profile, these devices are not without limitations. These include the need for a surgical procedure with its associated small but existing risks, the requirement for repeated procedures for battery replacement, and the inability to adjust heart rate and the resulting electrical activation sequence in the same effectiveness as the native pacemaker and cardiac conduction system.

In recent years, a number of innovative gene and cell therapy approaches have emerged as experimental platforms for the creation of potential future biological alternatives to implantable electronic devices.[30,31] These include gene therapy approaches aiming to augment the chronotropic response of existing pacemaking cells to neurohumoral stimulation (by overexpression of the β-adrenergic receptor)[32] or strategies attempting to convert quiescent cardiomyocytes into pacemaking cells (by shifting the balance between diastolic repolarization and depolarization currents). Strategies for achieving the latter goal focused either on decreasing the main background diastolic potassium current (Ik1 current)[33] or on augmenting diastolic depolarization currents (by overexpression of the hyperpolarization-activated, cyclic nucleotide-gated (HCN-2) encoded, pacemaker current, I_f).[34]

A possible alternative to the gene therapy approaches discussed above may be the use of cell therapy or tissue engineering. In the case of biological pacemakers, two conceptual strategies were suggested. The first involves a combined cell and gene therapy approach in which cells can initially be transfected *ex vivo* to express the required ionic channels. Proof of concept for this strategy was performed by Rosen's group using mesenchymal stem cells overexpressing the HCN-encoded pacemaker current (If).[35] We chose to use a different approach attempting to drive the differentiation of stem cells into the desired cardiomyocyte lineage (i.e., to generate cardiomyocyte with stable pacemaking properties). In both strategies, the *ex vivo* generated cells will then be used for *in vivo* grafting.

We chose to study the possibility of using the early-stage cardiomyocytes generated during the *in vitro* differentiation of the hESC for biological pacemaking due to their unique properties.[36] These include: (1) the presence of a large magnitude pacemaker (I_f) current as well as a high-density Na current, (2) a low-density background diastolic potassium current (due to the absence of almost any detectable I_{k1} current), (3) adequate positive and negative chronotropic responses to adrenergic and cholinergic stimulation, respectively, and (4) the fact that a mass of tissue (containing a few thousand cells in which spontaneous action potential is generated and propagated) is created allowing grafting of a whole functional unit, rather than isolated cells, thereby increasing the chance of capturing host cardiac tissue (because of issues related to source-sink mismatches).

To test the ability of the hESC-derived cardiomyocytes to function as a biological pacemaker, we established an animal model of slow heart rate in pigs by ablating their atrioventricular (AV) node, the major electrical conduction pathway between the atria and the ventricles. This resulted in complete dissociation between the atrial and ventricular electrical activities and generation of a slow ventricular rate, mimicking the clinical scenario of patients suffering from complete AV block, requiring the implantation of an electronic pacemaker. Following creation of AV block in these animals, we injected the spontaneously contracting EBs into the posterolateral left ventricular wall and monitored their electrocardiogram.

A few days following cell grafting, we could begin to detect episodes of a new ectopic ventricular rhythm. This new ectopic activity was identified in 11 out of the 13 animals studied, and in 6 of them it was characterized by sustained and long-term activity. To prove that this new rhythm was the result of the pacemaking activity of the transplanted cells, we subjected the animals to an additional electrophysiological mapping procedure. Electroanatomical mapping and pathological examination of these hearts confirmed that the source of this new rhythm was the transplanted cells.

More recently our results were corroborated by Xue *et al*.[37] Donor cardiomyocytes derived from hESCs, that were stably transfected to express the green fluorescent protein (GFP), were demonstrated to functionally integrate with otherwise-quiescent, recipient, ventricular cardiomyocytes *in vitro* and to induce rhythmic electrical activity. This phenomenon was also demonstrated *in vivo* following transplantation of the cells in the guinea pig left ventricle (as confirmed by optical mapping).

CELL THERAPY FOR TACHYARRHYTHMIAS

The same approaches that were used to increase the local excitability of the myocardium (by creating a biological pacemaker) could also theoretically be used to modify the myocardial electrophysiological substrate in an attempt to treat different tachyarrhythmias. The feasibility of this strategy was initially evaluated using a number of innovative gene therapy approaches. These studies demonstrated that overexpression of different potassium channels can be used to alter the action potential properties in cardiomyocytes *in vitro*[38–40] and even to suppress cardiac hyperexcitability in rabbit ventricular myocytes.[41] Gene delivery of different potassium channels was suggested as a method to accelerate cardiac repolarization and abbreviate the QT interval for the treatment of the long QT syndrome[42] and was also proposed as a way to reverse the downregulation of potassium channels in cardiomyocytes isolated from failing hearts.[40,43] A more localized *in vivo* application of this strategy was recently proposed by Donahue *et al.*[44] Using viral gene transfer, these investigators demonstrated that the AV nodal conduction properties could be modified by overexpression of $G\alpha_{i2}$, and that this approach represents a novel strategy for ventricular rate control for atrial fibrillation, mimicking the effects of beta-adrenergic antagonists.

An alternative strategy that can theoretically overcome some of the limitations of gene therapy may be the use of cell therapy and tissue engineering to manipulate the local myocardial electrophysiological properties. To assess the feasibility of this concept, we recently tested the ability of genetically engineered cells, overexpressing potassium channels, to modulate the localized cardiac electrophysiological properties. In this study, we studied the effects of adding engineered fibroblasts, transfected to express the voltage-gated potassium channel Kv1.3, on the electrophysiological properties of cardiomyocyte cultures.[45] A high-resolution MEA mapping technique was used to assess the electrophysiological and structural properties of primary neonatal rat ventricular cultures. The transfected fibroblasts were demonstrated to significantly alter the electrophysiological properties of the cardiomyocyte cultures. These changes were manifested by a significant reduction in the local extracellular signal amplitude and by the appearance of multiple local conduction blocks. The location of all conduction blocks correlated with the spatial distribution of the transfected fibroblasts as assessed by vital staining and all of the electrophysiological changes were reversed following the application of a specific Kv1.3 blocker, Charibdotoxin.

SUMMARY

Myocardial cell therapy is emerging as an attractive experimental strategy for a variety of cardiovascular disorders. Here we described our efforts in this field for three different applications: using hESC-derived cardiomyocytes for cell replacement for the treatment of heart failure, using the same cells for regenerating the pacemaking and conduction tissue for the treatment of bradyarrhythmias, and using engineered cells, overexpressing different ionic channels to modulate myocardial electrophysiological properties to suppress tachyarrhythmias. The potential of these approaches and experiments demonstrating proof-of-concept for their feasibility were detailed as well as the potential drawbacks and obstacles required to overcome before any of these strategies can become a clinical reality.

REFERENCES

1. COHN, J.N., M.R. BRISTOW, K.R. CHIEN, et al. 1997. Report of the National Heart, Lung and Blood Institute, special emphasis panel on heart failure research. Circulation **95:** 766–770.
2. LAFLAMME, M.A. & C.E. MURRY 2005. Regenerating the heart. Nat. Biotechnol. **23:** 845–856.
3. DIMMELER, S., A.M. ZEIHER & M.D. SCHNEIDER. 2005. Unchain my heart: the scientific foundations of cardiac repair. J. Clin. Invest. **115:** 572–583.
4. MURRY, C.E., L.J. FIELD & P. MENASCHE. 2005. Cell-based cardiac repair: reflections at the 10-year point. Circulation **112:** 3174–3183.
5. REINLIB, L. & L. FIELD. 2000. Cell transplantation as future therapy for cardiovascular disease: a workshop of the National Heart, Lung, and Blood Institute. Circulation **101:** 182–187.
6. TAYLOR, D.A., B.Z. ATKINS, P. HUNGSPREUGS, et al. 1998. Regenerating functional myocardium: improved performance after skeletal myoblast transplantation. Nat. Med. **4:** 929–933.
7. MENASCHE, P., A.A. HAGEGE, J.T. VILQUIN, et al. 2003. Autologous skeletal myoblast transplantation for severe postinfarction left ventricular dysfunction. J. Am. Coll. Cardiol. **41:** 1078–1083.
8. SOONPAA, M.H., G.Y. KOH, M.G. KLUG, et al. 1994. Formation of nascent intercalated disks between grafted fetal cardiomyocytes and host myocardium. Science **264:** 98–101.
9. KOH, G.Y., M.H. SOONPAA, M.G. KLUG, et al. 1995. Stable fetal cardiomyocyte grafts in the hearts of dystrophic mice and dogs. J. Clin. Invest. **96:** 2034–2042.
10. LEOR, J., M. PATTERSON, M.J. QUINONES, et al. 1996. Transplantation of fetal myocardial tissue into the infarcted myocardium of rat. A potential method for repair of infarcted myocardium? Circulation **94:** II332–II336.
11. ROELL, W., J. LUZ, W. BLOCH, et al. 2002. Cellular cardiomyoplasty improves survival after myocardial injury. Circulation **105:** 2435–2441.
12. LI, R.K., Z.Q. JIA, R.D. WEISEL, et al. 1999. Smooth muscle cell transplantation into myocardial scar tissue improves heart function. J. Mol. Cell. Cardiol. **31:** 513–522.

13. KLUG, M.G., M.H. SOONPAA, G.Y. KOH, *et al.* 1996. Genetically selected cardiomyocytes from differentiating embronic stem cells form stable intracardiac grafts. J. Clin. Invest. **98:** 216–224.
14. WANG, J.S., D. SHUM-TIM, J. GALIPEAU, *et al.* 2000. Marrow stromal cells for cellular cardiomyoplasty: feasibility and potential clinical advantages. J. Thorac. Cardiovasc. Surg. **120:** 999–1005.
15. TOMA, C., M.F. PITTENGER, K.S. CAHILL, *et al.* 2002. Human mesenchymal stem cells differentiate to a cardiomyocyte phenotype in the adult murine heart. Circulation **105:** 93–98.
16. JACKSON, K.A., S.M. MAJKA, H. WANG, *et al.* 2001. Regeneration of ischemic cardiac muscle and vascular endothelium by adult stem cells. J. Clin. Invest. **107:** 1395–1402.
17. ORLIC, D., J. KAJSTURA, S. CHIMENTI, *et al.* 2001. Bone marrow cells regenerate infarcted myocardium. Nature **410:** 701–705.
18. WEISSMAN, I.L., D.J. ANDERSON & F. GAGE. 2001. Stem and progenitor cells: origins, phenotypes, lineage commitments, and transdifferentiations. Annu. Rev. Cell. Dev. Biol. **17:** 387–403.
19. THOMSON, J.A., J. ITSKOVITZ-ELDOR, S.S. SHAPIRO, *et al.* 1998. Embryonic stem cell lines derived from human blastocysts. Science **282:** 1145–1147.
20. REUBINOFF, B.E., M.F. PERA, C.Y. FONG, *et al.* 2000. Embryonic stem cell lines from human blastocysts: somatic differentiation in vitro. Nat. Biotechnol. **18:** 399–404.
21. ITSKOVITZ-ELDOR, J., M. SCHULDINER, D. KARSENTI, *et al.* 2000. Differentiation of human embryonic stem cells into embryoid bodies compromising the three embryonic germ layers. Mol. Med. **6:** 88–95.
22. KEHAT, I., D. KENYAGIN-KARSENTI, M. SNIR, *et al.* 2001. Human embryonic stem cells can differentiate into myocytes with structural and functional properties of cardiomyocytes. J. Clin. Invest. **108:** 407–414.
23. LEV, S., I. KEHAT & L.GEPSTEIN. 2005. Differentiation pathways in human embryonic stem cell-derived cardiomyocytes. Ann. N. Y. Acad. Sci. **1047:** 50–65.
24. SNIR, M., I. KEHAT, A. GEPSTEIN, *et al.* 2003. Assessment of the ultrastructural and proliferative properties of human embryonic stem cell-derived cardiomyocytes. Am. J. Physiol. Heart Circ. Physiol. **285:** H2355–H2363.
25. KEHAT, I., A. GEPSTEIN, A. SPIRA, *et al.* 2002. High-resolution electrophysiological assessment of human embryonic stem cell-derived cardiomyocytes: a novel in vitro model for the study of conduction. Circ. Res. **91:** 659–661.
26. KEHAT, I., L. KHIMOVICH, O. CASPI, *et al.* 2004. Electromechanical integration of cardiomyocytes derived from human embryonic stem cells. Nat. Biotechnol. **22:** 1282–1289.
27. DRUKKER, M., G. KATZ, A. URBACH, *et al.* 2002. Characterization of the expression of MHC proteins in human embryonic stem cells. Proc. Natl. Acad. Sci. USA **99:** 9864–9869.
28. DRUKKER, M., H. KATCHMAN, G. KATZ, *et al.* 2005. Human embryonic stem cells and their differentiated derivatives are less susceptible for immune rejection than adult cells. Stem Cells **24:** 221–229.
29. BRADLEY, J.A., E.M. BOLTON & R.A. PEDERSEN. 2002. Stem cell medicine encounters the immune system. Nat. Rev. Immunol. **2:** 859–871.
30. ROSEN, M.R., P.R. BRINK, I.S. COHEN, *et al.* 2004. Genes, stem cells and biological pacemakers. Cardiovasc. Res. **64:** 12–23.

31. GEPSTEIN, L., Y. FELD & L. YANKELSON. 2004. Somatic gene and cell therapy strategies for the treatment of cardiac arrhythmias. Am. J. Physiol. Heart Circ. Physiol. **286:** H815–H822.
32. EDELBERG, J.M., W.C. AIRD & R.D. ROSENBERG. 1998. Enhancement of murine cardiac chronotropy by the molecular transfer of the human beta2 adrenergic receptor cDNA. J. Clin. Invest. **101:** 337–343.
33. MIAKE, J., E. MARBAN & H.B. NUSS. 2002. Biological pacemaker created by gene transfer. Nature **419:** 132–133.
34. QU, J., A.N. PLOTNIKOV, P. DANILO, et al. 2003. Expression and function of a biological pacemaker in canine heart. Circulation **107:** 1106–1109.
35. POTAPOVA, I., A. PLOTNIKOV, Z. LU, et al. 2004. Human mesenchymal stem cells as a gene delivery system to create cardiac pacemakers. Circ. Res. **94:** 952–959.
36. SATIN, J., I. KEHAT, O. CASPI, et al. 2004. Mechanism of spontaneous excitability in human embryonic stem cell derived cardiomyocytes. J. Physiol. **559:** 479–496.
37. XUE, T., H.C. CHO, F.G. AKAR, et al. 2005. Functional integration of electrically active cardiac derivatives from genetically engineered human embryonic stem cells with quiescent recipient ventricular cardiomyocytes: insights into the development of cell-based pacemakers. Circulation **111:** 11–20.
38. HOPPE, U.C., D.C. JOHNS, E. MARBAN, et al. 1999. Manipulation of cellular excitability by cell fusion: effects of rapid introduction of transient outward K+ current on the guinea pig action potential. Circ. Res. **84:** 964–972.
39. JOHNS, D.C., H.B. NUSS, N. CHIAMVIMONVAT, et al. 1995. Adenovirus-mediated expression of a voltage-gated potassium channel in vitro (rat cardiac myocytes) and in vivo (rat liver). A novel strategy for modifying excitability. J. Clin. Invest. **96:** 1152–1158.
40. NUSS, H.B., D.C. JOHNS, S. KAAB, et al. 1996. Reversal of potassium channel deficiency in cells from failing hearts by adenoviral gene transfer: a prototype for gene therapy for disorders of cardiac excitability and contractility. Gene Ther. **3:** 900–912.
41. NUSS, H.B., E. MARBAN & D.C. JOHNS. 1999. Overexpression of a human potassium channel suppresses cardiac hyperexcitability in rabbit ventricular myocytes. J. Clin. Invest. **103:** 889–896.
42. MAZHARI, R., H.B. NUSS, A.A. ARMOUNDAS, et al. 2002. Ectopic expression of KCNE3 accelerates cardiac repolarization and abbreviates the QT interval. J. Clin. Invest. **109:** 1083–1090.
43. ENNIS, I.L., R.A. LI, A.M. MURPHY, et al. 2002. Dual gene therapy with SERCA1 and Kir2.1 abbreviates excitation without suppressing contractility. J. Clin. Invest. **109:** 393–400.
44. DONAHUE, J.K., A.W. HELDMAN, H. FRASER, et al. 2000. Focal modification of electrical conduction in the heart by viral gene transfer. Nat. Med. **6:** 1395–1398.
45. FELD, Y., M. MELMAED-FRANK, I. KEHAT, et al. 2002. Electrophysiological modulation of cardiomyocytic tissue by transfected fibroblasts expressing potassium channels: a novel strategy to manipulate excitability. Circulation **105:** 522–529.

Adenylyl Cyclase Gene Transfer in Heart Failure

H. KIRK HAMMOND

University of California San Diego, La Jolla CA 92037 and VA San Diego Healthcare System, San Diego, California 92161, USA

ABSTRACT: The rationale for gene transfer of adenylyl cyclase type VI (AC_{VI}) for clinical congestive heart failure (CHF) is based on recent experimental studies that have extended from cultured cardiac myocytes to preclinical studies in animal models of CHF. Over the past several years substantial data have indicated an unexpected and pronounced favorable effect of AC_{VI} expression in cardiovascular disease. Preclinical studies have shown that increased cardiac AC content improves left ventricular function and attenuates deleterious remodeling in the failing heart, and reduces mortality in heart failure and in acute myocardial infarction. A brief review of the preclinical studies that have examined changes associated with increased AC expression in the heart is presented here.

KEYWORDS: gene therapy; contractile function; adenovirus; adenylyl cyclase

INTRODUCTION

Leaders in the field of clinical heart failure have identified adenylyl cyclase type VI (AC_{VI}) as a new target for heart failure therapeutics.[1,2] Since 1998 we have performed substantial preparatory studies anticipating the initiation of a clinical trial of AC_{VI} in patients with severe heart failure. The precise molecular mechanism by which AC_{VI} confers favorable effects in a variety of heart diseases is not well established. Integrative and multidisciplinary approaches, already under way, are likely to provide mechanistic insights in the future.

EFFECTS OF INCREASED CARDIAC AC_{VI} EXPRESSION

AC_{VI} Gene Transfer in Cultured Cardiac Myocytes

In the studies designed to explore the effects of AC_{VI} gene transfer on cardiac myocyte biology, we have used recombinant adenovirus to increase AC_{VI}

Address for correspondence: H. Kirk Hammond, Professor of Medicine, VA San Diego Healthcare System, San Diego, CA 92161. Voice: 858-552-8585; fax: 858-642-6413.
e-mail: khammond@ucsd.edu

expression in neonatal cardiac myocytes.[3] Cardiac myocytes with increased AC_{VI} expression responded to agonist stimulation with marked increases in cAMP production in proportion to protein expressed. Of particular note was that basal (unstimulated) cAMP levels were not at all affected by marked increases in AC_{VI} content.[3,4] This feature is quite different from what is observed after gene transfer of βAR or Gαs (the GTP-binding protein which links β-adrenergic receptor activation with stimulation of AC), which result in sustained activation and steady increases in intracellular cAMP.[5,6]

Cardiac-Directed AC_{VI} Expression—Transgenic Mice

To explore the consequences of long-term and high-level expression of AC_{VI} in the heart, we generated transgenic mice with cardiac-directed expression of AC_{VI}.[4] We were concerned that chronic high level expression of AC_{VI} would be deleterious to cardiac function, as was observed with long-term expression of the β-adrenergic receptor or Gαs—both of which were associated with short-term improvements in cardiac function but, eventually, caused heart failure.[5,6]

Mice with cardiac-directed AC_{VI} expression showed increased cardiac function (FIG. 1) and cardiac myocytes showed increased agonist-stimulated cAMP production. In contrast, basal cAMP and cardiac function were normal, and long-term transgene expression was not associated with abnormal histological findings or deleterious changes in cardiac structure and function.[4]

Cardiomyopathy and Increased Cardiac AC_{VI} Expression

Cardiac-directed expression of Gαq is associated with left ventricular dilation, reduced heart function, and impaired cAMP production, mimicking

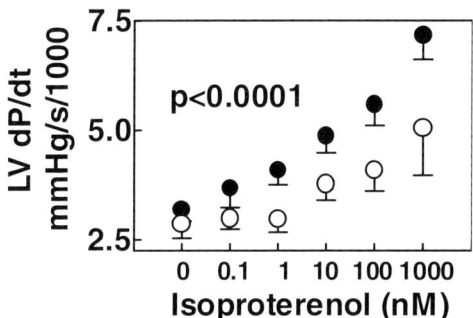

FIGURE 1. Hearts from transgenic mice were isolated and perfused and peak positive left ventricular pressure development (LV dP/dt) in response to isoproterenol was measured. Open circles, data from 6 transgene negative hearts; closed circles, data from 11 AC_{VI} positive hearts. Heart rate was unchanged (not shown).[4]

aspects of clinical heart failure. To determine if increased cardiac myocyte AC_{VI} content increases cardiac function in cardiomyopathy, we cross-bred AC_{VI} transgenic mice and mice with cardiomyopathy induced by cardiac-directed Gαq expression.[7] Cardiac-directed expression of AC_{VI} in this model of heart failure resulted in improved basal cardiac function *in vivo*. Left ventricular peak positive ($P < 0.005$) and negative ($P < 0.04$) dP/dt were increased, and cardiac myocytes showed increased cAMP production. Increased myocardial AC_{VI} content therefore improved cardiac function and responsiveness. Increased left ventricular function was facilitated by restoration of cAMP generating capacity in cardiac myocytes, left ventricular end-diastolic dimensions were decreased ($P<0.0001$). In subsequent studies we also found that cardiac hypertrophy was abrogated ($P<0.004$) and a marked improvement in survival ($P<0.0001$) was observed[8] (FIG. 2).

Abnormalities in calcium handling are dominant in the failing heart, and cardiac AC_{VI} was found to restore SERCA2a affinity for calcium and maximum velocity of cardiac calcium uptake by sarcoplasmic reticulum ($P = 0.012$) in murine dilated cardiomyopathy associated with Gαq.[9] The return to normal of SERCA2a affinity for calcium was associated with decreased phospholamban protein expression and increased phospholamban phosphorylation by PKA activation. These data suggest a mechanism by which AC_{VI}—unlike other signaling elements associated with increased cAMP generation—has a beneficial effect in the failing heart.

Exogenous Gene Transfer of AC_{VI}

Studies of transgenic mice provide data indicating that cardiac-directed expression of AC_{VI} may be beneficial in genetic cardiomyopathy. Two questions remain: (1) Can exogenous gene transfer provide an adequate amount of the transgene to evoke a favorable effect? (2) Is gene transfer of AC_{VI} effective in models of heart failure other than genetic cardiomyopathy?

Can gene AC_{VI} transfer provide increased global left ventricular function? We previously reported that intracoronary delivery of adenovirus vectors provides an efficient means to obtain gene transfer to the heart.[10] We then showed that intracoronary histamine increases the extent of gene transfer compared to the usual methods.[11] Using this delivery protocol, we asked whether we could alter left ventricular contractile function in normal pigs.[11] Animals were instrumented with high fidelity transducers in the left ventricle and flow probes to measure cardiac output. After recovery from surgery (10–12 days) animals underwent isoproterenol infusion and measurement of cardiac output and left ventricular dP/dt. Animals were studied again 12 days after gene transfer. Eighteen animals received intracoronary histamine (25 μg/min, 3 min) followed by intracoronary delivery of 1.4×10^{12} vp of an adenovirus encoding lacZ ($n = 8$) or AC_{VI} ($n = 10$). The vector was delivered by three separate infusions,

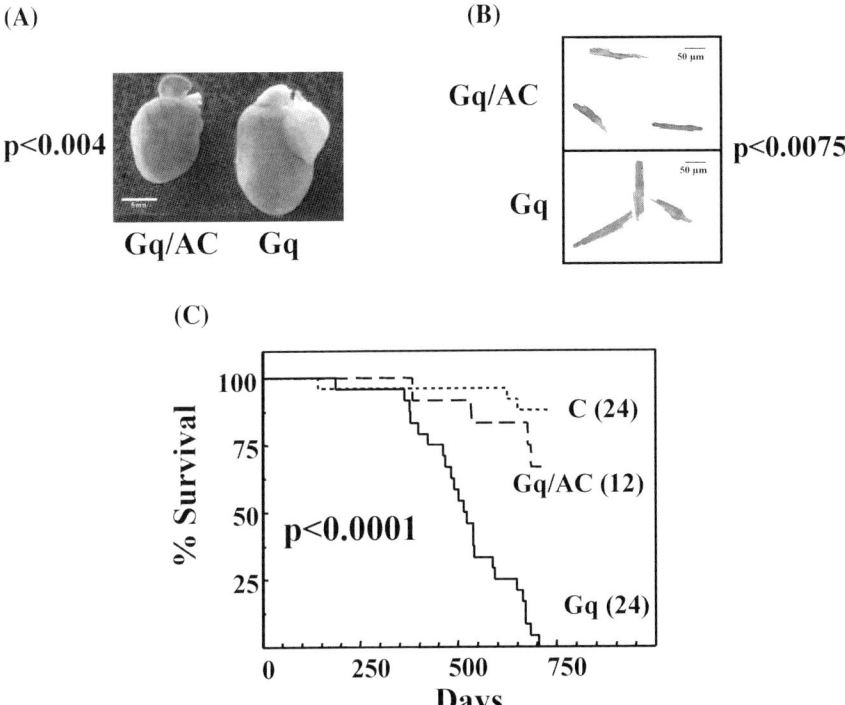

FIGURE 2. (A) Representative hearts from Gq/AC and Gq mice are shown. These hearts were obtained at 11 months of age—the time when mortality increases in Gq mice. These mice were killed electively for this photograph. Western blots of ventricular homogenates from these hearts confirmed increased expression of AC_{VI} and Gq proteins in the Gq/AC mouse and Gq protein in the Gq mouse (data not shown). (B) Representative cardiac myocytes isolated from Gq/AC and Gq mice are shown. These myocytes were obtained at 15 months of age—mice were killed electively for this photograph. Myocyte size was enlarged hearts from Gq animals, but was reduced to normal size by concurrent expression of cardiac AC_{VI} 160 X. (C) Kaplan–Meier curve showing mortality rate in Gq ($n = 24$), Gq/AC ($n = 12$), and Control mice ($n = 24$). Increased survival was associated with expression of cardiac AC_{VI} in cardiomyopathy ($P < 0.0001$). There was no difference in mortality between Gq/AC and Control mice. These data indicate a pronounced favorable effect on survival associated with cardiac-directed AC_{VI} expression in Gq cardiomyopathy.[8]

one in each major coronary artery, with the proportions of the total virus delivered: 50% LAD, 20% LCx, and 30% RCA. Gene transfer of AC_{VI} without precedent histamine was ineffective. Gene transfer of lacZ had no influence on isoproterenol-stimulated left ventricular dP/dt or cardiac output. In contrast, animals that had received intracoronary adenovirus encoding AC_{VI} with precedent histamine showed marked increases in left ventricular contractile function (FIG. 3 A) and cardiac output in response to isoproterenol infusion. In additional studies we demonstrated that increased left ventricular function due

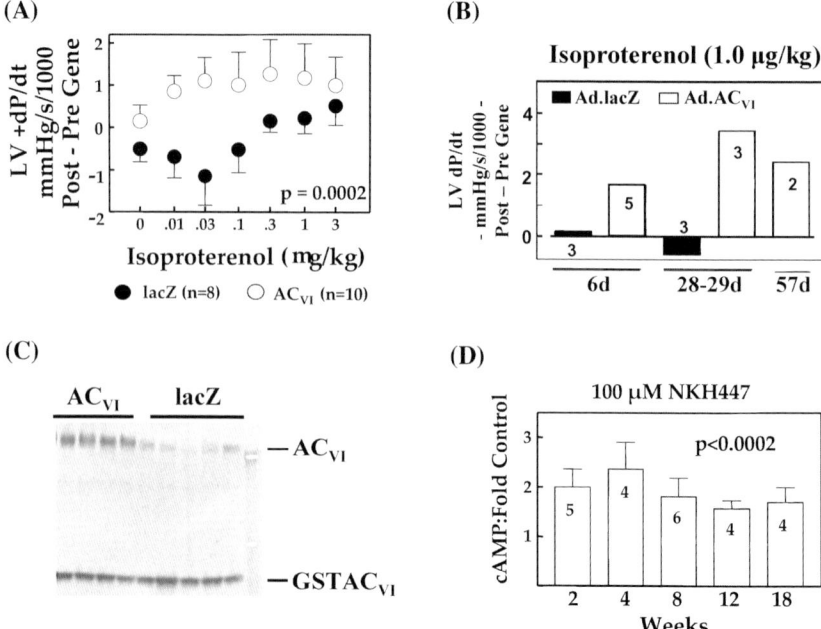

FIGURE 3. (**A**) Data from conscious pigs before and 12 days after intracoronary delivery of 1.4×10^{12} vp adenovirus encoding AC_{VI} (red) or lacZ (blue). The y axis of the graph displays the post gene values minus the pre gene values. Peak positive LV dP/dt in response to doses of infused isoproterenol was measured. Studies were repeated 2–3 times both before and again 12 days after gene transfer (blinded analysis). Gene transfer was preceded by intracoronary histamine infusion. Data indicate that intracoronary gene transfer of AC_{VI} can increase left ventricular function. (**B**) The onset and duration of the physiological effect was studied before and 6, ~30, and 57 days after gene transfer of AC_{VI} or lacZ. The y axis displays the difference in contractility between post- and pregene values. Peak positive LV dP/dt response to isoproterenol (1.0 μg/kg) was measured. Gene transfer of lacZ was not associated with changes in LV dP/dt 6 days or 28 days later. In contrast, AC_{VI} gene transfer was associated with increased LV function within 6 days that increased by 29 days and was still substantial 57 days later. Numbers associated with bars denote animals studied at each time point. Blinded analysis. (**C**) Ten to 14 days after gene transfer, LV AC_{VI} protein content was increased twofold ($P < 0.0007$) ($n = 4$ or 5 per group, as shown). Sucrose gradient centrifugation was used for left ventricular membrane preparation. GST-AC_{VI} was used to evaluate protein loading in each lane. (**D**) Left ventricular samples from pigs receiving gene transfer 2–18 weeks prior showed persistent increased cAMP generation compared to control animals, documenting a prolonged duration of effect of the transgene. NKH447 is a water-soluble forskolin analog that directly stimulates adenylyl cyclase independently of β-adrenergic receptors and Gsα. Numbers associated with bars denote animals studied at each time point.[11]

to gene transfer of AC_{VI} was associated with a twofold increase in left ventricular AC_{VI} protein (FIG. 3 C). A corresponding twofold increase in cAMP generation was also documented, an effect that persisted for the entire 18 weeks of the study[11] (FIG. 3 D). Finally, gene transfer was associated with increases in left ventricular function within 6 days that increased by 29 days and were still substantial 57 days later[11] (FIG. 3 B).

AC_{VI} Gene Transfer in Pacing-Induced Heart Failure

To replicate the strategy envisioned for a future clinical study, we delivered the transgene in an adenovirus vector by intracoronary injection in animals with severe heart failure. To achieve this, pigs underwent pacemaker and left ventricular pressure transducer implantation.[12] Physiological and echocardiographic studies were performed 13 days later, and pacing was initiated (220 bpm). Seven days later, isoproterenol-stimulated left ventricular dP/dt (a measure of contractile function) was reduced ($P < 0.0002$ versus prepacing) documenting left ventricular dysfunction. Pigs then received intracoronary Ad.AC_{VI} (1.4×10^{12} vp; $n = 7$) or saline (PBS; $n = 9$) (randomized, blinded) preceded by an intracoronary infusion of nitroprusside (50 µg/min, 6.4 min) to increase gene transfer.[13] Pacing was continued for 14 days and final studies performed. The *a priori* key end point was change in left ventricular dP/dt during isoproterenol infusion (pre-Ad.AC_{VI} value minus value 14 days later). Pigs receiving Ad.AC_{VI} showed less fall in both peak positive left ventricular dP/dt ($P = 0.0014$; FIG. 4 A) and peak negative left ventricular dP/dt ($P = 0.0008$). Serial echocardiography showed that Ad.AC_{VI} treatment was associated with reduced left ventricular dilation. AC-stimulated cAMP production was increased in left ventricular samples from Ad.AC_{VI}-treated pigs ($P = 0.006$; FIG. 4 B) and gene transfer was confirmed by PCR. These data indicated that AC_{VI} gene transfer attenuates deleterious left ventricular remodeling in pacing-induced heart failure.[12] However, the question remains as to whether or not increased AC_{VI} expression in the presence of severe LV failure can actually *increase* LV function or *reverse* adverse LV remodeling. Furthermore, can AC_{VI} gene transfer have favorable effects in models of heart failure more akin to the types of congestive heart failure (CHF) encountered in clinical settings?

Regulated Expression of Cardiac AC_{VI} in Ischemia-Based CHF

A primary method used to test efficacy has been cross-breeding mice harboring the gene of interest and mice with genetically induced heart failure. In this paradigm, when heart failure is prevented, the candidate gene is said to have "rescued" the failing heart. However, this strategy does not represent treatment since heart failure is never present. No transgene has yet been shown to improve function of a failing heart using this approach. To address this shortcoming, we asked whether activation of cardiac AC_{VI} expression would have favorable effects in the failing heart. Mice with cardiac-directed and regulated (tet-off) expression of AC_{VI} underwent coronary artery ligation to induce heart failure. Five weeks later, heart function was severely impaired,

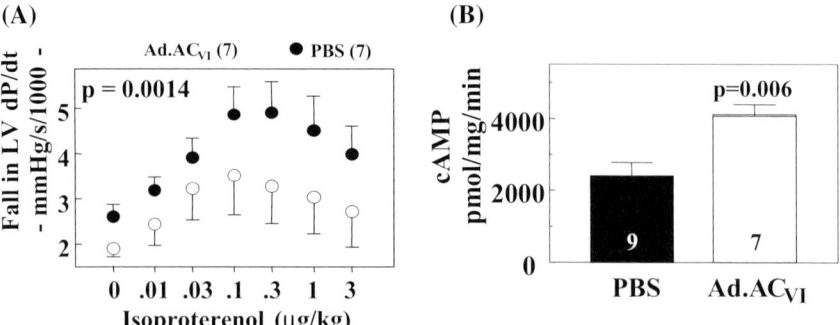

FIGURE 4. (**A**) Left ventricular peak +dP/dt. The y axis represents mean values before pacing *minus* mean values obtained after 21 days of continuous pacing. PBS or Ad.AC$_{VI}$ was given after 7 days of pacing, after documentation of heart failure. Pigs that received intracoronary Ad.AC$_{VI}$ (red circles) had less decrement in LV +dP/dt (less fall in contractile function) than pigs that received intracoronary PBS (blue circles). This was observed through a wide range of infused isoproterenol concentrations and also was evident when AC was directly stimulated with NKH477 (data not shown). Peak negative LV dP/dt was also increased by Ad.AC$_{VI}$ (data not shown). (**B**) Left ventricular cAMP generation. Samples of the left ventricle from animals that had received Ad.AC$_{VI}$ showed increased cAMP generation in response to AC stimulation with NKH477 (10 μM), a water-soluble forskolin analog that directly stimulates adenylyl cyclase independently of β-adrenergic receptors and Gsα. Bars represent mean values (net stimulation, i.e., basal subtracted), error bars denote SEM; numbers on bars denote number of animals per group.[12]

confirming heart failure. We then activated transgene AC expression in one group (AC-On), but not the other (AC-Off). Five weeks later AC expression increased contractile function (and relaxation) of the failing heart. Heart samples showed increased AC$_{VI}$ content and cAMP generation.[14] These data indicate that the use of regulated transgene expression in a clinically relevant model of heart failure provides a powerful and rigorous test of the efficacy of a candidate gene for heart failure treatment. This approach also enables determining the consequence of transgene manipulation in heart failure in a time-sensitive manner.

Effects of Increased Cardiac AC$_{VI}$ in Acute Myocardial Infarction

The use of β-adrenergic receptor stimulating agents, which increase intracellular cAMP, may cause sustained myocardial ischemia due to increased myocardial oxygen demand, or induce ventricular arrhythmias. Whether increased cardiac content of AC$_{VI}$ has a deleterious effect on myocardial ischemia is unknown. However, it is reasonable to expect that increased cAMP generation and hence contractile force, with attendant exacerbation of oxygen demand: supply imbalance would have detrimental consequences in the setting of myocardial infarction by increasing border zone injury and extending infarct size. We therefore performed proximal left coronary ligation in transgenic mice with cardiac-directed expression of AC_{VI} and their transgene negative littermates. We then assessed survival, infarct size, left ventricular size and function, myocardial apoptosis, and incidence of arrhythmias 1 to 7 days after myocardial infarction. Surprisingly, mice with increased AC_{VI} expression had increased survival (AC_{VI}: 74%; Control: 41%; $P = 0.004$; $n = 34$ both groups). Infarct size and myocardial apoptotic rates were similar in AC_{VI} and Control mice. However, AC_{VI} mice showed less left ventricular dilation ($P = 0.0001$) and better left ventricular function ($P < 0.03$). In acute myocardial infarction, increased cardiac AC_{VI} content attenuates adverse LV remodeling, preserves left ventricular contractile reserve and thereby reduces mortality.[15]

Transcriptional Regulation and AC_{VI}

The translational physiological studies reviewed indicate that cardiac-directed expression of AC_{VI} increases stimulated cAMP production, improves heart function, and increases survival in cardiomyopathy. In contrast, pharmacological agents that increase intracellular levels of cAMP have detrimental effects on cardiac function and survival. We wondered whether effects that are not direct consequences of increased cAMP might be responsible for these salutary outcomes associated with AC_{VI} expression. Studies on isolated cardiac myocytes were performed to elucidate the molecular mechanisms for these physiological changes.

Stimulation of cardiac myocytes with isoproterenol and forskolin (to increase cAMP generation) produced effects on gene transcription that were directionally opposite to that seen in the same cells after AC_{VI} gene transfer whether unstimulated or stimulated with the same agents (TABLE 1). For example, while phospholamban, $\beta_1 AR$ and ANF expression were increased by isoproterenol stimulation, they were decreased by AC_{VI} gene transfer. Thus, AC_{VI} expression appears to affect gene expression in a manner not recapitulated by cAMP generation alone.

TABLE 1. Cultured neonatal cardiac myocytes underwent gene transfer with adenovirus encoding AC_{VI} or were stimulated with isoproterenol (Iso; 10μM) or forskolin (fsk; 100 μM). Gene expression of selected genes was evaluated using Northern blotting.[a]

	Fsk or Iso Stimulation	AC_{VI} Gene transfer
PLB mRNA	↑	↓
β1AR mRNA	↑	↓
ANF mRNA	↑	↓

[a]PLB, phopsholamban; β1AR, β1-adrenergic receptor; ANF, atrial natriuretic factor. AC_{VI} Gene transfer vs. stimulation of cAMP generation

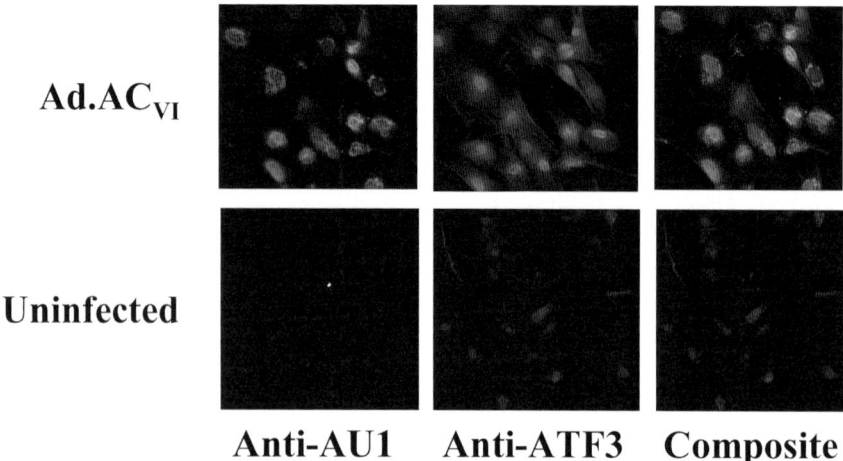

FIGURE 5. ATF3 protein localization after AC_{VI} gene transfer. Immunofluorescence staining with anti-AU1 antibody for the expression of AC_{VI} (green) and anti-ATF3 antibody (red) showed localization of AC_{VI} transgene in cell membrane and nuclear localization of ATF3 in cardiac myocytes overexpressing AC_{VI} (top row). Sparse amounts of endogenous AC_{VI} and ATF3 are seen (bottom row). Reference 16

In further studies[16] we found that gene transfer of AC_{VI} downregulated mRNA and protein expression of phospholamban, an inhibitor of SERCA2a, and that the CRE-like element in the phospholamban promoter was critical for downregulation. Furthermore, AC_{VI} gene transfer was associated with increased expression of ATF3 protein, a suppressor of transcription, which binds to the phosholamban promotor and reduces its activity with subsequent reduced phospholamban expression[16] (FIG. 5). These findings indicate that AC_{VI} has effects on gene transcription that are not directly dependent on cAMP generation.

One of the elements of cardiac-directed AC expression that has been difficult to reconcile in the context of clinical heart failure trials is how such a strategy is protective when most other therapies that increase cAMP have been harmful. Studies of transcriptional regulation are likely to provide important insights. Favorable effects on heart function conferred by AC may not depend directly on cAMP generation, but may reflect instead alterations in transcription of genes that influence contractile function.[9,16–18] Previous work has emphasized the importance of events distal to cAMP generation that are important determinants of left ventricular contractility. Reduced expression of phospholamban,[16] increased expression of SERCA2a, increased myofilament sensitivity to calcium, and alterations in calcium handling[9] are examples of changes that may affect contractility that do not directly or exclusively require changes in cAMP generation.

SUMMARY

The precise molecular mechanisms by which AC_{VI} confers protection to the failing heart are unknown, but sufficient evidence indicates that the deleterious effects associated with other agents that increase intracellular stores of cAMP are circumvented by AC_{VI}. Several logical speculations can be rendered to provide possible explanations for these differences: effector rather than receptor-based gene transfer, reduced cAMP generation *via* inhibitory pathways that are simultaneously influenced by increased AC_{VI} expression, or effects of AC_{VI} on transcription of genes that alter contractile function. The answers to these important questions require additional studies in this evolving field. Preclinical data regarding the relative safety and efficacy of increased AC_{VI} expression in the heart are sufficiently broad and consistent to warrant the initiation of rigorously conducted clinical trials of AC_{VI} gene transfer in patients with stable but severe heart failure.

ACKNOWLEDGMENT

This work was supported by NIH grants P01 HL66941 and HL081741 and a Merit Review Award from the Department of Veteran's Affairs

REFERENCES

1. FELDMAN, A.M. 2002. Adenylyl cyclase: a new target for heart failure therapeutics. Circulation **105**: 1876–1878.
2. SESTI, C. & R.A. KLONER. 2004. Gene therapy in congestive heart failure. Circulation **110**: 242–243.
3. GAO, M., P. PING, S. POST, *et al*. 1998. Increased expression of adenylylcyclase type VI proportionately increases ß-adrenergic receptor-stimulated cAMP in neonatal rat cardiac myocytes. Proc. Natl. Acad. Sci. USA **95**: 1038–1043.
4. GAO, M., N.C. LAI, D.M. ROTH, *et al*. 1999. Adenylylcyclase increases responsiveness to catecholamine stimulation in transgenic mice. Circulation **99**: 1618–1622.
5. IWASE, M., M. UECHI, D.E. VATNER, *et al*. 1997. Cardiomyopathy induced by cardiac Gsα overexpression. Am. J. Physiol. **272**: H585–H589.
6. ENGELHARDT, S., L. HEIN, F. WIESMANN, *et al*. 1999. Progressive hypertrophy and heart failure in beta1-adrenergic receptor transgenic mice. *Proc. Natl. Acad. Sci.* **96**: 7059–7064.
7. ROTH, D.M., M.H. GAO, N.C. LAI, *et al*. 1999. Cardiac-directed adenylyl cyclase expression improves heart function in murine cardiomyopathy. Circulation **99**: 3099–3102.
8. ROTH, D.M., H. BAYAT, J.D. DRUMM, *et al*. 2002. Adenylyl cyclase increases survival in cardiomyopathy. Circulation **105**: 1989–1994.
9. TANG, T., M.H. GAO, D.M. ROTH, *et al*. 2004. AC type VI corrects cardiac sarcoplasmic reticulum calcium uptake defects in cardiomyopathy. Am. J. Physiol. **287**: H1096–H1112.

10. GIORDANO, F., P. PING, M.D. MCKIRNAN, et al. 1996. Intracoronary gene transfer of fibroblast growth factor-5 increases blood flow and contractile function in an ischemic region of the heart. Nat. Med. **2:** 534–539.
11. LAI, N.C., D.M. ROTH, M.H. GAO, et al. 2000. Intracoronary delivery of adenovirus encoding adenylyl cyclase VI increases left ventricular function and cAMP-generating capacity. Circulation **102:** 2396–2402.
12. LAI, N.C., D.M. ROTH, M.H. GAO, et al. 2004. Intracoronary adenovirus encoding AC VI increases left ventricular function in heart failure. Circulation **110:** 330–336.
13. ROTH, D.M., N.C. LAI, M.H. GAO, et al. 2004. Nitroprusside increases gene transfer associated with intracoronary delivery of adenovirus. Human Gene Ther. **15:** 989–994.
14. LAI, N.C., M. SAITO, T. TANG, et al. 2005. Activation of cardiac adenylyl cyclase type VI expression in the presence of severe heart failure increases LV systolic and diastolic function. Circulation **112:**(Suppl II) II–67.
15. TAKAHASHI, T., N.C. LAI, D.M. ROTH, et al. 2005. Increased cardiac adenylyl cyclase expression is associated with increased survival after MI. Circulation **114:** 388–396.
16. GAO, M.H., T. TANG, T. GUO, et al. 2004. AC type VI gene transfer reduces phospholamban expression in cardiac myocytes via activating transcription factor 3. J. Biol. Chem. **279:** 38797–38802.
17. YUE, P., C.S. LONG, R. AUSTIN, et al. 1998. Post-infarction heart failure in the rat is associated with distinct alterations in cardiac myocyte molecular phenotype. J. Mol. Cell. Cardiol. **8:** 1615–1630.
18. LOWES, B.D., E.M. GILBERT, W.T. ABRAHAM, et al. 2002. Myocardial gene expression in dilated cardiomyopathy treated with beta-blocking agents. N. Engl. J. Med. **346:** 1357–1365.

Genetic Engineering and Therapy for Inherited and Acquired Cardiomyopathies

SHARLENE DAY,[a] JENNIFER DAVIS,[b] MARGARET WESTFALL,[b,c] AND JOSEPH METZGER[c]

[a]*Department of Internal Medicine, University of Michigan, Ann Arbor Michigan, 48103, USA*

[b]*Department of Molecular and Integrative Physiology, University of Michigan, Ann Arbor Michigan, 48103, USA*

[c]*Department of Surgery, University of Michigan, Ann Arbor Michigan, 48103, USA*

ABSTRACT: The cardiac myofilaments consist of a highly ordered assembly of proteins that collectively generate force in a calcium-dependent manner. Defects in myofilament function and its regulation have been implicated in various forms of acquired and inherited human heart disease. For example, during cardiac ischemia, cardiac myocyte contractile performance is dramatically downregulated due in part to a reduced sensitivity of the myofilaments to calcium under acidic pH conditions. Over the last several years, the thin filament regulatory protein, troponin I, has been identified as an important mediator of this response. Mutations in troponin I and other sarcomere genes are also linked to several distinct inherited cardiomyopathic phenotypes, including hypertrophic, dilated, and restrictive cardiomyopathies. With the cardiac sarcomere emerging as a central player for such a diverse array of human heart diseases, genetic-based strategies that target the myofilament will likely have broad therapeutic potential. The development of safe vector systems for efficient gene delivery will be a critical hurdle to overcome before these types of therapies can be successfully applied. Nonetheless, studies focusing on the principles of acute genetic engineering of the sarcomere hold value as they lay the essential foundation on which to build potential gene-based therapies for heart disease.

KEYWORDS: myofilament regulation; troponin I; gene delivery; sarcomere; gene-based therapies

Address for correspondence: Joseph M. Metzger, Department of Molecular and Integrative Physiology and Internal Medicine, University of Michigan, 1301 E. Catherine St., Ann Arbor MI 48109-0622. Voice: 734-647-6460; fax: 734-647-6461.
e-mail: metzgerj@umich.edu

INTRODUCTION

Heart disease claims more lives in the United States each year than the next four leading causes of death combined, accounting for one death every 35 s.[1] Coronary heart disease is the most prevalent form of cardiovascular disease, affecting 13 million Americans and claiming the lives of 40% of those who experience a coronary ischemic event in a given year.[1] Heart failure is similarly a highly prevalent and fatal condition that affects 5 million Americans and carries a 1-year mortality rate of 20%. These are staggering statistics, particularly in view of the considerable advances that have been made in medical, device, and surgical therapies for heart disease in the last decade. Clearly there is a continued need to develop novel therapies for cardiovascular diseases that go beyond contemporary medicine. Some investigators contend that we may have reached somewhat of a plateau with conventional treatments and predict a shift in emphasis toward gene-based therapy.[2]

Designing molecular therapies that target the ischemic or failing heart requires an understanding of the mechanisms that govern myocardial contractility and relaxation under both normal and pathological conditions. Acute myocardial ischemia alters key aspects of cardiac cell metabolism that, in turn, result in impaired contractility. Prominent among these is intracellular acidification caused by lactate formation during anaerobic glycolysis and by hydrolysis of high-energy phosphate compounds.[3] When blood flow to the myocardium is acutely compromised, cardiac muscle intracellular pH drops precipitously (from 7.0 to ~6.2), directly depressing myocardial force[4] (FIG. 1 A). This

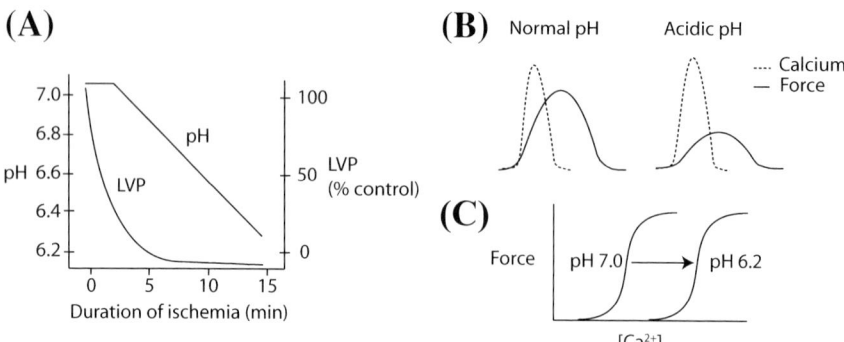

FIGURE 1. *Effects of acidosis on force and calcium.* (**A**) Graphic representation of the precipitous drop in both left ventricular pressure and pH during cardiac ischemia. Adapted from Orchard and Kentish 1990. *Am. J. Physiol.* **258**: C967–C981. (**B**) Effects of acidic pH on force and the Ca^{2+} transient in adult cardiac muscle. Force declines when intracellular pH drops, but the Ca^{2+} transient remains unchanged or may even increase. Thus, there is an uncoupling of excitation and contraction. (**C**) Acidic pH desensitizes the myofilaments to calcium, resulting in a marked rightward shift in the force-Ca^{2+} relationship.

depression in contractility occurs despite an unchanged or even increased intracellular Ca^{2+} transient, indicating a disruption of normal excitation–contraction coupling (FIG. 1 B). The basis for this phenomenon is an uncoupling of the response of the contractile proteins to activating calcium. This is manifest in a marked rightward shift in the force-Ca^{2+} relationship under acidic conditions (FIG. 1 C). In adult cardiac preparations, the pCa (-log $[Ca^{2+}]$) required for 50% maximal activation falls by an average of $\sim$0.12 pCa units for each 0.1 unit drop in pH.[5] In contrast, the contractile function of neonatal heart muscle is less affected than adult myocardium by acidic pH, $\sim$ 0.04 pCa unit per 0.1 unit drop in pH.[5-7] Developmentally regulated transitions in the isoform expression profile for the myofilament protein troponin I (TnI) correlate with shifts in the pH-mediated alteration in the force-Ca^{2+} relationship noted for neonatal and adult myocardium.[8] Thus, elucidation of key structural and functional characteristics of TnI isoforms could form the basis for new molecular therapies to improve contractile function during cardiac ischemia.

The importance of the myofilaments in regulation of cardiac function is further underscored by elucidation of the genetic underpinnings of a broad spectrum of cardiac muscle diseases over the past two decades. Primary inherited cardiomyopathies represent an increasingly recognized cause of "idiopathic" heart failure and are phenotypically categorized into three distinct clinical subtypes: hypertrophic (HCM), dilated (DCM), and restrictive (RCM) cardiomyopathies. While clinical classification of these cardiomyopathies is based predominantly on morphologic and hemodynamic characteristics, many structurally divergent cardiomyopathies share common genetic loci. Mutations in genes encoding contractile, cytoskeletal, calcium cycling, and metabolic proteins have been associated with a variety of cardiomyopathic phenotypes. Of these, sarcomeric gene mutations are the most prevalent and well characterized to date, with over 11 genes identified as causal for multiple cardiomyopathic subtypes[9] (FIG. 2). Since the anatomic and functional changes associated with primary cardiomyopathic diseases are also observed in acquired forms of heart failure (i.e., chronic ischemia, hypertension, diabetes, or valvular disorders), it is likely that altered sarcomere function plays an important role in the pathogenesis of acquired cardiomyopathies as well. Therefore, genetic or molecular strategies that target the sarcomere would be expected to have broad therapeutic benefit.

TnI ISOFORMS AND ACIDOSIS

TnI is the inhibitory subunit of the troponin complex that toggles between actin (diastole) and troponin C (systole) in a Ca^{2+}-dependent manner within the sarcomere.[10] There are two isoforms of TnI that are expressed in the heart at different times during development. Typically, the slow skeletal troponin I isoform (ssTnI) is expressed during the embryonic and early postnatal period.

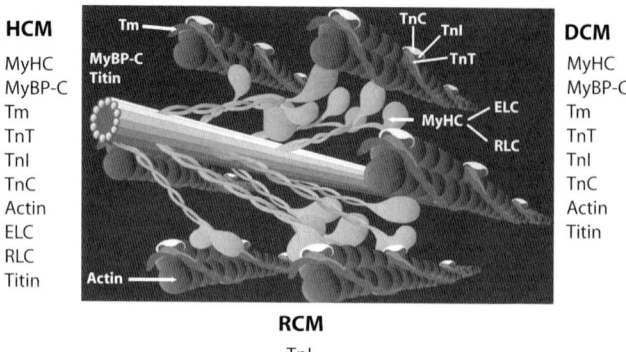

FIGURE 2. Identification and sarcomeric localization of genetic loci harboring mutations linked to inherited cardiomyopathies.

Shortly after birth, there is a transition in expression to the cardiac isoform (cTnI) that persists throughout adult life.[11,12] This TnI isoform transition correlates with the shift in the force-Ca^{2+} relationship in response to changes in pH.[8] In the adult cTnI-expressing heart, contractility is severely depressed during acidosis, largely due a decrease in the sensitivity of the myofilaments to Ca^{2+}. In contrast, the neonatal ssTnI-expressing heart demonstrates less of a decrease in myofilament Ca^{2+} sensitivity in an acidic pH environment compared to the adult heart, and consequently, contractile function is relatively preserved.[8] Although early studies showed a correlation between TnI isoform expression and myofilament pH sensitivity, the direct role played by TnI isoforms in these developmental responses was obscured by concurrent changes in other thin filament proteins over a similar time period.

Genetic engineering of TnI has clearly elucidated its isoform-dependent role in pH-mediated contractile dysfunction. Replacement of cTnI with ssTnI in adult cardiac myocytes using adenoviral-mediated gene transfer results in a marked enhancement of myofilament Ca^{2+} sensitivity at acidic pH.[6] These data are supported by transgenic mouse studies in which replacement of native cTnI with a ssTnI transgene increases papillary muscle tension development during acidosis.[13] Further studies using chimeras of cTnI and ssTnI provide evidence that this pH sensing domain localizes to the carboxyl terminus of cTnI.[14,15] More recently, we have identified a key residue, histidine at position 132 in mouse ssTnI, that uniquely confers acidic pH resistance of the Ca^{2+}-activated myofilament apparatus.[16] Adenoviral gene transfer of a modified ssTnI molecule, in which alanine was substituted for histidine at position 132 (H132A), into adult cardiac myocytes converts the ssTnI to the cTnI phenotype in terms of isometric, Ca^{2+}-activated tension at acidic pH.[16] Similarly, substituting histidine for alanine at codon 164 in cTnI (A164H) by gene transfer results in a modest gain of Ca^{2+}-activated tension at neutral pH, an effect that is accentuated at acidic pH.[16] These data suggest that TnI isoform dependence of pH sensitivity may relate to unique biochemical properties of this histidine residue. Owing to its imidazole side chain, histidine is deprotonated and hydrophobic at neutral pH, and protonated and hydrophilic at acidic pH. Thus the positive charge on histidine during intracellular acidosis could weaken interactions between TnI and arginine or lysine residues in actin, or strengthen interactions with glutamate or aspartate residues in troponin C (TnC), or both (FIG. 3 A). Any of these possibilities would tend to favor a stronger TnI-TnC association, and thus maintenance of contractile activation under acidic pH conditions.

ENGINEERING THE SARCOMERE FOR THE ISCHEMIC AND FAILING HEART

Myocardial ischemia can result in immediate and profound contractile failure, which often persists even after blood flow and intracellular pH have been restored. Existing pharmacological therapies for heart failure associated with ischemia are limited, often carry undesirable proarrhythmic side effects, and increase energy demand in the already metabolically compromised heart.[17,18] Therefore, a genetic-based approach focusing on the sarcomere to improve cardiac function during ischemia could offer an attractive alternative.

Intracellular acidosis is a prominent component of cardiac ischemia and contributes to contractile dysfunction and myocellular injury. Direct enhancement of myocardial function under acidic pH conditions may be advantageous during ischemia. Based on the cellular characterization studies in isolated myocytes, the genetically engineered cardiac TnI molecule, A164H, appears to be a promising therapeutic candidate to test in the ischemic heart. Indeed, recent studies demonstrate a protective effect of this cTnI variant under a variety of pathophysiological conditions in the whole heart *ex vivo* and *in vivo*.[16] Transgenic mice were generated in which ~80–85% of native cTnI was stoichiometrically replaced with cTnI A164H. Mouse hearts were retrograde perfused with an acidic buffer in the context of an *ex vivo* isovolumic heart preparation. Transgenic cTnI A164H mouse hearts were far more resistant to acidosis than nontransgenic controls, demonstrating improved systolic and diastolic performance. *In vivo* hypoxia and acute coronary ischemia studies yielded similar results; improved cardiac contractility in cTnI A164H transgenic mice under both conditions. We recently proposed that direct augmentation of sarcomeric Ca^{2+} activation under acidic pH conditions could account for the results described here.

During global ischemia and subsequent reperfusion in isolated hearts, cTnI A164H hearts demonstrated markedly improved myocardial recovery, attributable to both better contractility and a blunting of postischemic contracture.[16] In addition, transgenic replacement with cTnI A164H was associated

(A)

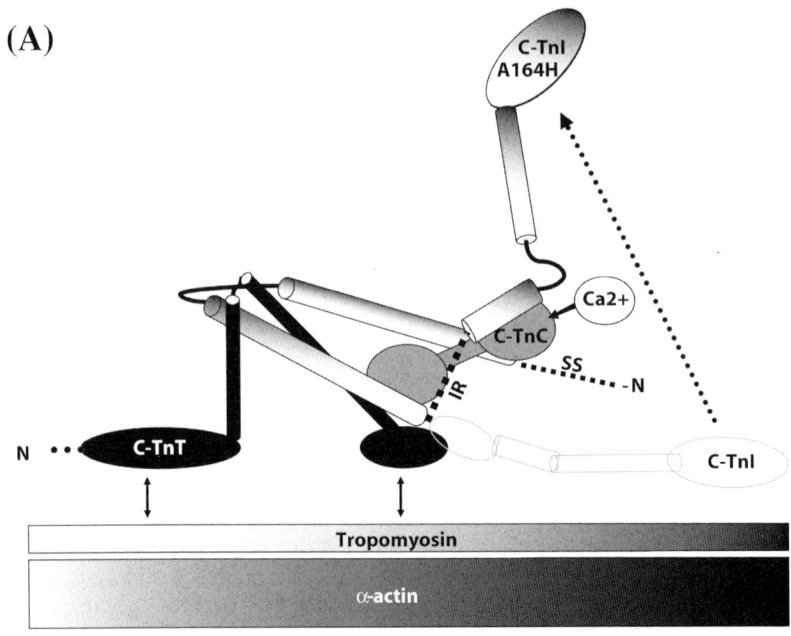

(B)

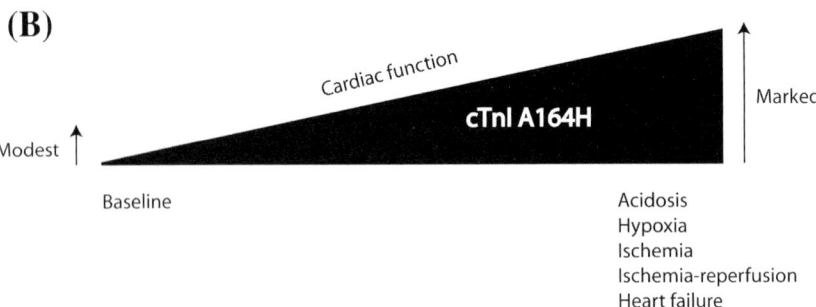

FIGURE 3. *Proposed biochemical and functional effects of cTnI A164H.* (**A**) Schematic representation of the troponin complex and its interactions based on the troponin core crystal structure of Maeda and colleagues (TAKEDA S., A. YAMASHITA, K. MAEDA & Y. MAEDA. 2003. Structure of the core domain of human cardiac troponin in the Ca (z+)-saturated form. Nature **424**: 35–41.). Cardiac troponin I (cTnI) A164H may stabilize the open confirmation, through strengthened interactions with TnC or weakened interactions with actin, or both. These effects are predicted to be greatest at acidic pH when histidine is protonated and hydrophilic. (**B**) Summary of the effects of TnI A164H replacement on cardiac function. The observed improvement in cardiac performance is most pronounced under pathophysiological conditions.

with a significant decrease in ventricular arrhythmias. These beneficial effects of cTnI A164H in the postischemic heart were surprising, given that pH is restored quite rapidly after the onset of reperfusion. Potential pH-independent mechanisms to explain improved cardiac function during reperfusion include better recovery of energetic substrates, or attenuation of the Ca^{2+} overload state characteristic of the postischemic heart. ^{31}P-NMR spectroscopy studies provide evidence that cTnI A164H hearts may be operating in a more economical manner in terms of high-energy phosphate utilization, both under baseline conditions and during reperfusion. Furthermore, cTnI A164H hearts demonstrated important adaptations in Ca^{2+} handling that may have occurred by virtue of a reduced requirement for intracellular activating Ca^{2+}. Collectively, these changes may contribute to improving performance in cTnI A164H transgenic hearts during ischemia–reperfusion.[16]

The A164H substitution in cTnI was also associated with an augmentation in the function of failing mouse hearts after myocardial infarction. Transgenic mice expressing cTnI A164H demonstrated improved systolic function and an attenuated ventricular remodeling and hypertrophic response. Additionally, adenoviral gene transfer of cTnI A164H into failing human cardiac myocytes obtained at the time of cardiac transplantation improved contractility and relaxation and restored a more favorable force–frequency response. Taken together with the above experimental results demonstrating the beneficial effects of the cTnI A164H protein in the acute settings of acidosis, hypoxia, ischemia, and ischemia–reperfusion, these data support the concept that genetic engineering of the sarcomere could offer a viable strategy for treating ischemic heart disease and heart failure. Sarcomere gene-based therapy represents a promising new approach for redressing heart disease, and could stand alone, or perhaps complement other emerging genetic therapies targeting signaling pathways or calcium homeostasis.[19]

SARCOMERE DYSFUNCTION IN INHERITED CARDIOMYOPATHIES

HCM

HCM is the most prevalent inherited cardiovascular disorder, affecting 1 in 500 individuals.[20] HCM carries an overall annual mortality rate of 1%, but accounts for over a quarter of sudden cardiac deaths in young competitive athletes.[21] HCM is phenotypically heterogenous, but is generally characterized by increased left ventricular wall thickness, primarily involving the interventricular septum. Dynamic left ventricular outflow tract obstruction occurs in 30–50% of patients and can exacerbate symptoms of breathlessness and chest pain.[22] The histopathological hallmarks of HCM include myocyte disarray, myocyte hypertrophy, and interstitial fibrosis.

Over 400 mutations in 11 different sarcomeric genes have been identified as causal for HCM, with mutations in β-myosin heavy chain (*MYH7*) and myosin binding protein C (*MYBPC3*) being the most prevalent.[9] Sarcomere mutations are identified in 30–70% of HCM patients, the frequency of which is highly dependent on the characteristics of the study population and the comprehensive nature of the genetic analysis.[23–25] The remaining cases may be due to other as yet unidentified mutations in sarcomere protein genes, or to mutations in other nonsarcomeric genes.[26] While each particular sarcomere gene mutation likely influences the clinical phenotype, establishing genotype–phenotype correlations is confounded by the vast number of mutations and phenotypic diversity of HCM. For example, certain mutations have been associated with a particularly malignant phenotype (*MYH7* R403Q and R719W), and others with a more benign clinical course (*MYH7* L908V, G256E, and V606M, and several *MYBPC3* mutations).[25,27] However, these associations are derived largely from pedigree analyses and may overestimate the correlation in more unselected populations.[23,24] Gene dosage does appear to influence the severity of the HCM phenotype. Patients who are homozygous for a mutation or compound heterozygous for different mutations (2–5% of the HCM population) are diagnosed at a younger age, have more hypertrophy, and carry a poorer prognosis than do patients with only one mutant allele.[23,28] Other proposed important influences on HCM phenotype include environmental factors and genetic modifiers.[25,29]

Significant advances have been made in elucidating the molecular basis for HCM through the use of a variety of experimental biochemical, cellular, and animal models. Collectively, these models suggest that sarcomere gene mutations act via a dominant negative mechanism resulting in a change of function at the molecular level. Biophysical studies indicate that most HCM-linked mutations directly heighten myofilament Ca^{2+} sensitivity causing increased force production at lower $[Ca^{2+}]_i$. The magnitude of change in Ca^{2+} sensitivity results in a corresponding increase in contractility and an impairment of relaxation in the intact cell.[30] Increased myofilament Ca^{2+} sensitivity is the primary cause of slowed relaxation kinetics seen in the unloaded cardiomyocyte, and likely contributes to diastolic dysfunction in the whole heart. While the pathways leading from altered Ca^{2+} sensitivity to myocardial remodeling are incompletely understood, there is evidence to support mechanisms involving altered Ca^{2+} homeostasis,[31,32] remodeling of the cardiac action potential,[33] increased energetic demands,[34,35] and activation of hypertrophy signaling pathways.[25]

DCM

DCM affects fewer individuals (∼1 in 2800) than HCM, but carries a worse prognosis with only 50% survival at 5 years after diagnosis.[1] DCM is inherited in about 35% of cases, most commonly in an autosomal dominant fashion.[25] DCM is characterized by ventricular wall thinning and dilation and impaired contractile function. The histopathological findings are often nonspecific, revealing myocyte hypertrophy, myocyte degeneration, and interstitial fibrosis. The first identified mutations linked to DCM were in genes encoding for cytoskeletal proteins.[36] This led to the hypothesis that the pathogenesis of DCM may be related to impaired force transmission between the contractile apparatus, the extracellular matrix, and the sarcolemmal membrane. However, subsequent identification of mutations in genes (25 genetic loci to date) encoding proteins with diverse functions suggested the existence of several pathways that could independently lead to DCM. Seven of the loci linked to DCM encode for sarcomeric proteins actin, β-MHC, α-MHC, titin, cTnT, cardiac troponin C (cTnC), and α-tropomyosin (Tm).[9,37,38] In recent biochemical studies, DCM-causing mutations in Tm, TnT, and TnC uniformly result in decreased myofilament Ca^{2+} sensitivity and depressed myofibrillar function after thin filament reconstitution.[39,40] These changes are quantitatively opposite to those resulting from HCM-associated thin filament mutations, suggesting that distinct changes in myofilament activation may account, at least in part, for the divergent clinical phenotypes observed in DCM compared to HCM.

RCM

RCM is the least common inherited cardiomyopathy (∼5% of all cardiomyopathies) but carries the worst prognosis.[25] Idiopathic RCM typically presents early in childhood and frequently results in early transplantation or sudden cardiac death. RCM is characterized by decreased myocardial compliance and diastolic dysfunction, but normal to near-normal systolic function and myocardial wall thickness. Extensive interstitial fibrosis is a common histopathological finding.[41] A recent study identified six different mutations (L144Q, R145W, A171T, K178E, D190G, and R192H) in the cTnI gene that were linked to both RCM and HCM phenotypes within the same families.[42] Many of these family members presented with early heart failure, and patients with the L144Q, D190G, and R192H cTnI mutations all died of sudden cardiac death before the fourth decade of life. The molecular basis for RCM has not been well characterized, although biochemical studies using reconstituted contractile systems from two different laboratories indicate that RCM mutations in cTnI result in a potent increase in myofilament Ca^{2+} sensitivity of force generation and ATPase activity.[43,44] The degree of myofilament Ca^{2+} hypersensitivity resulting from these cTnI mutations is quantitatively greater than that observed in similar previous experiments using exclusively HCM-causing cTnI mutations (R145G, R145Q, R162W, ΔK183, S199N, G203S, and K206Q). These data suggest that the magnitude of change in myofilament Ca^{2+} sensitivity may be a stimulus for the differentiation of distinct HCM or RCM pathways. However, the association of the same cTnI mutation with either HCM or RCM within the same family also suggests that additional genetic or environmental factors are important in modifying the disease phenotype.

GENETIC ENGINEERING FOR INHERITED CARDIOMYOPATHIES

There are a number of genetic therapies for heart failure that have been tested in a variety of animal models, most targeting components of calcium handling or the adrenergic signaling cascade.[19,45,46] Interruption of hypertrophic signaling pathways has also been achieved in animal models of pressure overload hypertrophy.[47–49] Similarly directed sarcomeric-based therapies may also remediate the functional and structural remodeling processes associated with inherited cardiomyopathies. The sarcomere maintains stoichiometric proportions between each protein constituent. Introduction of an exogenous gene encoding a sarcomere protein into an individual myocyte *in vitro*, or into the whole heart *in vivo*, results in stoichiometric replacement rather than overexpression of the contractile protein, such that the total amount of the targeted protein remains unchanged.[50,51] Endogenous myofilament turnover lays the framework for the development of sarcomere gene transfer approaches for inherited cardiomyopathies. Exogenous expression of a wild-type allele could in principle "compete off" a mutant allele of the same gene, thereby limiting the effective mutant gene dosage. Alternatively, introduction of a functionally complementary sarcomere gene allele might be able to counter the effects of a particular mutant allele on force production or propagation. For example, "normalization" of myofilament Ca^{2+} sensitivity might be achieved by introducing a sarcomeric variant that heightens Ca^{2+} sensitivity into a heart expressing a DCM-linked sarcomere mutation associated with reduced Ca^{2+} sensitivity and vice versa. These sarcomere gene-based therapeutic approaches, while theoretically promising, await further experimental study.

SUMMARY

The myofilaments play a central role in the regulation of cardiac function in acquired and inherited forms of human heart disease. Contractile dysfunction during cardiac ischemia is directly attributable to an uncoupling of the response of the contractile proteins to activating calcium. TnI is an important mediator of this response, and expression of different TnI isoforms during cardiac development are largely responsible for the divergent effects of acidic pH observed in neonatal versus adult myocardium. Recent studies highlight the importance of a single C-terminal amino acid (A164 in cTnI and H132 in ssTnI) in regulating cardiac function during acidosis, ischemia, and heart failure. Mutations in genes encoding a number of sarcomere proteins trigger various forms of inherited cardiomyopathies, including hypertrophic, dilated, and restrictive subtypes. Thus, altered sarcomere function forms the pathogenetic basis of a broad spectrum of cardiac muscle diseases, and provides an appealing target for gene-based therapies. The capability of the sarcomere to incorporate exogenous proteins and maintain stoichiometric proportions would facilitate such therapeutic approaches. Further studies focusing on sarcomere genetic engineering in the cell and whole organ, as well as on development of safe and efficient vector systems for gene delivery into the cardiac myocyte *in vivo*, will lay the foundation for new gene-based therapies for common acquired and inherited forms of heart disease.

ACKNOWLEDGMENTS

This work was supported by grants from the NIH and the American Heart Association.

REFERENCES

1. THOM, T., N. HAASE, et al. 2006. Heart disease and stroke statistics–2006 Update. A Report From the American Heart Association Statistics Committee and Stroke Statistics Subcommittee Circulation.
2. MITK, A.M. 2006. Do lackluster trial findings mean new avenues are needed for heart research? JAMA **295**: 611–612.
3. KATZ, A. 2001. Physiology of the Heart. Lippincott Williams and Wilkins. Philadelphia.
4. ORCHARD, C.H. & J.C. KENTISH. 1990. Effects of changes of pH on the contractile function of cardiac muscle. Am. J. Physiol. **258**: C967–C981.
5. SOLARO, R.J., J.A. LEE, J.C. KENTISH & D.G. ALLEN 1988. Effects of acidosis on ventricular muscle from adult and neonatal rats. Circ. Res. **63**: 779–787.
6. WESTFALL, M.V., E.M. RUST & J.M. METZGER 1997. Slow skeletal troponin I gene transfer, expression, and myofilament incorporation enhances adult cardiac myocyte contractile function. Proc. Natl. Acad. Sci. USA **94**: 5444–5449.
7. WESTFALL, M.V., F.P. ALBAYYA, I.I. TURNER & J.M. METZGER 2000. Chimera analysis of troponin I domains that influence Ca^{2+}-activated myofilament tension in adult cardiac myocytes. Circ. Res. **86**: 470–477.
8. REISER, P.J., M.V. WESTFALL, S. SCHIAFFINO & R.J. SOLARO 1994. Tension production and thin-filament protein isoforms in developing rat myocardium. Am. J. Physiol. **36**: H1589–H1596.
9. NHLBI PROGRAM FOR GENOMIC APPLICATION. 2006. Genomics of Cardiovascular Development, Adaptation, and Remodeling. Harvard Medical School. Ref Type: Electronic Citation
10. WESTFALL, M.V. & J.M. METZGER 2001. Troponin I isoforms and chimeras: tuning the molecular switch of cardiac contraction. News Physiol. Sci. **16**: 278–281.
11. SAGGIN, L., L. GORZA, S. AUSONI & S. SCHIAFFINO. 1989. Troponin I switching in the developing heart. J. Biol. Chem. **264**: 16299–16302.

12. HUNKELER, N.M., J. KULLMAN & A.M. MURPHY. 1991. Troponin I isoform expression in human heart. Circ. Res. **69:** 1409–1414.
13. WOLSKA, B.M., K. VIJAYAN, G.M. ARTEAGA, *et al.* 2001. Expression of slow skeletal troponin I in adult transgenic mouse heart muscle reduces the force decline observed during acidic conditions. J. Physiol. **536:** 863–870.
14. WESTFALL, M.V., I.I. TURNER, F.P. ALBAYYA & J.M. METZGER 2001. Troponin I chimera analysis of the cardiac myofilament tension response to protein kinase A. Am. J. Physiol. **280:** C324–C332.
15. WESTFALL, M.V., F.P. ALBAYYA & J.M. METZGER 1999. Functional analysis of troponin I regulatory domains in the intact myofilament of adult single cardiac myocytes. J. Biol. Chem. **274:** 22508–22516.
16. DAY, S.M., M.V. WESTFALL, *et al.* 2006. Histidine button engineered into cardiac troponin I protects the ischemic and failing heart. Nat. Med. **12:** 181–189.
17. TEERLINK, J.R. 2005. Overview of randomized clinical trials in acute heart failure syndromes. Am. J. Cardiol. **96:** 59G–67G.
18. BAYRAM, M., L.L. DE, M.B. MASSIE & M. GHEORGHIADE. 2005. Reassessment of dobutamine, dopamine, and milrinone in the management of acute heart failure syndromes. Am. J. Cardiol. **96:** 47G–58G.
19. HOSHIJIMA, M. 2005. Gene therapy targeted at calcium handling as an approach to the treatment of heart failure. Pharmacol. Ther. **105:** 211–228.
20. MARON, B.J. 2002. Hypertrophic cardiomyopathy: a systematic review. JAMA **287:** 1308–1320.
21. MARON, B.J. 2003. Sudden death in young athletes. N. Engl. J. Med. **349:** 1064–1075.
22. NISHIMURA, R.A. & D.R. HOLMES JR. 2004. Clinical practice. Hypertrophic obstructive cardiomyopathy. N. Engl. J. Med. **350:** 1320–1327.
23. RICHARD, P., P. CHARRON, L. CARRIER, *et al.* 2003. Hypertrophic cardiomyopathy: distribution of disease genes, spectrum of mutations, and implications for a molecular diagnosis strategy. Circulation **107:** 2227–2232.
24. VAN DRIEST, S.L., S.R. OMMEN, *et al.* 2005. Sarcomeric genotyping in hypertrophic cardiomyopathy. Mayo Clin. Proc. **80:** 463–469.
25. AHMAD, F., J.G. SEIDMAN & C.E. SEIDMAN. 2005. The genetic basis for cardiac remodeling. Annu. Rev. Genomics Hum. Genet. **6:** 185–216.
26. BLAIR, E., C. REDWOOD, *et al.* 2001. Mutations in the gamma(2) subunit of AMP-activated protein kinase cause familial hypertrophic cardiomyopathy: evidence for the central role of energy compromise in disease pathogenesis. Hum. Mol. Genet. **10:** 1215–1220.
27. CHARRON, P., O. DUBOURG, *et al.* 1998. Clinical features and prognostic implications of familial hypertrophic cardiomyopathy related to the cardiac myosin-binding protein. C Gene Circ. **97:** 2230–2236.
28. HO, C.Y.,H.M. LEVER, *et al.* 2000. Homozygous mutation in cardiac troponin T: implications for hypertrophic cardiomyopathy. Circulation **102:** 1950–1955.
29. MARIAN, A.J. 2002. Modifier genes for hypertrophic cardiomyopathy. Curr. Opin. Cardiol. **17:** 242–252.
30. MICHELE, D.E., C.A. GOMEZ, K.E. HONG, *et al.* 2002. Cardiac dysfunction in hypertrophic cardiomyopathy mutant tropomyosin mice is transgene-dependent, hypertrophy-independent, and improved by beta-blockade. Circ. Res. **92:** 255–262.
31. FATKIN, D., B.K. MCCONNELL, *et al.* 2000. An abnormal Ca(2+) response in mutant sarcomere protein-mediated familial hypertrophic cardiomyopathy. J. Clin. Invest. **106:** 1351–1359.

32. SEMSARIAN, C., I. AHMAD, et al. 2002. The L-type calcium channel inhibitor diltiazem prevents cardiomyopathy in a mouse model. J. Clin. Invest. **109:** 1013–1020.
33. KNOLLMANN, B.C., P. KIRCHHOF, et al. 2003. Familial hypertrophic cardiomyopathy-linked mutant troponin T causes stress-induced ventricular tachycardia and Ca2+-dependent action potential remodeling. Circ. Res. **92:** 428–436.
34. SPINDLER, M., K.W. SAUPE, et al. 1998. Diastolic dysfunction and altered energetics in the alphaMHC403/+ mouse model of familial hypertrophic cardiomyopathy. J. Clin. Invest. **101:** 1775–1783.
35. JAVADPOUR, M.M., J.C. TARDIFF, I. PINZ & J.S. INGWALL 2003. Decreased energetics in murine hearts bearing the R92Q mutation in cardiac troponin T. J. Clin. Invest. **112:** 768–775.
36. FATKIN, D. & R.M. GRAHAM. 2002. Molecular mechanisms of inherited cardiomyopathies. Physiol. Rev. **82:** 945–980.
37. KAMISAGO, M., S.D. SHARMA, et al. 2000. Mutations in sarcomere protein genes as a cause of dilated cardiomyopathy. N. Engl. J. Med. **343:** 1688–1696.
38. DAEHMLOW, S., J. ERDMANN, et al. 2002. Novel mutations in sarcomeric protein genes in dilated cardiomyopathy. Biochem. Biophys. Res. Commun. **298:** 116–120.
39. CHANG, A.N., K. HARADA, M.J. ACKERMAN & J.D. POTTER. 2005. Functional consequences of hypertrophic and dilated cardiomyopathy-causing mutations in alpha-tropomyosin. J. Biol. Chem. **280:** 34343–34349.
40. MIRZA, M., S. MARSTON, et al. 2005. Dilated cardiomyopathy mutations in three thin filament regulatory proteins result in a common functional phenotype. J. Biol. Chem. **280:** 28498–28506.
41. KUSHWAHA, S.S., J.T. FALLON & V. FUSTER. 1997. Restrictive cardiomyopathy. N. Engl. J. Med. **336:** 267–276.
42. MOGENSEN, J., R. KUBO, et al. 2003. Idiopathic restrictive cardiomyopathy is part of the clinical expression of cardiac troponin I mutations. J. Clin. Invest. **111:** 209–216.
43. GOMES, A.V., J. LIANG & J.D. POTTER. 2005. Mutations in human cardiac troponin I that are associated with restrictive cardiomyopathy affect basal ATPase activity and the calcium sensitivity of force development. J. Biol. Chem. **280:** 30909–30915.
44. YUMOTO, F., Q.W. LU, et al. 2005. Drastic Ca2+ sensitization of myofilament associated with a small structural change in troponin I in inherited restrictive cardiomyopathy. Biochem. Biophys. Res. Commun. **338:** 1519–1526.
45. HAGHIGHI, K., K.N. GREGORY & E.G. KRANIAS. 2004. Sarcoplasmic reticulum Ca-ATPase-phospholamban interactions and dilated cardiomyopathy. Biochem. Biophys. Res. Commun. **322:** 1214–1222.
46. SZATKOWSKI, M.L., M.V. WESTFALL, et al. 2001. In vivo acceleration of heart relaxation performance by Parvalbumin gene delivery. J. Clin. Invest. **107:** 191–198.
47. ROTHERMEL, B.A., T.A. MCKINSEY, R.B. VEGA, et al. 2001. Myocyte-enriched calcineurin-interacting protein, MCIP1, inhibits cardiac hypertrophy in vivo. Proc. Natl. Acad. Sci. USA **98:** 3328–3333.
48. SUSSMAN, M.A., H.W. LIM, N. GUDE, et al. 1998. Prevention of cardiac hypertrophy in mice by calcineurin inhibition. Science **281:** 1690–1693.
49. ZHANG, R., M.S. KHOO, Y. WU, et al. 2005. Calmodulin kinase II inhibition protects against structural heart disease. Nat. Med. **11:** 409–417.

50. ROBBINS, J. 2000. Remodeling the cardiac sarcomere using transgenesis. Annu. Rev. Physiol. **62:** 261–287.
51. MICHELE, D.E., F. ALBAYYA & J.M. METZGER 1999. Thin filament protein dynamics in fully differentiated adult cardiac myocytes: toward a model of sarcomere maintenance. J. Cell. Biol. **145:** 1483–1495.

Nanomedicine Opportunities in Cardiology

GREGORY LANZA,[a] PATRICK WINTER,[a] TILLMANN CYRUS,[a] SHELTON CARUTHERS,[a,b] JON MARSH,[a] MICHAEL HUGHES,[a] AND SAMUEL WICKLINE[a]

[a]*Washington University School of Medicine, St. Louis, Missouri 63110, USA*
[b]*Philips Medical Systems, Cleveland, Ohio 44143, USA*

ABSTRACT: Despite myriad advances, cardiovascular-related diseases continue to remain our greatest health problem. In more than half of patients with atherosclerotic disease, their first presentation to medical attention becomes their last. Patients often survive their first cardiac event through acute revascularization and placement of drug-eluting stents (DES), but only select coronary lesions are amenable to DES placement, resulting in the use of bare metal or no stent, both of which lack the benefit of antirestenotic therapy. In other patients, transient ischemic attacks (TIAs) and stroke constitute the initial presentation of disease. In these patients, the diagnostic and therapeutic options are woefully inadequate. Nanomedicine offers options to each of these challenges. Antiangiogenic paramagnetic nanoparticles may be used to serially assess the severity of atherosclerotic disease in asymptomatic, high-risk patients by detecting the development of plaque neovasculature, which reflects the underlying lesion activity and vulnerability to rupture. The nanoparticles can locally deliver antiangiogenic therapy, which may acutely retard plaque progression, allowing aggressive statin therapy to become effective. Moreover, these agents may be useful as a quantitative marker to guide atherosclerotic management in an asymptomatic patient. In those cases proceeding to the catheterization laboratory for revascularization, nanoparticles incorporating antirestenotic drugs can be delivered directly into the wall of lesions not amenable to DES placement. Targeted nanoparticles could help ensure that antirestenotic drugs are available for all lesions. Moreover, displacement of antiproliferative agents from the intimal surface into the vascular wall is likely to improve rehealing of the endothelium, improving postprocedural management of these patients.

KEYWORDS: nanoparticle; angiogenesis; restenosis; thrombolysis

Address for correspondence: Prof. Gregory M. Lanza, M.D., Ph.D., Med and Biomed Engineering, WUSTL, 4003 Kingshighway Bldg., St. Louis, MO 63130. Voice: 314-454-8813; fax: 314-454-5265.
e-mail: greg@cvu.wustl.edu

INTRODUCTION

Cardiovascular disease (CVD), principally heart disease and stroke, continues to be the nation's leading killer for both men and women across all racial and ethnic groups. Nearly 1 million or 42% of all American deaths are due to CVD, and these victims were not simply the elderly. Approximately 160,000 individuals between the ages of 35 and 64 years died.[1] Current techniques for early medical detection and treatment are limited and their effectiveness in actually preventing heart attacks is debatable. In one retrospective study, 86 of 326 individuals received physical examinations within a 7-day period prior to death from heart attack, and their physicians predicted none to have a myocardial infarction. As tragic as this death toll is, even more grievous are the 57 million American survivors who daily struggle with the complications of CVD. Moreover, the direct medical and lost productivity costs to society are staggering, approximately $274 billion each year and growing annually. Although changes in environmental exposures, reduction in tobacco use, adjustments in diet, and increased physical activity can all improve patient health, the progression of CVD is relentless in Western societies. New paradigms to detect and treat CVD in asymptomatic patients are needed in order to prevent the first presentation of symptoms from being the last. Improved and safer approaches to coronary and intracranial revascularization are still required, despite the myriad of advances in the last 10 years.

No single technology offers a solution for all problems. However, rapid evolution of molecular biology, cell biology, genomics, and proteomics combined with discoveries in material sciences and bioengineering have created many new cadres of "nanotools" to address these challenges. Pharmaceutical nanoparticles have emerged as multifaceted systems capable of identifying and characterizing early disease before the gross anatomical manifestations are easily apparent with a variety of clinically relevant imaging modalities. Moreover, targeted particles can deliver therapeutics preferentially to sites of pathologic disease by recognizing and binding to unique biochemical signatures. The synergy of biomarker imaging and therapy is a powerful adjunctive paradigm to current medical practice, which offers a rich palette of approaches to address cardiovascular problems from a new perspective.

LIGAND-DIRECTED PERFLUOROCARBON NANOPARTICLES

Perfluorocarbon (PFC) nanoparticles are unusual lipid-encapsulated colloidal emulsions with nominal sizes between 200 nm and 250 nm. The core of the emulsion particle (98 vol%) comprises perfluorochemicals, which have twice the specific gravity of water and offer excellent safety profiles in pharmaceutical formulations.[2] The fluorine-carbon bonds of these compounds render them both chemically and biologically inert. Chemically stable, nonmetabolizable, and intrinsically nontoxic, perfluorochemicals have seen use in varied human applications including blood replacement, liquid breathing, ocular fluid replacement, MR imaging, CT imaging, ultrasound imaging, and percutaneous transluminal cardiac angioplasty (PTCA), with many products approved or in development.

For imaging, the perfluorocarbon core of the nanoparticles provides inherent acoustic contrast relative to blood and tissues due primarily to a speed-of-sound that is one-half to one-third that of water.[2–4] Moreover, this echo contrast effect can be augmented by further decreases in the speed-of-sound imparted by heating.[5] For traditional proton MR imaging, the high surface area of nanoparticles increases the ionic relaxivity of each atom of gadolinium by three- to sixfold due to the slowed rotational effects, while increasing the payloads of paramagnetic metals from a few to 100,000 per particle greatly amplifies the signal, that is, the molecular or particular relaxivity.[6–8] As with ultrasound, the perfluorocarbon core of the particle can contribute to the MR signal through ^{19}F imaging and spectroscopy.[9–11] The high concentration of ^{19}F at sites targeted with nanoparticles in combination with the negligible amount of fluorine in the surrounding tissues creates a unique and inherent second marker. In addition, the fluorine signal provides a confirmation of nanoparticle delivery as well as the quantity of particles delivered within a voxel or region independent of the local tissue environment.

As site-targeted agents for medical applications, *in vivo* stability and prolonged circulatory clearance offers many advantages. Liquid PFC nanoparticles minimize rapid systemic destruction, clearance, and coalescence without the addition of surface polyethylene glycol groups or surfactant cross-linking, which frequently complicate targeting efforts, interfere with drug transport, or mask surface components such as metal chelates or bioactive agents.

ASSESSING AND TREATING ATHEROSCLEROSIS IN ASYMPTOMATIC PATIENTS WITH PERFLUOROCARBON NANOPARTICLES

Perhaps one of the most active areas of cardiovascular research of immediate clinical significance is the quest to identify, quantify, and treat vulnerable and unstable plaque. For some time it has been recognized that thrombosis associated with plaque rupture is the principal cause of acute coronary syndromes and strokes, and that these events occur more often than not in asymptomatic vascular regions with approximately 50% diameter stenosis. Until recently, the dogma has been that a single complex lesion was responsible for the clinical event. But the diffuse nature of arterial tree inflammation renders many lesions within a vascular bed equally susceptible to extrinsic mechanical forces modulated by sympathetic tone or direct proteolytic degradation of the fibrous cap. Although multiple sites of rupture are uncommon as a cause of sudden coronary death, luminal fibrin from multiple ruptures are frequent and associated with plaque hemorrhage and superficial macrophages.[12–14] These sites of intimal fissuring, demarcated by accumulated surface fibrin, are suggested to be responsible for the rapid angiographic progression of vascular stenosis in patients.[15] In fact, accumulated surface fibrin may be a critical hallmark of lesion instability, and the sensitive and specific detection of fibrin by nanoparticle technology may define important strategies for the prevention of plaque progression and its sequellae. We[7] have previously reported and demonstrated the use of fibrin-specific paramagnetic nanoparticles for detecting fibrin with MRI, while others have used small paramagnetic peptides.[16,17] However, plaque rupture is a late manifestation of atherosclerotic plaque progression and further techniques are required to assess and treat the disease earlier in its natural progression in order to achieve any meaningful clinical impact.

One signature of atherosclerosis is the proliferation of an angiogenic vasculature, which frequently develops disproportionately from the vasa vasorum in response to the metabolic activity of plaque cellular constituents.[18–22] Extensive neovascular proliferation has been spatially localized to atherosclerotic plaque, and in particular, to "culprit" lesions clinically associated with unstable angina, myocardial infarction, and stroke. In addition, plaque angiogenesis has been suggested to promote plaque growth, intraplaque hemorrhage, and lesion instability. The interplay between angiogenesis and plaque development was explored by Moulton *et al.*[23] in Apo E $^{-/-}$ mice treated with antiangiogenic therapy for 4 months (20 to 36 weeks): TNP-470, a water-soluble fumagillin analogue, or endostatin (30 mg/kg every other day, 1.68 g/kg total dose).[23] Reduction in plaque angiogenesis and diminished atheroma growth were noted despite persistent elevation of total cholesterol levels. TNP-470 and its parent compound, fumagillin, directly inhibit endothelial cell proliferation by covalently binding to methionine aminopeptidase 2 specifically, which catalyzes the cleavage of N-terminal methionine from nascent polypeptides.[24–26] Unfortunately, chronic, high doses of TNP-470 administered systemically have caused neurocognitive side effects in humans.[27,28]

Site-targeted nanoparticles offer the opportunity for local drug delivery in combination with molecular imaging, which can provide noninvasive confirmation of targeting, spatial localization of drug distribution, and quantification of therapeutic payload accumulated at the site. This concept was initially demonstrated *in vitro* using doxorubicin and paclitaxel nanoparticles to inhibit the proliferation of vascular smooth muscle cells.[29] At that time, we proposed that targeted perfluorocarbon nanoparticles could deliver chemotherapeutic agents through a novel mechanism we called "contact facilitated lipid exchange." Subsequent studies using confocal microscopy have illustrated the exchange of fluorescent-labeled phospholipids from the outer surfactant layer of the particle to the target cell membrane.[30]

Using a hyperlipidemic New Zealand White rabbit model, we initially demonstrated the antiangiogenic effectiveness of $\alpha_v\beta_3$-targeted fumagillin nanoparticles administered as a single dose,[31,32] which was several orders of magnitude less than used systemically in the ApoE model.[23] In that study, hyperlipidemic rabbits (~80 days on diet) were injected via the ear vein with $\alpha_v\beta_3$-targeted fumagillin nanoparticles ($n = 5$), $\alpha_v\beta_3$-targeted nanoparticles without fumagillin ($n = 6$), or nontargeted fumagillin nanoparticles ($n = 6$) at 1.0 mL/kg. Four hours after nanoparticle injection, rabbits were reimaged to assess the magnitude and distribution of signal enhancement. Multislice, T_1-weighted, spin-echo, fat-suppressed, black-blood images of the entire abdominal aorta from the renal arteries to the diaphragm (TR = 380 msec, TE = 11 msec, 250 × 250 μm inplane resolution, 5 mm slice thickness, number of signals averaged = 8) were acquired. After treatment, all rabbits were converted to normal rabbit chow (Purina Mills). One week later, the extent of $\alpha_v\beta_3$-integrin expression in each animal was reassessed by injection of integrin-targeted paramagnetic nanoparticles (1.0 mL/kg; no drug) and noninvasive imaging as described earlier. MRI signal enhancement from the aortic wall was averaged over all imaged slices using a custom, semiautomated segmentation program previously described.[33] Signal enhancement in the aortic wall was measured for each individual animal using all properly segmented slices. The percentage enhancement in MRI signal was calculated slice-by-slice in the 4-h postinjection images relative to the average preinjection MRI signal.

Consistent with the early stage of atherosclerosis in this animal model, T_1-weighted, black-blood images showed no gross evidence of plaque development in terms of luminal narrowing or wall thickening when compared to previous experiments using age-matched, nonatherosclerotic rabbits.[33] MRI signal enhancement in the aortic wall following injection of $\alpha_v\beta_3$-targeted nanoparticles, both with and without fumagillin, displayed a patchy distribution, with typically higher levels of angiogenesis occurring near the diaphragm. Nontargeted nanoparticles produced less extensive MRI enhancement of the neovasculature at much lower levels with a similar heterogeneous distribution, consistent with previous reports. The average MRI signal enhancement per slice integrated across the entire aortic wall was identical for $\alpha_v\beta_3$-targeted nanoparticles with (16.7 ± 1.1%) and without (16.7 ± 1.6%) fumagillin. Nontargeted nanoparticles, however, provided less signal enhancement, presumably representing nonspecific accumulation and/or delayed washout within the tortuous microvasculature.[34]

One week after nanoparticle treatment, the residual expression of $\alpha_v\beta_3$-integrin was assessed as a marker of angiogenic activity within the aortic wall. Preinjection scans were collected, followed by injection of $\alpha_v\beta_3$-targeted paramagnetic nanoparticles (no drug) and contrast enhancement imaging 4 h post injection. The preinjection aortic wall signal intensities for all groups at treatment and at the 1-week follow-up were identical, confirming that the paramagnetic nanoparticles administered 1 week prior were no longer detectable. MRI aortic wall signal enhancement 1 week following $\alpha_v\beta_3$-targeted fumagillin nanoparticle treatment was markedly reduced (2.9 ± 1.6%; $P < 0.05$) in both spatial distribution as well as intensity. By comparison, MRI

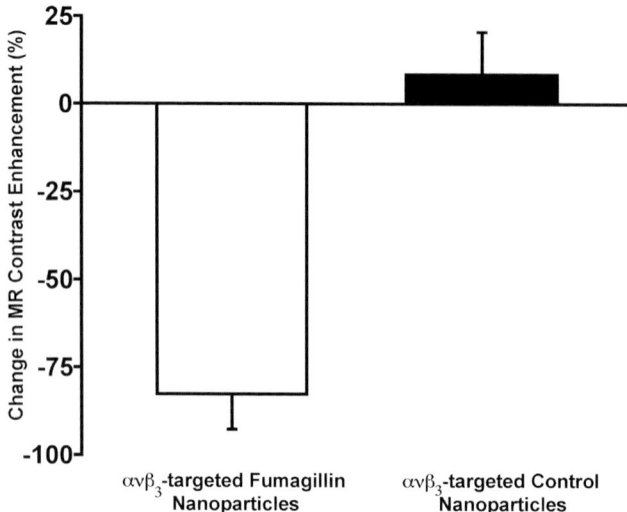

FIGURE 1. MRI aortic wall signal enhancement with $\alpha_v\beta_3$-targeted paramagnetic nanoparticle (no drug) 1 week following treatment with $\alpha_v\beta_3$-targeted fumagillin or control (no drug) nanoparticles.

signal enhancement 1 week after treatment with $\alpha_v\beta_3$-targeted nanoparticles lacking fumagillin was undiminished (18.1 ± 2.1%) (FIG. 1). Treatment with nontargeted fumagillin nanoparticles did not significantly diminish $\alpha_v\beta_3$-integrin levels as determined by MRI signal enhancement 1 week after treatment, although a numerical decrease was observed (12.4 ± 0.9%).

In this study, the total dose of fumagillin administered as a single injection in $\alpha_v\beta_3$-targeted nanoparticles was >10,000 times lower than the cumulative oral dose of TNP-470 reported by Moulton *et al.* Reduced $\alpha_v\beta_3$-integrin expression as determined by MRI molecular imaging and corroborated by decreased $\alpha_v\beta_3$-integrin positive vessel density supported the potential reduction in dosage and increase in efficacy of chemotherapeutic agents using targeted nanomedicine approaches. Incorporation of fumagillin into paramagnetic nanoparticles allowed both aortic expression of $\alpha_v\beta_3$-integrin and local drug delivery to be assessed and quantified concomitantly and noninvasively. Moreover, the initial magnitude of the aortic signal response among hyperlipidemic rabbits receiving $\alpha_v\beta_3$-targeted paramagnetic nanoparticles was correlated with the degree of change in MRI enhancement measured 7 days later with $\alpha_v\beta_3$-targeted paramagnetic nanoparticles (without drug). These data illustrate the concept of "rational drug dosing," which provides noninvasive measures of treatment dosimetry and allows follow-up of response.

For asymptomatic patients, nanomedicine approaches offer the ability to quantitatively interrogate the severity and distribution of disease more directly, to locally treat pathology with minimal doses, and to follow up response to treatment noninvasively when there are no clinical symptoms or meaningful measures with which to titrate treatment efficacy.

NANOMEDICINE APPROACH TO CORONARY REVASCULARIZATION

Far too often the progression of atherosclerosis to acute coronary syndromes presents the need for acute revascularization. Fortunately, continuous advances from balloon angioplasty, bare-metal stents, and drug-covered stents such as heparin-coated stents, to the more recent, new class of drug-eluting stents (DES), have expanded our armamentarium for reopening stenotic vessels while preventing vascular reocclusion. Within the last few years, the use of conventional balloon angioplasty and bare-metal stent implantation, which were associated with clinical restenosis rates of 32–42% and 19–30%, respectively,[35–37] have been improved with the local deposition of a pharmacologic agent to suppress neointimal proliferation. Current DES have reduced the rate of angiographic restenosis to below 9% and diminished the frequency for repeat revascularization to below 5%.[38,39] Unfortunately, DES cannot be routinely used for all lesions. In some situations, vessel tortuosity or the distal location of lesions prevents manipulation of the relatively inflexible DES. In other cases, the vessel diameter at the culprit lesion is too small for stent placement. As a result many lesions, in whole or part, do not receive the local antirestenotic therapy after revascularization.

Moreover, despite the clear success of DES, the incidence of late instent thrombosis has arisen as an infrequent but serious complication of delayed endothelial healing.[40] To avoid acute thrombosis, aggressive dual (and occasionally triple) antiplatelet therapy is employed for 6 months to a year. We now recognize that some patients are nonresponders to one or more of the drugs.[41–43] In other instances, thrombosis presents when antithrombotic drugs are withheld secondary to bleeding complications or the need for emergent surgery. Late instent thrombosis has been linked to fatal outcomes,[40] and the risk can persist up to 30 months after DES implantation.[42,43] We anticipate that targeted local delivery of antirestenotic drugs such as paclitaxel or rapamycin into the stretch-injured arterial wall rather than the intimal surface will permit better healing and recovery of the endothelium. More rapid endothelial repair of the injured wall should substantially diminish the incidence of thrombosis and reduce the long-term requirement for aggressive antiplatelet therapy.

Moreover, DES are now known to elicit unwanted effects on vessel healing and local endothelium-dependent vasomotor responses 6 months after implantation in the vessel distal to the intervened segment.[44] Although still limited, data on the effect of sirolimus on vasomotor response are accumulating in animal models and patients alike. Swine coronary artery segments exposed to sirolimus for 48 h showed severe impairment of endothelial function.[45] In patients, exercise-induced coronary vasoconstriction was noted in vessel segments adjacent to DES but not bare-metal stents.[46] The mechanism for this effect is unclear. Higher rates of restenosis proximal to stent placement compared with the distal edge support an asymmetric downstream effect.

We use a nanomedicine approach to address restenosis in lesions not amenable to current DES stent technology by intramural targeting and anchoring of rapamycin nanoparticles to the $\alpha_v\beta_3$-integrin, present on smooth muscle and other plaque components (e.g., macrophages, T cells). In previous studies, we demonstrated that ligand-directed perfluorocarbon nanoparticles could penetrate balloon-injured vessel walls and target intramural biomarkers, including tissue factor,[47] collagen III, and integrins.[48] We have recently reported that integrin-targeted PFC nanoparticles can provide effective intramural delivery of rapamycin and inhibit vascular stenosis following balloon overstretch injury. In these studies, femoral arteries of 12 rabbits on atherogenic diets for 3 weeks were subjected to balloon stretch injury via a catheter approach from the left common carotid artery. Using a double-balloon technique, paramagnetic $\alpha_v\beta_3$-nanoparticles with rapamycin were administered to one artery while the contralateral vessel received targeted nanoparticles without drug or saline. Two weeks after nanoparticle treatment, plaque development was determined by MR angiography and by microscopic morphometric quantification. Routine MR angiograms were indistinguishable between control and targeted-vessel segments. Microscopic analysis of serial vascular sections 2 weeks after injury revealed that the intimal plaque to lumen area ratio of vessels treated with $\alpha_v\beta_3$-targeted rapamycin nanoparticles were significantly ($P < 0.05$) less ($\sim$50%) than arteries receiving targeted nanoparticles without drug or saline (FIG. 2). Scanning electron microscopy of the intima performed 24 h after injury and treatment with $\alpha_v\beta_3$-targeted rapamycin nanoparticles demonstrated their binding to the underlying matrix and cells. Immunofluorescent imaging of the vessel wall $\sim$2 h after treatment demonstrated that the nanoparticles had penetrated into the media and adventitia, consistent with the MR images previously obtained. Although early, the results suggest that $\alpha_v\beta_3$-integrin-targeted nanoparticles can provide effective intramural therapy and may be a tool to extend the use of antirestenotic drugs to all revascularized sites with or without adjunctive stent placement.

NANOMEDICINE APPROACH TO THROMBOLYSIS

Stroke is the third leading cause of death in the United States and often results in functional impairment and long-term disability among survivors.[49] Clinical trials have demonstrated that thrombolytic treatment such as tissue plasminogen activator (t-PA) can reduce or reverse ischemia in patients treated within the first 3 h of onset.[50] However, intravenously administered thrombolytic agents are associated with an increased incidence of intracerebral hemorrhage and expanding stroke. This serious risk frequently delays the receipt of aggressive thrombolytic therapy until intracranial bleeding can be ruled out

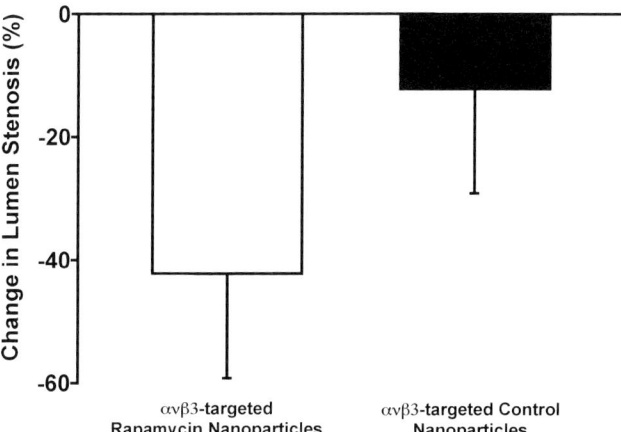

FIGURE 2. Microscopic analysis of serial vascular sections 2 weeks after injury revealed that the intimal plaque to lumen area ratio of vessels treated with $\alpha_v\beta_3$-targeted rapamycin nanoparticles were significantly ($P < 0.05$) less than arteries receiving targeted nanoparticles without drug or saline.

by CT study of the head. As a result of these delays, the window of opportunity to ameliorate neural damage is lost, and the personal and societal losses are magnified.

The advent of perfluorocarbon nanoparticles to specifically deliver drug payloads to intravascular sites of interest presents a unique opportunity to target clot-dissolving therapeutics to cerebral sites of embolism while decreasing the risk of hemorrhagic complications and increasing the effectiveness of thrombolytic therapy. We have previously demonstrated targeting of liquid perfluorocarbon nanoparticle emulsions to thrombi *in vitro* and *in vivo*,[51] with concomitant enhancement of acoustic reflectivity from the targeted surfaces. Acoustic reflectivity enhancement of surfaces targeted with the nanoparticles arises because of the acoustic impedance mismatch between the adherent layer of nanoparticles and the surrounding media. We have recently demonstrated that nanoparticles modified with thrombolytic enzyme (streptokinase) can be targeted onto plasma clots and effect rapid dissolution in the presence of plasminogen. In this series of experiments, acellular thrombi were produced from citrated human plasma combined with 500 mM calcium chloride and thrombin. Since this study was conducted *in vitro*, targeting of the nanoparticles to fibrin was accomplished using a three-step process in which biotinylated antifibrin antibody (NIB 1H10[52]), avidin, and biotinylated nanoparticle emulsions (with or without streptokinase, depending on treatment group) were combined sequentially with interval washings of unbound reagents. Acoustic microscopy was performed on targeted and control samples using a broadband, 25-MHz immersion transducer (Panametrics V324, Waltham, MA, USA) operated in pulse-echo mode. A computer-controlled pulser receiver was used to generate insonifying pulses and amplify the received echoes. The transducer was affixed to a three-axis, computer-controlled, motorized gantry. Radiofrequency (RF) data were acquired, digitized to 8 bits at 500 MHz for 2,048 point records, and stored to disk at every site as the transducer was scanned over each sample in a rectangular grid with 100-μm resolution. In preparation for scanning, each sample was sealed within a chamber having a cellophane acoustic window, and which was filled with phosphate buffered saline (PBS). The sample chamber was submerged within a 37°C water bath, and the sample was scanned to yield a baseline measurement. The chamber was then emptied of PBS through an injection port and refilled with either plasminogen in PBS buffer (3 U/mL) or PBS alone. Scans were then performed at 15-min intervals for 3 h, and spatial registration was maintained at all times.

RF data were analyzed to assess temporal changes in clot morphology and backscatter. A sliding Hamming window (0.2 μsec duration) was applied and moved over the data in 2-nsec steps. The sum of the squared values within each segment, a quantity proportional to the reflected energy, was used as input to a peak-detection algorithm (implemented in LabVIEW, National Instruments Corp., Austin, TX, USA) and used to determine the arrival time of the echo from the thrombus surface. A similar technique was used to detect the echo from the nitrocellulose substrate in the same waveform. The difference between the echo arrival times of the clot surface and substrate determined the profile of the clot, and these values were used to generate surface plots for visualization of the sample volume. Backscatter was quantified by first applying a rectangular window to each waveform to isolate the reflection from the targeted surface, and then by calculating the log spectral difference with respect to the reflection from a steel plate. The average value within the usable bandwidth (10–30 MHz) was recorded in dB for each point in the scan, and this value was used to generate a C-scan image of the integrated backscatter from the sample surface.

The detected clot volume was dramatically decreased ($P < 0.05$) for clots treated with fibrin-targeted streptokinase nanoparticles and exposed to plasminogen in buffer (FIG. 3). Treatment with fibrin-targeted streptokinase nanoparticles incubated in saline or fibrin-targeted nanoparticles without streptokinase incubated with plasminogen in buffer had no thrombolytic effect. The time to complete lysis varied with small changes in the synthesis process of the streptokinase nanoparticle formulations. Initial conjugates had to be left overnight for complete dissolution while more optimized agents formed later completely dissolved clots *in vitro* within an hour, often less than 15 min. Fibrin clot dissolution occurred from inside to outside. In some replicates, the clot measured at 1 h was a hollow fibrin shell, which immediately collapsed with slight motion. None of the control clots revealed morphologic or acoustic changes.

The measurements presented here suggest that fibrin-targeted streptokinase nanoparticles could be used to promote local thrombolysis of plasma clots *in vivo*. We have previously shown that fibrin-targeted nanoparticles can

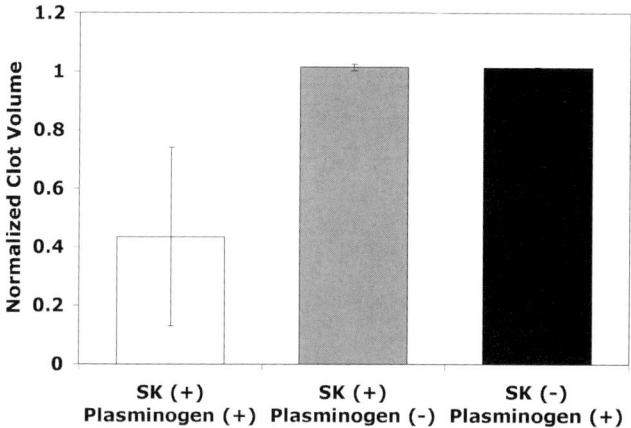

FIGURE 3. Mean normalized clot volume following 2-h treatment with fibrin-targeted nanoparticles streptokinase-modified or control perfluorocarbon nanoparticles incubated with plasminogen or saline.

penetrate and acoustically enhance acute intravascular thromboses in dogs. Moreover, we have found that perfluorocarbon nanoparticles are constrained to the vasculature due to their nominal size, even in "leaky" vascular beds such as tumor neovasculature. Collectively, those results suggest that fibrin-targeted streptokinase nanoparticles could be used early in acute stroke or unstable angina with limited extravascular effects.

SUMMARY

Nanomedicine is a new evolving field referred to by many names, which promises to significantly enhance the tools available to clinicians to address some of the serious challenges responsible for profound mortality, morbidity, and numerous societal consequences. Unlike the simple pharmaceutics of the past, nanomedicine agents are typically three-dimensional, multicomponent systems, which require interdisciplinary expertise to produce and use. In this review, we have briefly introduced the opportunities associated with targeted perfluorocarbon nanoparticles in early atherosclerosis, in acute revascularization, and in thrombolytic therapy. The potential impact of these three concepts is enormous but pales in comparison with the advancements likely to evolve in this field over the coming decades.

ACKNOWLEDGMENTS

This research was supported by the NIH grants (HL-42950, HL-59865, HL-78631, NO1-CO-37007, and EB-01704), SCAI/Bracco Diagnostics, Inc.-ACIST Fellowship Program, and the American Heart Association. Philips

Medical Systems (Cleveland, OH, USA) provided valuable equipment, software, and engineering support.

REFERENCES

1. ANONYMOUS. 2005. American Heart Association, Vol. 2005.
2. LANZA, G., K. WALLACE, M. SCOTT, et al. 1996. A novel site-targeted ultrasonic contrast agent with broad biomedical application. Circulation **94:** 3334–3340.
3. MATTREY, R.F. 1994. The potential role of perfluorochemicals (pfcs) in diagnostic imaging. Artif. Cells Blood Substit. Immobil. Biotechnol. **22:** 295–313.
4. HALL, C.S., G.M. LANZA, J.H. ROSE, et al. 2000. Experimental determination of phase velocity of perfluorocarbons: applications to targeted contrast agents. IEEE Trans. Ultrason. Ferroelec. Freq. Contr. **47:** 75–84.
5. HALL, C., J. MARSH, M. SCOTT, et al. 2001. Temperature dependence of ultrasonic enhancement with a site-targeted contrast agent. J. Acous. Soc. AM. **110:** 1677–1684.
6. LANZA, G., C. LORENZ, S. FISCHER, et al. 1998. Enhanced detection of thrombi with a novel fibrin-targeted magnetic resonance imaging agent. Acad. Radiol. **5**(Suppl 1): s173–s176.
7. FLACKE, S., S. FISCHER, M. SCOTT, et al. 2001. A novel MRI contrast agent for molecular imaging of fibrin: implications for detecting vulnerable plaques. Circulation **104:** 1280–1285.
8. WINTER, P., S. CARUTHERS, X. YU, et al. 2003. Improved molecular imaging contrast agent for detection of human thrombus. Mag. Reson. Med. **50:** 411–416.
9. YU, X., S.-K. SONG, J. CHEN, et al. 2000. High-resolution MRI characterization of human thrombus using a novel fibrin-targeted paramagnetic nanoparticle contrast agent. Mag. Reson. Med. **44:** 867–872.
10. LANZA, G.M., P.M. WINTER, A.M. NEUBAUER, et al. 2005. $^{1}H/^{19}F$ magnetic resonance molecular imaging with perfluorocarbon nanoparticles. Curr. Top. Dev. Biol. **70:** 57–76.
11. CARUTHERS, S.D., A.M. NEUBAUER, F.D. HOCKETT, et al. 2006. In vitro demonstration using 19f magnetic resonance to augment molecular imaging with paramagnetic perfluorocarbon nanoparticles at 1.5 tesla. Invest. Radiol. **41:** 305–312.
12. KOLODGIE, F.D., R. VIRMANI, A.P. BURKE, et al. 2004. Pathologic assessment of the vulnerable human coronary plaque. Heart **90:** 1385–1391.
13. VIRMANI, R., F.D. KOLODGIE, A.P. BURKE, et al. 2005. Atherosclerotic plaque progression and vulnerability to rupture: angiogenesis as a source of intraplaque hemorrhage. Arterioscler. Thromb. Vasc. Biol. **25:** 2054–2061.
14. SCHAAR, J.A., J.E. MULLER, E. FALK, et al. 2004. Terminology for high-risk and vulnerable coronary artery plaques. Report of a meeting on the vulnerable plaque, June 17 and 18, 2003, Santorini. Greece. Eur. Heart J. **25:** 1077–1082.
15. OJIO, S., H. TAKATSU, T. TANAKA, et al. 2000. Considerable time from the onset of plaque rupture and/or thrombi until the onset of acute myocardial infarction in humans: coronary angiographic findings within 1 week before the onset of infarction. Circulation **102:** 2063–2069.

16. BOTNAR, R.M., A. BUECKER, A.J. WIETHOFF, et al. 2004. In vivo magnetic resonance imaging of coronary thrombosis using a fibrin-binding molecular magnetic resonance contrast agent. Circulation **110**: 1463–1466.
17. BOTNAR, R.M., A.S. PEREZ, S. WITTE, et al. 2004. In vivo molecular imaging of acute and subacute thrombosis using a fibrin-binding magnetic resonance imaging contrast agent. Circulation **109**: 2023–2029.
18. KAHLON, R., J. SHAPERO & A.I. GOTLIEB. 1992. Angiogenesis in atherosclerosis. Can. J. Cardiol. **8**: 60–64.
19. FAN, T.P., R. JAGGAR & R. BICKNELL. 1995. Controlling the vasculature: angiogenesis, anti-angiogenesis and vascular targeting of gene therapy. Trends Pharmacol. Sci. **16**: 57–66.
20. SUEISHI, K., Y. YONEMITSU, K. NAKAGAWA, et al. 1997. Atherosclerosis and angiogenesis. Its pathophysiological significance in humans as well as in an animal model induced by the gene transfer of vascular endothelial growth factor. Ann. N. Y. Acad. Sci. **811**: 311–322; 322–324.
21. MOULTON, K. 2002. Plaque angiogenesis: its functions and regulation. Cold Spring Harb. Symp. Quant. Biol. **67**: 471–482.
22. MOULTON, K.S. 2001. Plaque angiogenesis and atherosclerosis. Curr. Atheroscler. Rep. **3**: 225–233.
23. MOULTON, K.S., E. HELLER, M.A. KONERDING, et al. 1999. Angiogenesis inhibitors endostatin or tnp-470 reduce intimal neovascularization and plaque growth in apolipoprotein e-deficient mice. Circulation **99**: 1653–1655.
24. KLEIN, C.D. & G. FOLKERS. 2003. Understanding the selectivity of fumagillin for the methionine aminopeptidase type II. Oncol. Res. **13**: 513–520.
25. RODRIGUEZ-NIETO, S., M.A. MEDINA & A.R. QUESADA. 2001. A re-evaluation of fumagillin selectivity towards endothelial cells. Anticancer Res. **21**: 3457–3460.
26. LIU, S., J. WIDOM, C.W. KEMP, et al. 1998. Structure of human methionine aminopeptidase-2 complexed with fumagillin. Science **282**: 1324–1327.
27. TRAN, H.T., G.R. BLUMENSCHEIN JR., C. LU, et al. 2004. Clinical and pharmacokinetic study of TNP-470, an angiogenesis inhibitor, in combination with paclitaxel and carboplatin in patients with solid tumors. Cancer Chemother. Pharmacol. **54**: 308–314.
28. HERBST, R.S., T.L. MADDEN, H.T. TRAN, et al. 2002. Safety and pharmacokinetic effects of TNP-470, an angiogenesis inhibitor, combined with paclitaxel in patients with solid tumors: evidence for activity in non-small-cell lung cancer. J. Clin. Oncol. **20**: 4440–4447.
29. LANZA, G.M., X. YU, P.M. WINTER, et al. 2002. Targeted antiproliferative drug delivery to vascular smooth muscle cells with a magnetic resonance imaging nanoparticle contrast agent: implications for rational therapy of restenosis. Circulation **106**: 2842–2847.
30. CROWDER, K.C., M.S. HUGHES, J.N. MARSH, et al. 2005. Sonic activation of molecularly-targeted nanoparticles accelerates transmembrane lipid delivery to cancer cells through contact-mediated mechanisms: implications for enhanced local drug delivery. Ultrasound Med. Biol. **31**: 1693–1700.
31. LANZA, G.M., D.R. ABENDSCHEIN, X. YU, et al. 2002. Molecular imaging and targeted drug delivery with a novel, ligand-directed paramagnetic nanoparticle technology. Acad. Radiol. **9**(Suppl 2): S330–S331.
32. LANZA, G.M., P. WINTER, S. CARUTHERS, et al. 2004. Novel paramagnetic contrast agents for molecular imaging and targeted drug delivery. Curr. Pharm. Biotechnol. **5**: 495–507.

33. WINTER, P.M., A.M. MORAWSKI, S.D. CARUTHERS, *et al.* 2003. Molecular imaging of angiogenesis in early-stage atherosclerosis with alpha(v)beta3-integrin-targeted nanoparticles. Circulation **108:** 2270–2274.
34. WILSON, M.W., J.M. LABERGE, R.K. KERLAN, *et al.* 2002. MR portal venography: preliminary results of fast acquisition without contrast material or breath holding. Acad. Radiol. **9:** 1179–1184.
35. JAEGERE PD, P., R. DOMBURG RV, H. NATHOE, *et al.* 1999. Long-term clinical outcome after stent implantation in coronary arteries. Int. J. Cardiovasc. Interv. **2:** 27–34.
36. KIMURA, T., T. TAMURA, H. YOKOI, *et al.* 1994. Long-term clinical and angiographic follow-up after placement of palmaz-schatz coronary stent: a single center experience. J. Interv. Cardiol. **7:** 129–139.
37. KEANE, D., A.J. AZAR, P. DE JAEGERE, *et al.* 1996. Clinical and angiographic outcome of elective stent implantation in small coronary vessels: an analysis of the benestent trial. Semin. Interv. Cardiol. **1:** 255–262.
38. SERRUYS, P.W., P.A. LEMOS & B.A. VAN HOUT. 2004. Sirolimus eluting stent implantation for patients with multivessel disease: rationale for the arterial revascularisation therapies study part II (ARTS II). Heart **90:** 995–998.
39. SERRUYS, P.W., E. REGAR & A.J. CARTER. 2002. Rapamycin eluting stent: the onset of a new era in interventional cardiology. Heart **87:** 305–307.
40. ONG, A.T., E.P. MCFADDEN, E. REGAR, *et al.* 2005. Late angiographic stent thrombosis (last) events with drug-eluting stents. J. Am. Coll. Cardiol. **45:** 2088–2092.
41. WENAWESER, P. & O. HESS. 2005. Stent thrombosis is associated with an impaired response to antiplatelet therapy. J. Am. Coll. Cardiol. **46:** CS5–CS6.
42. MCFADDEN, E.P., E. STABILE, E. REGAR, *et al.* 2004. Late thrombosis in drug-eluting coronary stents after discontinuation of antiplatelet therapy. Lancet **364:** 1519–1521.
43. RODRIGUEZ, A.E., J. MIERES, C. FERNANDEZ-PEREIRA, *et al.* 2006. Coronary stent thrombosis in the current drug-eluting stent era: insights from the eraci iii trial. J. Am. Col. Cardiol. **47:** 205–207.
44. HOFMA, S.H., W.J. VAN DER GIESSEN, B.M. VAN DALEN, *et al.* 2006. Indication of long-term endothelial dysfunction after sirolimus-eluting stent implantation. Eur. Heart J. **27:** 166–170.
45. JEANMART, H., O. MALO, M. CARRIER, *et al.* 2002. Comparative study of cyclosporine and tacrolimus on coronary endothelial function. J. Heart Lung Transplant. **21:** 990–998.
46. TOGNI, M., S. WINDECKER, R. COCCHIA, *et al.* 2005. Sirolimus-eluting stents associated with paradoxic coronary vasoconstriction. J. Am. Coll. Cardiol. **46:** 231–236.
47. LANZA, G., D. ABENDSCHEIN, C. HALL, *et al.* 2000. Molecular imaging of stretch-induced tissue factor expression in carotid arteries with intravascular ultrasound. Invest. Radiol. **35:** 227–234.
48. CYRUS, T., D.R. ABENDSCHEIN, S.D. CARUTHERS, *et al.* 2006. MR three-dimensional molecular imaging of intramural biomarkers with targeted nanoparticles. J. Cardiovasc. Magn. Reson. **8:** 535–541.
49. HINCHEY, J.A. & C. BENESCH. 2000. Thrombolytic therapy in patients with acute ischemic stroke. Arch. Neurol. **57:** 1430–1436.
50. GROUP, T.N.I.O.N.D.A.S.R.-P.S.S. 1995. Tissue plasminogen activator for acute ischemic stroke. The National Institute of Neurological Disorders and Stroke rt-PA Stroke Study Group. N. Engl. J. Med. **333:** 1581–1587.

51. LANZA, G.M., K.D. WALLACE, M.J. SCOTT, *et al.* 1996. A novel site-targeted ultrasonic contrast agent with broad biomedical application. Circulation **95:** 3334–3340.
52. RAUT, S. & P. GAFFNEY. 1996. Evaluation of fibrin binding profile of two antifibrin monoclonal antibodies. Thromb. Haemost. **76:** 56–64.

Effects of Synchronized Cardiac Assist Device on Cardiac Energetics

AMIR LANDESBERG,[a] AVSHALOM SHENHAV,[a] RONA SHOFTY,[a]
EUGENE KONYUKHOV,[a] CARMIT LEVY,[a] OSCAR LICHTENSTEIN,[a]
RAFAEL BEYAR,[a] HENK E.D.J. TER KEURS,[b] GIORA LANDESBERG,[c]
MARCO CABRERA,[d] WILLIAM STANLEY,[d] AND GERALD M. SAIDEL[d]

[a]*Department of Biomedical Engineering and Bruce Rappaport School of Medicine, Technion, Israel Institute of Technology, Haifa, Israel*

[b]*Department of Medicine, Physiology and Biophysics of the Faculty of Medicine, University of Calgary, Alberta, Canada*

[c]*The Faculty of Medicine and Hadassah Hospital, Hebrew University, Jerusalem, Israel*

[d]*Department of Biomedical Engineering, Department of Pediatrics and Department of Physiology and Biophysics, Case Western Reserve University, Cleveland, Ohio, USA*

ABSTRACT: A novel physiological cardiac assist device (PCAD), the LEVRAM assist device, which is synchronized with the failing heart ejection, was developed to improve the failing heart systolic and diastolic functions and cardiac energetics. The PCAD uses a single short cannula, which is inserted into the beating left ventricle (LV) by means of a specially designed device. Blood is ejected from the PCAD into the LV after the opening of the aortic valve and augments the cardiac stroke work. The same amount of blood is withdrawn from the LV into the PCAD, through the same cannula, during the diastole. The study aims to test the effects of the PCAD on cardiac energetics and coronary blood flow. Adult normal sheep were anesthetized and the heart was exposed by left thoracotomy. Pressures transducers (Millar Instruments, Inc., Houston, TX) were inserted into the LV and aorta. LV volume was measured by sonocrystals (Sonometrics Corp., London, Ontario, Canada) and impedance catheter (CD Lycom, Argonstrat 116 Zoetermeer, 2718 SP The Netherlands). Flowmeters (transonic) measured the cardiac output (CO) and the coronary arteries (left anterior descending (LAD) and circumflex) flows. A thin cannula was inserted into the coronary sinus and the oxygen content of the LV and the coronary sinus were determined (AVOXimeter-1000). Pressure-volume loops, myocardial energetics, and coronary flow were measured. The displaced PCAD volume was 11 mL. Four different levels of assist were studied by changing the frequency of

Address for correspondence: Prof. Amir Landesberg, M.D., Ph.D., Department of Biomedical Engineering, Technion, IIT, Haifa 32000 Israel. Voice: 972-4-829-4143; fax: 972-4-8294599.
 e-mail: amir@bm.technion.ac.il

Ann. N.Y. Acad. Sci. 1080: 466–478 (2006). © 2006 New York Academy of Sciences.
doi: 10.1196/annals.1380.035

the assist: (1) assist beat after three successive regular beats [1:4], (2) assist every third beat [1:3], (3) alternate assist and normal beat [1:2], and (4) continuous assist [1:1]. Cardiac output (CO) and stroke volume (SV) increased proportionally with increasing frequency of assist. Systolic mechanical efficiency of the PCAD was above 90%. Simultaneously, the PCAD decreased the end-diastolic volume (EDV; diastolic unloading). The PCAD increased coronary flow and decreased cardiac arterial–venous O_2 difference. We conclude that the PCAD efficiently augments CO and stroke work, decreases preload, and decreases the coronary arterial–venous O_2 difference; all these may expedite cardiac reverse remodeling, and promote recovery of function and eventual easy explanation of the device.

KEYWORDS: heart failure; ventricular assist device; reverse remodeling; cardiac mechanics; excitation–contraction coupling; coronary flow

INTRODUCTION

Chronic heart failure (CHF) is among the leading causes of death in the industrialized world. Long-term survival is short. The 5-year mortality rate of patients with CHF is 75% for men and 62% for women. Mortality rate of patients with decompensated (end stage IV) heart failure is 60% per year. Cardiac transplantation is the only treatment that promises substantial longevity and quality of life. However, heart donors are scarce and less than 3,000 donor organs are annually available worldwide.[1] Consequently, most end-stage CHF patients seek an effective "alternative to transplant" with mechanical ventricular assist devices (VADs).[2–7] As demonstrated in FIGURE 1 A, all presently available VADs support the circulation by using a mechanical pump to reroute the blood from the failing ventricle into the aorta.[2–8] These devices bypass and continuously unload the failing heart. The application of the available assist devices in severe heart failure normalizes hemodynamics, improves organ dysfunction, provides a reasonable quality of life,[4,8–10] and demonstrates meaningful survival benefit.[8] The Rematch study[8] has shown that the pulsatile assist devices (such as Heart Mate VE, Thoratec Corp., Pleasanton, CA) improve survival and the quality of life when compared to optimal medical management. Based on the Rematch study, the FDA has approved (November 2002) marketing of the HeartMate VE for "destination therapy;" that is, as a permanent support for end-stage patients who are not eligible for heart transplantation.

While present VADs reduce myocardial energy consumption, the continuously unloaded failing heart undergoes rapid atrophy and fibrosis in the majority of cases. Most patients become fully dependent on the implanted VAD, and only a small minority of patients demonstrate reverse remodeling and recovery that allows device explanation.[4,8,9] Mueller and Hetzer[11] have suggested that the major contributing factors for the consequent fibrosis and deterioration in

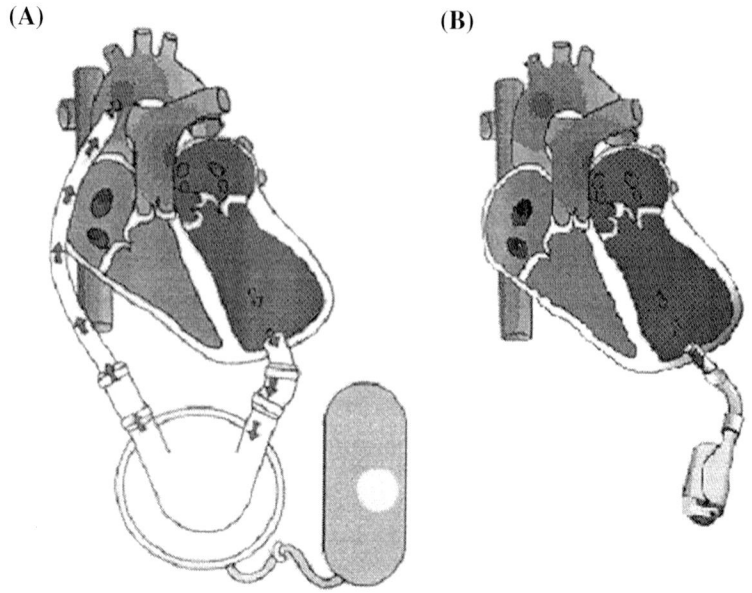

FIGURE 1. (A) VAD. (B) PCAD.

the native heart function are the duration and magnitude of unloading by the VADs. The longer the unloading of the ventricle and the lower the maximal left ventricular (LV) pressure below 60 mmHg, the greater the deterioration of cardiac performance.

The VADs usage is presently limited mainly to patients with severe end-stage heart failure (stage IV), as a "bridge to transplantation," or less frequently as "destination therapy," when full replacement of cardiac function is required. The mean survival of patient with the VAD based on the Rematch study is 408 days.[8] However, patients at an earlier stage of heart failure (stage III) with a life expectancy of a couple of years also suffer from a poor quality of life and require augmentation of the cardiac function during mild exercises. Thus it is desired to boost the native heart function at the earlier stage (stage III), and relieve the loading condition imposed on the heart, improve myocardial perfusion, and allow myocardial recovery (reverse remodeling).

The novel physiological cardiac assist device (PCAD) discussed here introduces (FIG. 1B) a new concept of an assist/therapeutic device that favorably works in synchrony with the native failing heart dynamics rather than bypassing the failing ventricle. Our recent studies[12] have established the mechanical feasibility of the device in animal models with acute (cardiogenic shock) and CHF.[12]

The PCAD's unique novelty is that it uses a single small (5 cm long and 1 cm in diameter) cannula, which is inserted into the failing ventricle, without the need for a bypass connection to the aorta (FIG. 1 B). Moreover, the PCAD supports both the systolic and diastolic functions of the heart. Blood is displaced from the PCAD into the LV through the cannula immediately after the opening of the ventricle outlet valve. Thus it augments the systolic function by adding external work during the ejection phase of the contraction. During early diastole, immediately after the aortic valve closure, the PCAD withdraws blood from the LV back into the PCAD. This unloading of the ventricle continues during diastole, after the opening of the mitral valve. The ventricle assists in pulling the blood back into the PCAD during the relaxation phase. Augmentation of the CO and unloading during the diastole alleviate the preload, reduce the LV end-diastolic volume (EDV), and is thus expected to decrease the myocardial energy consumption.[13–15] The PCAD mode of operation is practically analogous to the implantation of billions of healthy cardiac myocytes into the ventricular tissue, performing about a quarter of the cardiac external work by ejecting approximately one quarter of the stroke volume (SV) during the systolic ejection phase. Moreover, unlike the native heart that passively returns to its EDV, the PCAD provides active recoil and actively unloads the ventricle during the diastole, thereby improving diastolic function.

The aims of the study reported here were: (1) to use the assist/therapeutic devices as a means for studying the effects of changes in the loading condition on energy consumption, and thereby to improve our understanding of the regulation of cardiac energy conversion; and (2) to examine the effects of the PCAD on cardiac mechanics, energetics, and coronary flow.

METHODS

Mature normal sheep (2+ years and ~80 kg) were anesthetized and maintained so by isoflurane (1.5%). Fentanyl (10 μg/kg/h), pancuronium (12.5 μg/kg/h), and midazolam (0.1 mg/kg/h) were added upon need. Two pressure transducers (Millar) were inserted through the carotid arteries into the LV cavity and aortic arch. The heart was exposed through left thoracotomy. An additional pressure transducer (Millar) was inserted into the left auricle. A dissection was made between the ascending aorta and the pulmonary trunk, and a flowmeter (transonic) was placed around the ascending aorta. (Two flowmeters (transonic) were placed around the common (right) brachiocephalic and the proximal aortic arch to monitor the CO in some cases, where the sheep had a very short ascending aorta before this bifurcation). Two additional flowmeters (transonic) were placed around the two main coronary arteries—the circumflex and the left anterior descending (LAD) arteries—to monitor cardiac coronary flow for the calculation of energy consumption. Six sonocrystal transducers (Sonometrics) were implanted in the LV wall to measure LV dimensions and to assess LV volume. An impedance catheter (CD Lycom) was inserted into the LV cavity for additional direct measurement of the LV volume.

TABLE 1. Effects of the different levels of assist (1:4, 1:3, alternating-1:2, or continuous-1:1) on cardiac mechanics and energetics.[a]

Assisted beats Ratio	Baseline	1:4				Baseline	1:3		
		1	2	3	Assist		1	2	Assist
Event No. (Baseline 1 or Assist)	32–33		34–35			23–24		25–26	
Event No. (Baseline 2)	36–37					27–28			
EDV	155	150	155	155	155	155	159	156	155
LV_SV	42	39	43	43	40	43	41	44	41
Total SV	42	39	43	43	64	43	41	44	54
Pend Sys[mmHg]	80	80	80	80	89	80	80	80	90
LV Work [Joule]	0.44	0.41	0.45	0.45	0.47	0.45	0.43	0.45	0.49
Total External Work	0.44	0.41	0.45	0.45	0.63	0.45	0.43	0.45	0.64
Heart rate2[pls/sec]	115.4		115.4			115.4		115.4	
Card.Out.1[L/min]	4847		5164			4962		5347	
delta CO [%]			6.5					7.8	
mean LV work	0.444		0.447			0.454		0.462	
mean EW	0.444		0.489			0.454		0.513	
delta EW [%]			10.2					13	
Coronary flow	168		158			162		188	
Aortic O2	10.7		10.7			11		10.85	
Venus O2	8.1		8.05			8.45		8.6	
O2 consumption	436.8		418.7			413		423	
Delta O2 consumption			−18.1					9.9	

[a] The effects of the assisted beat on the successive normal beats were evaluated. For example, when the assist was instituted after every three normal beats (1:4 mode), we separately evaluated the cardiac mechanical indices in each of the normal beats (denoted by '1', '2', and '3' – in the second row). The coronary flow was measured in the circumflex artery while the venous O_2 content was measured in the coronary sinus.

continued.

TABLE 1. Continued.

Assisted beats Ratio	Baseline	1:2 Baseline	1:2 1	1:2 Assist	Baseline	1:1
Event No. (Baseline 1 or Assist)	17–18	19–20			28–29	30–31
Event No. (Baseline 2)	21–22				32–33	
EDV	145		140	145	152	147
LV.SV	38		36	36	40	39
Total SV	38		36	48.5	40	49
Pend Sys[mmHg]	82		82	91	80	90
LV Work [Joule]	0.41		0.39	0.43	0.42	0.46
Total External Work	0.41		0.39	0.58	0.42	0.58
Heart rate2[pls/sec]	118			118	116.5	116.5
Card.Out.1[L/min]	4484			4986	4660	5700
delta CO [%]				11.2		22.5
mean LV work	0.411			0.411	0.422	0.463
mean EW	0.411			0.486	0.422	0.582
delta EW [%]				18.2		37.8
Coronary flow	162			185	162	176
Aortic O2	11			11.45	10.7	11.1
Venus O2	8.45			9.35	8.15	8.85
O2 consumption	413.1			388.5	413.1	396
Delta O2 consumption				−24.6		−17.1

EDV=end-diastolic volume; LV–SV=Left ventricle shortening as assessed from the pressure-LV volume loops by the sonocrystals (Sonometrics); Total–SV=The volume ejected out of the LV as measured by the aortic flowmeters (transonic); $P_{end-Sys}$=End-systolic pressure; LV-work=The work that is done by the LV during the systole, evaluated from the systolic pressure and the LV shortening. Total external work=The work done upon the peripheral circulation, evaluated from the systolic pressure and the total ejected volume. Mean LV work and mean EW are the mean works during the various assist modes, taking into account the normal and the assisted beats.

A catheter was inserted into the coronary sinus through the azygos vein (which drains into the coronary sinus in sheep) and the azygos vein was ligated to assure that the blood samples originated from the coronary system.

Oxygen content of the LV and the coronary sinus were measured using the AVOXimeter-1000 oxymeter. The oxygen consumption was calculated by multiplying arterial–venous oxygen content difference by mean coronary arterial blood flow. Oxygen consumption was measured at a steady state, after reaching stable CO and pressure-volume loops for at least 4 min. All measurements were averaged per single heartbeat in order to avoid heart rate-related changes.

Following the implantation of all the transducers, a purse-string was prepared around the apex of the LV and a small cannula (5 cm long and 10 mm in diameter) was inserted into the LV cavity via the apex, using a specially designed cannulation tool. This tool allows fast (less than 15 sec) and safe cannulation in all the experiments with beating hearts. The implanted cannula was connected to the PCAD after filling the displacement chamber of the PCAD with normal saline. The volume displaced by the PCAD was measured by an encoder attached to the pusher plate of the PCAD.

The effects of four levels of assist were studied by changing the rate of the PCAD displacement. At baseline there was practically no assist as the device displaced blood back and forth into the LV once every 10 or more normal beats. This low frequency of displacement during baseline was required to prevent clot formation due to stagnation within the device. The four levels of assist were: (1) once every four beats (1:4), (2) assist every third beat (1:3), (3) alternating assist and normal beats (1:2), and (4) continuous assist, every beat (1:1). The volume displaced was constant (11 mL). After every change in the rate of the assist, we waited until a steady CO and pressure-volume loops were observed for at least 4 min. Thereafter, blood samples were obtained for oxygen content measurements from both the artery and the coronary sinus. Only short-term, less than 10 min, effects of PCAD operation were evaluated since each period of assist was followed by a 10-min stabilization period without assist (return to baseline). All data were continuously acquired by Lab-View data acquisition system, at a sampling rate of 1 kHz.

RESULTS AND DISCUSSION

The effects of assist every third beat on the mechanical performances are presented in FIGURE 2. Note the increase in the aortic flow and ventricular pressure, in the assisted beats.

The results are summarized in TABLE 1. Each sequence of several minutes of assist was preceded by a sequence of several minutes of normal (baseline) contractions without an assist. Thus the effects of the assist were compared with the baseline performances without an assist.

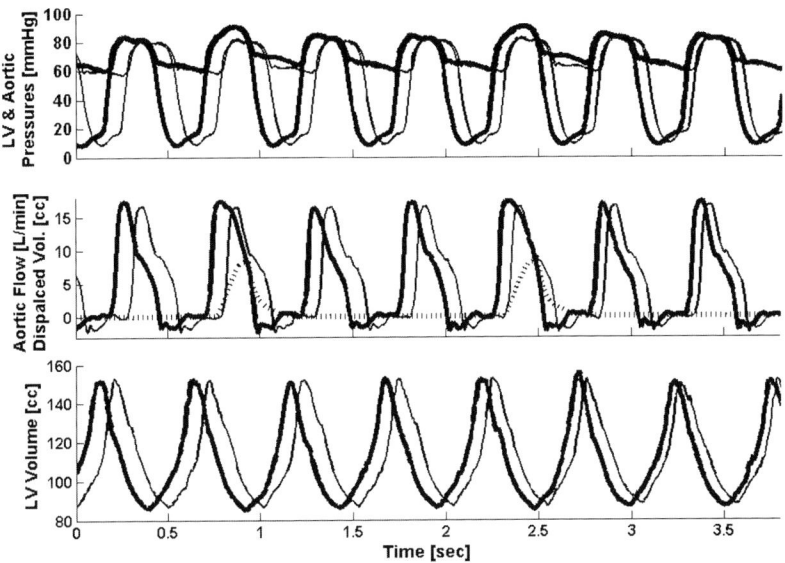

FIGURE 2. The effects of assist every third beat on cardiac mechanics. The tracing during the assist (bold lines) are compared with the base line without an assist (thin lines). The profile of the assist is described in the second row (dashed line).

We have also evaluated the effects of the assisted beats on the normal beats that followed them; for example, when the assist was activated after every three normal beats (1:4 mode) we also evaluated the cardiac mechanical indices in each of these normal beats (denoted by '1', '2', and '3' –second row, TABLE 1).

The cardiac SV ejected from the LV into the aorta was derived by integrating the aortic flow. There was a conspicuous increase in the SV in the assisted beat, and the cardiac SV is larger than the ventricle shortening; for example, the total SV was 49 mL during continuous assist while the base line total SV was 40 mL. The LV–SV during the continuous assist phase was 39 mL and the PCAD provided the additional 10 mL (TABLE 1). According to the conservation of mass law, the SV is the sum of the volume displaced into the ventricle by the PCAD and the ventricle contraction.

The following significant effects of the PCAD on the cardiac mechanics were observed:

- The first beat after the assisted beat (label '1' in the Table) had the smallest EDV. The decrease in the EDV after an assisted beat resulted from active blood withdrawal from the LV back into the device during the diastole (diastolic unloading by the device). There was a decrease of 5 mL in the EDV during continuous assist within a few minutes.

- The first beat after the assisted beat had the smallest SV. This was due to the decrease in the EDV in that beat and the Frank–Starling Law of the heart. The drop in the SV increased as the frequency of assist decreased. The total-SV during 1:4 assist was 54 in the assisted beat and it decreased to 39 mL in the successive first unassisted beat (TABLE 1).
- Shortening during the assisted beat was decreased by 1mL (in the 1:1 mode) to 3 mL (in the 1:4 mode). This decrease in the LV shortening resulted from the increase in the LV pressure. Thus the decrease in the LV shortening was relatively small compared to the increase in the total cardiac SV. As anticipated,[12] this phenomenon relates to the cardiac force–velocity relationship.
- There was a conspicuous increase in the total SV by 8 mL to 10 mL. Hence most of the blood volume displaced by the device appeared as added SV.
- There was a significant increase in the end-systolic pressure by 9 mmHg to 10 mmHg during the assist. This increase in the systolic pressure is especially large in the normal healthy animal, and is significantly smaller in the CHF model and during continuous assist.[12] In the CHF model the increase in the CO is associated with a decrease in the systemic resistance. In contrast to the animal with heart failure, the normal animal does not need an increase in the CO. In the setting of heart failure we encounter inadequate CO and high peripheral resistance. The physiological response to improvement in the CO is a decrease in the total peripheral resistance. Hence there is a significant larger increase in the CO than in the blood pressure in the setting of chronic heart failure.[12]
- As shown in FIGURE 3, there was a significant increase in the CO; the increase was proportional to the level of the assist. During continuous assist the CO increased by 1.05 l/min or 22.5%. During assist of 1:2, the CO increased by half (0.5 l/min or 11.2%). At the lower levels of assist, where the ratio of assisted beats to normal beats was 1:3 and 1:4, the increase in the CO was a third and a quarter of the increase in the CO during continuous assist.
- A significantly larger effect was observed in the external work. The external work increased by 37% during the continuous assist (TABLE 1, FIG. 2). The increase in the stroke work was proportional to the level of the assist. The increase in the external work is larger than the increase in the CO since the external work is determined by the SV and the systolic pressure, while the changes in the CO reflect only the changes in the SV.
- As we have shown before, the results suggest that most of the mechanical energy introduced by the device emerge as added external work. Thus the mechanical efficiency of the device, the ratio of the added external work to the device work, is above 90%.
- The assist increased the coronary flow (FIG. 4). The increase in the coronary flow relates to the increase in the aortic pressure and the decrease

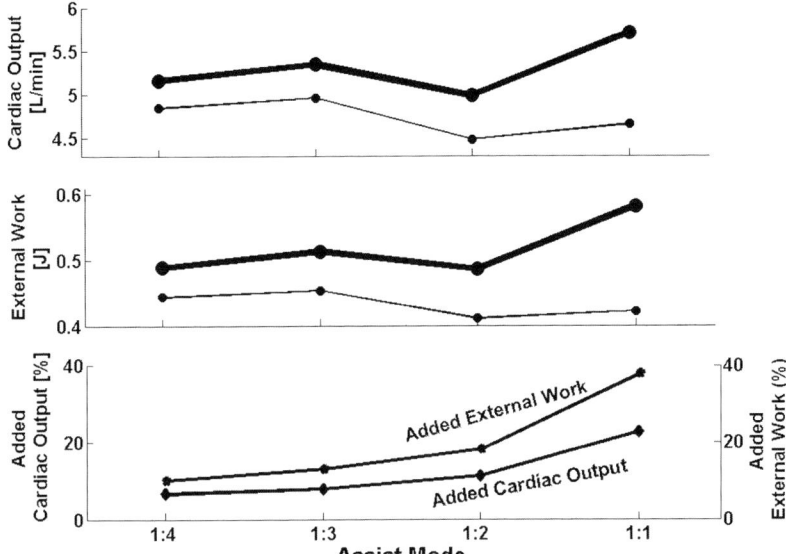

FIGURE 3. The effects of the frequency of the assist (assist beat every four, three, two beats, or continuous assist) on the CO (upper plot) and external work (middle). The assisted contraction (bold lines) is compared with the base line without an apparent assist (thin lines). The increase in the CO and the external work were proportional to the frequency of the assist (bottom trace).

in the ventricle diastolic pressure during the assist. It may also reflect an increase in the ventricular wall dynamics and augmentation of the "intramyocardial pump"; the squeezing and expansion effects of myocardial wall motion on the coronary vessels and interstitial fluid.
- The assist increased the oxygen content in the coronary sinus, and decreased the arterial–venous O_2 difference (FIG. 4). Thus, although there was an increase in the coronary flow during the assist, the oxygen consumption decreased due to the decline in the arterial–venous O_2 difference. These two effects, the increase in the coronary flow and the increase in the venous O_2 content, imply that the device improves myocardial wall perfusion and increases the coronary O_2 reserve.

Limitations of the present study include:

1. Only relative short-term assists, for less than 10 min, were instituted (although we have tested various levels of assist). Thus the long-term effects of supporting the circulation, unloading the LV, and working in a physiological mode were not studied.
2. The effects of the assist were measured in normal healthy sheep without heart failure. Significant larger effects are expected in the failing heart, based on our previous studies.[12]

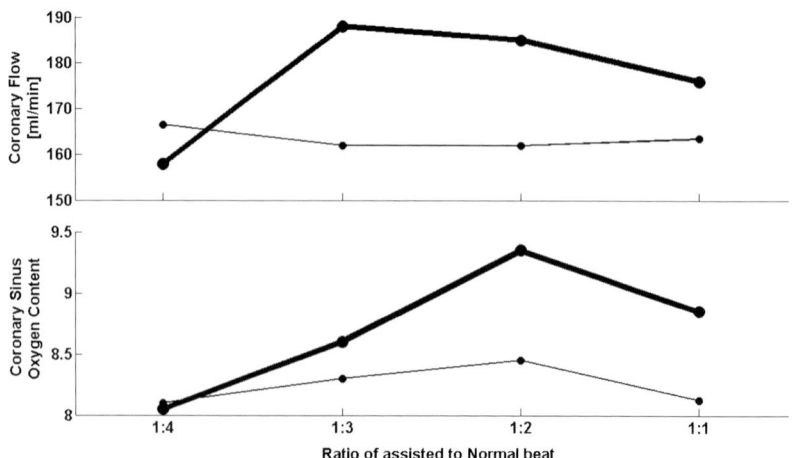

FIGURE 4. The effects of the frequency of the assist procedure (assisted beat every four, three, two beats, or continuous assist) on the coronary flow and the coronary sinus oxygen content. The assist increased the coronary oxygen reserve by increasing the coronary flow and decreasing the arterial–venous O_2 difference. The measurements during assisted contractions (*bold lines*) are compared with the baseline without an assist (*thin lines*).

3. Further studies are needed to test the utility of this assist mode in expediting cardiac reverse–remodeling.

The effects of the assist device on cardiac reverse remodeling is determined by the effects of the device on the cardiac loading conditions, the cellular control of contraction and energy consumption, coronary perfusion, and the provided circulatory support. The circulatory support is associated with reduction in the humoral and neural stimuli of heart. Based on the above results, it is anticipated that the suggested assist mode will promote cardiac reverse remodeling, while keeping the heart working against physiological loadings.

SUMMARY

The PCAD is based on a unique mode of operation whereby a small pulsatile but valveless device works in cadence with the native heart dynamics. The PCAD is connected to the heart by a single small cannula with opposite flows within the cannula during diastole and systole. The PCAD significantly improves the cardiac systolic and diastolic functions. It increases the CO (+22%) and the stroke work (+37%) with a smaller increase in the systolic pressure (12.5%). The improvement in the systolic function is associated with a decrease in the EDV and a decrease in the cardiac energy consumption (−4% within several minutes). The PCAD improves the cardiac coronary oxygen reserve by increasing the coronary flow and decreasing the arterial–venous O_2 difference. The results reported here substantiate the anticipated benefits of using the device to support the circulation. The PCAD improves the balance between oxygen supply and the mechanical demands.

ACKNOWLEDGMENTS

The study was supported by H. & R. Sohnis Cardiology Research Fund and a grant from the United States Israel Binational Science Foundation (BSF Research Project No. 2003399).

REFERENCES

1. HOSENPUD, J.D., L.E. BENNETT, B.M. KECK, et al. 2000. The Registry of the International Society for Heart and Lung Transplantation: seventeenth official report. J. Heart Lung Transplant. **19:** 909–931.
2. GOLDSTEIN, D.J., M.C. OZ & E.A. ROSE. 1998. Implantable left ventricle assist device. N. Engl. J. Med. **339:** 1522–1533.
3. MOSKOWITZ, A.J., A.D. WEINBERG, M.C. OZ & D.L. WILLIAMS. 1998. Quality of life with an implantable left ventricle assist device. Ann. Thorac. Surg. **64:** 1764–1769.
4. MANCINI, D.M., A. BENIAMINOVITZ, H. LEVIN, et al. 1998. Low incidence of myocardial recovery after left ventricular assist device implantation in patients with chronic heart failure. Circulation **98:** 2383–2389.
5. WIESELTHALAR, G.M., H. SCHIMA, M. HIESMAYR, et al. 2000. First clinical experience with the DeBakey VAD continuous axial flow pump for bridge to transplantation. Circulation **101:** 356–359.
6. DEROSE, J.J. & R.K. JARVIK. 2000. Axial flow pump. In Cardiac Assist Devices. D.J. Goldstein & M.C. Oz, Eds.: 359–373. Futura Pub. NY.
7. RICHENBACHER, W.E. & W.S. PIERCE. 1997. Assisted circulation and the mechanical heart. In Heart Disease. E. Braunwald, Ed.: 534–547. W.B. Saunders. Philadelphia, PA.
8. ROSE, E.A., A.C. GELIJNS, A.J. MOSKOWITZ, et al. 2001. Long term use of left ventricular assist device for end stage heart failure. N. Engl. J. Med. **345:** 1435–1443.
9. YACOUB, M.H. 2001. A novel strategy to maximize the efficacy of left ventricular assist devices as a bridge to recovery. Euro. Heart J. **22:** 534–540.
10. SHAPIRO, P.A. 2000. Quality of life issues associated with the use of left ventricular assist devices. In Cardiac Assist Devices. D.J. Goldstein & M.C. Oz, Eds.: 121–135. Futura Pub. NY.
11. MUELLER, J. & R. HETZER. 2000. Left ventricular recovery during left ventricular assist device support. In Cardiac Assist Devices. D.J. Goldstein & M.C. Oz, Eds.: 121–135. Futura Pub. NY. 121–135.
12. LANDESBERG, A., E. KONYUKHOV, R. SHOFTI, et al. 2004. Augmentation of dilated failing left ventricular stroke work by a physiological cardiac assist device. Ann. N. Y. Acad. Sci. **1015:** 379–390.

13. SUGA, H. 1990. Ventricular energetics. Physiol. Rev. **70:** 247–277.
14. LANDESBERG, A. 1996. End systolic pressure-volume relation based on the intracellular control of contraction. Am. J. Physiol. **270:** H338–H349.
15. LANDESBERG, A. & S. SIDEMAN. 2000. Force-velocity relationship and biochemical to mechanical energy conversion by the sarcomere. Am. J. Physiol. **278:** H1274–H1284.

Index of Contributors

Ahammer, H., 301–319
Antzelevitch, C., 268–281
Aronheim, A., 97–109
Austin, T.M., 334–347

Balaban, R.S., 140–153
Banerjee, I., 76–84
Barker, R.J., 49–62
Baudino, T.A., 76–84
Bers, D.M., 165–177
Beyar, R. 207–215, 466–478
Borg, T.K., 76–84
Bossuyt, J., 165–177
Boyden, P.A., 248–267
Burton, R.A.B., 301–319

Cabrera, M.E., 120–139, 466–478
Caruthers, S., 451–465
Chen, M., 362–375
Cleemann, L., 154–164
Cyrus, T., 451–465

Dantzig, J.A., 1–18
Davis, J., 437–450
Day, S., 437–450
Despa, S., 165–177

Field, L.J., 34–48
Foley, A.C., 85–96

Garfinkel, A., 376–394
Gavaghan, D., 301–319
Gepstein, L., 207–215, 415–425
Ghatnekar, G.S., 49–62
Goldman, Y.E., 1–18
Gourdie, R.G., 49–62
Grau, V., 301–319
Greenstein, J.L., 362–375
Gupta, R.W., 85–96
Gurev, V., 320–333
Guzzo, R.M., 85–96

Hammond, H.K., 426–436
Hasin, T., 97–109

Hooks, D.A., 334–347
Hughes, M., 451–465
Hunter, A.W., 49–62
Hunter, P.J., 334–347

Itzhaki, I., 207–215

Janowski, E., 154–164
Jourdan, J., 49–62

Kagaya, Y., 248–267
Karma, A., 376–394
Keeling, S.L., 301–319
Kehat, I., 97–109
Kohl, P., 301–319
Konyukhov, E., 466–478
Korol, O., 85–96

Lab, M.J., 282–300
Lakatta, E.G., 178–206
Landesberg, A., 235–247, 466–478
Landesberg, G., 466–478
Lanza, G., 451–465
Lee, J., 301–319
Levy, C., 235–247, 466–478
Lichtenstein, O., 466–478
Liu, T.Y., 1–18
Lyashkov, A., 178–206

Maleckar, M.M., 320–333
Maltsev, V.A., 178–206
Markwald, R.R., 19–33
Marsh, J., 451–465
McCulloch, A.D., 348–361
Mercola, M., 85–96
Metzger, J., 437–450
Miura, M., 248–267
Morad, M., 154–164

Nickerson, D.P., 334–347
Noble, D., 395–414

O'Quinn, M., 49–62

Plank, G., 301–319
Price, G., 248–267
Pullan, A.J., 334–347

Qu, Z., 376–394

Razeghi, P., 110–119
Rhett, M.J., 49–62
Rodríguez, B., 395–414
Rosenbaum, D.S., 216–234
Rubart, M., 34–48
Ruknudin, A., 178–206

Saidel, G.M., 466–478
Sands, G.B., 334–347
Sasse, P., 154–164
Satin, J., 63–75, 207–215
Saucerman, J.J., 348–361
Schiller, J., 207–215
Schneider, J.U.R.E., 301–319
Schroder, E.A., 63–75
Shenhav, A., 466–478
Shiferaw, Y., 376–394
Shofty, R., 466–478
Sideman, S.A., xi–xxiii
Sirenko, S., 178–206
Smaill, B.H., 334–347
Smith, N.P., 301–319
Stanley, W.C., 120–139, 466–478

Stuyvers, B.D.M., 248–267
Sugai, Y., 248–267

Taegtmeyer, H., 110–119
Tanskanen, A., 362–375
Ter Keurs, H.E.D.J., 248–267, 466–478
Trayanova, N.A., 301–319, 320–333, 395–414
Trew, M.L., 334–347

Vinogradova, T., 178–206
Visconti, R.P., 19–33

Wakayama, Y., 248–267
Wan, X., 216–234
Wei, Y., 63–75
Weiss, J.N., 376–394
Westfall, M., 437–450
Wickline, S., 451–465
Wilson, L.D., 216–234
Winslow, R.L., 362–375
Winter, P., 451–465

Yaniv, Y., 235–247
Yekkala, K., 76–84
Yu, X., 120–139

Zhou, L., 120–139
Zhu, C., 49–62
Zhu, W., 178–206